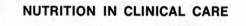

NUTRITION IN CLINICAL CARE

McGRAW-HILL BOOK COMPANY

A Blakiston Publication

New York St. Louis San Francisco Auckland
Bogotá Düsseldorf Johannesburg London
Madrid Mexico Montreal New Delhi Panama Paris
São Paulo Singapore Sydney Tokyo Toronto

NUTRITION
IN CLINICAL CARE

ROSANNE BEATRICE HOWARD M.P.H., R.D.

Director of Nutrition Training in the
Developmental Evaluation Clinic
Children's Hospital Medical Center
Boston, Massachusetts

NANCIE HARVEY HERBOLD M.S., R.D.

Assistant Professor of Foods and Nutrition
Department of Nutrition
Simmons College
Boston, Massachusetts

This book was set in Baskerville by Progressive Typographers.
The editors were Mary Ann Richter and Henry C. De Leo;
the designer was Anne Canevari Green;
the production supervisor was Angela Kardovich.
The drawings were done by Gail L. Kass, with photographs by Carolin Dick.
Picture on inside front cover courtesy of Christopher Murphy.
R. R. Donnelley & Sons Company was printer and binder.

**NUTRITION
IN CLINICAL CARE**

2 3 4 5 6 7 8 9 0   D O D O   7 8 3 2 1 0 9

Supported in part through the U.S. Department of Health, Education,
and Welfare: Maternal and Child Health Service (Project 928).

Library of Congress Cataloging in Publication Data
Main entry under title:
Nutrition in clinical care.

   Includes index.
   1. Diet therapy. 2. Nutrition. 3. Food—
Composition. 4. Nursing. I. Howard, Rosanne
Beatrice. II. Herbold, Nancie Harvey.
[DNLM: 1. Nutrition. 2. Diet therapy. QU145
H851c]
RM216.N84   613.2′8   77-23908
ISBN 0-07-030545-5

NOTICE

To

Mother, Beatrice M.;
and the John E. Howard Family,
John, Eleanor, Johnny, Joe, Steve

Rosanne Beatrice Howard

Rick for his patience
and my Family

Nancie Harvey Herbold

There are no special diets only special people

Madge L. Myers

CONTENTS

PART ONE
FOOD: ITS NUTRITIVE SUBSTANCES AND PHYSIOLOGICAL EFFECTS

PART TWO
FOOD AND THE HUMAN ENVIRONMENT

LIST OF CONTRIBUTORS

Christine E. Cronk, M.S.
Anthropologist
Developmental Evaluation Clinic
Children's Hospital Medical Center
Boston, Massachusetts

Roberta Duyff, M.S., R.D.
Nutrition Education Consultant
New York, New York

Linda Fetters, M.S., R.P.T.
Assistant Professor
Simmons College
Boston, Massachusetts

Edith L. Getchel, M.S., R.D.
Director of Nutrition Services
Children's Hospital Medical Center
Boston, Massachusetts

Shirley R. Goldstein, M.S., R.D.
Associate Director of Dietetics
Beth Israel Hospital
Boston, Massachusetts

Susan K. Golovin, M.Ed., R.D.
Nutrition Consultant
San Francisco, California

Roberta Ruhf Henry, R.D.
Dialysis Nutrition Coordinator for
    Special Research
National Dialysis Study
Peter Bent Brigham Hospital
Boston, Massachusetts

Nancie Harvey Herbold, M.S., R.D.
Assistant Professor of Foods and
    Nutrition
Department of Nutrition
Simmons College
Boston, Massachusetts

Jean Hine, M.S., R.D.
Section Head, Nutrition Section
Waisman Center
University of Wisconsin
Madison, Wisconsin

Rosanne Beatrice Howard, M.P.H., R.D.
Director of Nutrition Training in the
    Developmental Evaluation Clinic
Children's Hospital Medical Center
Boston, Massachusetts

T. Howard Howell, D.D.S.
Instructor in Periodontology
Harvard Dental School
Boston, Massachusetts

Carol Hum, M.S., R.D.
Nutrition Consultant
Montreal, Canada

Patricia A. Kreutler, Ph.D.
Assistant Professor
Chairman, Department of Nutrition
Simmons College
Boston, Massachusetts

Dorothy M. MacDonald, B.S., R.N.
Senior Surgical Clinic Nurse
Children's Hospital Medical Center
Boston, Massachusetts

Mary Alice Marino, R.D.
Nutritionist
Inborn Errors of Metabolism Clinic
Children's Hospital Medical Center
Boston, Massachusetts

Margaret L. Mikkola, R.D.
Research Dietitian
Arteriosclerosis Center
Massachusetts Institute of Technology
Cambridge, Massachusetts

Christine Adamow Murray, M.S., R.D.
Research Nutritionist
Nutrition Support Team
Children's Hospital Medical Center
Boston, Massachusetts

Ruth Palombo, M.S., R.D.
Assistant Director for Patient Services
Frances Stern Nutrition Center
Tufts New England Medical Center
Boston, Massachusetts

Peggy L. Pipes, M.S., M.P.H., R.D.
Assistant Chief Nutrition Section
Clinical Training Unit
Child Development and Mental Retardation Center
Lecturer, School of Home Economics
University of Washington
Seattle, Washington

Richard R. Schnell, Ph.D.
Director of Psychology Training
Developmental Evaluation Clinic
Children's Hospital Medical Center
Boston, Massachusetts

Grace Shen, Ph.D.
Nutrition Director
Clinical Research Center
Children's Hospital Medical Center
Boston, Massachusetts

Carol Stollar, M.Ed., R.D.
Nutritionist
Frances Stern Nutrition Center and
    The Rehabilitation Institute
Tufts New England Medical Center
Boston, Massachusetts

Robert M. Suskind, M.D.
Associate Professor of Pediatrics and Clinical
    Nutrition
Associate Program Director Clinical Research Center
Department of Nutrition and Food Science
Massachusetts Institute of Technology
Cambridge, Massachusetts

Robert W. Telzrow, M.D.
Instructor in Pediatrics
Department of Pediatrics
University of Washington
School of Medicine
Seattle, Washington

Nancy S. Wellman, M.S., R.D.
Nutrition Division Director
The Mailman Center for Child Development
University of Miami
Miami, Florida

FOREWORD

One of the joys of practicing applied nutrition in a large city such as Boston with an abundance of academically oriented health care institutions is that its assembly of health professionals permits a deep study of vexing nutritional problems from many different perspectives. The contributors to this book are products of such an environment.

The reward for the practitioner comes in the applications which can be developed to help patients. It is in the marshalling of the facts toward the worthy end of improving human health and happiness by nutritional means that this book excels. The scientific underpinnings of nutrition as a health science are woven into discussions of clinically relevant problems from the viewpoint of the practitioner. The usual trap of the textbook is that it is either all light (or theory) or all heat (or practice). This book strikes a happy medium, as those who wrote these chapters do in their treatment of the patient. The reader will be pleased, as we were in leafing through the book, at the real-life flavor it has.

It is with great pleasure that we recommend this book to the reader. The esteemed colleagues and good friends who have put so much of their own expertise into writing it are fine clinical nutritionists. We trust that those who master the contents of this text will follow in their competent footsteps in their own later careers.

Johanna Dwyer, D.Sc., R.D.
Associate Professor
Tufts University School of Medicine
Director, Frances Stern Nutrition Center
Tufts New England Medical Center
Boston, Massachusetts

Mary Ellen Collins, M.Ed., R.D.
Director of Dietetics
Peter Bent Brigham Hospital
Boston, Massachusetts

PREFACE

This book has been planned to provide the student with the information from which a nutrition-centered health care practice can be established. The book is divided into three major areas. The first part considers Food: Its Nutritive Substances and Physiological Effects, setting forth the biochemical principles needed to understand the complex interactions of food within the human body. These basic principles are expanded in the second section, where Food and the Human Environment are considered, followed by the third study area which addresses The Consequences of Disease on Nutritional Status.

Since the science of nutrition can be abstract and impersonal, the study of scientific facts needs to be tempered with a value-level application. This then adds relevancy to the facts and increases the possibility of their application. With this in mind, each chapter has been designed to give the student the information needed to understand the relevance of each nutrient to health, followed by a clinical analysis which will involve the student in the solution of concrete problems, leading to a deeper working understanding that cannot be acquired in didactic lectures, reading, or memorizing facts. Through this case study approach, the student will learn to apply theory to the practical situation—to the patient, thereby integrating nutrition into the health care delivery system.

At the beginning of each chapter, certain key words have been identified to facilitate learning; and questions, along with a case study, are included at the end of the chapter to encourage the development of the student's own nutrition-expertise. Case study discussions are located in the Appendix.

The study of nutrition is an applied study. Nutrients operate within a complex organism—the human body. To be effective, nutrition educators must apply the scientific facts to the human need. This is the purpose of this book.

ACKNOWLEDGMENTS

We wish to acknowledge the support and encouragement of our special and helpful friends Basil Petrou, Gail L. Kass, and Carolin and Dr. Macdonald Dick. Thanks also go to our respected colleagues Dr. Allen Crocker, Dr. Patricia A. Kreutler, Jeanette Epstein, Carol Hum, Christine Murray, Christine Cronk, Dr. Frank Davidoff, Mary Alice Marino, Edith Getchel, Richard Schnell, Anita Wilson, Margarite Queneau, Thalia Metalides, Alice Shea, Marie Cullinane, Marguerite Moran, Sue Cullen, Roberta Judge, Margaret Donovan, Yoline Gabriel, Carol Higgins, Rainy Broomfield, and Allen Liechan. Finally, we wish to thank our willing students Mary Sereda, Katie Graham, and Ann Jones.

Rosanne Beatrice Howard
Nancie Harvey Herbold

PART ONE

FOOD : ITS NUTRITIVE SUBSTANCES AND PHYSIOLOGICAL EFFECTS

This section presents the principles of nutrition, which can be overwhelming to the student who is exposed for the first time to the biochemical theory on which the study of nutrition is based. The anxiety experienced by the new student is a common phenomenon, often compounded by the student's failure to understand the relevancy of biochemical principles to patient care. Let us assure you that, as in all other areas of study, you will master these principles with some work, greatly enhanced by an open attitude. Let us further assure you that this study area is relevant, for it is upon these basic principles that your future practice of clinical nutrition will eventually be established.

CHAPTER 1

NUTRITION: AN APPLIED SCIENCE

Rosanne B. Howard

KEY WORDS
Food Ways
Present-Day Nutritional Concerns
Nutritional Education
Behavioral Change
Preventive Nutrition

To each present situation, people bring their past experiences and define it in those terms—and so knowledge of the past role of food helps our understanding of nutrition in our present society.

Food is not only basic to survival but has been pertinent to the development of the human race. The quality of life has been dependent on the quality of food. It all started a few million years ago around the middle Pleistocene epoch when our distant anthropoid cousins were constrained to become hunters under the spur of ecological change.

This adaptation from a food scavenger of roots, fruits, and other vegetable foods to a hunter made it possible for the early hominids to accommodate to environmental changes. By becoming omnivorous, humanlike apes evolved to apelike humans as they increased their capacity for survival.

It seems clear that man survived the climatic changes of the middle Pleistocene by a new behavioral adaptation that affected fundamentally and irrevocably his psychosocial character; it was his change in food finding behavior among other things that finally made man, and that . . . helps to justify our recognition of the change from Australopithecus the apeman to Homo the man.[1]

The transition from food-gathering herbivore to hunter not only produced a change in diet but automatically implied group cooperation, since hunting could be carried out only by the strongest young males. Cooperative hunting and sharing the proceeds of the hunt with females and infants became the trademark of the human condition among primates.

Herein lies the anthropological and social significance of food as part of our cultural heritage. Food sharing and cooperation brought prehistoric humans together in a very intimate way in a situation that probably even encouraged speech. Our distinctly human act of hospitality, of inviting friends to dinner, is based to an extent on those earlier advantages of sharing. Food, so essential to survival, provided the incentive for socialized behavior around which society formed.

Throughout all societies, food and eating have been looked upon as symbolizing friendliness and interpersonal acceptance, and the withholding of food as rejection or punishment. Since history has been recorded, famine and the fear of hunger have plagued humankind and the most pressing human problem has been the securing of food to satisfy this hunger. Food has been used as a means of political subjugation and often its availability has been the determining factor in the outcome of wars. According to a retrospective study of hunger by Keys and his coworkers that included wartime observations of starvation and the reported experiences of explorers, hunger becomes completely overpowering and incites baseness in human behavior. This human response to hunger is the same regardless of time and place.[2]

Before humans learned to cultivate the land, satiety was dependent on whatever plants or animals inhabited the locality, giving rise to the vast range of geographical distinction among food preferences. Whatever was edible was eaten. The extent to which primitive peoples explored their food environment can be illustrated by their discovery of the remedial properties and the narcotic effect of certain herbs, roots, and leaves. Early societies were known to chew coca leaves, smoke Indian hemp, and drink tea, cocoa, and coffee.[3] For centuries the Chinese people held the belief that the plant ginseng was a panacea for disease. Remnants of these ancient beliefs can still be found in our present culture. An appreciation of this ecological framework, a human-land interaction, helps toward an understanding of current cultural influences on food use.

From the beginning, societies developed patterns around the conduct of food activities. These standardized practices, known as *food ways*, are unique to each individual society, having evolved from different environmental factors and having been incorporated into the

society to maintain the viability of the group. Food ways are part of our cultural heritage and are inculcated from birth, as the child is either placed to the breast or given a bottle.

Culture enters into the food experience, shaping and choosing the significant factors for defining the experience.[4]

Thus, culture determines *what* will be recognized as food, *when* we should have an appetite, and for *what* we should be hungry.

Because of the general American societal mixtures, there is no one cultural pattern that exists in its pure form. But whatever the potpourri, food habits develop from culturally determined values, attitudes, and beliefs. The cultural significance of food habits predates the concept of nutrition, a twentieth-century science which has helped us to define the food that humans need in order to grow and maintain health.

NUTRITION, A SCIENCE

The early knowledge of nutrition consisted of anecdotal observations that go as far back as Hippocrates, the father of medicine (460–370 B.C.), who is said to have paid strict attention to the diet of his patients as a feature of his therapeutic regimens. However, little of a scientific nature was accomplished in the development of nutrition or any science until the latter part of the eighteenth century. It was at this time that Antoine Laurent Lavoisier measured in guinea pigs and in his laboratory assistant the amount of body heat lost, oxygen consumed, and carbon dioxide expired. He concluded that respiration is a combustion process similar to the process utilized in a flame. Lavoisier's measurements taken in fasting and resting states essentially represent basal metabolism, a concept fundamental to the development of nutritional science, and are the reason that Lavoisier is known as the father of nutrition.

During the nineteenth century, consider-

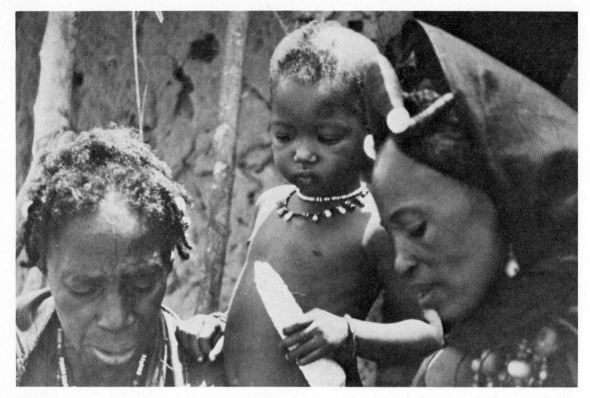

Figure 1-1
Cultural evolution of food habits. "Food ways" are passed from one generation to another. (Photo courtesy of Jane McCotter O'Toole.) Bamako, Mali, West Africa.

able work was done on energy exchange and on the nature of major foodstuffs, and the energy value of a large number of foods was determined. Leiberg, Rubner, Atwater, Voit are but some of the names of researchers whose work began to bring the science of nutrition to an age. However, the progress was slow until chemical methodology had developed to the point that relatively purified foodstuffs could be isolated. Prior to 1910, vitamins and minerals had not been identified.

F. G. Hopkins (1906) in England recognized the relationship between accessory food factors, now known as *vitamins,* and the dietary deficiency syndromes known for many years and described by James Lind in his *Treatise on Scurvy* (1753). In 1912, the accessory food factors were named *vitamines* by Casimir Funk. He

propounded the theory that beriberi, scurvy, pellagra, and possibly rickets were caused by *deficiency,* or the lack of special substances. He called these special substances *vitamins—vita,* the factors essential for life, and *amines,* because he thought that the antiberiberi factor he was attempting to isolate was an amine.

The vitamin hypothesis prompted new vistas of exploration and technology and by 1913 McCollum and Davis had discovered vitamin A. The continuing isolation and synthesis of vitamins and minerals is the matrix around which nutrition has developed as a field of scientific study that is closely interwoven with medicine, anatomy, physiology, chemistry, bacteriology, and agriculture.

Nutrition as we know it today is "the science that interprets the relationship of food to the functioning living organism."[5] It has been recognized as an independent field of study since 1926 with the appointment of Mary Swatz Rose as professor of nutrition at Columbia University.

NUTRITION: PRESENT-DAY CONCERNS

Advances in the science of nutrition heralded in the field of food technology, which has created improved methods of producing, preserving, and processing food. The fortification of milk with vitamins A and D, the iodization of salt, and the enrichment of flour, cornmeal, cereals, and bread are but a few illustrations. Despite these modern food processes, despite the restoration, fortification, or enrichment of nutrients, nutrients can be lost with poor manufacturing techniques. Many questions about the continued availability of nutrients, especially the trace elements, in processed and fabricated foods are now being raised among health professionals.

In the United States the marriage of food technology and the science of nutrition, along with a great deal of capital and ingenuity, has resolved the problem of our food supply. However, these same solutions have provoked concern over the adulteration of our food supply with residues of fertilizers and with additives to preserve, flavor, color, or thicken food. As far back as 1970, it was estimated that 5 lb of additives per person per year were ingested by an average citizen. Although the use of additives has guaranteed our food supply, and has probably made it safer than ever before in history, the cumulative effects are as yet unknown and their relationship to allergies, cancer, birth defects, and interactions with drugs and diets needs to be fully investigated.

Modern food technology has led to the development of many new products and convenience foods, reflected in the 8000 items that line the shelves of the average large supermarket. The consumer is now faced with many food choices which, when carefully examined, may offer little variation. Consumer compliance and acceptance of foods, and the failure to demand from the food industry a wholesome, unadulterated food supply, are prime examples of the need for consumer education. Only after consumer education has been successful and has produced resultant changes in consumer food preferences can we expect action by the food industry toward increasing the nutritional value of the food offered to the consumer.

Fat- and sugar-rich foods, commonly known as "junk" foods or "snack" foods, have become increasingly popular. Some experts estimate that snack foods are close to comprising 30 percent of the daily caloric intake, with 6.5 lb of various potato chip products consumed per person per year.[6] This has prompted them to consider even the fortification of some of these same junk foods.

The spiraling use of junk foods and the excess consumption of sugar and fat, combined with the sedentary life style, has led to the "overweight society," a product of the imbalance between essential and energy-yielding nutrients. Weight is a problem that now plagues 20 to 40 million of our citizens and knows no barriers of age, race, or income level.

With increased weight many of our citizens face an increased risk of coronary heart disease, a disease with an alarming incidence rate in our population. Many questions are now asked about the relationship of dietary fat, cholesterol, sugar, and fiber to the etiology of this disease.

Recently, low-fiber diets have been implicated in the growing incidence of lower bowel disease and cancer of the colon in our population. The focus on fiber relates to its role in promoting gastrointestinal motility and viscosity of the gastrointestinal contents, its interaction with bile acids, and its effects on the microbial flora, fecal bulk, and the time of passage of food through the intestine. Canned fruit juices, vegetable soups, and white bread are a few examples of the bland, low-roughage foods that permeate our food supply. The fact

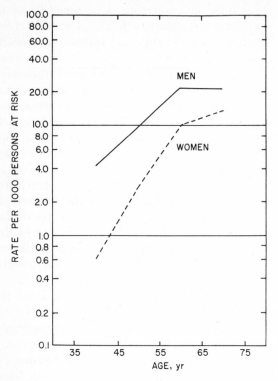

Figure 1-2

Increasing incidence of coronary heart disease. Average annual incidence rate of initial events of coronary heart disease by age and sex, Framingham Study, 16-year follow-up. (From Arteriosclerosis, U.S. Dept. Health, Education, and Welfare Publ. no. (NIH) 72-219, June 1971, p. 301.)

that foods such as these do not promote gastrointestinal motility but cause intestinal stasis is suggested as the causative factor in lower bowel disease.

The increasing use of refined carbohydrate is associated with the prevalence of dental caries, endemic to our population and found in all economic strata. It is figured that 100 lb of sugar disappear for each person per year. The problem of highly refined, sugar- and fat-rich foods is compounded by the fact that these foods are popularized in fast-food chains and restaurants across the nation, with the prediction that $74 billion will be spent annually in restaurants by 1980.[6]

The fact that more people eat in restau-

rants is a function of our industrialized life style and of the change in family structure, with the working mother an emerging phenomenon. It is estimated that in the period from 1947 to 1965, there was an increase of 131 percent in the number of mothers added to the work force, and that by 1975, 39 percent of these women were mothers of preschool children.[7] The working mother and the urbanization of life has had a significant impact on family meals and consequent food habits. For the most part the working mother's family has relied heavily on restaurants, day-care centers, and school lunch and breakfast programs, so that the formation of early food habits now emanates from influences other than those of the home. Convenience foods, such as frozen dinners and packaged mixes, have become a sine qua non to the American family as meals are eaten on the run.

Another present-day concern is our per capita meat consumption of 186 pounds per year,[8] which may reflect a belief emanating from our frontier ancestors that eating meat from strong animals conferred strength. We appear to continue to subscribe to this notion, as meat high in saturated fat and cholesterol remains at the center of the American meal table despite its identification as a risk factor in cardiovascular disease. Furthermore, this overuse of animal protein may come to be viewed as irresponsible in the face of global food shortages and malnutrition in the third-world nations.

In the future, food scarcity may be more persistent as negative ecological trends gain momentum yearly in poor countries. The prospects are for ever-increasing dependence on North American grain stores. Since it takes approximately 5 lb of grain to produce 1 lb of meat, grain is siphoned away from human consumption.[9]

Before children born today in developing countries reach their fifth birthdays, approximately 75 million youngsters will die of malnutrition and associated illnesses.[10]

For our nation the implication is clear: we need a comprehensive nutritional policy to assure adequate food production and maintenance of quality for our global commitments as well as domestic needs. In this regard one idea has been to create a federal office that will be responsible for nutritional planning. The government's reluctance to develop a federal food and nutrition office has caused much debate within the U.S. Senate's Select Committee on Nutrition and Human Needs.[11] This committee was established in response to the discovery of malnutrition in America during the 1960s by a Senate subcommittee headed by Senator Robert Kennedy. Originally mandated to solve the problem of hunger and malnutrition in the 20 to 30 million so-identified Americans, it then broadened its scope to consider the effectiveness of federally subsidized food programs. Presently, the existing programs are tied to different special-interest groups, each oriented toward its own narrow goals, and as a consequence federal food policy has developed piecemeal.

For the most part, our nutritional problems are ones of excess or imbalance, rather than deficiency, and can be found in all socioeconomic groups. However, in poverty pockets (Appalachia, the Deep South, urban ghettos), malnutrition is found polarized in blacks, Indians, Mexican Americans, Puerto Ricans, and the elderly. The hunger in America discovered by the Senate subcommittee was confirmed by the Ten-State Nutrition Survey conducted from 1968 to 1970. A combination of subsistence income, a poor policy of food distribution, and ignorance has brought many of our citizens to the state of nutritional risk reflected in the incidence of iron-deficiency anemia seen in young children and pregnant women. That malnutrition exists in pregnant women and young children is an alarming fact in face of an increasing body of knowledge indicating that malnutrition during pregnancy, infancy, and early childhood may have serious effects on growth and brain development.

The allure of food cults and quackery has further compounded the nutritional status of our citizens. Deutsch concluded in his exposé of food cures that fake food cures are perhaps the biggest public health problem in America today, since scarcely anyone is free from false beliefs about food.[12] Misinformation about food is often promulgated by the media, and this in turn influences children's food habits. It has been estimated that nearly 44 million children under 12 years of age who watch a moderate amount of TV see 21,300 commercials in one year. The effectiveness of this advertising can be seen in the aisles of the supermarkets, as children pressure parents for a particular product, or on the breakfast tables across the nation, each replete with several different brands of cereal, many with dubious nutritional value.

We have advanced in isolating nutrients and in applying technology to the production and processing of food, but we have progressed little in the area of adequate food distribution and the effective application of the science of nutrition to individual needs. Satisfying these latter unmet needs is necessary in order to bring about the behavioral changes and the formation of good food habits that are necessary for the improved health of the population. With the escalating cost of health care and without strong evidence to support a concomitant improvement in our nation's health, greater emphasis must be placed on preventive health services, including preventive nutrition. The goal of *preventive nutrition* is to achieve a balance between the nutrients needed for health and those which must not be eaten to excess, so as to prevent nutrition-related diseases.

Nutrition educators must broaden their scope—away from pathology and therapy, and toward normal nutrition in its most positive aspects.

Efforts should focus on the establishment and protection of nutritional health rather than on crisis intervention. It is needed regardless of income, location, or cultural, social, or economic practices or level of education. Nutrition education must be a continuing process through the life cycle as new research brings new knowledge.[13]

To accomplish this goal, nutrition must be applied—a science applied to the human need.

NUTRITION, AN APPLIED SCIENCE

Nutrition education is a multidisciplinary process that involves the transfer of information, the development of motivation and the modification of food habits where needed. It must form the bridge that carries appropriate information from the research and development laboratories to the public, the ultimate user. During transport, nutrition educators and their counterparts in related professions must apply their skills and knowledge to adapt the information so it can be applied to a variety of everyday situations and then package it for distribution in a variety of ways, whether directly to the intended user or indirectly through intermediate agents.[14]

A subcommittee of the Intra-Agency Committee on Nutrition Education has proposed four basic concepts of nutritional education:

1   Nutrition is the food you eat and how the body uses it.
   •   We eat food to live, to grow, to keep healthy and well, and to get energy for work and play.
2   Food is made up of different nutrients needed for growth and health.
   •   All nutrients needed by the body are available through food.
   •   Eating many kinds and combinations of food can lead to a well-balanced diet.
   •   No food, by itself, has all the nutrients needed for full growth and health.
   •   Each nutrient has specific uses in the body.
   •   Most nutrients do their best work in the body when teamed with other nutrients.

3   All persons, throughout life, need the same nutrients, but in varying amounts.
   •   The amounts of nutrients needed are influenced by age, sex, body size, activity, and state of health.
4   The way that food is handled influences the amount of nutrients in the food, as well as its safety, appearance, and taste.
   •   Handling means everything that happens to food while it is being grown, processed, stored, and prepared for eating.

These concepts can help to launch a nutrition education program. However, any attempt to apply the science of nutrition must take into consideration that humans are part of a dynamic sociopolitical system buffeted by the environmental resources (climate, soil, water, energy) in the land around them. People, whether in an affluent nation or an undeveloped country, have certain basic needs to which nutritional science must be applied, for it is from these needs that food habits develop.

Food habits of an individual are the characteristic and repetitive acts that he performs under the impetus of the need to provide himself with nourishment and simultaneously to meet an assortment of social and emotional goals. By the choices he makes, which become habit on repetition, he strives to achieve such satisfactions as security, comfort, status, pleasure, and enhancement of his ego.[15]

Since food habits are learned in response to a need and are not genetically determined, nutrition education is possible. The concern of the nutrition educator is the way in which people learn and how this learning can affect behavioral change.

Behavioral change as an integral part of nutrition education is a complex process, and as such is best achieved through the combined efforts of a health-care team. A multidisciplinary team of physician, nurse, nutritionist, and behavioral scientist, with other members as needed (physical therapist, dentist, speech therapist, home economist, etc.), working together yet from different vantage points, formulate a plan of nutrition intervention while considering the total person, with a discipline to relate to each individual need. By focusing on the level of need, the health professional can apply the science of nutrition at that level to effect behavioral change. There is no one way to change food behavior. Each program must be individually tailored to the human need.

According to Maslow, human needs are ordered in a hierarchical pattern, and as one level is reasonably satisfied the next level emerges.[16] This theoretical pattern can be a useful guide for the nutrition educator who is attempting to understand human motivation. Approaching the individual at his or her level of need may bring about the desired change (see Table 1-1).

THE NURSE AND NUTRITION, AN APPLIED SCIENCE

The influential role that the nurse has for the patient and the role of nutrition in health and treatment of disease mean that they both share

common territory in patient care. Implied herein is the nurse's role as a nutrition educator, whereby he or she becomes a food therapist replete with the knowledge of food ways. To be an effective food therapist, the nurse must have an understanding of food as it relates to human needs and must incorporate the role of a food expert into that of being a nurse.

By being the food experts, we should know and be interested in everything about food as it relates to people, chemically, physiologically, biochemically, economically—everything from the source to use and what happens to it in us.[17]

This is a chain which connects all the factors that influence our food intake and ultimately our nutritional status, with each link permanently and irreversibly linked to the next. A knowledge of all these links is a prerequisite to the application of the science of nutrition.

Changes in food consumption patterns develop within the context of a cultural evolution. This evolution is responsive to human-land interactions and may change the food itself in some instances, as occurs with food processing. In other instances this evolution affects the response to food as a function of life style. These changes exert both positive and negative effects, which must be interpreted for the patient. These effects are ever-changing, and it is essential that you as nutrition educator maintain credibility by being well-informed, so that your patient can learn to rely on you and your nutritional information.

TABLE 1-1 CONSCIOUS ACTION ARISES FROM NEEDS

Basic human needs: order of priority	Nutrition focus
Basic physiological needs (food, water, oxygen, sleep)	Food for sustenance
Safety and security	Food for growth and maintenance
Belonging and social activity	Food for social reinforcement
Esteem and status	Food for prestige
Self-realization and fulfillment	Food for optimum productivity and well-being
Need to know and understand	Nutritional education

STUDY QUESTIONS

1 What is the cultural significance of food?

2 List all of the present-day nutritional concerns around which we must base a nutritional education program.

3 Explain the statement "nutrition is an applied science."

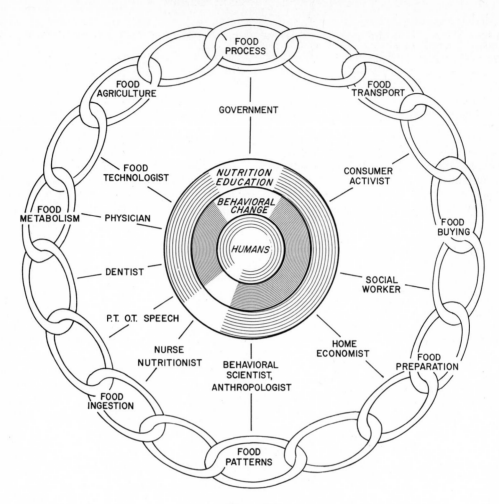

Figure 1-3
The interconnecting chain of food factors influencing nutritional educa-
tion. This chain connects all factors that influence food intake and ulti-
mately man's nutritional status.

REFERENCES

1 B. Campbell, *Human Evolution,* Aldine Publishing Company, Chicago, 1966, p. 235.
2 A. Keys, J. Brozek, A. Henschel, O. Mclkelser, and H. L. Taylor, *The Biology of Human Starvation,* vols. 1 and 2, University of Minnesota Press, Minneapolis, 1950.
3 E. V. McCollum, *A History of Nutrition,* Riverside Press, Cambridge, Mass., 1957, p. 4.
4 D. Lee, "Cultural Factors in Dietary Choice," *American Journal of Clinical Nutrition,* **5** March–April 1957, p. 166.
5 R. Pike and M. Brown, *Nutrition: An Integrated Approach,* 2d ed. John Wiley and Sons, Inc., New York, 1975, p. 1.
6 L. M. Henderson, "Nutritional Problems Growing Out of New Patterns of Food Consumption," *American Journal of Public Health,* **62,** September 1972, 1198.

7 Christian Beals, "The Case of the Vanishing Mommy," *The New York Times,* July 4, 1976, p. 28.

8 A. Berg, *The Nutrition Factor,* The Brookings Institution, Washington, D.C., 1973, p. 64.

9 Ibid., p. 65.

10 Ibid.

11 Select Committee on Nutrition and Human Needs, *Towards a National Nutrition Policy,* U.S. Government Printing Office, Washington, D.C., 1975.

12 R. M. Deutsch, *The Nuts among the Berries: An Exposé of America's Food Fads,* Ballantine Books, New York, 1961.

13 "American Dietetic Association Position Paper on Nutrition Education for the Public," *Journal of American Dietetic Association,* **62,** 1973, p. 429.

14 R. Leverton, "Commentary: What Is Nutrition Education?," *Journal of American Dietetic Association,* **64,** 1974, p. 17.

15 Helen H. Gift, Marjorie B. Washbon, Gail G. Harrison, *Nutrition, Behavior and Change,* Prentice-Hall, Inc., Englewood Cliffs, N.J., 1972, p. 29.

16 A. H. Maslow, "A Theory of Human Motivation," *Psychological Review,* **50,** 1943, pp. 370–396.

17 Madge L. Meyers, "Fact and Fantasy in the Practice of Clinical Dietetics: Ninth Martha F. Trulson Memorial Lecture," *Abstracts of the 58th American Dietetic Annual Meeting,* October 1975, p. 123.

CHAPTER 2

THE ADEQUATE DIET—THE PRUDENT DIET

Roberta Duyff

KEY WORDS
Food Additive
Nutrification
Enrichment
Fortification
Nutrient Density
Nutrient Labeling
Recommended Dietary Allowances

INTRODUCTION

An adequate diet is one that provides all the necessary nutrients in amounts needed by the body for optimum health. While specific eating practices may range widely from individual to individual, the nutrient needs of most Americans can be met by following the requirements of two standards: the recommended dietary allowances (RDA) and the basic four food groups. Health professionals must interpret these guidelines for clients, and in doing so must consider the numerous factors that may affect the nutrient quality of the food selected. These influences include:

Food processing
Food consumption patterns
Food purchasing
Food handling and preparation

This chapter will consider these influences and their effect on the nutrient content of food and diet, to better enable the health professional to determine the effect of these influences on dietary standards.

FOOD PROCESSING

Technological advances in food processing methods have increased the number of available food products. In the early 1900s approximately 800 items were supplied to retail stores while today over 8000 products are stocked on grocery shelves. Although the modern supermarket carries many nonfood items, a large percentage of the consumer's spending options are for edible goods. Consumers must discern which processing methods and food products will meet personal and family needs and which will influence their own diets in a positive way.

The term *processing* covers a wide variety of physical steps to which food is subjected prior to consumption. Washing produce, cooking a garden vegetable at home, or refining wheat at a mill are all forms of processing; however, the term commonly refers to industrial processing before purchase. Processing foods through *preservation* techniques, the use of *additives,* and *nutrification* have both advantages and disadvantages.

> *Advantages:* storage time increased
> preparation time and effort decreased
> food safety ensured
> overall product appeal improved
> nutritional value improved
> food changed into edible form
>
> *Disadvantages:* nutrients destroyed
> cost increased
> quality changed, decreasing the overall product appeal
> individuals subjected to unknown risk factors

From a nutritional standpoint, three aspects of processing must be considered: (1) the trade-off between increased availability of food and the loss of nutrients, (2) the degree of nutrient loss (e.g., home preparation often results in greater losses than commercial processing does), and (3) the relative importance of the loss (e.g., ascorbic acid is destroyed in pasteurization of milk, but milk does not contain significant quantities of the nutrient).[1]

Preservation Methods

Since most foods do not have a long storage life, processing methods have been developed to retain the nutrient value, aesthetic qualities, and functional properties of foods while reducing the possibility of microbial spoilage. There are five commonly used methods of preservation: *canning, freezing, freeze-drying, drying,* and *dehydrating.* Another, *irradiation,* is now undergoing research.

Preserved foods aid the consumer by providing a varied diet throughout the year. With the use of processed foods, seasonal changes in the food supply need not impose a major shift in one's dietary pattern. Processing allows foods to be transported over a wide geographical area as well as to be stored at home for longer periods of time. Some processing may be purely a convenience to consumers. For instance, dried and freeze-dried foods are excellent for backpacking, when refrigeration is not available.

While some nutrients are lost in the course of preservation, overall quality can remain high. In fact, preserved produce may provide more nutrients than fresh produce that has been improperly handled during storage and preparation.

Additives

Food additives are used in food processing. They are defined as substances added to food either directly for a functional purpose (*intentional food additives*) or unintentionally during some phase of production, processing, storage, or packaging (*incidental food additives*). Those added purposely are expected to:

> Improve nutritional value
> Enhance flavor
> Maintain appearance, palatability, and wholesomeness
> Impart and maintain a desired consistency
> Control acidity or alkalinity
> Impart a desired and characteristic color
> Serve as maturing and bleaching agents in milling and baking
> Maintain quality in processed foods, e.g., curing agents and anticaking agents

While many additives are recognized as harmless components of food if eaten in moderation, the public has expressed increasing concern over the use and safety of many additives. A list has been compiled of additives that are generally recognized as safe (GRAS) for moderate use in food processing without serious health hazard (e.g., ascorbic acid to nutrify and to prevent browning in cut fruits and vegetables, lecithin to emulsify mayonnaise, and alum to produce crispness in pickles). Currently some commonly used additives (particularly coloring agents, nitrates, and nitrites) are under debate for being potentially deleterious to health.

While the Food and Drug Administration (FDA) and businesses share the responsibility of ensuring the safety and proper use of additives by means of research and by removal of an additive from the market if necessary, the consumer's role should be to:

Keep informed about food additives, using reliable information sources

Communicate concerns to the government and industry

Read package labels, understanding the function of additives included

Consume a varied diet to minimize exposure to any one additive

Nutrification

Nutrification is both a form of processing and a type of food additive. Nutrification encompasses *enrichment* and *fortification* of conventional foods and *formulation* of new foods, all methods that can increase the nutritional value of food.

Enrichment is the adding of nutrients to foods to replace those that have been lost or removed through processing. These nutrients are usually added in amounts up to or exceeding original levels. Most enrichment is done to foods made with grain. Milling, which removes the germ and outer layers of grain, causes the loss of several nutrients, including iron, thiamine, riboflavin, and niacin. Enrichment replaces these nutrients in the product. However, it does not add back all of the trace elements that are lost in processing.

Although enrichment of bakery bread was made mandatory in 1943 for the duration of World War II, no such federal legislation currently exists. This early law, however, set a precedent for today's voluntary enrichment by some manufacturers, as well as for several state laws which mandate enrichment in some bread and cereal products. Since enrichment is not required in many states, consumers may be unaware of the added food quality it provides unless they are educated to look for an enrichment statement on a product label. In particular, foods considered as staples, such as rice and bread, should be enriched since they play such an important role in the daily diet.

Fortification is the addition of nutrients not normally present in a food. Nutrients that are used to fortify foods are those which generally are consumed in less than adequate amounts by sectors of the population. Examples include vitamin D added to milk, iodine added to table salt, vitamin C added to fruit-flavored drinks, and vitamin A added to margarine.

Improving the quality of conventional food is done in a careful and systematic fashion. Industry is encouraged to follow guidelines which ensure the effectiveness and safety of fortification. In 1973 the Council on Foods and Nutrition of the American Medical Association (AMA) and the Food and Nutrition Board of the National Research Council (NRC) recommended the nutritional improvement of conventional foods that meet the following critieria:[2]

1 The food is commonly consumed.
2 The added nutrient is:
   a Below desirable levels of intake in diets
   b Important to the overall diet
   c Safe, not creating a dietary imbalance or, through excessive intake, not resulting in toxicity
   d Stable during normal storage and usage
   e Physiologically available from food
3 The additional cost is reasonable.

The addition of iron for enrichment and fortification has been controversial. Although pregnant and menstruating women and growing children need increased amounts of iron, the problem may not be solved by simply adding iron to foods. Both biological and technological problems must be faced. Not all iron compounds are bioavailable (i.e., in a form readily available to the body). Ferric phosphates, for instance, have limited or no bioavailability, according to research findings. Other compounds, like ferrous gluconate, ferrous sulfate, ferrous lactate, and reduced iron, have limited availability in comparison to natural iron. Addition of iron has also caused an undesirable color and flavor in foods.[3] Another consideration is that the foods to be fortified may not necessarily be consumed by the population at risk. Further research is necessary if iron deficiencies are to be made up by simple enrichment or fortification measures.

Formulation   Supermarket shelves are filled with an ever-increasing number of formulated or "engineered" food items. These foods are complex mixtures of ingredients designed for a particular dietary use; both scientific and technological knowledge are employed in food processing to obtain products with predictable color, texture, odor, flavor, and nutritional quality. The products usually resemble existing, more natural products.[4] Such items include egg substitutes which have had the cholesterol and many saturated fats removed; meat substitutes, made of a soybean base, that resemble hot dogs, ground beef, or bacon; dairy substitutes made with vegetable oils, like nondairy creamers and margarine; and meal-replacement beverages and bars which have little or no resemblance to existing foods. In many developing nations where protein consumption is low, engineered foods with a soybean base have been developed to be a protein substitute (e.g., Incaparina).

The nutritional composition of engineered foods is a controversial issue. While many of these items have been formulated to meet specific dietary needs, others have been developed purely to offer a convenience or to develop a new "taste" in the consumer. Although nutrients used to fortify the product often make a significant dietary contribution, other important nutrients, such as trace elements, may be lacking.

In order to ensure the nutritional quality of formulated foods, the AMA's Council on Foods and Nutrition and the NRC's Food and Nutrition Board have established relevant guidelines:[5]

1   Formulated foods are significant to the diet if they contribute 5 percent or more of any recommended nutrient or energy requirement or if they act as substitutes for other foods.
2   Unless developed for a specific dietary reason, the substitute products should contain similar nutrients to those foods that they are formulated to resemble.
3   The quantity of protein and fat should be nutritionally appropriate to the food and its use.
4   Foods which are meal replacers should provide 25 to 50 percent of the actual or estimated RDA.
5   The caloric content should be determined by the intended use.

Food processing is essential to the complex food production and marketing system in the United States. Careful selection of processed food can enhance the overall quality of the diet. Consumers need particular guidance in the appropriate use of processed food and an understanding of its nutrient value.

FOOD CONSUMPTION PATTERNS

The effect of industrialization and urbanization on family structure is reflected in the emerging food ways, or habits, of many American families, who rely heavily on fast-food chains, high-energy snack foods, and convenience dinners. With the technological age promoting speed and efficiency, people have learned to eat quickly—standing at lunch counters and sitting behind the wheel of a car. Parents can even be seen feeding babies hastily, spooning a mouthful in before the first is swallowed. In addition, eating patterns are influenced by a host of sociological and psychological factors which transcend a conscious recognition of the health value of food. (See Chap. 10.)

Food at Home

The three-meals-a-day pattern has undergone changes in the last few years. The pattern which many people follow is that of little or no breakfast, a light lunch, and a large evening meal containing the bulk of the day's energy supply. Studies show that "gorging" at one time of the day results in single high glucose levels and continuous higher levels of free fatty acids in the serum. Smaller, more frequent meals result in lower levels.[6] However, the overall contribution of snacks should not be overlooked, as they can provide significant dietary components when chosen wisely. The concern over this food style is its nutritional adequacy, since foods high in energy and low in nutrients may be selected. Erratic eating patterns may also affect the utilization of nutrients. There is growing evidence of natural body rhythms that suggests better utilization of protein during the morning than at other times.[7,8]

In the past heavy breakfasts were important for those involved in strenuous activity. However, a more sedentary life style and the many pressures on people's time have dictated changes in early morning eating patterns, for which there are several solutions. For example, for those in a hurry, prepared items like cheese and crackers can help to supply nutritional needs.

Depending upon a person's life style, a midday meal may be light or heavy. Regardless of its size, the meal should be balanced nutritionally and should fill the social and psychological needs of the individual. Bag lunches are often carried to the office and school. With careful thought these meals can fill the requirements from all four food groups; e.g., either a peanut butter sandwich, an apple, and a carton of milk from the cafeteria or vending machine, or a ham and cheese sandwich and a can of fruit juice, can make a balanced lunch.

For most people, the evening meal is the largest of the day. Again, it should include a well-balanced selection of food. If lunch was large, this meal should be lighter. For the elderly and the bedridden, eating a larger lunch and smaller dinner is often recommended, and it may also be well advised for sedentary populations. No one pattern is recommended for dinner, as cultural patterns dictate many equally nutritious meals.

Table 2-1 provides guidelines to be considered in planning the family's daily meals and snacks.

Fast-Food Chains

Fast food is becoming a way of life in the United States. Most fast-food service has been aimed at two populations, young families and college students.

The nutritional quality of the food may be a problem if the food is consumed frequently and regularly. In general the meals are high in energy content and lack several essential nutrients. (See Table 2-2.) Studies indicate that the average take-out lunch consisting of a hamburger, french fried potatoes, and a milkshake provides about 800 kcal (3360 kJ). This combination of foods may lack vitamin A, vitamin C, iron, several trace elements, and dietary fiber. Additionally, there are excessive quantities of energy, fat, salt, and sugar. When soft drinks rather than dairy products are consumed as the beverage, the meals are also low in calcium and riboflavin.[9,10,11]

Well-balanced meals can be planned from a fast-food menu. Substitution of milk for a

TABLE 2-1 GUIDELINES FOR PLANNING MEALS AND SNACKS

1 Food patterns should be planned to provide *recommended servings from each of the four food groups* (milk, meat, bread, and fruits and vegetables) and should allow for sufficient energy needs.

2 *Outside food sources* of the family like school lunch programs and restaurants should be considered as part of the food budget and total dietary program.

3 *Snacks and beverages* supplement nutrient needs. Those high in nutrients but low in calories should be readily available to members of the household.

4 *Special dietetic needs* like fat- or calorie-restrictive diets or mechanical difficulties in eating should be considered in the overall planning in order to satisfy the appropriate physical, social, and psychological needs.

5 *Aesthetic qualities* make a meal more appetizing. Variety of color, texture, flavor, temperature, and shape is important.

6 *Planning a week ahead* allows consumers to cut food costs.

7 The *size of the group to be fed* is an important consideration. A balanced diet cannot be eaten if there is an insufficient quantity of food. Too much food, on the other hand, may be a waste.

8 The *age of individuals* in the group is important. Young children eat less, and growing teenagers and those involved in strenuous activity may need more. Although the elderly require the same nutrients as younger adults, their caloric needs are lower.

9 *Food likes and dislikes* of family members influence the entire family's food patterns. Consideration of preferences and the provision of alternative foods when necessary helps to ensure adequate dietary consumption.

milkshake or soft drink will provide important nutrients without excessive energy. Including tomato and lettuce on the hamburger or adding a serving of cole slaw can help provide dietary fiber as well as vitamins A and C. Likewise, a slice of cheese will provide additional protein, B vitamins, and calcium.

Snacks

Between-meal eating is part of the American food style. Snack foods such as potato chips, pretzels, nuts, crackers, and spreads now gross $2 billion per year.[12] Coffee breaks and the omnipresent vending machine are part of this pattern. Both the ubiquitousness of food and the increased purchasing power of children and adults contribute to between-meal eating. Although consumers generally do not regard snacking as an important part of the day's diet, snack foods do contribute significantly to the total diet. A recent study of teenagers' snacking patterns from the Ten-State Nutrition Survey showed that 23 percent of the day's total calories were consumed between meals. The average nutrient intake from snacks met

TABLE 2-2 NUTRIENT CONTENT OF A TYPICAL FAST-FOOD MEAL

Food	Energy Kcal	kJ	Protein	Vitamin A	Vitamin C	Thiamine	Riboflavin	Niacin	Calcium	Iron
¼ lb cheeseburger	414	1739	41	5	5	15	37	36	7	21
French fried potatoes	215	903	5	†	15	7	2	13	†	2
Chocolate milkshake	317	133	17	†	†	5	33	2	40	5
	946	2775	63%	5%	20%	32%	72%	51%	47%	28%

* Expressed as percent of U.S. RDA for adults and children over age 4 years.

† Supplies less than 2% of the U.S. RDA (recommended dietary allowances) for these nutrients.

Source: J. Goldberg, "The Fast Food Phenomenon," *Family Health,* April 1975, p. 39.

or exceeded the RDA for protein, calcium, ascorbic acid, and thiamine. Intake of iron, vitamin A, and riboflavin was also significant.[13]

Since snack patterns are not only a way of life but play a significant nutritional role in the diet, nutritional educators should utilize this phenomenon and help people toward healthful snacks. Snacks which should be encouraged are those which supply nutrients, not merely calories, such as fruit, vegetables, crackers and cheese, peanut butter, nuts, whole-grain breads, milk, and milk products. Individuals who need to watch their weight should take special care to consume foods high in nutrients but low in calories, such as raw vegetables or skim milk products.

Beverages

In the day's total food pattern, beverages also play an important role. They satisfy thirst, supply nutrients, and fill psychological and social needs. While some beverages like milk and fruit and vegetable juices are excellent sources of nutrients, others provide few, if any, and may in fact be detrimental to one's health.

Like food patterns in general, the pattern of beverage consumption is changing, with the consumption of soft drinks replacing coffee and milk. Soft drinks, which are fast becoming the national beverage, provide only calories. When consumers purchase low-caloric beverages, they do not even get calories for the money spent; moreover, such beverages use varying amounts of sugar substitutes with unknown long-term effects. The increased consumption of soft drinks is now causing concern over the alteration of the normal ratio of calcium to phosphorus in the diet, because of the high phosphate content of these beverages.

Soft drinks can have a negative effect on the diet since they displace nutrients. They may also pose a threat to weight and dental health because of their sugar content. In addition, coffee, tea, cocoa, and cola beverages contain high levels of caffeine, theophylline, and theobromine. These substances are central

nervous system stimulants and may also act as excessive stimulants to the cardiovascular system.

Intake of alcoholic beverages can be a problem. Nutritionally, these beverages contribute more in calories than in nutrients. Each gram of ethanol provides 7.1 kcal (29.8 kJ). Alcohol may, in fact, displace other more nutritious foods in the diet because of cost problems and because the alcohol causes a sense of satiety. Chronic alcohol consumption may interfere with the digestion and absorption of nutrients like thiamine, riboflavin, pyridoxine, folate, and zinc.

Intake of beverages should not be overlooked when one is assessing diets since it can provide many important dietary constituents. The dietary requirement of eight glasses of liquid per day is partially met by beverages. Consumers should be sure that the selection and quantity of their beverages will aid them in obtaining an adequate daily nutrient intake.

FOOD PURCHASING

Affluence, change in life style, and the availability of a more diversified food supply have changed American patterns of food consumption. Since 1900, a notable change has occurred: sugar, protein, and fat intake have increased sharply while consumption of grain has decreased drastically.

The food expenditure patterns of families are influenced by many demographic factors. Among the most significant are family size and regional differences in food costs:

Family size   Large families and those with growing children and teenagers generally must spend more for food.

Regional differences in food costs   Traditionally costs of food are highest in the Northeast while they are less in the South. Food purchased near its source of production is generally less expensive than food which must be transported. Home gardening and home preparation of food also save the cost of producers' and processors' services.

While food has always been a major budget item for many Americans, recent increases in food costs have made the expenditure even more significant. In 1960, food represented 16 percent of the budget, and by 1974 inflationary costs had escalated the food budget to an average of 30 percent and to over 38 percent for low-income people.[14] The rise is also reflected in the price of menu items in restaurants. Since the average American spends approximately 30 percent of the food budget outside the home,[15] restaurant expenses must now be considered in planning wise use of the food dollar.

Adjustment in the expenditure for food must be based on the following factors:[16]

What foods are selected?

Where does the family buy food?

How much food is prepared at home?

Is some food produced at home?

How carefully does the family plan and make purchases?

What importance does the family place on food in relation to other family needs?

While most individuals need to be cognizant of food expenditures, those with low incomes need to be even more selective in their purchasing in order to meet basic nutrient needs. Because of their limited purchasing power, a limitation in food choice is a characteristic of the poor.

Out of necessity, many of the poor have learned to put up with some degree of dreary monotony in eating most of the time.

An occasional feast, however, can be symbolically important. Welfare recipients who buy steaks and chops when the check is received and then eat skimpily toward the end of the month demonstrate behavior that is typical of many poor cultures around the world—the feast or famine custom of eating all you can hold when food is available and doing without when it isn't.[17]

As health professionals help families toward a more appropriate use of the food dollar, they must recognize both the limitation of resources and the psychological significance of food. Candy, potato chips, and liquor may be devices that are helping an individual to cope with life in a bleak, inner-city ghetto. Here middle-class values are inappropriate and should not interfere in counseling relationships. However, the health professional should attempt to motivate the individual toward the wise use of the food dollar, using the person's own value system and focusing on what he or she feels is important and on what benefits will be derived from using a food budget.

Although federally subsidized food programs like food stamps and the special supplemental food program for women, infants, and children (see Chap. 14) have been developed to increase the purchasing power of the poor, they do not fill the gap, as evidenced by the incidence of malnutrition found by the Ten-State Nutrition Survey. Only with a planned program of consumer education that includes directives for economical shopping and help in understanding consumer information (nutrient labeling, universal product coding, open dating) can the food dollar be used effectively.

Good nutrition begins with wise and careful purchasing behavior. With knowledge of the dynamics of the food market and skill in discerning quality products, and through nutrient labeling, open dating, and universal product coding, the consumer can purchase food that fits physical, social, and economic needs.

Economical Shopping

Most consumers are anxious to get the most for their food dollar. For many, careful shopping is the only way they can purchase an adequate supply of food. Supermarket psychology, however, is geared toward increasing sales. Meat counters often stretch across the ends of aisles so that customers will keep confronting meat, a high-profit item. Aisles themselves are often long without breaks in the middle; consumers must walk the full length for a single item, passing shelves stocked with goods as they go. Cereals advertised on children's television are placed at youngsters' eye level. Store specials are also carefully placed at the ends of aisles so that they have prominence. Fresh produce is the first section that many shoppers encounter. These are items with special appeal because the consumer sees the food itself rather than a package; they are also high-profit items. A few simple suggestions can help to protect consumers from impulse shopping and allow them to cut costs and ultimately to shop wisely (see Table 2-3).

Labeling

A product label is one form of consumer education. The information provided on many foods can help a shopper to determine the contents and cost of the product, compare it to similar items on the shelf, understand how to use it, and learn how to save money on the item. All products must carry the following information on a package label:

Common name of the product

Name and address of the manufacturer, packer, or distributor

TABLE 2-3 GUIDELINES FOR ECONOMICAL SHOPPING

1 *Shopping lists*   A consumer who plans food purchases ahead will not only eliminate unnecessary food purchases but will save time, energy, and transportation costs by not having to return to the supermarket. Also, studies indicate that shopping when hungry increases impulse buying.

2 *Store brands*   Often the store brand of a specific item will cost 5 to 10 percent less than similar name-brand products. Comparison shopping will provide the answer.

3 *Newspaper advertisements*   Purchasing "specials" listed in weekly newspapers can provide savings. Although consumers were encouraged by nutrition educators in the past to take advantage of specials at many stores each week, limits on time and transportation costs may make this kind of shopping less economical.

4 *Coupons*   Coupons, available through magazine and newspaper advertisements, direct mailings, and package labels, offer reduced prices on specific items, but they are useful only if the items are needed.

5 *Unit pricing*   Comparison shopping is facilitated in some states by unit pricing. This system allows consumers to compare the price on like quantities of specific products. On the shelf under each product the price per pound, serving, cup, etc. is given, rather than the price per package.

6 *Quantity purchases*   If adequate storage is available and if money can be tied up in food, the purchase of large quantities of food at one time can be a saving. However, buying a larger container is not a saving if the food is unused and ultimately discarded.

7 *Economy foods*   By purchasing inexpensive cuts of meat, dried or evaporated milk, and less expensive produce like green beans and peas, the consumer can spend less in the supermarket for equally nutritious foods.

8 *Seasonal produce*   Purchasing vegetables and fruits in season can reduce the food expenditure. If possible, it is wise to purchase large quantities for freezing or canning when they are in season, and to cook foods that are in season.

9 *Limitation of convenience foods*   The consumer can generally save money by preparing food at home rather than purchasing the same item prepared. The cost of preparation is included in the price of convenience items like frozen dinners.

10 *Frequency of shopping*   Research indicates that consumers spend less on food by shopping once or twice a month rather than once a week or more frequently.

11 *Food-buying cooperatives*   Another way to save money on food is to become involved in a food cooperative, a nonprofit food outlet operated by its members. Consumers invest their time and energy to help the cooperative in exchange for being able to buy food at wholesale prices.

Variety, style, and packaging medium
Net weight or volume
Ingredients

When a manufacturer chooses to use nutritional labeling, the amounts of eight nutrients—protein, vitamins A and C, niacin, riboflavin, thiamine, calcium, and iron—must be included on the nutrient panel. These nutrients are expressed as percentages of the U.S. RDA. Examples of those not required but helpful to consumers to know are cholesterol, fats, sodium, and potassium. When stated on the label, cholesterol and polyunsaturated and saturated fats are listed in milligrams and grams, respectively, per serving, while sodium and potassium are expressed in percentages of the U.S. RDA. (See Fig. 2-1.)

Nutritional labeling can be a useful tool in nutrition education. A label can help consumers to identify the dietary quality of specific foods and compare them with similar items. By reading labels, patients on therapeutic diets can decide which foods are appropriate for their daily consumption. The patients must be instructed that not all nutrients are listed on all labels.

By creating a consumer awareness, nutrient labeling also pressures industry into monitoring and improving the nutritional quality of food. While this may force industry to be continually cognizant of the nutrient value of food, there is also the concern that the food supply could become overfortified with some nutrients while those not listed on a panel could be forgotten. For this reason, a regulation was passed requiring that any food that contained added vitamins or minerals at a level of 50 percent or more of the U.S. RDA would be classified as a *dietary supplement;* supplements containing 150 percent or more of the U.S. RDA would be considered *drugs.*

Open Dating and Universal Product Coding

Open dating is a system for informing consumers of the age and freshness of a packaged

Figure 2-1

Food label with nutritional labeling and universal product coding. The food label has both mandatory information (common name of product, name and address of manufacturer, style, net weight, and ingredients) and voluntary information (nutritional labeling, storage instructions, recipe, and universal product code, which is in the lower right hand corner.)

MRS. O'LEARY'S

small curd

COTTAGE CHEESE

4% MILKFAT MINIMUM

net wt. 16 oz. (1 lb.)

NUTRITION INFORMATION
(per serving)
Serving size = ½ cup
Servings per container = 4

CALORIES.........120	CARBOHYDRATE..3 gm
PROTEIN.......15 gm	FAT.............5 gm

PERCENTAGE OF U.S. RECOMMENDED DAILY ALLOWANCES (U.S. RDA)

PROTEIN.........30	NIACIN.............0
VITAMIN A.........4	CALCIUM.............6
VITAMIN C.........0	IRON.............0
THIAMINE (B₁).....0	VITAMIN B₁₂......10
RIBOFLAVIN (B₂)...10	PHOSPHORUS......15

INGREDIENTS: CULTURED SKIM MILK, MILK, CREAM, SALT, LOCUST BEAN GUM, GUAR GUM AND DEXTROSE.

FRIENDLY DAIRY FOODS, INC. HOMETOWN, U.S.A. 87654

STORE IN REFRIGERATOR

COTTAGE CHEESE SALAD

Arrange lettuce on plate; top with cottage cheese, peach slices, pineapple, and fresh grapes.

12345 67890

food. For example, manufacturers may use the packaging date or pull date to express the age of their product.[18] Consumers should understand that a product will maintain the freshness indicated by the date only if it has been properly handled and stored. A date cannot guarantee quality.[19]

Universal product coding (UPC) (see Fig. 2-1) is a new addition to many grocery labels. Its purpose is to cut costs for the retailer and ultimately for the consumer, to simplify storage, inventory, and ordering of merchandise, to speed check-out, and to reduce errors at check-out. The codes are standard ten-digit numbers with a machine-readable bar code that represents price, product, size, manufacturer, and the nature of the contents.[20] This code is read by a scanning device at the check-out counter. A computerized receipt identifies the product, manufacturer, price, and weight.

FOOD HANDLING AND PREPARATION

Although the food industry influences the quality of food from the farm to the retail store, the consumer's domestic handling of the purchased food strongly affects its overall quality. Proper methods of *storage, sanitation,* and *cooking* are necessary.

Storage to Maintain Food Quality

Most food items can maintain quality in nutritional value, taste, texture, and appearance only for a finite period of time. Storage times and temperatures that are longer and higher, respectively, than optimal will result in deterioration in many foods. Other factors that may cause food spoilage include exposure to oxygen, moisture, and bacterial growth. For each product, the life and method of storage is specifically determined. All, however, must be properly covered or in suitable containers to protect against contamination and off-flavor.

All foods deteriorate over time. For instance, fats change through the chemical reactions of oxidation and hydrolysis. Protein molecules break down, causing textural changes and loss of functional properties like thickening and whipping qualities. Pigments change color as they oxidize, and some vitamins are lost through deterioration.[21]

The following losses, however, occur prematurely if food is not stored properly:[22]

> *Loss of nutrient value,* such as vitamin loss and protein breakdown
>
> *Spoilage by microorganisms, enzymatic action, or insect infestation*
>
> *Loss of aesthetic qualities* such as color, flavor, aroma, texture, or general appearance
>
> *Loss of functional properties* such as leavening activity in baking powder, thickening power in sauce mixes, or the "set" in instant puddings

Refrigeration is the preferred method for storing many fresh foods, including produce, dairy products, and all fresh meat, fish, poultry, and eggs. Food that requires refrigeration should be kept at approximately 40°F (5°C); since bacteria, yeasts, and molds grow rapidly at 50 to 120°F (10 to 49°C), an unrefrigerated product may become contaminated in as little as 3 to 4 h. Milk requires immediate refrigeration since exposure to sunlight also destroys riboflavin. Vegetables stay crisper when they are refrigerated and tightly covered. Refrigeration is also necessary for fats and oils since temperatures of 80°F (27°C) can cause rancidity. During the summer and when the refrigerator is heavily filled, the temperature should be set lower because nutrient losses are greater at these times.[23]

To maintain the quality of frozen food, the temperature inside freezers must be held at 0°F (−18°C) or lower. Most freezing compartments within refrigerators do not reach these low temperatures; therefore, storage periods in them should be short. Separate freezer units, however, generally do hold food at 0°F (−18°C) but should preferably be set even lower for long-term freezing.

Products stored at room temperature should be kept in cool, dry areas. Moisture and heat are perfect conditions for bacterial growth. To protect against contamination by insects and rodents, foods should also be well sealed. Root and tuber vegetables can be stored at room temperatures not exceeding 70°F (21°C); higher temperatures cause rapid deterioration.

Sanitation in Food Handling

To minimize the incidence of food-borne illnesses (see App. Table A-8), food must also be handled properly. While food in the United States is among the safest in the world, many reported instances of food poisoning occur each year and a great many others go unreported. In 1974, 456 outbreaks of food poisoning were reported, involving 15,489 individual cases. At that time bacteria caused 61 percent of these food illnesses. Chemicals caused 29 percent; parasites, 8 percent; and viruses, another 3 percent of the illnesses. In this period there were 14 resulting deaths.[24] Most of these illnesses could have been prevented if food had been handled properly.

Proper handling of food in the store is necessary for its safety. Consumers should find stores that maintain high standards of quality and cleanliness. The consumer can also follow simple rules of domestic food sanitation to eliminate the possibility of transmitting food-borne illness. Table 2-4 lists important guidelines.

Cooking Methods

Cooking enhances the palatability, digestibility, and safety of many food items. Preparation methods, however, also affect nutritional value, color, texture, taste, smell, and, ultimately, acceptability. Normal home cooking may result in high vitamin and mineral losses.

Overcooking or overheating a product can destroy its nutritive value, texture, color, and flavor. Nutrient loss primarily occurs in the water-soluble vitamins (the B complex vitamins and ascorbic acid) through leaching. Even proper cooking methods cause some nutrient loss, and overcooking may make that loss excessive.

Just as products should not be overcooked, they also should not be undercooked. Sufficiently high temperatures are necessary to destroy microorganisms. For example, meat, fish, and poultry should be cooked in order to

---

TABLE 2-4   RULES FOR SANITATION IN FOOD HANDLING

1   The refrigerator should be kept at 40 to 45°F (5 to 8°C).
2   Cooked foods should be refrigerated immediately. They should not be allowed to cool on the counter before being put in the refrigerator as this provides an ideal medium for bacterial growth.
3   Frozen foods should be thawed in the refrigerator, not on the counter.
4   Produce should be washed before it is eaten.
5   Foods that are kept at room temperature should be in proper containers to protect them from insects, rodents, and dirt.
6   Anyone having an infectious illness (e.g., a cold) or sores on the hands should not prepare food.
7   Cans that have a leak or that bulge should be discarded *without tasting* the contents.
8   Products made with mayonnaise or cream fillings should be refrigerated.
9   Hands, counter, and cooking equipment should be clean before food preparation begins.
10   A utensil should not be returned to a bowl after being licked.
11   After use, dishes, utensils, and cooking equipment should be washed in hot soapy water and carefully rinsed.
12   Hands should be washed by anyone using the toilet or blowing his or her nose.

destroy parasites, bacteria, and viruses that may be present. Cooking destroys salmonellae. Pork in particular should be adequately cooked in order to eliminate the possibility of trichinosis. Legumes may carry toxic substances that are destroyed by cooking.

When preparing produce for cooking, the nutrient content can be retained in four ways:

1 By cutting the produce into larger rather than smaller pieces. The greater the exposed surface areas in cooking, the greater the loss of nutrients.

2 By scrubbing produce when possible rather than peeling it. The outer coat of many produce items (e.g., potatoes, apples, carrots) contains abundant supplies of nutrients and fiber.

3 By using the least amount of liquid possible in cooking. Water-soluble vitamins are a particular problem since they are lost in the cooking water. The nutrient-containing liquids that remain after cooking should be saved for gravies and soups.

4 By using a shorter cooking time. Covering the pot will decrease the cooking time since the steam increases the temperature. Exceptions are vegetables like cabbage and onions that have a high sulfur content. The sulfur flavor of these vegetables becomes quite pronounced and less palatable if they are covered during cooking.

DETERMINATION OF DIETARY ADEQUACY

Many guides have been developed to aid consumers in making wise decisions in their food consumption patterns, and with further research these guides will continue to be adjusted and updated. Ultimately, it is up to the consumers to be aware of these changes. Only then can they make informed food choices that reflect sound nutrition principles. Two guide-

TABLE 2-5   A COMPARISON OF INTERNATIONAL NUTRIENT STANDARDS FOR SELECTED NUTRIENTS

| | | | | | Fat-soluble vitamins | | | | | |
| | | | | | Vitamin A | | Vitamin D | | | Vitamin E |
Standard	Sex/ Age	Weight, kg	Kcal (kJ)	Protein, g	μ	RE*	μg	IU	IU	mg d-α-tocopherol
Recommended intakes of nutrients, FAO/WHO†	Male Adult	65	3000 (12,600)	37	750		2.5			
1974 recommended dietary allowances, USA‡	Male 23–50	70	2700 (11,340)	56		1000		0	15	
1975 Recommended daily nutrient intake, Canada§	Male 19–35	70	3000 (12,600)	56		1000	100			9

* RE: Retinol equivalents

† H. S. Mitchel, H. J. Rynbergen, L. Anderson, and M. V. Diblle, *Nutrition in Health and Disease*, J. B. Lippincott Co., Philadelphia, 1976, p. 296.

lines have been developed to aid health professionals and consumers choose diets to meet nutrient needs:

Recommended dietary allowances
Basic four food groups

Recommended Dietary Allowances

The recommended dietary allowances (RDA) represent nutritional standards for planning and assessing dietary intake. They are defined by the Food and Nutrition Board of the National Research Council (NRC) as "levels of intake of essential nutrients considered to be adequate to meet the nutritional needs of practically all healthy persons."[25] (See App. Table A-1.) These guidelines are appropriately used only for normal, healthy members of the American population. Since their development in 1943, the allowances have been continually updated in accordance with the most current scientific research. Every five years new data

are reviewed and both the RDAs and background information on nutrients and their functions are revised.

Other countries (e.g., Canada) have also developed their own standards as a means of improving nutritional status; standards have also been issued by the Food and Agriculture Organization (FAO) (see Table 2-5). Differences between these standards relate to using minimal vs maximal nutrient needs (the latter provide a margin of safety), and reflect nutrient needs based on differing life styles and environments. The Canadian recommendations are similar in philosophy to those of the United States. The guidelines established by the FAO are set for minimum daily requirements and reflect the needs of a moderately active population.[26]

Determination of the RDAs Nutrient allowances are based on the most current and valid scientific evidence available. Ideally, recommendations consider (1) the *average* nutrient re-

TABLE 2-5 *(continued)*

	Water-soluble Vitamins						Minerals					
Ascorbic acid, mg	Folacin, μg	Niacin, mg	Riboflavin, mg	Thiamine, mg	Vitamin B6, mg	Vitamin B12, μg	Calcium, mg	Phosphorus, mg	Iodine, μg	Iron, mg	Magnesium, mg	Zinc, mg
30	200	19.8	1.8	1.2		2.0	400–500			5–9		
45	400	18.0	1.6	1.4	2.0	3.0	800	800	130	10	350	15
30	200	20.0	1.8	1.5	2.0	3.0	800	800	150	10	300	10

‡ Food and Nutrition Board, *Recommended Dietary Allowances*, rev. ed., 1974, National Research Council Publications, National Academy of Sciences, Washington, D.C.

§ Information Canada, Ottawa, KIA OS9, *Dietary Standard for Canada*, Catalog H58-26, 1975.

quirements of a representative segment of healthy people for each age group, (2) the statistical *variability* of people, and (3) the possible *increased requirement* above the average in order to meet the needs of almost all healthy Americans.[25] A variety of research procedures are used to determine nutrient requirements. These include balance studies, biochemical measurements of nutrients, and clinical evaluations.

Scientific knowledge is well established for some nutrients, while relatively little data are available for others. Protein (see Chap. 3) is an example of a nutrient for which data are rather extensive. Establishing caloric needs is relatively easy since a close relationship exists between energy intake and energy expenditure. The study of vitamin A, however, has been limited, and only two major studies have been considered in determining its allowance.

In the United States norms, a margin of safety is added for all nutrients except calories. A margin of safety is an "extra" that allows for differences in nutrient requirements among individuals. This allowance is approximately the average requirement plus an added 30 to 50 percent. The RDAs are guidelines are not specific nutrient requirements for individuals, and failure of individuals to meet the RDAs does not connote a deficiency state.

Method of expression The RDAs are grouped to apply to varying age, sex, and weight groups and reflect the increased needs of pregnancy and lactation.

For most nutrients, the RDAs are expressed in metric measures. (The metric system is the internationally accepted standard of measure, and with the passage of the 1975 Metric Conversion Act, voluntary conversion to the metric system will be assisted through a national policy.) Since the *joule* is the unit of measure in the metric system, kilocalories are now expressed also as kilojoules. One kilocalorie (*kcal*) equals 4.2 kilojoules (kJ). Historically many RDAs have been expressed in metric measure. For example, protein requirements

are listed in grams while thiamine, ascorbic acid, calcium, and iron are expressed in milligrams. Both vitamins D and E are expressed in international units (IU).

Influences on the RDA The following factors influence the recommendations of nutrients for individuals: physiological state (growth, pregnancy, lactation), body size, sex, physical activity, environmental temperature, age, and illness and the presence of intestinal parasites.

Although *activity levels* will differ among individuals, the RDA for calories has been set to meet the needs of typically sedentary activity levels in the United States. Because of the high incidence of obesity and overweight in the United States, there is no need to include a margin of safety for calories.

Although much of the United States climate is temperate, the extreme *temperatures* found in some areas may influence nutrient needs. Prolonged exposure to cold temperatures increases requirements for calories while exposure to higher temperatures lowers these requirements due to reduced activity and energy expenditure.

As people *age,* requirements for most nutrients do not change; however, energy need is decreased because of a lowered basal metabolic rate and reduced activity levels.

When a person is fighting *illness, surgical stress, or intestinal parasites,* nutrient requirements need to be adjusted to accommodate for metabolic loss.

Interpretation and Use of the Recommended Dietary Allowances

As a tool for guiding nutrient intake, RDAs should be interpreted with these considerations:

1 RDAs are expressed in groupings by age, sex, and weight, with special recommendations for pregnant and lactating women.

2 RDAs do not designate a particular diet.

They guide nutrient intake, not food intake.

3 RDAs are provided on the basis of daily intake. Fat-soluble vitamins are stored in the body, so that larger amounts may be consumed one day and used later; the average daily value is provided by the RDA.

4 RDAs are not designed for therapeutic needs (states of illness, stress, surgery).

5 Evidence is inadequate on which to base some allowances, such as those for adolescents, older adults, or users of contraceptives. RDAs do not completely represent the nutrient needs of these groups.

6 RDAs are appropriately used to evaluate diets of groups of people and not individual diets. When these data are coupled with clinical and biochemical evidence, dietary deficiencies can be identified. Many researchers have used *two-thirds* of the RDA as the breaking point between an adequate and an inadequate diet, which means that when the intake of a nutrient is two-thirds below the RDA, the diet may be deficient. Since the RDA is a somewhat arbitrary tool that is periodically revised on the basis of current research, *two-thirds of the RDA* must be used cautiously to express dietary adequacy.

7 RDAs do not establish the percentage of calories to be consumed from carbohydrate, fat, and protein.

8 The RDA level of protein must be exceeded in order to have adequate intakes of vitamin B_6, iron, and zinc.

9 RDAs are not established for all nutrients known to be essential to man (e.g., trace minerals).

Food Group Classification

Food grouping systems are used throughout the world to translate nutritional needs such as those established by the RDAs into practical guidelines for food intake. Food groups are designed so that individuals fulfilling the specified criteria will consume necessary quantities of essential nutrients.

Basic Four Food Groups

The grouping of specific foods is determined first and foremost by nutrient content, and then reflects availability of food, food patterns, and local nutrition problems. However, at the present time both the United States and Canada use the basic four food groups system (See Fig. 2-2). The basic four classifies foods into the following four groupings: *milk, meat, fruit and vegetables,* and *grain*. This system also establishes the requirements for portion size and number of servings (see Table 2-6).

Foods are grouped according to their similarity in nutrient content and have a high *nutrient density;* i.e., a high proportion of nutrients to the amount of calories supplied. Foods with a high *caloric density* have a high proportion of calories for the amount of nutrient provided.

Foods that are high in fats, oils, or sugar and low in other nutrients are classified outside the four food groups. These include sugar, potato chips, soft drinks, cakes, candy, jam, syrup, salad dressings, oil, butter, and margarine. These foods have a high caloric density and a low nutrient density.

Basic four as an evaluation tool The basic four food groups system was primarily designed as an easy tool for the evaluation of a day's meal pattern for normal, healthy individuals. It was not designed to be an absolute measure of dietary quality. It is a simple, rough estimate that allows consumers and health professionals to check the intake of essential foods in order to plan a diet which offers the basic nutrient requirements for optimal health.

There are times, however, when adjustments need to be made. As an example, pregnant and lactating women require more than the usually recommended intake of foods from the meat and milk groups, while infants and small children require smaller amounts of food than called for in the guideline. At the present

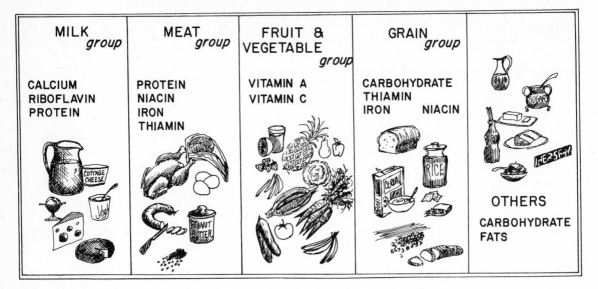

Figure 2-2

Food groups. Food is classified into groups on the basis of nutrient content. By consuming recommended servings from the four groups with high nutrient density most individuals can be adequately nourished. Foods from the other groups provide calories but few nutrients.

time the basic four is a good system for a consumer's quick and easy dietary evaluation.

Limitations of the basic four   The following points should be considered when using food groups:

1   The high amounts of iron required by pregnant, lactating, and premenopausal women cannot be met by the basic four food groups.

2   Strict adherence to the basic four guideline without accompanying foods of high caloric density (e.g., gravies, condiments, etc.) may result in an energy intake that is lower than the RDA for some individuals.

3   The guideline for protein-rich foods is high, providing excess protein in order to supply adequate quantities of vitamin B_6, iron, and zinc.

4   Ready-to-eat processed and fabricated foods that are consumed in industrialized societies, like formulated fruit drinks and breakfast bars, cannot be classified into a food group because they may not follow the nutrient pattern of any one food group. In addition, they do not provide trace elements that are present in naturally occurring foods.

5   Overprocessing destroys nutrients in a given food; thus, a food may no longer represent a serving from any food group. For example, potato chips cannot be included in the vegetable group.

6   Combinations of foods like casseroles and pizzas make group classification difficult. They should often be classified into two or more groups.

7   Some foods are omitted from the basic four altogether because there is no classification for "empty-calorie" foods like sugar and oils.

8   It may be difficult to utilize the basic four when assessing the diet of ethnic groups (e.g., Chinese-American).

TABLE 2-6 BASIC FOUR FOOD GROUPS WITH NUTRIENT PATTERN AND RECOMMENDED QUANTITY

Group	Nutrients	Quantity	Comments
Milk	Calcium Protein Phosphorus Riboflavin	*Servings:* Three or more for children, four or more for teenagers, two or more for adults *Serving size equals:* 8 oz milk or yogurt 1 oz cheese 1½ cup cottage cheese, ice cream, or custard	Butter is not included in this group as it is a fat and does not contain other essential nutrients
Meat	Protein B vitamins Iron	*Servings:* Two or more *Serving size equals:* 3 oz meat, poultry, or fish 2 eggs 2 tbsp peanut butter ½ cup lentils or beans	Legumes, nuts, and soy extenders can be substituted for meat although the protein has a lower biological value than meat has. These foods can be combined with animal or grain products to increase protein quality
Vegetable and fruit	Vitamin A Vitamin C Carbohydrate (fiber) Iron	*Servings:* Four or more *Serving size equals:* ½ cup vegetable or fruit 4 oz citrus juice 1 medium size fruit ½ cup dark green or yellow vegetables	One serving daily should be vitamin C–rich (e.g., citrus fruits). Vitamin A–rich foods (e.g., leafy green and yellow vegetables) should be consumed 3–4 times/wk
Grain	Carbohydrate (fiber) B vitamins Iron	*Servings:* Four or more *Serving size equals:* 1 slice bread ½ cup cereal	Whole grain and enriched products are recommended grain foods

While food grouping systems have limitations, they are still an invaluable tool in nutrition counseling and education. It is essential to be flexible, understanding that a wide variety of food combinations can satisfy a person's nutrient requirements.

Basic four scoring system The basic four is a simple guideline for evaluating a patient's diet that can be used both by health professionals and by patients themselves. This is done by recording all food intake for a 24-h period or longer and then scoring the diet using the basic four food group as a guideline. Generally a 3- or 7-day record provides more information than a single day's about meal patterns and a better picture of food intake (see Chap. 15).

Once the intake of food has been recorded, it should be compared with the quantity suggested by the four food groups. Table 2-7 is an example of a scoring system used to rate diets. The amount of each item consumed is recorded in one column. One point is recorded for *each full serving consumed.* Table 2-7 lists serving sizes. A score is then determined for each food group, and a grand total is assigned for the diet. The optimum scores are 12, 13, and 14 for adults, children, and teenagers, respectively.

Within the milk group each age group has different requirements; as a result the total possible points to be earned varies. The fruit and vegetable group also has special scoring requirements. In order to receive a possible 4 points in this group, one serving each of vitamin A–rich and vitamin C–rich foods must be consumed, for which a maximum of 2 points is given, with all other vegetables contributing another possible 2 points. Using this food pattern summary, data on the caloric and nutrient intake may be easily gathered.

TABLE 2-7 SCORING SYSTEM FOR A FOOD RECORD

Food group	Serving size	Amount consumed	Total no. servings consumed	Total possible points	Score for food group
Milk	2 cups adults			2	
	3 cups children			3	
	4 cups teenagers			4	
	4 cups pregnancy and lactation			4	
Cheese	1 oz cheddar				
	1½ cup cottage				
Yogurt	8 oz				
Ice cream	1½ cups				
Others					
Meat					
Meat, fish, poultry	3 oz				
Eggs	2			3	
Nuts or legumes	½ cup				
Others					
Fruits and vegetables					
Vitamin C–rich	½ cup fruit or vegetable juice			1	
	1 medium-size fruit				
Vitamin A–rich	½ cup dark green or yellow fruit			1	
Others				2	
Grain					
Bread	1 slice				
Cereal	½ cup			4	
Others					
Others					
Sweets					
Fats and oils					
Soft drinks				0	
Coffee, tea					
Alcohol					
Total points					

Optimum score					
Children				13	
Teenagers				14	
Adults				12	
Pregnancy and lactation				14	

Food Composition Tables as a Tool for Evaluating Diets

Food composition tables, giving the approximate nutrient content of foods, are a necessary tool for evaluating diets. Tables are expressed in either 100-g portions of a food, the edible portion of 1 lb of food, or portions commonly consumed. Energy is expressed as calories, and nutrients are generally indicated using metric measure or international units (or retinol equivalents for vitamin A). The values represent the average nutrient content of food items throughout the year and throughout the United States. An average is taken from research on a variety of weighed samples. Actual analysis is completed by government, universities, and industry.

When using composition tables for dietary evaluation, nutrient values must be considered in proper perspective. They are estimates and not the exact nutrient content of specific foods.

1 Growing conditions (e.g., sunlight, soil, climate) affect the nutrient content of the same variety of a food.
2 There is variability in a plant food, depending upon maturity, variety, season, and plant part.
3 Storage, processing, and preparation influence nutrient values.
4 The total amount of the nutrient listed may not be biologically available to an individual.

Examples of available food composition tables include:

Composition of Foods: Raw, Processed, and Prepared, USDA Handbook No. 8, United States Department of Agriculture, Washington, D.C., December 1963.

Nutritive Value of American Foods in Common Units, USDA Handbook No. 456, United States Department of Agriculture, Washington, D.C., November 1975.

C. Church and H. Church, *Food Values of Portions Commonly Used,* J. B. Lippincott Co., Philadelphia, 1975.

THE ADEQUATE DIET—THE PRUDENT DIET

The adequate diet for our population must now become the "prudent diet" to combat many of our diet-related diseases and conditions such as coronary heart disease, obesity,

---

CASE STUDY 2-1

P is a 28-year-old graduate student on a limited income who shares an apartment with three roommates. Because of an erratic study schedule and social activities there is little thought given to meal planning. This is further complicated by lack of income and inadequate storage facilities. Most of P's meals are consumed on the run from vending machines or fast-food chains. His typical dietary pattern includes:

9:00 A.M.	*1 cup black coffee and sugar*
10:30 A.M.	*1 cup black coffee and sugar*
1:00 P.M.	*3 slices of pizza, 12 oz Coke, 1 candy bar*
5:00 P.M.	*12 oz beer*

7:00 P.M.	*1 hamburger (3 oz beef, roll, 1 tbsp mayonnaise, and mustard)* *12 oz Coke* *Bag of potato chips*

Case Study Questions

1 Score this diet according to the basic four food groups. What groups are missing?
2 What recommendations would you make to improve the adequacy of this diet?
3 What suggestions would you make for economical shopping?

---

and now perhaps even cancer. The prudent diet will still contain foods from the basic four food groups but now more skim milk will be suggested, and from the meat group fish and poultry will be encouraged, with eggs kept to a maximum of three times per week. Vegetables and fruit and whole-grain breads and cereals will be emphasized for fiber, and combinations of these foods may be used to supply future protein needs and help to preserve dwindling protein reserves. The future of our health now depends on the adequate diet's becoming the prudent diet.

Basic four food group	*Prudent diet*
Milk	skim milk
Meat	chicken, fish, eggs 3x/wk
Fruits and vegetables	increase
Breads and cereals	whole-grain
Other	less sugar
	less fat

Study Questions

1 Are fortified, enriched, and engineered foods a benefit or detriment to the diet? Explain.

2 What information can the label provide for the consumer?

3 What steps must be taken to reduce possibilities of food-borne illness?

4 For what purpose is the RDA used? What are its limitations?

5 In what way is the basic four food groups system an appropriate tool for dietary evaluation?

REFERENCES

1 Institute of Food Technologists' Expert Panel on Food Safety and Nutrition and the Committee on Public Information, "The Effects of Food Processing in Nutritional Values," Chicago, October 1974.

2 Food and Nutrition Board, "Improvement of the Nutritive Quality of Foods," *Journal of American Medical Association,* August 27, 1973, p. 63.

3 Anonymous, "Problems in Iron Enrichment and Fortification of Foods," *Nutrition Reviews,* February 1975, p. 46.

4 Ibid., p. 65.

5 Ibid., p. 63.

6 W. M. Bortz, P. Howat, and W. L. Holmes, "The Effect of Feeding Frequency on Diurnal Plasma Free Fatty Acids and Glucose Levels," *Metabolism,* February 1969, p. 120.

7 R. J. Wurtman, "Biologic Rhythms in the Body," *Technical Review,* March 1968, p. 3.

8 R. J. Wurtman, C. M. Rose, C. Shou, and F. F. Larin, "Daily Rhythms in the Concentrations of Various Amino Acids in Human Plasma," *New England Journal of Medicine,* July 25, 1968, p. 171.

9 J. Goldberg, "The Fast Food Phenomenon," *Family Health,* April 1975, p. 39.

10 H. Appledorf, "Nutritional Analysis of Food from Fast Food Chains," *Food Technology,* April 1974, p. 50.

11 L. F. Chem and P. A. LaChance, "An Area of Concern: The Nutritive Profile of Fast Food Combinations," *Food Product Development,* October 1974, p. 40.

12 J. M. Coon and J. C. Ayres, "Safety of Foods," chap. 11 in J. Mayer (ed.), *U.S. Nutrition Policies of the Seventies,* W. H. Freeman and Co., San Francisco, 1973.

13 J. A. Thomas and D. L. Call, "Eating between Meals—A Nutrition Problem Among Teenagers?" *Nutrition Reviews,* May 1973, p. 137.

14 Anonymous, "Food Takes More of Needy Budgets," *Community Nutrition Institute Week,* May 1, 1975, p. 8.

15 C. K. Sherk, "Changes in Food Consumption Patterns," *Food Technology,* **25,** September 1971, p. 914.

16 B. Peterkin, "Food Plans and Family Budgeting," *Family Economic Review,* May 1975, p. 3.

17 H. H. Gift, M. B. Washbon, and G. Harrison, *Nutrition Behavior and Change,* Prentice-Hall, Inc., Englewood Cliffs, N.J., 1972, p. 104.

18 F. J. McEwen, "Consumer Problems in Relation to the Food Industries," chap. 16 in J. Mayer (ed.) *U.S.*

Nutrition Policies in the Seventies, W. H. Freeman and Co., San Francisco, 1973.

19 E. F. Taylor, "Guide to Buying—Open Dating and Price per Unit," *Shopper's Guide,* 1974 Yearbook of Agriculture, USDA, Washington, D.C., 1975.

20 Health and Consumer Product Department, "Looking Ahead to Automation in the Supermarkets," *Dow Dairy,* Fall, 1975.

21 Institute of Food Technologists' Expert Panel on Food Safety and Nutrition and the Committee on Public Information, "Shelf Life of Foods," Chicago, August 1974.

22 Ibid.

23 B. C. Hobbs, *Food Poisoning and Food Hygiene,* 2d ed., Edward Arnold, Ltd., London, 1968.

24 Center for Disease Control, "Foodborne and Waterborne Disease Outbreaks," USHEW, Public Health Service, Atlanta, 1976.

25 Food and Nutrition Board, *Recommended Dietary Allowances,* rev. ed., National Research Council Publications, National Academy of Sciences, Washington, D.C. 1974.

26 J. A. Campbell, "Approaches in Revising Dietary Standards—Canadian, U.S., and International Standards Compared," *Journal of American Dietetic Association,* February 1974, p. 175.

CHAPTER 3

PROTEIN

Ruth Palombo

KEY WORDS
Conjugated Proteins
Peptide Bonds
Essential Amino Acids
Nonessential Amino Acids
Transamination
DNA (Deoxyribonucleic Acid)
RNA (Ribonucleic Acid)
Deamination
Decarboxylation

INTRODUCTION

The controversy over protein requirements has sparked a lively debate in both the scientific and popular literature.[1,2] Today the subject of protein nutrition is a major political, economic, and social issue. The potential problem of world hunger cannot be taken lightly. Are we facing a protein crisis? We are warned of a grain deficit of 85 million tons in developing countries by 1985 if food production does not increase.[3] We can speculate on ways to develop, use, and redistribute the world's agricultural resources. Yet we have no national plan developed nor are we focusing our scientific and technical knowledge toward meeting the increased needs for food production around the world.

Although protein is available from many sources, each nation usually has a particular protein food or food combination which serves as its dietary staple. In the United States this food has traditionally been meat. Americans are very fond of meat, and with increasing affluence people consume more meat. Even in families with low incomes, a major part of the food budget is spent on meat, poultry, and fish, with little money left for other foods such as dairy products, fruits, and vegetables.[4] Consumers in the United States are very sensitive to meat prices. Evidence of this was the 1973 nationwide boycott of meat touched off by rising meat prices. Yet as food prices rise, many people have begun questioning whether they should change their eating practices; that is, eat less meat and more of alternative protein sources.[5]

Consumption of protein has generally been high in the United States, with inadequate intakes being a problem in only a few cases.[6,7] Sixty years ago cereals supplied 36 percent of our available protein and meat only 30 percent; in 1971, cereal products provided 18 percent, while meat, fish, and poultry supplied 42 percent. These shifts in consumption of meat and cereal products represent major changes in the source of dietary proteins in the American diet.[8]

In addition to the current controversy over the use of protein, the confirmed role of protein in growth and the maintenance of body tissue, and its newly discovered role in the body's immune defense system, make the knowledge of protein essential to the student who will establish a nutrition-centered health practice.

FUNCTIONS OF PROTEINS

Proteins have a wide range of specialized functions and characteristics. They are necessary for:

1 Growth
2 Maintenance and repair of body tissues
3 Energy supply

Yet, despite the diversity of functions, proteins have some common characteristics. Proteins are large organic molecules of which simpler compounds called *amino acids* are the basic structural unit. When proteins are broken down (hydrolyzed), they split into these amino acids. All proteins contain the elements carbon, hydrogen, nitrogen, and oxygen. Many proteins contain sulfur and phosphorus and some also contain metallic components such as iron, zinc, and copper. Each gram of protein supplies 4 kcal (17 kJ) when metabolized. However, it is the presence of nitrogen that makes protein unique and differentiates it from fat and carbohydrate, the other energy-yielding nutrients in our diet.

When we eat, food proteins supply our bodies with amino acids for synthesis of body proteins and nitrogenous compounds. During normal tissue turnover some amino acids are released and are reused for synthesis of body protein. Other products of amino acid metabolism such as urea, creatinine, and uric acid are excreted in the urine. Nitrogen is also lost through many body secretions, excretions, sweat, feces, sloughed skin, hair, and nails. Therefore, in order to replace these losses, dietary proteins which supply amino acids and nitrogen are necessary throughout the life cycle, even when growth has stopped.

The human body is approximately 18 to 20 percent protein by weight. Protein provides the structural framework for our bodies. Muscles contain about 45 percent of this protein and the skeleton about 18 percent. Skin and adipose tissues contain about 10 and 4 percent respectively of the body's total protein.[9]

CLASSIFICATION OF PROTEINS

Proteins can be classified in many ways. One common method is to describe proteins as either simple or conjugated. *Simple proteins* consist of only amino acids. Upon hydrolysis, they yield only amino acids. There are no nonprotein constituents in simple proteins. *Conjugated proteins* consist of simple proteins plus a prosthetic group (nonprotein constituent). Upon hydrolysis, conjugated proteins are broken down into amino acids and other substances. Examples of conjugated proteins are nucleoproteins (protein and RNA or DNA), lipoproteins (protein and lipid), glycoproteins (protein and carbohydrate), and metaloproteins (protein and metal such as zinc, copper, or iron). Another way to group proteins is according to function (see Table 3-1).

CLASSIFICATION OF AMINO ACIDS

The general formula for the amino acids found in protein can be represented as the following:

$$
\underset{\text{Side chain}}{R} - \underset{\underset{H}{|}}{\overset{\overset{NH_2}{|}}{C}} - \underset{\text{Carboxyl group}}{COOH}
$$

Amino group

TABLE 3-1   CLASSIFICATION OF PROTEIN BY FUNCTION

Classification	Body location	Example	Function
Structural proteins	Skin, cartilage, bone	Collagen	Principal substance in connective tissue
Contractile proteins	Skeletal muscle	Actin, myosin	Muscle contraction
Antibodies	Blood plasma, spleen, lymphatic cells	Alpha globulins	Disease protection
Blood proteins	Blood plasma	Albumins	Control osmotic pressure of blood Maintain the buffering capacity of blood pH
	Blood	Fibrinogen	Blood clotting
	Blood	Hemoglobin	Transports oxygen from lungs to all parts of the body
Hormones	Endocrine or duct-less glands (thyroid, pancreas, parathyroid, adrenals, pituitary)	Insulin	Regulates carbohydrate metabolism
		Growth hormone	Stimulates overall protein synthesis and growth
Enzymes	Throughout body—nearly 2000 different enzymes known; each highly specific in function		Biological catalysts; proteins which allow chemical reactions to proceed at their proper rate
	Stomach	Pepsin	Protein digestion
	Pancreas	Trypsin and chymotrypsin	Protein digestion
Nutrient proteins		Meat, fish, chicken, milk, cheese, eggs, peanut butter, nuts, soybeans, tofu, dried peas and beans	Sources of amino acids required by man and other animals
Viruses	Microscopic infective agents	Smallpox, measles	Cause disease
Nucleoproteins	Cell nucleus	DNA	Determines and transmits hereditary characteristics; carries genetic (hereditary) code

As indicated, the amino acid is formulated from a carbon chain (carbon skeleton), and the amino and radical groups are then added. Since the amino group is on the carbon adjacent to the carboxyl group (the alpha carbon), the amino acids having this formula are known as alpha-amino acids. All amino acids have a free carboxyl group (COOH) and a free amino group (NH_2) on the alpha carbon atom. Amino acids differ from each other according to their unique side chains or R groups. There are 20 different amino acids which serve as the building blocks of protein. Amino acids are usually grouped according to their chemical nature. The classification is as follows:[10]

1   Monoamino monocarboxylic: glycine, leucine, alanine, isoleucine, valine
2   Hydroxyl-containing: serine, threonine
3   Sulfur-containing: cystine, cysteine, methionine
4   Aromatic: tyrosine, phenylalanine
5   Heterocyclic: proline, hydroxyproline, histidine, tryptophan
6   Diamino monocarboxylic (basic): arginine, lysine
7   Monoamino dicarboxylic (acidic): glutamic acid, aspartic acid

Amino acids are joined together in proteins by linkages called *peptide bonds:*

These linkages are formed by the attachment of the carboxylic carbon of one amino acid to the nitrogen of another amino acid. At the same time, a molecule of water is eliminated.

In protein molecules, the amino acids are linked together in long chains called *polypeptides.* (A *peptide* is two or more amino acids linked together; a *polypeptide* is many amino acids linked together.) Polypeptides are large molecules which may consist of hundreds of amino acids in the form of a helix or spiral. Some proteins consist of only one polypeptide chain; some contain two, three, or more. The specific function of each protein depends on its constituent amino acids and the arrangement of the amino acids in the polypeptide chain. The number, kind, and sequence of the amino acids (known as the *primary structure*) in each polypeptide chain of each protein is genetically determined by DNA (deoxyribonucleic acid) on the chromosomes (see "Protein Synthesis," below). Each polypeptide chain has its own unique characteristics:

1   Specific molecular weight
2   Specific chemical composition
3   Definite amino acid sequence
4   Definite three-dimensional shape

The molecular weights of proteins vary from 5000 to 1 million. Most polypeptide chains contain 100 to 300 amino acids and have a molecular weight of 12,000 to 36,000.[11]

DETERMINANTS OF PROTEIN REQUIREMENTS

Nitrogen Balance

Determining nitrogen balance provides a gross measure of protein utilization. This determination is based on the assumption that nitrogen equilibrium occurs in adults when the diet supplies adequate protein for (1) synthesis of tissues (such as hair and nails) and (2) replacement of endogenous losses in the urine, feces, sweat, and sloughed epithelial cells. Theoretically, the formula for nitrogen balance is:

Nitrogen balance = dietary nitrogen intake
 − (urinary + fecal + skin losses of nitrogen)

$$B = I - (U + F + S)$$

Measuring the amount of nitrogen eaten in food and comparing this to the amount excreted in the feces helps to determine nitrogen balance. A *positive nitrogen balance* indicates that the body is retaining nitrogen, while a *negative balance* signifies that more nitrogen is being excreted than consumed. When the nitrogen in the food consumed equals what is excreted, nitrogen balance is zero and the body is in *nitrogen equilibrium.* Nitrogen balance is affected by physiological state, energy requirements, and diet.

Physiological state   Childhood growth periods, pregnancy, and lactation are characterized by a marked positive nitrogen balance. When an individual is under severe stress from infection, fever, surgical trauma, or starvation, protein is depleted from the tissues, resulting in negative nitrogen balance. There is no evidence at present to indicate that the normal stresses of daily living increase our nutrient needs.

Energy requirements   The body's energy needs take first priority. If calories (joules) from fat and carbohydrate are inadequate, protein and amino acids from the diet and from tissue breakdown are used for energy. Energy, not nitrogen, becomes the limiting factor when food intake is low. Diets used in nitrogen balance studies must be adequate in fat and carbohydrate in order to spare protein for its unique functions.

Diet   Nitrogen balance depends on the amounts and proportions of essential amino acids in the diet plus the total nitrogen intake. For an adult, finding that the body is in ni-

trogen equilibrium would probably mean that the diet is adequate.

Essential and Nonessential Amino Acids

Protein requirements vary, depending on the composition of the protein eaten. Therefore, the central problem in protein nutrition is our requirement for specific types, amounts, and proportions of amino acids rather than protein per se.

The proteins in the human body are made up of 20 amino acids in varying combinations. Each protein has its own unique amino acid composition. Eight of these amino acids cannot be synthesized by the body in large enough quantities to meet body needs. These amino acids, because they must be supplied by food, are known as the *essential amino acids.* They are

Tryptophan	Valine
Leucine	Threonine
Isoleucine	Methionine
Lysine	Phenylalanine

Histidine is an essential amino acid for infants.[12] Histidine was thought to be nonessential for adults; however, a recent study suggests that this may not be the case,[13] and further studies must be done to clarify the essentiality of histidine for adults.

In order for our bodies to carry out protein synthesis, all eight essential amino acids must be present simultaneously and in the proper proportions. This means that if one essential amino acid is missing in the diet or present in a disproportionately small quantity, protein synthesis will slow down or stop completely. When a food is low in one or more of the essential amino acids, the utilization of all amino acids is reduced in the same proportion as the "limiting" amino acid.

The *nonessential* or *dispensable amino acids* can be produced by the body if there is an adequate source of nitrogen as well as carbon, hydrogen, and oxygen. The nonessential amino acids are as important as the essential amino acids in growth and body metabolism. The terms *essential* and *nonessential* refer only to how they are supplied to the body; i.e., the carbon skeleton of the essential amino acids cannot be formed in the human body and must be supplied by our diets.

After the requirement for essential amino acids has been met, the requirement for additional nitrogen can be met by any protein-containing foods in our diet, or by nitrogenous compounds such as urea or amino acids from the metabolic pool. The carbon skeletons for the nonessential amino acids can arise from intermediary products of fat and carbohydrate metabolism. Nonessential amino acids may be formed when a carbon skeleton combines with a free amino group derived from another amino acid or from ammonia. The process by which an amino group is transferred from one amino acid to another is called *transamination*. The availability of the nonessential amino acids depends on the proper functioning of these conversion systems. In diseases in which protein formation is disturbed, such as liver disease or protein malnutrition, the failure to form nonessential amino acids may increase the severity of the illness.[14]

Our diet is the usual source of nonessential amino acids and nitrogen. When the nonessen-tial amino acids in the diet are low, they must be formed in adequate quantities from the products of intermediary metabolism in order to allow the most efficient usage of the essential amino acids. Therefore protein synthesis is determined by the supply of essential amino acids, as well as by the rapidity and efficiency of production of nonessential amino acids. Both the essential and nonessential amino acids must be present simultaneously and in the proper proportions for protein synthesis to proceed efficiently. For example the protein in cereal is better utilized when milk is consumed with it.

Recommended Protein Allowances

There is no universal agreement on the optimal amount of protein needed in the diet.[15] In general, the protein requirements are less than the quantities consumed by most Americans.

Adults

The Food and Nutrition Board of the National Research Council advocates a daily protein allowance of 0.8 g/kg of ideal body weight for adults. The 1974 recommended dietary allowance (RDA) for protein is based on the following criteria:[16]

0.47 g protein/kg body weight per day—average maintenance requirement for nitrogen, estimated from nitrogen balance studies; not for growth

+

0.14 g protein/kg body weight per day—30% over maintenance requirement to account for individual variability

---

0.6 g protein/kg body weight per day—allowance for high-quality protein; to cover needs of almost all healthy individuals in the U.S. (95% population)

+

0.2 g protein/kg body weight per day—additional allowance for U.S. diet, which contains a combination of high-quality and lower-nutrient-quality proteins; 75% efficiency of utilization assumed

---

Total 0.8 g protein/kg body weight per day—RDA for protein for adults

For a "reference" man weighing 70 kg, the RDA is 56 g of protein per day (0.8 g × 70 = 56), a decrease from the 1968 RDA of 65 g. For a reference woman weighing 58 kg, the RDA is 46 g of protein per day (0.8 g × 58 = 46), a decrease from the 1968 RDA of 55 g. These reduced protein recommendations have been criticized as being "incompatible with sound nutritional planning."[17] Protein foods contain a variety of nutrients, including B_6 and some trace elements. Adequate intakes of these nutrients may be difficult to obtain within the current RDAs for protein and energy.[18] Deficiency of these nutrients is unusual since most Americans consume more protein than the current recommendations. However, problems with these nutrients might occur in institutions where personnel are required to keep costs down as well as meet the recommended allowances.[19] Since protein is one of the more expensive dietary components, it is often held within the recommendation.

It should be emphasized that the controversy revolves around the potentially inadequate intake of other nutrients found in protein, not the recommendation for protein per se. The current RDAs for protein more than cover the maintenance requirement for nitrogen equilibrium, individual variation, and variable utilization of mixed proteins in the American diet. However, since our knowledge of the availability, essentiality, and balance of trace elements and other less-studied nutrients is uncertain, it seems wise to plan diets around protein levels which we know are compatible with health from epidemiological studies, even though they may contain more protein than necessary to maintain nitrogen equilibrium.[20] When protein intake is limited because of poor food selection or inadequate income, the additional calories often come from low-nutrient fats, sugars, and alcohol, components which already comprise a large proportion of the American diet and are contributory to our major health problems of obesity, heart disease, and dental caries.

Infants

Protein allowances for infants are based on normal growth rates, changes in body composition, and the amount of milk protein that will result in satisfactory growth. We know from clinical experience that the protein in human milk is adequate for a breast-fed infant who feeds completely at the breast of a well-nourished woman. During the first year of life, the protein content of the body increases from 11 to 14.6 percent. This increase in body protein is approximately 3.5 g per day during the first 4 months and 3.1 g per day during the next 8 months.[21] The recommended protein allowance (RDA) is 2.2 g/kg body weight per day for infants up to age 6 months and 2.0 g/kg body weight for infants age 6 months to 1 year.[22]

During early infancy, the most rapid postnatal growth period, an unusually high proportion of protein intake is used for growth. Beyond infancy, as the growth rate decreases, children and adults use an increasing proportion of their protein intake for maintenance (nongrowth) needs.

The low-birth-weight infant has an increased requirement for both energy and protein, because of a potentially more rapid growth rate which is comparable to that of the fetus rather than that of a mature infant. The formula must have a energy and nutritional content greater than that of human milk.[23] The estimated protein requirement for low-birth-weight infants is 3 to 4 g/kg body weight per day.[24,25] (See Chap. 26.)

Children and Adolescents

Studies on the nitrogen and protein requirements of children and adolescents are limited. The allowances for individuals aged 1 to 18 years are calculated from data on growth rates[26] and body composition.[27,28] The RDAs for children and adolescents are found in the Appendix.

Pregnancy

Throughout pregnancy, an additional 30 g of protein per day is now recommended. The Food and Nutrition Board increased the protein allowances from the 1968 RDA of 10 additional grams per day because of (1) recent nitrogen balance data suggesting that efficiency of protein utilization during pregnancy is lower than was previously thought, and (2) epidemiological evidence that protein intakes of healthy pregnant women tend to be higher than estimated needs.[29]

The additional protein allowance during gestation provides for the needs of the developing fetus and surrounding tissue, maintenance protein requirements of the mother, and an adjustment for efficiency of dietary protein utilization. It is widely accepted that 925 g of protein is deposited in the fetus and surrounding tissue during pregnancy, at the rate of 0.6, 1.8, 4.8, and 6.1 g/day during the successive quarters of gestation.[30]

There are potential risks to mother and infant from low protein and inadequate food intakes. However, it is difficult to isolate the separate effects of protein and energy, since low protein intakes are often associated with low caloric intakes. When calories (joules) are inadequate, protein is used for energy needs and not for its unique functions of growth, repair, and body maintenance.

Lactation

During lactation, the RDA for protein is 66 g per day, an increase of 20 g per day for the average woman.[31] The additional dietary protein requirement during lactation can be better understood if we look at the amount of breast milk secreted and its protein content.

Average daily milk secretion is approximately 850 ml, with an upper range of about 1200 ml. Human milk contains about 1.2 percent protein.[32] Therefore, 850 ml of human milk contains 10 g of protein; 1200 ml contains 15 g. On the basis of this argument, the RDA for protein during lactation should be adequate for nearly all women.

The Elderly

The protein requirements of the elderly are not well documented. The evidence to date does not suggest that the protein requirements of the elderly are quantitatively different from those of other adults. However, impaired digestion, which frequently occurs in old age, may increase nutrient requirements.

DIETARY SIGNIFICANCE OF PROTEIN

Evaluation of Protein Quality

The quality of a protein is determined by its amino acid composition, which defines a protein's ability to sustain growth and maintain body tissue. Therefore, biological evaluation, based on nitrogen retention in the body, is the usual method of assessing protein quality. For human studies, procedures have been developed which use nitrogen balance or growth as indices of nitrogen retention. Nitrogen retention may also be measured by direct analysis of the animal body. Procedures used to describe biological evaluation are summarized in Table 3-2. Common terms associated with the quality of protein are *protein efficiency ration* (PER), *biological value* (BV),[33] and *net protein utilization* (NPU). For example, an egg has a PER of 3.92,[34] a BV of 93.7,[35] and an NPU of 93.5,[36] which indicates that it is a high-quality protein.

Availability of Dietary Protein

Both the quality and quantity of consumed protein are important. The quantity of protein in the diet is influenced by the total amount of food eaten as well as by the protein concentration in the food selected. The concentration of protein in food can be calculated by multiplying the nitrogen content of the food by the factor 6.25, since the nitrogen content in most protein foods is approximately 16 percent of the total grams of protein present in the food. This value is for crude protein because a small quantity of nonprotein nitrogen is present as

TABLE 3-2 METHODS OF BIOLOGICAL EVALUATION

Procedure	Calculation formula	Experimental conditions	Study design	Comments	
				Advantages	Disadvantages
1 Protein efficiency ratio (PER)	$\dfrac{\text{Weight gain, g}}{\text{Protein intake}}$	Standardized dietary conditions: adequate caloric intake; adequate protein intake—not excess	Small animals (laboratory rats), human infants	Simplest method. Requires measure of protein intake and weight gain. Inexpensive, quick	Weight gain may not be proportional to gain in body protein
2 Biological value (BV)	$\dfrac{\text{Nitrogen retained}}{(\text{Dietary N} = \text{urinary N} + \text{fecal N})}$ $\dfrac{\text{Nitrogen absorbed}}{(\text{Dietary N} - \text{fecal N})}$	Protein must be fed at or below maintenance level for maximum efficiency of utilization; BV is determined by nitrogen balance	Laboratory animals, humans	Represents proportion of absorbed nitrogen retained; this is amount of nitrogen body actually uses	No allowance for incomplete nitrogen absorption; i.e., that proportion of nitrogen absorbed by digestive tract
3 Net protein utilization (NPU)	$\dfrac{\text{Nitrogen retained}}{\text{Nitrogen intake}}$ or BV × digestibility	Standardized dietary conditions: adequate caloric intake; adequate protein intake—not excess; NPU is determined by amino acid pattern	Humans—NPU obtained by nitrogen balance Animals—NPU measured by nitrogen balance or by direct body analysis	Measures both biological value of absorbed amino acid mixture and digestibility of food protein; represents proportion of food nitrogen absorbed; is directly related to dietary intake of nitrogen	

well as the nitrogen from protein and amino acids.[37] For example, an egg contains approximately 7 g of protein[38] and approximately 1.12 g of nitrogen ($1.12 \times 6.25 = 7$).

Energy intake also influences protein availability. When the body's energy needs are not met by carbohydrate and fat, protein will be used for energy. Therefore, rehabilitation of a malnourished individual requires increasing the intake of both protein and calories.

The availability of amino acids is also affected by incomplete digestion and absorption. This seems to be a problem only with proteins of vegetable origin. Possible explanations are the high fiber content of the diet, and the inhibitors of digestive enzymes which are present in some foods and which must be inactivated by heating. The excessive heat treatment that is sometimes used in the manufacture of dry milk powder, fish protein concentrates, and oil seed meals may also decrease the availability of amino acids, particularly lysine

and the sulfur amino acids. Home cooking and commercial canning procedures have little or no effect on the availability of amino acids.[39]

Sources and Nutritional Value of Dietary Protein; Complete and Incomplete Proteins

Dietary protein may be derived from both animal and vegetable sources. The protein content of foods varies widely, as seen in Table 3-3.

Complete proteins contain all eight essential amino acids in approximately the correct proportions. Complete proteins—meat, fish, poultry, eggs, and dairy products (milk, cheese, yogurt)—come from animal sources. They have a high biological value, which enables small quantities of these foods to meet our daily protein requirements. For example 6 oz of meat, fish, or poultry plus 8 oz of milk

TABLE 3-3 PROTEIN CONTENT OF SOME COMMON FOODS

Food	Household measure	Protein content, g*	Cholesterol content, mg†	Biological value‡ (BV)	Net protein utilization§ (NPU)
Whole milk	8 oz	9	34	84.5	81.6
Cheddar cheese	1 oz	7	28	70.6	69.8
Rice	1 cup	4.1	0	64	62.7
Lentils, cooked	1 cup	15.6	0	44.6	29.7
Lima beans, cooked	1 cup	13	0	66.5	51.5
Soybeans, cooked	1 cup	19.8	0	72.8	61.4
Sunflower seeds (hulled seeds)	⅓ cup	11	0	69.6	58.1
Beef, lamb, pork	3 oz	23	80–90	74.3	66.9
Chicken	3 oz	20	63	74.3	72.9
Fish	3 oz	22	50–70	76	79.5
Egg	1 large	7	252	93.7	93.5

* USDA, Consumer and Food Economics Division, Agricultural Research Service, "Nutritive Value of Foods," *Home and Garden Bulletin No. 72,* Washington, D.C., 1970.

† R. M. Feeley, P. E. Criner, and B. K. Watts. "Cholesterol Content of Foods," *Journal of American Dietetic Association,* **61:** 134, August 1972.

‡ FAO, Food Policy and Food Service, Nutrition Division, *Amino-Acid Content of Foods and Biological Data on Proteins, FAO Nutritional Studies No. 24,* Rome, Italy, 1972.

§ Ibid.

will generously cover the 46 g of protein recommended for the adult woman.

Incomplete proteins—vegetables, grains, and legumes—also contain all eight essential amino acids but are low in one or more of them. The terminology *incomplete* may be misleading since proteins of plant origin are not lacking in types of amino acids but rather are deficient in quantity and proportion. Vegetable proteins are less complete than animal proteins—not incomplete. They are not as well used in the body as animal proteins are and cannot support satisfactory growth unless combined with other foods. In diets composed primarily of plant foods, the amino acids most frequently low are lysine, isoleucine, tryptophan, cysteine, and methionine.[40]

Protein Complementarity

The correction of amino acid deficiencies in plant proteins is made through a process called protein complementarity. By combining two different proteins, the essential amino acids which are low (limiting) in one food are present or complemented in the other food eaten with it, thereby improving the biological value of the protein. By eating a variety of plant proteins with complementary amino acid patterns, individuals can consume the correct quantity and proportion of amino acids without depending on animal proteins. Some good plant protein combinations are beans and rice, beans and wheat, or legumes and rice.[41]

Individuals who consume no animal foods are known as *vegans*. These vegetarians must plan their diets very carefully to include plant proteins that mutually supplement each other. Vegan parents must be particularly judicious in selecting foods for their infants and small children. Vegetable proteins have a lower biological value, are less readily digested, and are more difficult to chew than animal proteins. These problems, coupled with rapid growth, which causes an increased need for protein in infants and young children, may result in protein-calorie deficiencies.[42] For infants, soy formulas must be well processed to inactivate the enzyme inhibitors present in raw soybeans and must be supplemented with small amounts of L-methionine for improved protein quality.[43] Individuals on vegan diets must also be careful to get an adequate intake of vitamin B_{12}, a vitamin found exclusively in animal protein and important in the prevention of pernicious anemia (see Chap. 6).

An alternate way of improving the biological value of plant protein is to include small quantities of animal foods such as fish, eggs, or dairy products along with the vegetable proteins. Good protein mixtures would be cereal with milk, bread with cheese, or a bean and cheese casserole. Vegetarians who include eggs and dairy products are known as *lacto-ovo vegetarians;* those who include only dairy products are known as *lacto-vegetarians.* When small amounts of animal foods are eaten, vegetarians can be better assured of getting the correct supply of amino acids.

THE BODY'S USE OF PROTEIN

Protein Digestion

Amino acids are the end products of protein digestion as well as being the basic structural units of protein. Protein digestion begins in the stomach. The acid environment of the stomach (which is due to the secretion of hydrochloric acid by the stomach mucosa) activates the enzyme pepsin. Pepsin begins to break down the protein into large protein derivatives called proteoses and peptones. There is another special enzyme in the stomach, called rennin, which coagulates milk and begins to digest casein, the protein in milk. Rennin slows down the passage of milk from the stomach and changes the casein to a form that can be acted on by pepsin. Rennin is a particularly important enzyme for infants whose main source of dietary protein is milk. When this enzyme is deficient, milk then passes too quickly through the stomach, causing the infant to be milk-intolerant.

The next modification of protein occurs in the small intestine. Pancreatic juices containing the protein-splitting enzymes trypsin and chymotrypsin are secreted from the pancreas into the small intestine. These enzymes continue to break down protein (native protein, proteoses, and peptones) from the stomach to produce polypeptides. The polypeptides are then broken down into their constituent amino acids in the small intestine by the peptidases, a mixture of carboxypeptidase (an enzyme from the pancreatic juice) and aminopeptidase and dipeptidase (enzymes found in the intestinal juices). The carboxypeptidases split the terminal peptide bond at the carboxyl end of the polypeptide chain; the aminopeptidase splits the terminal peptide bond at the free amino end of the chain. Once food proteins are converted into their constituent amino acids by the enzymatic cleavage of the peptide linkages and the mechanical action of the digestive organs, they are ready for absorption by the intestinal mucosa. This absorptive process is an active one and requires energy, provided by adenosine triphosphate (ATP). Once the amino acids are absorbed, they are carried to the liver via the portal vein and are utilized through various metabolic processes.

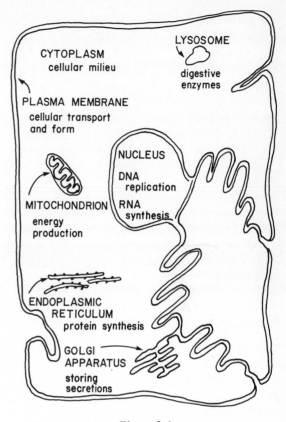

Figure 3-1

The function of cell components as related to protein metabolism.

Protein Metabolism

Protein Synthesis (Anabolism)

Amino acids from the amino acid pool leave the liver and are transported throughout the body to be used for growth, repair, and maintenance of body tissues, and formation of special compounds (enzymes, hormones, plasma proteins). An adequate supply of both essential and nonessential amino acids is needed for protein synthesis. If essential amino acids are not supplied via the diet to the cell, synthesis cannot take place. However, when the supply of nonessential amino acids is inadequate they can be synthesized in the cell through a process called transamination. (See "Essential and Nonessential Amino Acids," above.) Once the essential and nonessential amino acids are present in the cell, synthesis of specific body proteins will be genetically controlled by DNA (deoxyribonucleic acid) located in the cell nucleus. The genetic information for the amino acid sequence (the primary structure of the protein) is stored in DNA. This information is carried by messenger RNA (ribonucleic acid) to the site of protein synthesis, the cell cytoplasm, where specific protein is produced. (See "Genes," in Chap. 12.)

Catabolism

Catabolism (metabolic breakdown) of amino acids involves the processes of deamination and decarboxylation. *Deamination*, the removal of the nitrogen portion (—NH₂) of the amino acid to form alpha-keto amino acids, occurs for

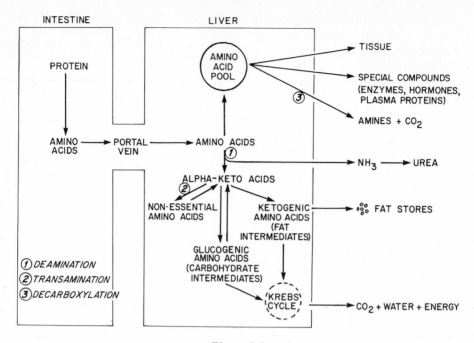

Figure 3-2

Sites of protein metabolism. (1) Deamination; (2) Transamination; (3) Decarboxylation.

the most part in the liver, although it can occur in the kidney and other organs of the body. Ultimately the nitrogen portion of the amino acid is converted to ammonia and finally to urea, which is excreted in the urine. The deaminated ketoacids may be converted to nonessential amino acids by transamination, or oxidized for needed energy through the Krebs cycle. According to the nature of the carbon skeleton, the oxidized ketoacids become either ketogenic amino acids or glycogenic amino acids. If energy is not required the amino acids are converted to fat and stored in the body.

Decarboxylation, a reaction that involves the splitting off of CO_2 from the carboxyl group of the amino acid to form amines, occurs in tissues such as the kidney, liver, or intestinal flora. An example of this reaction is the decarboxylation of hydroxytryptophan to form 5-hydroxytryptamine or serotonin, a neuro-

transmitter necessary for central nervous system function. (See Chap. 22.)

Fig. 3-2 summarizes the sites of protein utilization.

CLINICAL APPLICATIONS

Protein Requirements and Disease

States of protein deficiency can be differentiated into clinical entities: kwashiorkor (protein malnutrition) and marasmus (protein-calorie malnutrition) (see Chap. 16). These states of malnutrition decrease resistance to disease and retard growth. In developing countries, the combined effects of infection and protein deficiency contribute to the high mortality rates. Diarrhea, measles, and respiratory infections are more severe and often fatal in children with protein malnutrition. In hospitalized patients, therapy is poorly tolerated and recovery from surgery or trauma is complicated when the patient is malnourished.

In certain disease states, and with stress or trauma, protein requirements are increased because the body is catabolizing protein and nitrogen is being lost. A state of negative nitrogen balance results, lean body mass decreases, and body weight declines. Initially, when protein is withdrawn from the cells, a normal concentration of plasma proteins is maintained. However, with increasing protein depletion, plasma proteins are reduced.

The most common biochemical tests for determination of protein nutriture, and their normal values, are total serum protein (6.0 to 8.0 g/100 ml) and serum albumin (3.5 to 5.5 g/100 ml).[44] Another biochemical measure being used to assess protein status is the creatinine-height index. The excretion of creatinine is reduced during states of malnutrition.[45] (See Chap. 15.)

Clinical treatment for protein-depleted patients involves the provision of extra dietary protein along with sufficient calories. It has been estimated that as much as 2 to 3 g of protein/kg of body weight may be necessary in severe pathological states when nitrogen losses are extensive.[46] In other milder states and during convalescence, a protein intake of 0.6 to 1.2 g/kg of body weight has been found to be adequate.[47]

In disease states involving the kidney or liver, protein intake may need to be curtailed because of the body's inability to handle the waste products of protein metabolism.

Table 3-4 lists some common conditions that alter protein requirements.

TABLE 3-4 PATHOLOGICAL CONDITIONS ALTERING PROTEIN REQUIREMENTS

Condition	Increased	Decreased
Sepsis	X	
Fever	X	
Trauma—injury	X	
Fractures	X	
Burns	X	
Gastrointestinal disorders (ileostomy, colostomy, diarrhea and other malabsorption states, ulcerative colitis)	X	
Respiratory infections	X	
Parasitic infections	X	
Bacterial infections	X	
Viral infections	X	
Hepatic coma		X
Liver disease	X	
Massive hepatic necrosis		X
Proteinuria	X	
Renal disease (glomerulonephrosis)	X	
Renal failure, acute and chronic		X
Cancer	X	
Marasmus (protein-calorie malnutrition)	X	
Kwashiorkor (protein malnutrition)	X	
Pain	X	
Anxiety or other psychological stress	X	
Profuse sweating	X	

Protein Requirements and Exercise

Exercise or heavy work does not significantly increase one's need for protein.[48] Athletes are often attracted to expensive high-protein diets and concentrated protein supplements such as high-protein drinks or powders in order to increase their body size and strength.[49] Buying these foods is an unnecessary expense since performance is not improved. In addition, excess protein can cause dehydration unless large amounts of water are consumed to help the body excrete the metabolic by-products of protein metabolism. Also, large quantities of animal protein increase the quantity of saturated fat and cholesterol ingested (see Table 3-3).

FUTURE AVAILABILITY OF PROTEIN

We are living at a time when people are questioning how to best meet our nutrient needs. World population continues to rise and food production becomes more sophisticated. However, there still seems to be a lag in applying technology to solving food problems in developing countries. Further research is needed in order to define protein requirements more precisely and to advance solutions for meeting world protein needs.

In affluent countries of the world, such as the United States, substantial quantities of animal protein will continue to be eaten, even though there seems to be a growing awareness of the ecological wastefulness and potential health risks of eating large quantities of meat. As developing countries improve their living standards and enlarge their populations, the demand for animal protein will probably increase. However, because of the limits of the earth's agricultural capacity and animal resources and the high cost of animal foods, animal protein will probably never make significant nutritional contributions to the diets of most of the world's people.

In the future, we can look forward to many exciting changes in the types of protein foods available. There will probably be an increased utilization of fish and fish protein concentrates, algae and microorganisms, oilseed meals, and textured soy proteins, and use of synthetic amino acids, especially lysine and methionine, to improve the quality of legume and cereal protein mixtures. These new foods will add greater variety to our diets and help conserve the earth's limited food resources.

CASE STUDY 3-1

Past History
S. G. is a 15-month-old boy who is brought to the community health center by his parents for a routine check-up. Until age 10 months, the time of the child's last clinic visit, S. G. was in good health and growing along the 10th percentile for both height and weight (height = 70 cm; weight = 8.25 kg). His parents had reported at that time that S. G. was feeding well at the breast and taking solids, consisting primarily of grains and vegetables. At approximately 10 months, S. G. began to teethe, and Mrs. G. decided to wean the child from the breast to a cup. The G.'s are strict vegetarians who eat no animal foods. S. G. is being raised on a diet similar to his parents'.

Present
S. G.'s current weight and height are 7.5 kg and 70 cm. Since the 10-month visit, he has lost weight and has not grown. Currently, S. G. is eating grains, vegetables, nuts, and seeds; no animal foods or soy products are included in the diet. The nurse is concerned that the child is not eating enough and is failing to thrive as a result.

Case Study Questions
1 *What would you tell the parents about protein requirements of infants and young children?*

2 *What practical dietary recommendations would you suggest to assure a more adequate protein intake for the child?*

3 *What would you tell the parents about the relationship between caloric intake and protein utilization?*

STUDY QUESTIONS

1 Identify three factors that affect nitrogen balance. When does positive nitrogen balance occur? When does negative nitrogen balance occur?

2 Explain the importance of essential and nonessential amino acids in protein synthesis.

3 Why are protein requirements increased during pregnancy and lactation?

4 Describe two methods for improving the biological value of plant protein. Identify appropriate food combinations for each. What problems might a child encounter if no animal foods are consumed?

5 Describe the interrelationship between protein nutrition and disease. Identify two pathological states where (a) protein requirements are increased and (b) protein requirements are decreased.

REFERENCES

1 N. S. Scrimshaw, "Shattuck Lecture—Strengths and Weaknesses of the Committee Approach: An Analysis of Past and Present Recommended Dietary Allowances for Protein in Health and Disease (Part One)," *New England Journal of Medicine,* **294**(3): 136–142, January 1976.

2 N. S. Scrimshaw, "Shattuck Lecture—Strengths and Weaknesses of the Committee Approach: An Analysis of Past and Present Recommended Dietary Allowances for Protein in Health and Disease (Part Two)," *New England Journal of Medicine,* **294**(4): 198–203, January 1976.

3 D. Morgan, "UN Reports Warn of Global Food Crisis By '85," *Boston Sunday Globe,* June 20, 1976.

4 USDA Consumer and Food Economics Institute, Agricultural Research Service, "Dietary Levels of Households in the United States, Seasons of Year 1965–55," *Household Food Consumption Survey, 1965–66, Report No. 18,* Washington, D.C., 1974.

5 M. Pines, "Breaking the Meat Habit," in C. Lerza and M. Jcobson (eds.), *Food for People Not Profit,* Ballantine Books, New York, 1975.

6 "10 State Nutrition Survey, 1968–1970, V, Dietary," *DHEW Publication No. (HSM) 72-8133,* Health Services and Mental Health Administration, Center for Disease Control, Atlanta.

7 "Hanes Study—Preliminary Findings of the First Health and Nutrition Examination Survey, United States, 1971–1972, Dietary Intake and Biochemical Findings," *DHEW Publication No. (HRA) 74-1219-1,* Health Resources Administration, National Center for Health Statistics, Rockville, Md., 1974.

8 *Food Consumption, Prices, Expenditures, 1971 Supplement to Agricultural Economic Reports, No. 138,* Economic Research Service, Washington, D.C., tables 1, 38, 39.

9 A. A. Albanese and L. A. Orto, "The Proteins and Amino Acids," in R. S. Goodhart and M. E. Shils

(eds.), *Modern Nutrition in Health and Disease,* 15th ed., Lea and Febiger, Philadelphia, 1973, p. 28.

10 R. L. Pike and M. L. Brown, *Nutrition: An Integrated Approach,* 2d ed., John Wiley and Sons, Inc., New York, 1975, pp. 49–52.

11 A. L. Lehninger, *Biochemistry,* 2d ed., The Johns Hopkins University School of Medicine, Worth Publishers, Inc., New York, chap. 3.

12 S. E. Snyderman, A. Boyer, E. Roitman, L. E. Holt, Jr., and P. H. Prose, "The Histidine Requirement of the Infant," *Pediatrics,* **31**: 786–801, May 1963.

13 R. L. Pike and M. L. Brown, op. cit., p. 860.

14 A. A. Albanese and A. Orto, op. cit., p. 40.

15 A. E. Harper, P. R. Payne, and J. C. Waterlow, "Human Protein Needs," *Lancet,* **1**: 1518, June 1973.

16 *FNB-NRC (Food and Nutrition Board, National Research Council, Committee on Dietary Allowances) Recommended Dietary Allowances,* National Academy of Sciences, Washington, D.C., 1974, p. 47.

17 D. H. Calloway, "Recommended Dietary Allowances for Protein and Energy," *Journal of American Dietetic Association,* **64**: 161, February 1974.

18 Ibid.

19 Ibid.

20 Ibid.

21 S. Fomon, *Infant Nutrition,* 2d ed., W. B Saunders Company, Philadelphia, 1974, chap. 6.

22 FNB-NRC, op. cit., pp. 37–48.

23 S. G. Babson, "Feeding the Low Birthweight Infant," *Fetal and Neonatal Medicine,* **79**: 694–701, October 1971.

24 M. Davidson, S. Z. Levine, C. H. Bauer, and M. Dann, "Feeding Studies in Low Birthweight Infants," *Journal of Pediatrics,* May 1967, pp. 695–713.

25 L. E. Holt and S. E. Snyderman, "The Feeding of Premature and Newborn Infants," *Pediatric Clinics of North America,* **13**(4): 1103–1115, November 1966.

26 M. L. Hathaway, "Heights and Weights of Children in the United States," *USDA Home Economics Research Report No. 2,* U.S. Government Printing Office, Washington, D.C., 1957, p. 131.

27 E. M. Widdowson and J. W. T. Dickerson, "Chemical Composition of the Body," in C. L. Comar and F. Bronner (eds.), *Mineral Metabolism,* vol. II, pt A, Academic Press, New York, 1963, pp. 1–247.

28 S. Fomon, op. cit., pp. 118–151.

29 FNB-NRC, op. cit., pp. 37–48.

30 F. E. Hytten and I. Leitch, *The Physiology of Human Pregnancy,* 2d ed., F. A. Davis Co., Philadelphia, Blackwell Scientific Publications, Oxford, 1971, pp. 1–599.

31 FNB-NRC, op. cit., pp. 37–48.

32 WHO (World Health Organization), "Nutrition in Pregnancy and Lactation," Report of a WHO Expert Committee, *WHO Technical Report, series 302,* WHO, Geneva, 1965, p. 54.

33 H. H. Mitchell, "A Method of Determining the Biological Value of Protein," *Journal of Biological Chemistry,* **58:** 873–922, January 1924.

34 FAO (Food and Agriculture Organization) of the United Nations, Food Policy and Food Science Service, Nutrition Division, "Amino-Acid Content of Foods and Biological Data on Proteins," *FAO Nutritional Studies, No. 24,* Rome, Italy, 1972, p. 180.

35 Ibid.

36 Ibid.

37 FAO/WHO (Food and Agriculture Organization/World Health Organization), "Protein Requirements. Report of a Joint FAO/WHO Expert Group," *FAO Nutrition Meetings Report Series 37,* Food and Agriculture Organization of the United Nations, 1965, p. 41.

38 USDA, Consumer and Food Economics Division, Food and Agriculture Organization of the United Nations, *Home and Garden Bulletin 72,* Washington, D.C., 1970, p. 9.

39 FAO/WHO, op. cit., p. 24.

40 F. M. Lappe, *Diet for a Small Planet,* Ballantine Books, New York, 1975, pp. 80, 81.

41 Ibid., p. 81.

42 FAO/WHO, op cit., p. 24.

43 S. Fomon, op. cit., pp. 387–390.

44 J. Wallach, *Interpretation of Diagnostic Tests,* Little, Brown and Co., Boston, 1970, p. 9.

45 Committee Report, "Assessment of Protein Nutritional Status," *American Journal of Clinical Nutrition,* **23**(6), 807–819, June 1970.

46 FAO/WHO, op cit., p. 30.

47 H. S. Soroff, E. Pearson, and C. P. Artz, "An Estimation of the Nitrogen Requirements for Equilibrium in Burned Patients," *Surgery, Gynecology, and Obstetrics,* **112:** 159–172, February 1961.

48 N. J. Smith, *Food for Sport,* Bull Publishing Co., Palo Alto, Cal., 1976, chap. 1, pp. 16–20.

49 Ibid., chap. 3, p. 48.

CHAPTER 4

CARBOHYDRATE

Carol Stollar

KEY WORDS
Monosaccharides
Disaccharides
Polysaccharides
Glycogen
Fiber
Gluconeogenesis
Glycogenolysis
Glycolysis

INTRODUCTION

Changing patterns in carbohydrate consumption—an increase in the use of highly refined carbohydrate (milled, bleached flour) and an excessive sugar intake—are products of our technological age that are provoking nutritional concern. Now being examined are cause-effect relationships between the lack of fiber in the American diet and the incidence of lower bowel disease, atherosclerosis, obesity, and cancer; and between excessive sugar intake and dental caries. A knowledge of carbohydrate, its food sources, and its metabolism is essential for health professionals who are working toward preventing the above disorders and treating other disease states such as diabetes mellitus, malabsorption, allergies, and inborn errors of metabolism such as galactosemia. Even to counteract the food misinformation of the low-carbohydrate, quick-weight-loss reduction diet a knowledge of carbohydrate is necessary. This chapter will provide the student with the information to be a competent, well-informed nutrition educator in all areas requiring a basic knowledge of carbohydrate.

Definition of Carbohydrate

Carbohydrate is the term used to describe any of various neutral compounds of carbon, hydrogen, and oxygen, most of which are formed by green plants. As sugars, starches, and cellulose, carbohydrate is the major energy source in the human diet, comprising 45 to 55 percent of the energy in the American diet and up to 80 to 90 percent of the calories (joules) in the diets of those in the developing nations where vegetation is lush and livestock production and refrigeration are limited.

Carbohydrate and its potential energy originate in chlorophyll-containing plants, which synthesize carbohydrate from carbon dioxide and water, using energy from the sun in a process known as photosynthesis:

$$6H_2O + 6CO_2 \xrightarrow{\text{light}} C_6H_2O_6 + 6O_2$$

Water   Carbon dioxide   Sugar   Oxygen

The carbohydrate formed consists of carbon, hydrogen, and water, and so the term *carbohydrate* indicates somewhat the basic chemical composition. However, the term gives no real indication of the chemical structure and the implied formula excludes many members of this class. The term *saccharide* is more appropriate since it allows for classification into monosaccharides, disaccharides, and polysaccharides.

CLASSIFICATION OF CARBOHYDRATES

Carbohydrates are divided into three main groups according to the number of *saccharides,* or *sugar units,* comprising the basic structure. They are:

Monosaccharides The simplest form of carbohydrate, consisting of a single sugar. (Single)

Disaccharides A more complex form of carbohydrate, consisting of two sugars or two monosaccharides. (Double)

Polysaccharides The most complex carbohydrate, consisting of many units of one or more monosaccharides. (Many)

Monosaccharides

The structure of a simple sugar or monosaccharide is a carbon chain:

$$-C-C-C-C-C-C-C-C-$$

with hydrogen and oxygen atoms attached singly or in groups known as aldehydes (an alcohol that has been oxidized and contains a C—H group) or ketones (a compound containing a C=O group)

Glucose
(an aldose)

Fructose
(a ketose)

According to the number of carbons present in the basic structure, the monosaccharides are grouped as follows:

Trioses	3 Carbons
Tetroses	4 Carbons
Pentoses	5 Carbons
Hexoses	6 Carbons
Heptoses	7 Carbons

The hexoses are nutritionally the most important of the monosaccharides.

Hexoses (Six-Carbon Sugars)

The four monosaccharides in the hexose group are glucose, fructose, galactose, and mannose.

Glucose The most abundant monosaccharide, glucose is found in a natural state in many fruits, such as ripe grapes (known therefore as grape sugar), plums, dates, and figs. It is also a constituent of disaccharides (sucrose, lactose, maltose), of the polysaccharides, and of glycogen, starch, and cellulose. Glucose is the form in which carbohydrate is used by the body—the form that is transported in the bloodstream and oxidized in the cell for energy. Glucose is present in the systemic venous blood, when a person is resting after a meal, in the following concentrations:

Whole blood 60 to 100 mg/100 ml
Plasma 65 to 110 mg/100 ml

There are no clinically significant sex or age differences in blood glucose concentrations except that values are low (30 mg/100 ml) in the newborn and tend to be somewhat higher than average in the elderly.

Glucose is also known as *dextrose* because it is the dextrorotatory form of the molecule (which means that in a chemical reaction this compound rotates a plane of polarized light toward the right). Dextrose is produced commercially by the hydrolysis of starch (hydrolysis is a chemical process of decomposition involving the splitting of a chemical bond and the addition of the elements of water). The product formed is dextrose (corn syrup), which is often added to cow's milk in order to modify it for infant feeding. Dextrose is also used in intravenous therapy along with water and electrolytes.

Fructose Fructose, known also as *fruit sugar,* is found in its natural state in many fruits, including apples and pears, and in honey, and is a constituent of sucrose and the polysaccharide inulin. It is the sweetest of the monosaccharides. In the human body it is found only in seminal fluid. Fructose in food can be used directly for energy or can be converted to glucose derivatives.

Fructose is also called *levulose* as it is the levorotatory form of the molecule (which means that as an optically active molecule it rotates a plane of light to the left).

Galactose Galatose is found in nature only in a combined form. In the human body it is a constituent of lactose (milk sugar), certain glucoproteins, and the complex glycosides of nervous tissue. Galactose is converted to glucose in the liver. During lactation, the human body converts glucose to galactose in the mammary tissue for the synthesis of the lactose component of breast milk.

Milk is the primary source of this sugar.

Legumes also contain galactose which, after digestion, may be available to the human body. (These food sources are of note in planning a diet for a child with galactosemia, an inborn error of metabolism that necessitates the removal of all food sources of galactose. See Chap. 26.)

Pentoses (Five-Carbon Sugars)

Among the important pentoses are arabinose, xylose, ribose, 2-deoxy-D-ribose, and xylulose. Arabinose and xylose are examples of naturally occurring pentoses found in foods; nuts are a good source. Ribose and deoxyribose are synthesized in the body and are integral components of the nucleic acids ribonucleic acid (RNA) and deoxyribonucleic acid (DNA). Ribose is also part of coenzymes derived from the vitamins niacin and riboflavin.

The body is capable of synthesizing its own supply of pentose from glucose by way of the pentose shunt (pentose phosphate pathway) and from glucuronic acid. Normally the body produces glucuronic acid (a monosaccharide derivative) from glucose.

The pentose phosphate pathway is important as an alternative pathway for glucose oxidation. This route does not require adenosine triphosphate and about 30 percent of glucose metabolism in liver cells takes place by this mechanism.

Xyloses may appear in the urine after the ingestion of large amounts of certain fruits such as cherries and plums, causing a condition known as alimentary pentosuria. As a result of a benign inborn error of metabolism (a familial type of pentosuria), xylulose is excreted in the urine independently of the nature of the diet.

Xylose can be used as an indicator of carbohydrate malabsorption. A known amount (25 g) is ingested and its appearance in the urine is then monitored. When less than 4.5 g is excreted in 5 h (if the patient has normal renal function), impaired carbohydrate absorptive capacity is indicated.

Disaccharides

A disaccharide is composed of two monosaccharides which are joined together by a glycosidic linkage with the release of one molecule of water. For example:

Monosaccharide + monosaccharide $\longrightarrow$
disaccharide + water

$$C_6H_{12}O_6 + C_6H_{12}O_6 \longrightarrow$$
Glucose   Glucose

$$C_{12}H_{22}O_{11} + H_2O$$
Maltose   Water

The disaccharides include sucrose (glucose and fructose), maltose (glucose and glucose), and lactose (glucose and galactose).

Sucrose Sucrose (glucose and fructose) is the common granulated *table sugar,* known also as beet, cane, or invert sugar. It is obtained from sugar cane, sugar beets, and the sap of maple trees. Many fruits and vegetables such as bananas, dates, ripe pineapple, green peas, and sweet potatoes contain sucrose in its natural state. Many food products are now processed with large amounts of sugar; consequently, sucrose now comprises about 15 to 20 percent of our total calories in our daily food intake. It has been estimated that slightly over 100 lb of sugar is used per person per year in the United States.

Lactose Lactose (glucose and galactose) or *milk sugar,* is the sugar found in milk and is unique to mammals. Lactose comprises about 7½ percent of the total content of human milk and 4½ percent of cow's milk. When milk products are fermented, or milk sours, much of the lactose is converted to lactic acid, which gives sour milk and yogurt their characteristic flavor. In cheesemaking, the whey (the fluid part of soured milk) is removed and, since lactose is soluble in the whey, the hard, ripened cheeses (cheddar, Swiss, mozzarella) that are made from the curds contain only trace amounts of lactose.

Lactose is hydrolyzed to glucose and galactose in the cells of the intestinal mucosa. When the enzyme lactase is absent or deficient, symptoms of cramping and flatulence may occur (see p. 64).

Maltose Maltose (glucose and glucose), or *malt sugar,* is not present in a natural state but is produced by the action of the amylase enzymes on polysaccharides like starch and glycogen. It is of little dietary significance except for its contribution to the process of beer making, in which the action of the enzyme diastase on grain (starch) produces the first step in alcohol production. Cereals, corn syrup, and baby foods produced by hydrolysis of cereal grains contain some maltose.

Sweetness of Sugar

The sweetness of sugar is perceived on the tip of the tongue. Humans are conditioned to enjoy this taste from infancy, since sugar is added to infant cereals and baby foods.

The sweetness of various sugars is measured by a subjective sensory test, in which individuals are asked to judge the relative sweetness of the sugars at differing concentrations. Sucrose is usually used as the standard of

TABLE 4-1 COMPARISON OF SWEETNESS OF SUGARS AND OTHER SWEETENERS

Sugar or sweetener	Degree of sweetness
Sucrose	100
Lactose	39
Maltose	46
Sorbitol	50
D-Mannose	59
Galactose	63
D-Glucose	69
D-Fructose	114
Sodium cyclamate*	1500–3100
Saccharin*	24,000–35,000

Scale: Compared to sucrose = 100

* These are designated as artificial sweeteners.

Source: Adapted from L. W. Aurand and A. E. Woods, *Food Chemistry,* Avi Publishing Company, Westport, Conn., 1973.

comparison and is given a value of 100 (see Table 4-1). Since taste is a highly individualized response influenced by many factors, including genetic predisposition and environmental conditioning, the amount of sugar sweetness is subject to individual variation.

Polysaccharides

Polysaccharides are complex carbohydrates composed of large numbers of monosaccharide units linked together. Polysaccharides can be divided into two groups—those that have a function in energy storage and those that have structural roles.

Storage function: starch (plants)
                       glycogen (animals)
                       dextran
                       inulin
Structural function: cellulose
                       hemicelluloses
                       pectin
                       agar, alginates, and
                       carageen
                       lignin

Storage Forms

Starch   Starch is a storage form of carbohydrate in plants where it acts as a food reserve, freeing monosaccharides as they are needed. It is the most significant source of carbohydrate in the human diet. The basic structure of the starch molecule is composed of glucose units, which range in number from 250 to 1000 units per molecule. These monosaccharide units are arranged in a straight chain such as is found in amylose or in a branched-chain configuration as in amylopectin. Starch from most sources is a mixture of amylose and amylopectin.

Starch granules differ in size and shape and are completely insoluble in cold water. However, with moist heat the starch grains swell, breaking the cell wall and making it more digestible. As starch cooks, it thickens because of the gel-like quality of amylopectin.

Starch is found in plant seeds, particularly cereal grains, and in tubers, fruits, and roots. Legumes and nuts also contain significant amounts of starch. The use of starch differs around the world according to local sources. In the United States, wheat, oats, rye, barley, corn, potatoes, and rice are important. In other countries, millet, sweet potato, taro, breadfruit, cassava, and plantain are staples.

The digestion of starch to maltose is accomplished in the body by the digestive enzyme α-amylase, found in the saliva (where starch digestion begins) and in the pancreatic juice present in the small intestine (where starch digestion is completed). *Dextrins* are the intermediate products of starch digestion.

$$Starch \rightarrow Dextrins \rightarrow Maltose \rightarrow Glucose$$

Dextrins are utilized in baby foods, breakfast cereals, and malt mixtures.

Glycogen   The animal equivalent of starch, glycogen consists of branched-chain polysaccharides of great and varying length. The human body stores glycogen in small amounts in the liver and muscle tissue where it serves as a source of glucose when needed for energy and helps to maintain blood glucose levels. Glycogen is of little importance as a dietary source of carbohydrate.

Dextrans   Dextrans are substances produced when certain bacteria grow on a sugar substrate. They are branched-chain polysaccharides but differ from glycogen and starch in the nature of their linkages. Dextrans form the substrate for the plaque on the surface of teeth that is implicated in the formation of dental caries. (See Chap. 23.)

Dextran is used intravenously in solution as a plasma expander after blood loss to increase blood volume through osmotic pressure. It is slowly utilized, remaining in the blood for 24 h or more.

Inulin   Inulin is a fructose-containing polysaccharide found in the Jerusalem artichoke. It can be utilized for energy. Inulin is filtered by the kidney but not reabsorbed and is therefore used to determine kidney function. This test is known as the *inulin clearance test.*

Structural Forms

These are polysaccharides such as cellulose, hemicellulose, and pectin that give rigidity and structure to plant cell walls.

Cellulose   Cellulose is the most plentiful organic compound in the world. It is found in the stems, roots, leaves, hulls, and seed coverings of plants. The human body does not have the digestive enzymes that are needed to split the specific linkages of glucose units which make up these long-chain polysaccharides. Thus, for the most part, cellulose stays whole in the digestive tract, lending bulk to the diet, stimulating peristalsis, moving food along through the intestine, and holding water in the fecal mass, all of which aids in elimination. It has been estimated that only 15 percent of cellulose undergoes bacterial breakdown in the large intestine.

Hemicellulose   Hemicellulose was a term originally applied to a mixture of nondigestible polysaccharides extracted from plants, since they were thought to be related to cellulose. More recently, chemical analysis has shown that these substances are not related to cellulose but are composed of polysaccharides of various sugars, including xylose, glucose, and mannose.

Hemicelluloses are present in whole wheat; carrots, cabbage, and other leafy vegetables; and common fruits, such as peaches, pears, apples, and melons. Hemicelluloses are considered to be the factor in dietary fiber that is associated with increasing stool bulk. Some 85 percent of hemicellulose may undergo bacterial breakdown in the large intestine, with end products of gases (carbon dioxide, methane).

Pectins   Pectins are nondigestible polysaccharides with a colloidal property that are often classified with hemicellulose. They are soluble in hot water, forming a gel. This property is utilized in preparing fruit jams and jellies and also makes them useful in certain drugs. For example, pectin is used with an adsorbent, kaolin, in the treatment of diarrhea. Pectin is found in the rind of citrus fruits and in the skin of apples.

Agar, alginates, and carageen   These are nondigestible polysaccharides found in seaweed and having properties that allow gel formation. Agar is used to make kosher gelatin since it contains no animal products and can be used under the Jewish dietary laws. Agar is also used as a culture medium on which bacterial growth can be studied (agar plate). Carageen and alginates are additives used to emulsify, stabilize, and thicken, especially in milk products such as ice cream and evaporated milk.

Lignin   Lignin is a woody substance closely bound to cellulose in plants and therefore is grouped with the polysaccharides. It lends fiber to the diet and is now being used in special high-fiber products such as bread.

Derivatives of Polysaccharides

Mucopolysaccharides   These heteropolysaccharides are found in combination with protein in body structures and secretions. They tend to be viscous in nature and are usually found in the substance surrounding connective tissues.

Hyaluronic acid is a mucopolysaccharide that assists in lubricating joints and is present as a gel-like substance filling the space between capillaries and cells in connective tissue. *Chondroitin* and *chondroitin sulfate* are mucopolysaccharides that form the matrix of cartilage and the intercellular substance of other connective tissues. *Heparin,* another derivative of polysaccharides, is the anticoagulant that helps to prevent fibrin clots. It also plays a role with lipoprotein lipase in clearing chylomicrons from plasma. It occurs in most cells as part of the granules in which histamine is stored.

THE FIBER CONTENT OF THE DIET

Both the dietary and crude fiber content of food must be considered in determining the fiber content of the diet.

Dietary Fiber

Dietary fiber consists of all parts of the plant cell wall that are resistant to the normal digestive enzymes of the small intestine. This includes lignin and most of the cellulose, hemicellulose, and pectin.

Crude Fiber

Crude fiber is the term used for the fiber left in plant food after it has been subjected to acid and alkali breakdown in the laboratory for nutrient analysis. The remaining amount of lignin, some cellulose, and a small amount of hemicellulose comprise the crude fiber value. These values are included in the fiber content stated in food composition tables, and the tables therefore greatly underestimate the amount of dietary fiber available. For example, after analysis, the amount of dietary fiber in whole-grain cereal may exceed the crude fiber content by 5 times.

Fiber exerts a special effect on intestinal function because of the following properties:

1 its ability to take up water and swell
2 its capacity to form a gel
3 its cation exchange properties
4 its ability to absorb organic molecules such as bile salts from the intestine (therefore affecting cholesterol metabolism)

These properties, in combination, alter fecal weight, change intestinal flora, bind various ions such as calcium, zinc, and iron, and speed

TABLE 4-2 FIBER CONTENT OF FOOD

A diet high in fiber would contain the following foods:

Type of food	Crude fiber, %
Bran	10.0–13.5
Whole grains	1.0–2.0
Nuts	2.0–5.0
Legumes (cooked)	1.5–1.7
Vegetables	0.5–1.5
Fruits (fresh)	0.5–1.5
Fruits (dried)	1.0–3.0

Fiber-free foods include all meat, fish, eggs, milk, cheese, fats, sugar, beverages, and alcoholic drinks.

transit time through the intestine. This special effect of fiber helps to maintain bowel regularity.

The fiber content of food varies with the age and type of the plant, and with the amount of processing. Whole grains are the best source of fiber because of the seed coat of the grain kernel, which is known as *bran*. Bran contains 6 percent cellulose, 24 percent hemicellulose, and 4 percent lignin. Refined grains have had the bran and germ removed in processing and therefore have a lower fiber content. Current crude fiber intake in the United States is estimated at a low of 3.5 g to a high of 11 g per day, with vegetarians consuming even more (see Table 4-2).

THE BODY'S USE OF CARBOHYDRATE

Functions

The functions of carbohydrate in the human body are important and varied:

1 It is a source of energy and potential energy.
2 It is a starting material for the synthesis of

other types of compounds in the body, such as fatty acids and certain amino acids.

3 It plays a role in the structure of many biologically important compounds: glycolipids, glycoproteins, heparin, nucleic acids.

As a source of energy, 1 g of carbohydrate equals 4.1 kcal (or approximately 17.2 kJ).

Glucose is the form of carbohydrate utilized by the body. The brain is especially dependent on a continuous supply of glucose, as are the red blood cells. After digestion and absorption, glucose is either oxidized or converted to glycogen and stored in the muscles, heart, and liver, while excess is converted to fat and stored as adipose tissue.

It is necessary to ingest carbohydrate in sufficient amounts at regular intervals because it is not stored in large amounts in the body. In persons weighing 70 kg, the following distribution is seen:

Sites of concentration	Amount, g
Muscle	245
Liver	108
Blood and extra-cellular fluid	17
Total	370 (× 4 kcal or 17.2 kJ per gram = 1480 kcal or 6216 kJ)

The amount of energy in this stored glycogen provides only enough calories (joules) for half a day for such a person if engaged in a sedentary occupation. The infant, whose liver is one-tenth the size of the adult liver, has much smaller glycogen reserves and is dependent on frequent feedings for an adequate glycogen supply.

When there is a limited supply of carbohydrate, adipose tissue is utilized and then protein stores, as the nonnitrogenous fraction of the protein is converted to energy. This is why carbohydrate has what is termed a *protein-sparing action*. An ample supply of carbohydrate allows the body to conserve protein for tissue maintenance and growth.

Digestion and Absorption

Digestion of carbohydrate is primarily a function of the small intestine, although some breakdown begins in the mouth. The final products of digestion of carbohydrate are glucose, fructose, and galactose (see Fig. 4-1).

Figure 4-1

The digestion of carbohydrate.

Mouth

Mechanical:	Carbohydrates are mechanically broken down by chewing and are mixed with other nutrients.
Chemical:	Saliva contains the enzyme salivary amylase (ptyalin), which begins to break cooked starch into dextrins and maltose.

Stomach

Mechanical:	Peristaltic action continues mixing carbohydrates with gastric juices.
Chemical:	Gastric juices contain no specific enzymes for digestion of carbohydrates. Hydrochloric acid counteracts the alkaline activity of salivary amylase and prevents further carbohydrate digestion.

Small Intestine

Mechanical:	Peristaltic action continues to move liquid-like, semidigested food mass (chyme) through the intestine.
Chemical:	Carbohydrate digestion is completed by amylase from the pancreas that continues the breakdown of all starch to maltose. Disaccharidase enzymes in the intestinal cell (sucrase, lactase, and maltase) break down their respective disaccharides.

$$\text{Sucrose} \xrightarrow{\text{sucrase}} \text{glucose and fructose}$$

$$\text{Lactose} \xrightarrow{\text{lactase}} \text{glucose and galactose}$$

$$\text{Maltose} \xrightarrow{\text{maltase}} \text{glucose and glucose}$$

The comparative rates of absorption of monosaccharides through the cells of the intestinal mucosa and into the portal bloodstream, in decreasing order of absorption, are as follows: galactose, glucose, fructose, mannose, and the pentoses. Very small amounts of glucose may be absorbed from the stomach. The main site of absorption is in the small intestine, particularly in the duodenum.

Sugars are absorbed by the following mechanisms:

1 *Diffusion*—the process whereby particles in solution randomly move from areas of high concentration to low, thus equalizing the concentration. This is dependent on the sugar concentration between the intestinal lumen, mucosal cells, and blood plasma. Mannose and the pentoses utilize this method.

2 *Active transport*—a process which requires energy to carry particles in solution from an area of lesser to an area of greater concentration. This process requires the use of an energy-dependent carrier system involving sodium to transport sugars through the mucosal cell. Glucose and galactose use this mode of transport.

There is a limiting rate of absorption of about 1 g/kg of body weight per hour. Approximately ½ to 1 h after a meal, the blood glucose reaches a maximum of 130 mg/100 ml, then decreases in 2 to 2½ h to approximately 70 to 90 mg/100 ml. (This blood glucose curve provides the basis of the glucose tolerance test that is used to diagnose underlying pathology of carbohydrate metabolism; see Chap. 20.) *Hypoglycemia* is the term used to indicate blood sugar levels below the normal range, while hyperglycemia indicates ranges above, and normoglycemia indicates levels within, the normal range.

At blood levels above 160 to 190 mg/100 ml, glucose cannot be reabsorbed by the kidney tubules and is therefore excreted in the urine; this level is called the *renal threshold*.

If blood glucose levels fall markedly, central nervous system signs and symptoms such as dizziness, convulsions, and loss of consciousness may occur. Sustained and profound hypoglycemia may cause irreversible brain damage since the brain has no stored glucose and is dependent on a constant supply.

Metabolism

The prime site of carbohydrate metabolism is the liver. Here glucose is carried after absorption and is stored as glycogen. Fructose and galactose are converted here to glucose, which in turn is stored as glycogen or used for energy. Other tissues of the body, including adipose, muscle, and renal tissue, are active sites of glucose metabolism. However, for the most part energy metabolism goes on in all cells of the body.

The first stage of glucose metabolism occurs in the cell cytoplasm. In this stage, called *glycolysis,* or glucose breakdown, the glucose molecule is split into smaller fragments and phosphorylated (i.e., phosphorus is added to glucose), yielding some energy and glucose 6-phosphate. This glycolytic pathway is known as the *Embden-Myerhof pathway.* The glucose 6-phosphate is then either converted to glycogen (a process known as *gluconeogenesis*) and stored (in the liver or muscle), or proceeds in the presence of oxygen to be converted to pyruvic acid (in the absence of oxygen, to lactic acid). Pyruvic acid then enters the mitochondria of the cell where the oxidative steps of the tricarboxylic acid cycle (*Krebs cycle*) take place, and carbon dioxide, water, and energy are formed (See Chap. 9, Fig. 9-7). Ninety percent of the energy derived from carbohydrate is metabolized in this matter.

Another pathway for glucose metabolism is the *pentose phosphate shunt* of the Embden-Meyerhof pathway, in which the glucose 6-phosphate is side-channeled to produce pentoses for nucleic acid synthesis and an important enzyme factor called *reduced niacin adenine dinucleotide phosphate* (NADPH), which is

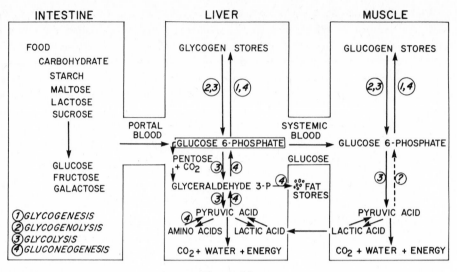

Figure 4-2

The sources and routes of carbohydrate utilization. (1) Glycogenesis; (2) Glycogenolysis; (3) Glycolysis; (4) Glucogenogenesis. (Adapted from A. Cantarow and M. Trumperer, Clinical Biochemistry, W. B. Saunders Co., Philadelphia, 1975.)

needed for the synthesis of fatty acids and steroids.

When energy demands for glucose have been satisfied, and the demand as an intermediate for other types of compounds (e.g., synthesis of nonessential amino acids) has been fulfilled, along with repletion of the storage reserves in tissues and in circulation, excess glucose is then converted to fat through the process of *lipogenesis* and the fat is stored in various tissues throughout the body.

When there is a need for glucose, glycogen stores in the liver are converted to glucose in the process of *glycogenolysis* and then released into the bloodstream. Glycogen stored in muscle can be used only for immediate local energy and is not available for circulation. If the work or exercise imposed on the body is

Figure 4-3

The metabolism of glucose within the cell.

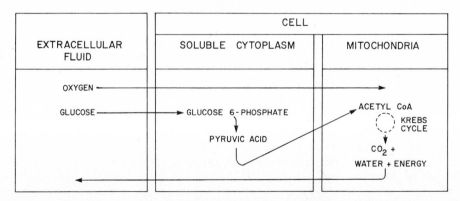

greater than the oxygen available, the anaerobic process of the Embden-Meyerhof pathway takes place and the glucose is then converted to lactic acid instead of pyruvic acid. The lactic acid is then transported to the liver and converted to glucose and returned to the exercising muscle.

Both protein and fat are noncarbohydrate sources of glucose. They are converted to glucose by the process of *gluconeogenesis* when energy is needed. Several hormones are crucial to the regulation and integration of the mechanisms for supplying glucose to the blood from the liver and its utilization by the tissues. Insulin, glucagon, epinephrine, thyroxine, and the pituitary hormones are the major influences on glucose metabolism (see Table 4-3).

DIETARY REQUIREMENTS AND SOURCE OF CARBOHYDRATES

Requirements

The daily requirement for carbohydrate in the diet has not been established by the National Research Council, although there is evidence that humans require at least 100 g per day to provide energy for the nervous system. When carbohydrate is the only source of energy in the diet, the fasting individual requires closer to 150 g per day to prevent tissue (muscle) breakdown.[1] Most adult Americans consume diets that provide 200 to 300 g of carbohydrate per day, which constitutes somewhere between 40 and 50 percent of the calories in our diet.

Dietary Sources

Both the nature and the amount of carbohydrate in the American diet has changed over the past 40 years. The total carbohydrate content of the diet has declined because of a decreased intake of flour and cereal products. Also, milk, fruit, and vegetable consumption has decreased, causing net losses in dietary carbohydrate. This in part reflects the change from the temporary increase in the use of carbohydrate during the depression years when cereals and potatoes were the more affordable entities. Since that time, increasing prosperity has led to the greater use of meat and dairy

TABLE 4-3   HORMONAL CONTROL OF CARBOHYDRATE METABOLISM

Hormone	Effect on carbohydrate metabolism	Effect on blood glucose levels
Insulin	Promotes glucose uptake by the cell Increases glycogen formation from glucose in the muscle Stimulates conversion of glucose to fat	Decreases
Glucagon	Stimulates glycogen breakdown and glyconeogenesis in the liver	Increases
Epinephrine	Accelerates glycogenolysis in the liver and muscles, causing a decrease in the glycogen content of these structures	Increases (and blood lactic acid increases)
Thyroxine	Accelerates liver glycogenolysis May increase glucose absorption from the small intestine	Increases
Hydrocortisone	Promotes gluconeogenesis in the liver	Increases
Growth hormone	Acts as an insulin antagonist, thereby depressing glucose utilization by the cell	Increases

products, which are also carriers of saturated fat.[2]

While the amount of carbohydrate has decreased, the type of carbohydrate consumed has changed markedly, with a precipitous rise in sugar consumption. Sugar now contributes 53 percent of the carbohydrate in our national food supply. This large proportion of sugar is related to the greater use of processed foods and soft drinks.

Ripening and processing cause changes in the nature of carbohydrate. In the ripening process in some plants, such as bananas, starch is changed to sugar; in others, such as corn, sugar may be changed to starch as the seed matures. Drying foods such as fruit and vegetables causes a relative increase in their carbohydrate content. Food processors have even modified starch to improve the functionality of a variety of food products. The starch is treated by adding small amounts of chemicals to a suspension of starch granules in water and then all the chemicals that have not reacted with the starch are removed during processing. This processing alters the properties of the starch; however, it does not alter its energy value or digestibility.[3] However, the use of modified food starch in baby foods has caused some concern over the inability of some infants to absorb the modified starch, with consequent diarrhea. It is estimated that over 150 million lb of modified starches are used yearly in salad dressings, fruit pie fillings, canned soups, gravies, frozen dinners, and baby foods.[4] In these products, the modified food starches serve as thickeners, fillers, moisture adsorbents, and carriers for fats, oils, and flavors.

It is apparent that the trend in carbohydrate consumption favors the consumption of carbohydrate in processed foods over that from fresh foods. For the most part, natural food sources of carbohydrate are cereal grains, fruits, vegetables, milk, and concentrated sweets (See Table 4-4).

In food composition tables, carbohydrate is usually listed as total carbohydrate with no differentiation between crude (unavailable) and dietary (available) carbohydrate, and no

TABLE 4-4 THE PERCENTAGE OF CARBOHYDRATE IN FOODS (AVERAGE)

Food	Percentage of carbohydrate
Sugar	99–96
Honey	82
Corn syrup	75
Flour (wheat)	72
Bread	50
Rice	80
Oatmeal	68
Dry corn, cold	85
Dry corn, sugar-coated	91
Bran	
Nuts	7–30
Vegetables:	
Legumes, cooked	20
Potatoes, cooked	15
Others	2.5–18
Fruits:	
Fresh	6–15
Canned in syrup	20–27
Dried	60–70
Milk	5

identification of whether the carbohydrate content is composed of monosaccharides, disaccharides, or polysaccharides. The carbohydrate content of fruit consists mainly of the monosaccharides glucose and fructose, with some disaccharides in the form of sugar, and the polysaccharides cellulose, hemicellulose, dextrins, and pectin. Vegetables have varying amounts of sucrose and starch, with small amounts of glucose and fructose. The root tuber and seed variety of vegetable (potatoes, sweet potatoes, beans, beets, carrots, squash) have a higher starch and sucrose content, while the leafy vegetables contribute appreciable amounts of cellulose and hemicellulose.[5]

CLINICAL APPLICATIONS

There are many normal (physiologic) conditions and abnormal conditions (disease states) which affect carbohydrate metabolism, as re-

TABLE 4-5 PHYSIOLOGICAL CONDITIONS ALTERING BLOOD GLUCOSE LEVELS

Condition	Increase	Decrease
Pain	× (transitory)	
Intense emotion	× (transitory)	
Brief strenuous exercise	× (transitory)	
Protracted strenuous exercise		×
Premature infants		×

TABLE 4-6 DISEASE STATES ALTERING BLOOD GLUCOSE LEVELS

Condition	Increase	Decrease
Stress (shock, burns, anaesthesia)	×	
Increased circulating adrenalin from injection or adrenalin-producing tumors	×	
Diabetes mellitus—insulin-dependent or resistant	×	
ACTH or adrenal steroid therapy	×	
Acute pancreatitis	×	
Wernicke's encephalopathy—thiamine deficiency	×	
Some central nervous system lesions— subarachnoid hemorrhage	×	
Insulin excess		×
Insulin overdose or overeffectiveness		
Oral antidiabetic agent overdose		
Pancreatic disorders		×
Islet cell tumor		
Pancreatitis		
Glucagon deficiency		
Extrapancreatic tumors—stomach, adrenal		×
Hepatic disease		×
Leucine sensitivity		
Any severe liver disease—cirrhosis, hepatitis, tumors, enzyme deficiencies, Von Gierke's galactosemia		
Poisons		
Endocrine disorders		×
Addison's disease and hypopituitarism		
Hypothyroidism		
Absorptive disturbances		×
Gastroenterostomy, postgastrectomy		×
Malnutrition		×
Ethanol-induced hypoglycemia		×
"Reactive" hypoglycemia		×
After alimentary hyperglycemia		
Latent diabetes		
Nervous, high-strung individuals		
Hypothalamic lesions		×

Source: Adapted from J. Wallach, *Interpretation of Diagnostic Tests*, 2d ed., Little, Brown and Company, Boston, 1974.

flected in altered levels of blood glucose (see Tables 4-5 and 4-6), the most common condition being diabetes mellitus (see Chap. 20). Presently, there is also some controversy regarding the role of carbohydrate in the causation of coronary heart disease[6-8] (see Chap. 17). Some of these conditions will require the dietary regulation of the type of carbohydrate, the amount of carbohydrate, or both. It is therefore important for the student to be able to differentiate between the various types of carbohydrate and their food sources.

Carbohydrate and Dental Caries

Glucose and, to lesser degrees, other disaccharides and monosaccharides play a role in the promotion of dental caries. Bacteria in the mouth utilize the sugar to produce an acid that invades the enamel of the teeth, causing caries (see Chap. 23).

Carbohydrate and Exercise

Research has shown that carbohydrate is the preferred energy source for the working muscles of a trained individual. The muscles must be worked to exhaustion 1 week prior to the athletic competition. A diet high in protein and fat should be eaten for 3 days; thereafter a high carbohydrate diet should be consumed until the day of the athletic event.[9] This promotes maximum glycogen stores, which enhances physical endurance.

Carbohydrate and Malabsorption Syndrome

Individuals who have an enzyme lack (disaccharidase deficiency) are unable to digest disaccharides. This causes a state of malabsorption that results in diarrhea, abdominal cramps, flatulence, and failure to thrive. Treatment involves the removal of disaccharides from the diet and supplementation to replace the missing foods. For example, the lactose-intolerant individual, who lacks the enzyme lactase, must avoid milk and milk products, and a milk-free formula or supplement must be provided to replace the missing nutrients (see Chap. 18).

STUDY QUESTIONS

1 Differentiate between a monosaccharide, a disaccharide, and a polysaccharide and give an example of each.

2 What are the main sources of carbohydrate in the American diet?

3 Describe the functions of dietary fiber and list important sources.

4 Trace the route of carbohydrate from ingestion to metabolism.

5 What is the recommended level of carbohydrate in the diet?

CASE STUDY 4-1

Susan, a 26-year-old active professional, arrives at the company health service with the chief complaint of general lethargy, abdominal pain, and constipation.

A physical examination revealed a normal healthy woman with a height of 5 ft 4 in and weight of 115 lb. Laboratory analysis and gastrointestinal x-ray series were normal. Present diet includes the following meal pattern:

Breakfast	*4 oz orange juice*
	1 English muffin with margarine
	coffee with milk and sugar
Midmorning	*coffee with milk and sugar*
	jelly doughnut
Lunch	*tuna fish sandwich*
	12 oz Coke
	1 candy bar

Dinner	*chicken breast*
	french fried potatoes
	squash
	chocolate cake
	coffee with milk and sugar

On the basis of the normal clinical and laboratory findings, the diagnosis of constipation was made and Susan was referred to the nutritionist for counseling.

Case Study Questions

1 *What types of carbohydrate are excessive in the diet? What types are negligible?*

2 *Outline a diet plan incorporating the type of carbohydrate sources that are lacking.*

3 *How does fiber promote intestinal function?*

REFERENCES

1 Agricultural Stabilization and Conservation Service, *Sugar Report No. 241,* U.S. Dept. of Agriculture, 1972.

2 American Medical Association, *Nutrients in Processed Foods: Fats, Carbohydrates,* Publishing Services Group, Inc., Acton, Mass., 1975, pp. 85–140.

3 *Toxicological Evaluation of Some Enzymes, Modified Starches and Certain Other Substances,* Publ. No. 1, World Health Organization, Food Additive Series, WHO, Geneva, 1972, pp. 7, 23–58.

4 American Medical Association, op. cit., p. 86.

5 Mervyn G. Hardinge, J. B. Swarner, and H. Crooks, "Carbohydrates in Foods," *Journal of the American Dietetic Association,* March 1965, pp. 197–204.

6 J. Yudkin and J. Roddy, "Levels of Dietary Sucrose in Patients with Occlusive-Atherosclerotic Disease," *Lancet,* **11:**6–8, 1964.

7 N. Zollner and F. Wolfram, "Sucrose in Human Nutrition," in *The Role of Sugar in Modern Nutrition, Naringsforskning,* vol. 17, suppl. 9, 1973, pp. 22–25.

8 "Sucrose, Starch and Hyperlipidemia," *Nutrition Reviews,* **33:**44–46, 1975.

9 P. O. Astrand, "Nutrition and Work Performance," *Federation Proceedings,* **26:**1772–1777, 1967.

CHAPTER 5

LIPIDS*

*Rosanne B. Howard
and
Nancie H. Herbold*

KEY WORDS
Saturated Fats
Unsaturated Fats
Essential Fatty Acids
Medium-Chain Triglycerides
Cholesterol
Phospholipid

INTRODUCTION

A growing incidence of coronary heart disease has prompted epidemiological surveys of risk factors among our population. Since increased levels of serum cholesterol and triglycerides have been identified as associated risk factors, much attention has been focused on dietary lipids and their role in the causation, treatment, and prevention of coronary heart disease. This growing concern over the type and amount of fat in the diet necessitates a knowledge of lipid function in the human body. In addition there are many conditions, such as biliary obstruction, hypothyroidism, nephrosis, and pancreatic disease, that have associated abnormalities in plasma lipid transport. Also, certain genetic diseases (Tay-Sachs, Gaucher's, Niemann-Pick disease), although not amenable to dietary treatment, have an inherent lipid storage disorder, which further demonstrates the need for health professionals to have an acquaintance with lipid metabolism.

In the human body, lipid has many important roles. Probably the most important quantitatively is that of fuel, since lipid provides twice the energy of carbohydrate and protein. One g of fat supplies 9.3 kcal (39.06 kJ), while one g of protein or carbohydrate provides 4.1 kcal (17.22 kJ). Lipid is not only an effective fuel source but is the body's storage form of energy, for, unlike carbohydrate and protein, it can be stored in almost unlimited quantity. All cells of the body, except for those of the central nervous system and the erythrocytes, are able to use fatty acids as a source of energy.

Besides providing a storehouse of energy, fat depots exert an insulating effect in the body and cushion the internal organs. Another important function of lipid is that of supplying compounds that cannot be synthesized by the human body, and the fat-soluble vitamins (A, D, E, and K), which are classified as lipids. Some compounds derived from lipids are im-

* The authors wish to acknowledge the research assistance of Nancy Keith, M.S., R.D.

portant building blocks of biologically active materials, for example, the prostaglandins, substances with hormone-like activity that cause many effects in the body. Other lipids that are compounded with proteins, namely lipoproteins, function as structural components of the cell membrane. In the diet, fats have a satiety effect, since fats are digested and absorbed more slowly than carbohydrate and protein.

This chapter considers these functions of lipids within the body and those lipids involved in clinically significant abnormalities.

DEFINITION OF LIPIDS

When lipids are liquid at room temperature, they are called *oils,* and when they are solid at room temperature, they are called *fats.* Fats and oils can be either visible or invisible to the human eye. The so-called *invisible fats* are those dispersed within a food, such as that within nuts and egg yolks, whereas the visible fats such as butter or vegetable oil are readily apparent to the consumer.

As a group, lipids comprise a heterogeneous collection (fats, oils, waxes, and related organic substances) that are related by the fact that they are poorly soluble in water but are soluble in organic solvents such as ethanol or ether. (This solubility property is utilized in extraction of lipids from tissues.) Lipids are also related by the fact that in their molecular structure there is usually a fatty acid or a fatty acid derivative. These fatty acids are similar to carbohydrate and contain the same elements— carbon, hydrogen, and oxygen—but there is less oxygen relative to the amounts of carbon and hydrogen in fatty acids than in carbohydrate. Table 5-1 summarizes the chemical reactions of lipids.

TABLE 5-1   CHEMICAL REACTIONS OF LIPIDS

Property	Reaction	Comments
Hydrogenation	Liquid oils become solid fats by the introduction of hydrogen. This hardening process is used commercially to produce solid cooking fats and margarine from liquid vegetable oils. In processing, the unsaturated bonds of the fatty acids become saturated by the hydrogen gas, in the presence of a catalyst (nickel, palladium, or platinum).	Since this processing affects the degree of saturation, this has significance in determining the vegetable-oil margarine appropriate for diets high in polyunsaturates. The harder the margarine, the less polyunsaturated, which inhibits the ability to alter serum cholesterol.
Iodine number	The iodine number is the amount of iodine that can be retained by 100 g of fat. It reflects the average number of double bonds or the degree of unsaturation of a lipid.	Vegetable oils have a high iodine number and animal fats have a low iodine number. Individuals on a diet lowering blood cholesterol would want to consume fats with a high iodine number, as they would be unsaturated fats.
Saponification (hydrolysis)	Occurs when a fat is hydrolyzed by alkali. Salts are formed (soaps) from the liberation of free fatty acids and glycerol.	Formation of insoluble soaps in the G.I. tract, whereby fat combines with calcium to form a soap which is excreted in the feces (steatorrhea).
Rancidity	Caused by hydrolysis or oxidation. Oxidation occurs when the double bonds are broken and form peroxides, aldehydes, ketones, and acids, which have an unpleasant odor and flavor. Oxidation requires oxygen and is accelerated by heat, light, moisture, and acids.	Rancidity may be slowed down by storing food in air-tight containers, and in green or brown containers which are light-proof. Vitamin E is a natural antioxidant which may be present in vegetable fat but not animal fat. Vitamin A can become inactivated in rancid fats.

TABLE 5-2 CLASSIFICATION OF LIPIDS ACCORDING TO PRESENCE IN THE BODY

I   Major constituents
   A   Fatty acids
   B   Fatty-acid derivatives
      1   Fatty acids with glycerol: glycerides
      2   Cholesterol esters
      3   Phospholipids: phosphatides (lecithin, cephalin), plasmalogens, sphingomyelins
      4   Glycolipids: cerebrosides, gangliosides
   C   Sterol alcohols
      1   Free cholesterol
      2   Bile acids
      3   Steroids
II   Minor constituents
   A   Fat-soluble vitamins: carotene, vitamins A, D, E, K
   B   Prostaglandins

Source: Adapted from Montgomery et al., *Biochemistry: A Case Oriented Approach,* C. V. Mosby Company, St. Louis, 1974, chap. 8.

CLASSIFICATION OF LIPIDS

Since lipids are such a heterogeneous group, classification is best conceptualized by considering only those lipids that are significant to human nutrition, and then grouping these lipids into two categories, major constituents and minor constituents, based on the amount of lipid present in body tissue (Table 5-2). The minor constitutents, fat-soluble vitamins and prostaglandins, are present in minute amounts, milligrams or less. Those in the major category, fatty acids, fatty acid derivatives, and sterols, are present in somewhat larger amounts (e.g., the average amount of cholesterol in serum ranges from 200 to 240 mg/100 ml).[1]

MAJOR CONSTITUENTS OF LIPIDS IN BODY TISSUE

Fatty Acids

Saturated and Unsaturated Fatty Acids

Fatty acids are the basic structural units of lipids. Fatty acids vary in the number of carbon atoms in the molecule and therefore vary con-

1   Carbon has a valence of four, which means that in a chemical reaction four atoms may attach to the carbon atom to form a compound.

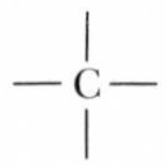

$$-\overset{|}{\underset{|}{C}}-$$

2   During a chemical reaction in which all the valence bonds of a fatty acid become filled with hydrogen, the compound formed is referred to as *saturated,* that is, *"saturated with hydrogen."*

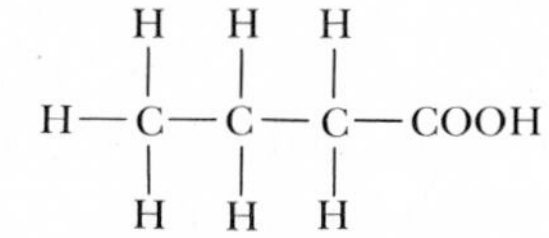

$$H-\overset{\overset{\textstyle H}{|}}{\underset{\underset{\textstyle H}{|}}{C}}-\overset{\overset{\textstyle H}{|}}{\underset{\underset{\textstyle H}{|}}{C}}-\overset{\overset{\textstyle H}{|}}{\underset{\underset{\textstyle H}{|}}{C}}-COOH$$

Saturated fat, butyric acid ($C_4 : O$)
(4 carbon atoms, 1 double bond,
found in butter)

3   In the carbon chain of the fatty acid, when there are two less hydrogen atoms attached to the carbon atom, the carbon atoms join their two available valence bonds and make a *mutual bond.* Adding this new mutual bond to an existing bond forms a *double bond,* thereby creating a state of *unsaturation,* which provides room for more hydrogen. It is the number of double bonds present along the carbon chain of the fatty acid that determines the degree of saturation. When there are many double bonds present in a fatty acid, there is more space available to combine hydrogen, and the fatty acid is known as *polyunsaturated.* When there is only one double bond in the fatty acid, it is known as *monounsaturated.*

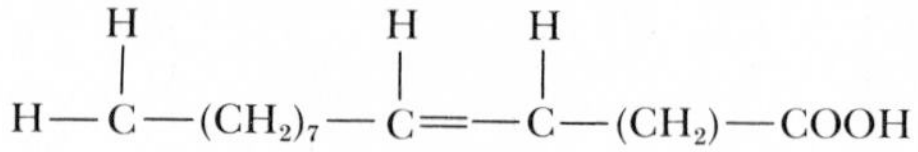

$$H-\overset{\overset{\textstyle H}{|}}{\underset{\underset{\textstyle H}{|}}{C}}-(CH_2)_7-\overset{\overset{\textstyle H}{|}}{C}=-\overset{\overset{\textstyle H}{|}}{C}-(CH_2)-COOH$$

Monounsaturated, oleic acid ($C_{18} : 1$)
(18 carbon atoms, 1 double bond
found in olive oil)

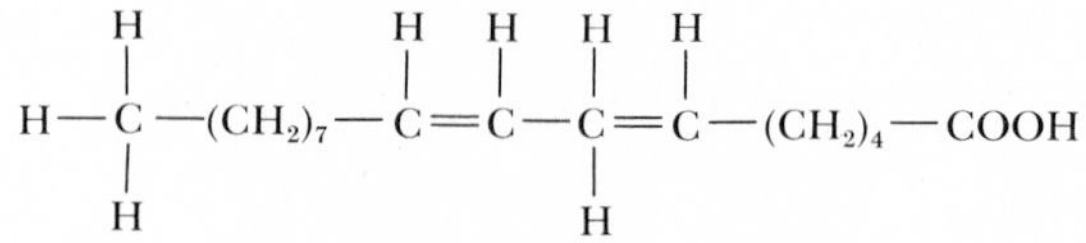

$$H-\overset{\overset{\textstyle H}{|}}{\underset{\underset{\textstyle H}{|}}{C}}-(CH_2)_7-\overset{\overset{\textstyle H}{|}}{C}=\overset{\overset{\textstyle H}{|}}{C}-\overset{\overset{\textstyle H}{|}}{\underset{\underset{\textstyle H}{|}}{C}}=\overset{\overset{\textstyle H}{|}}{C}-(CH_2)_4-COOH$$

Polyunsaturated, linoleic acid ($C_{18} : 2$)
(18 carbon atoms, 2 double bonds
found in vegetable oils)

Figure 5-1
The process of saturation of a fatty acid.

siderably in chain length, with most having an even number of carbon atoms and a straight chain. Fatty acids can be grouped according to chain length into short, medium, and long:

Short-chain fatty acids: 2 to 4 carbon atoms

Medium-chain fatty acids: 6 to 10 carbon atoms

Long-chain fatty acids: 12 to 26 carbon atoms

Fatty acids also vary in another important chemical characteristic, the degree of *saturation* or *unsaturation*. These terms describe the basic carbon chain and the degree to which it is filled with hydrogen. This is an important concept to understand since the degree of saturation of the lipid determines the effect within the body, namely, the effect on the serum cholesterol, since the position of unsaturation influences the breakup point of the chain in metabolism,

affecting the body's ability to modify the molecule and to metabolize the remaining fragments. Saturated fats raise the serum cholesterol, monounsaturated fats have no effect, and polyunsaturated fats lower the serum cholesterol.

An important characteristic of polyunsaturated fatty acids is the shape of the molecule. In unprocessed foods, polyunsaturated fatty acids normally occur in what is known as a *cis* configuration, which means that the fatty acid is folded back upon itself at each of the double bonds. During processing, the cis form may be converted to the unfolded or *trans* form and thereby acquires different nutritional properties. An example would be linoleic acid, which loses its effectiveness as an essential fatty acid during processing when converted from the cis to the trans form.

Tables 5-3 and 5-4 list the saturated and unsaturated fatty acids occurring in nature, along with their chemical formulas.

TABLE 5-3 SOME NATURALLY OCCURRING SATURATED FATTY ACIDS

Molecular formula	Common name	Systematic name	Chain length and unsaturation
$C_2H_4O_2$	Acetic		$C_2{:}0$
$C_3H_6O_2$	Propionic		$C_3{:}0$
$C_4H_8O_2$	n-Butyric		$C_4{:}0$
$C_6H_{12}O_2$	Caproic	n-Hexanoic	$C_6{:}0$
$C_8H_{16}O_2$	Caprylic	n-Octanoic	$C_8{:}0$
$C_9H_{18}O_2$	Pelargonic	n-Nonanoic	$C_9{:}0$
$C_{10}H_{20}O_2$	Capric	n-Decanoic	$C_{10}{:}0$
$C_{12}H_{24}O_2$	Lauric	n-Dodecanoic	$C_{12}{:}0$
$C_{14}H_{28}O_2$	Myristic	n-Tetradecanoic	$C_{14}{:}0$
$C_{16}H_{32}O_2$	Palmitic*	n-Hexadecanoic	$C_{16}{:}0$
$C_{18}H_{36}O_2$	Stearic*	n-Octadecanoic	$C_{18}{:}0$
$C_{20}H_{40}O_2$	Arachidic	n-Eicosanoic	$C_{20}{:}0$
$C_{22}H_{44}O_2$	Behenic	n-Docosanoic	$C_{22}{:}0$
$C_{24}H_{48}O_2$	Lignoceric	n-Tetracosanoic	$C_{24}{:}0$
$C_{26}H_{52}O_2$	Cerotic	n-Hexacosanoic	$C_{26}{:}0$
$C_{28}H_{56}O_2$	Montanic	n-Octacosanoic	$C_{28}{:}0$

* The most common saturated fatty acids in animal fats.

Source: Adapted from A. White, P. Handler, and E. Smith, *Principles of Biochemistry,* 5th ed., McGraw-Hill Book Company, 1973, New York, p. 60.

TABLE 5-4   SOME NATURALLY OCCURRING UNSATURATED FATTY ACIDS

Molecular formula	Common name	Systematic name	Chain length and unsaturation
$C_{16}H_{30}O_2$	Palmitoleic*	9-Hexadecenoic	C16:1
$C_{18}H_{34}O_2$	Oleic*	cis-9-Octadecenoic	C18:1
$C_{18}H_{34}O_2$	Elaidic	trans-9-Octadecenoic	C18:1
$C_{18}H_{34}O_2$	Vaccenic	11-Octadecenoic	C18:1
$C_{18}H_{32}O_2$	Linoleic*	cis,cis-9,12-Octadecadienoic	C18:2
$C_{18}H_{30}O_2$	Linolenic*	9,12,15-Octadecatrienoic	C18:3
$C_{18}H_{30}O_2$	Eleostearic	9,11,13-Octadecatrienoic	C18:3
$C_{20}H_{32}O_2$	Arachidonic	5,8,11,14-Eicosatetraenoic	C20:4

* The most common unsaturated fatty acids in animal fats.

Source: Adapted from A. White, P. Handler, and E. Smith, *Principles of Biochemistry*, 5th ed., McGraw-Hill Book Company, New York, 1973, pp. 58, 62.

Saturated fatty acids which have carbon chains with fewer than 10 even-numbered carbon atoms are liquid at room temperature, and the melting and boiling points rise as the chains get longer. Those fatty acids with more than 10 carbon atoms are solid at room temperature. Saturated fatty acids with 10 carbons or less are usually not present in animal fats. The most abundant saturated fatty acids in animal fats are myristic (C_{14}), palmitic (C_{16}), and stearic (C_{18}). Those saturated fatty acids with fewer than 12 carbons and those with more than 18 have little effect on serum cholesterol, while those in between, lauric (C_{12}), myristic (C_{14}), and palmitic (C_{16}), have the strongest effect of the saturated fatty acids in raising the serum cholesterol in the human body.[1,2] Animal fat (dairy products, meat) is the abundant source of saturated fatty acids.

All of the common unsaturated fatty acids are liquid at room temperature. Oleic, palmitoleic, linoleic, and linolenic acids are the most unsaturated fatty acids found in nature. They occur in the oils of vegetable and cereal products, such as soy, corn, cottonseed, and safflower oils.

Certain unsaturated fatty acids have been identified as essential to the body because of the fact that:

1   The body is unable to synthesize these fatty acids.

2   The absence of this fatty acid will cause a deficiency state.

Essential Fatty Acids (EFA)

There are two polyunsaturated fatty acids that cannot be synthesized in the human body and must be supplied by the diet. These *essential fatty acids* (EFA) are linoleic and arachidonic. However, arachidonic acid can be formed in the body from linoleic acid and therefore only linoleic acid is actually essential to man.

Essential fatty acids are necessary to maintain the function and integrity of the cellular and subcellular membranes in tissue metabolism. Linoleic acid derivatives are also necessary for prostaglandin synthesis. Prostaglandins are hormonelike compounds with many and varied functions in the human body. They are known to stimulate smooth-muscle contractions, reduce blood pressure, inhibit gastric secretions, and activate or antagonize other hormones.

When linoleic acid is not present in the diet, symptoms of deficiency appear:

Scaly skin

Sparse hair growth

Poor wound healing

Thrombocytopenia (decrease in blood platelets)

The analysis of blood serum, plasma, or erythrocytes for certain unsaturated fatty acids is used as a diagnostic means of recognizing a dietary deficiency of linoleic acid. Biochemical evidence of EFA deficiency includes a decrease in plasma lipids, arachidonic acid, and linoleic acid, and an increase in 5,8,11-eicosatrienoic, palmitoleic, and oleic acids.[3,4,5] A major change noted is an increase in the ratio of trienoic to tetraenoic fatty acids (triene/tetraene ratio) of more than 0.4, which is regarded as critical evidence of EFA deficiency.[6]

Essential fatty acid deficiency has been reported in hospitalized infants and adults who have been kept on fat-free total parenteral nutrition for several weeks.[7] Infants fed skim milk formulas for extended periods of time without fatty acid supplementation can also become fatty acid–deficient.[8] Once linoleic acid is added to the diet, symptoms of EFA deficiency disappear. To prevent fatty acid deficiency the National Research Council recommends an intake of 1 to 2 percent of the total calories as essential fatty acids.[9] Good sources of linoleic acid are corn, cottonseed, peanut, soybean, and safflower oils.

For infants, particular attention should be given to providing 1 to 3 percent of the calories as linoleic acid, because of the rapid growth period and limited body stores. It has been found that the average linoleic acid content of breast milk from United States mothers amounts to 4 to 5 percent of the total breast-milk calories. However, variations are found in other populations and are related to the mother's nutritional status and diet.[10]

Essential fatty acids appear to play a role in the regulation of cholesterol metabolism, especially cholesterol transport, its transformation into metabolic products, and the excretion of some of these products. It has been shown that a diet high in essential fatty acids reduces high levels of serum cholesterol in experimental animals and in humans.[11]

Fatty Acid Derivatives

Fatty acids are rarely found free in nature but are combined to other moieties by an ester linkage or an amide linkage, and the complex lipids thus formed can be considered fatty acid derivatives. (An *ester linkage* is a chemical bond that connects an alcohol and an acid of an ester, as in the formation of glycerides (see below). An *amide linkage* connects the alpha-carboxyl group of one amino acid to the alpha-amino group of another amino acid; this linkage becomes operative when fat and protein combine to form a lipoprotein.)

Fatty Acids with Glycerol (Glycerides)

Upon hydrolysis, simple lipids yield fatty acids and glycerol. Glycerol is a sweet viscous liquid that is closely allied to carbohydrate, which it can be converted to within the body. Glycerol contains three hydroxyl (OH) groups, which makes it an alcohol. When the acidic (COOH) groups of the fatty acids react with the alcoholic OH of glycerol, a neutral fat or glyceride results. This process, whereby a compound is formed from an alcohol and a fatty acid by the removal of water, is known as *esterification,* and the product formed is known as an *ester.*

These fatty acid esters of glycerol are known as *acylglycerol* (*acyl group* is the name for the fatty acid moiety in lipid esters) and are

Figure 5-2

The formation of a triglyceride. R_1, R_2, *and* R_3 *represent different or identical fatty acids.*

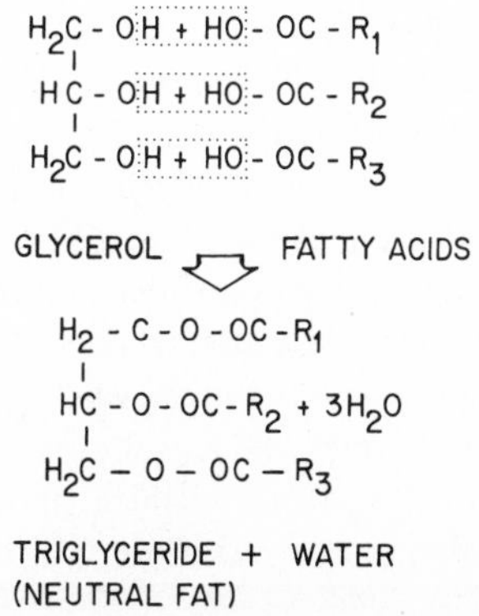

$$H_2C - O\!:\!H + HO\!:\!- OC - R_1$$
$$HC - O\!:\!H + HO\!:\!- OC - R_2$$
$$H_2C - O\!:\!H + HO\!:\!- OC - R_3$$

GLYCEROL ⇩ FATTY ACIDS

$$H_2 - C - O - OC - R_1$$
$$HC - O - OC - R_2 + 3H_2O$$
$$H_2C - O - OC - R_3$$

TRIGLYCERIDE + WATER
(NEUTRAL FAT)

commonly called *glycerides*. There are three general types of glycerides, mono-, di-, and triglycerides. The distinction between them depends on the number of glycerol alcohol groups esterified.

In the human body, monoglycerides are important in digestion and as metabolic intermediates, which is almost the exclusive role of diglycerides. Triglycerides are the major transport and storage form of fatty acids. The average triglyceride content of blood plasma is 140 to 225 mg/100 ml. These triglycerides for the most part contain long-chain fatty acids.

Recently, *medium-chain triglycerides* (MCT) —those triglycerides containing medium-chain fatty acids—have been used effectively in the treatment of patients with impaired absorption or digestion of fat (e.g., from biliary obstruction, pancreatic insufficiency, chronic pancreatitis, or cystic fibrosis). These triglycerides contain fatty acids with 8 and 10 carbon atoms and are a mixture of octanoic (C_8) and decanoic (C_{10}) fatty acids. A commercially prepared MCT product is made from coconut oil, which contains octanoic and decanoic acids. When the coconut oil is hydrolyzed, the octanoic and decanoic acids are esterified with glycerol and the resulting product, MCT Oil, contains 75 percent octanoic acid and 25 percent decanoic acid.

MCT derives its special effect from the fact that it is digested and metabolized differently from long-chain triglycerides. These medium-chain triglycerides are rapidly hydrolyzed and absorbed directly into the intestinal mucosa, requiring neither bile salts, chylomicron formation, nor lymphatic transport, and they travel directly to the liver. For example, in the condition known as abetalipoproteinenemia, absorption of long-chain fatty acids is impaired because of an inherited defect which interferes with the synthesis of low-density lipoproteins. MCT can be used as a dietary supplement to provide a source of dietary fat and energy. Currently, MCT is being used to induce ketosis in patients with intractable seizure disorders. Inducing a ketotic state has been shown to be somewhat effective in controlling certain types of seizures in patients who have not responded to drug therapy. (See Chap. 22.)

MCT now provides the fat component of several infant formulas used for children with defects in fat assimilation (Portagen and Pregestimil; Mead Johnson). Also, MCT is used as a source of readily absorbable calories, providing 8.3 kcal (34.8 kJ) per ml. It is a light yellow oil with a slightly acrid taste that is somewhat apparent only when it is added to foods during cooking or preparation.

Cholesterol Esters and Free Cholesterol

Although these compounds should be differentiated by strict classification we will consider them together because of their interrelating role within the body.

Cholesterol is an alcohol and is therefore capable of forming esters with fatty acids. Cholesterol esters contain fatty acids esterified to a 3-beta-hydroxyl group of a steroid ring. The fatty acid component of the ester usually has a long carbon chain and is frequently unsaturated. These cholesterol esters are the storage form of cholesterol and are found in the plasma, constituting two-thirds of the total cholesterol there. In fact, most of the cholesterol that accumulates in the walls of atherosclerotic arteries is esterified. Free or unesterified cholesterol exists in smaller amounts, for the most part in plasma lipoproteins and cell membranes.

Most cholesterol contained in the diet is present as the free sterol and is readily absorbable. It is only present in foods of animal origin, especially meats, glandular organs, egg yolk, whole milk, cheese, and fats. Plants do not have cholesterol but contain other sterols, known as phytosterols, which are poorly absorbed by the human body. These sterols, such as β-sitosterol, if fed in large quantities, are known to inhibit cholesterol absorption. This property is utilized clinically in patients with elevated serum cholesterol levels in an attempt to reduce cholesterol absorption.

In addition to the exogenous supply of

cholesterol from food sources, the human body synthesizes cholesterol and thus provides an endogenous supply. Cholesterol is synthesized in most tissues of the body (with the possible exception of the human brain), but primarily in the liver, which regulates cholesterol synthesis.[12] It is estimated that the body synthesizes approximately 1.5 to 2 g of cholesterol per day.[13] In the United States, we eat between 600 and 1200 mg of cholesterol per day and of this we absorb 300 to 400 mg per day or 50 percent of the dietary cholesterol. To further reduce the absorption, it is necessary to lower the intake of cholesterol to the range of 100 to 300 mg per day.[14] (See Chap. 17.)

The fact that the body can synthesize cholesterol has led to some confusion with respect to the effectiveness of low-cholesterol diets in reducing serum cholesterol. It should be noted that although synthesis continues in a normal person on a low-cholesterol and low-saturated-fat diet, the synthesis does not replace that which is taken away from the diet, so that the blood cholesterol level does become somewhat lower. Also, there are certain factors that influence the amount of cholesterol absorbed. They are as follows:[15,16]

The total amount of cholesterol per feeding

The frequency of ingestion

The type of dietary fat fed with cholesterol

Age

Past dietary intake

The body's efficiency in synthesizing cholesterol relates to its important functions within the human body. Cholesterol is a structural component of cell membranes and plasma lipoproteins and is converted in the liver to bile acids. Another important role is that it is a precursor to steroid and sex hormones. In the adrenals, cholesterol, perhaps as a sulfate, is the precursor for pregnenolone, which is the precursor for progesterone, testosterone, and the estrogens, and is also the precursor of the adrenocortical steroids such as aldosterone and cortisol. In the skin, cholesterol serves as the precursor of vitamin D when, on exposure to sunlight or ultraviolet irradiation, 7-dehydrocholesterol is converted to active vitamin D.

Phospholipids

Phospholipids are another class of compound lipids. They are composed of fatty acids, phosphoric acid, and a nitrogenous base. The functions of phospholipids in the body are:

1 Formation of structural elements within the cell
2 Synthesis of cholesterol
3 Carrier in the transport of fatty acids and protein

Phospholipids can be subdivided into three groups:

Phosphatides (lecithin, cephalin)
Plasmalogens
Sphingomyelins

We will focus our attention on the phosphatides and sphingomyelins, as they have the most dietary significance.

Phosphatides (lecithin, cephalin) Phosphatides are derivatives of glycerol phosphate. Upon hydrolysis (the splitting of a compound by the addition of water) phosphatides yield one molecule of phosphoric acid and two molecules of fatty acid. Usually the phosphoric acid is bound to a nitrogenous compound such as choline, in which case it is called phosphatidyl choline. Choline, a vitamin, must be supplied in the diet or synthesized in the body in order to form lecithin. *Lecithin* is composed of glycerol, fatty acid, and the nitrogenous base choline. It is a component of the erythrocyte plasma membrane and is distributed in the cells of the body. Egg yolks and soy beans are excellent sources of lecithin. Lecithin is produced commercially from soy beans for use as an emulsifying agent in such foods as mayonnaise and salad dressings.

Cephalins are another group of phosphatides that are found in egg yolks and animal tissues, especially brain. Cephalin is present in thromboplastin, which is needed in the blood clotting process.[17]

Sphingomyelins The sphingomyelins are found in the nerves and brain tissue and are components of the myelin sheath which acts as an insulator around the nerve fibers. Sphingomyelins are composed of:

Fatty acids
Phosphoric acid
Choline
Sphingosine

Niemann-Pick disease is a lipid-storage disorder of childhood that is due to the lack of sphingomyelinase, the enzyme needed for the breakdown of sphingomyelin. Because of the lack of this enzyme, sphingomyelin is not broken down, and hence is deposited in all organs and tissues of the body. This disease is fatal and many stricken children do not live beyond the age of three.[18]

Glycolipids

Glycolipids are composed of fatty acids, carbohydrate, and nitrogen. Included in this classification of glycolipids are cerebrosides and gangliosides.

Cerebrosides are found in high concentrations in the white matter of the brain and are a component of myelin. They are also found in lesser amounts in the blood serum, erythrocytes, spleen, and kidney. Cerebrosides are composed of:

Sphingosine
Fatty acids (22 to 24 carbon atoms)
Galactose

Gangliosides are also found in the brain and nerve tissue and are typical constituents of synaptic membranes. Gangliosides are composed of:

Sphingosine
Fatty acids (22 to 24 carbon atoms)
Glucose and galactose
Complex compounds containing an amino acid sugar

A number of diseases are caused by a deficiency of the ganglioside enzyme. In Tay-Sachs disease, one such disorder, a large amount of gangliosides is deposited in the gray matter of the brain. It is a disease of infancy and is generally fatal.[19]

THE BODY'S USE OF FAT

Fats play many important roles in human nutrition. Fats contained in the foods we eat are sources of energy, of essential fatty acids, and of fat-soluble vitamins. Food fats give flavor to our foods and help to delay the onset of hunger, as fat remains in the stomach longer than carbohydrate or protein. Fat deposits in the adipose tissue insulate the body and cushion the body's organs.

Fats provide twice as much energy as carbohydrate or protein does and therefore are the most concentrated source of energy available to the body. One gram of fat provides 9.3 kcal (39.06 kJ), compared to 4.1 kcal (17.22 kJ) from one gram of carbohydrate or protein. Fatty acids can be utilized as a source of energy by all the cells in the body except for the erythrocytes and cells of the central nervous system. Fat can be stored in the adipose tissue and therefore becomes a form of stored energy.

Digestion and Absorption of Fat

Glycerides

Fat digestion does not actually begin until the fat reaches the first section of the small intestine, the duodenum. The secretions which aid in the enzymatic breakdown of fats are:

1 The bile salts, produced by the liver and secreted by the gallbladder
2 Pancreatic lipases, produced and secreted by the pancreas
3 Enteric lipase, secreted by the walls of the intestine

Bile salts and the alkali from the intestinal fluid mix with the glycerine molecules to form an emulsion. The emulsifying process serves two purposes:[20]

1 It divides the fat into small globules, which increases the surface area open to enzymatic action.
2 It lowers surface tension, which in turn eases the penetration of enzymes.

Then pancreatic and enteric lipases break the fat into monoglycerides, diglycerides, fatty acids, and glycerol. Glycerol, monoglycerides, diglycerides, and medium-chain fatty acids (10 carbon atoms or less) are absorbed directly into the portal blood system from the intestine and are transported to the liver. Long-chain fatty acids (over 14 carbon atoms) are first esterified to form neutral fat within the mucosal wall of the intestine and then combine with cholesterol, phospholipids, and protein to form chylomicrons. The chylomicrons are absorbed from the intestine into the lymphatic system and are transported from the thoracic duct to the left subclavian vein, where they enter the venous blood and are carried to the liver. Sixty to seventy percent of dietary fat is absorbed via this route (see Fig. 5-3). The remainder, cholesterol and phospholipids, are absorbed by a different route.

Cholesterol

Once dietary cholesterol reaches the small intestine, the majority is esterified with fatty

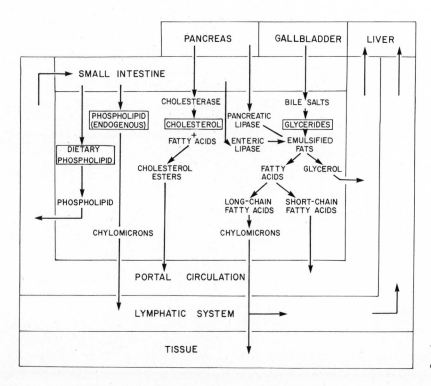

Figure 5-3
The various mechanisms of fat absorption.

acids by pancreatic cholesterol esterase. This esterified cholesterol is absorbed via the lymphatic system and converted to bile acids in the liver. When bile acids are needed for digestion they are excreted into the small intestine and reabsorbed with the digested fat. This process, which is known as the *enterohepatic cycle,* regulates cholesterol synthesis by negative feedback. It is this endogenous synthesis that makes dietary restriction of cholesterol not totally effective in regulating serum cholesterol levels. (See Fig. 5-3.)

Phospholipids

Phospholipids are ingested in food in the form of lecithin. They may also be synthesized by the small intestine. Dietary phospholipids can be absorbed directly into the portal system, while synthesized phospholipids are incorporated into chylomicrons and absorbed via the lymphatics. (See Fig. 5-3.)

Fat Absorption Test

Some fat is not absorbed but is excreted via the stool. An excretion of fecal fat above 6 g per day is a condition known as *steatorrhea.* Steatorrhea is caused by a malabsorption of fat due to defective breakdown and absorption.

Normal adults can absorb up to 300 g of fat daily. A fecal fat test is used in the diagnosis of many gastrointestinal disorders. The test involves the use of a high-fat diet: patients must consume a diet of 100 g of fat daily for 3 days prior to a stool collection. If the amount of fat in the collected stool exceeds 6 g (6 percent of the ingested fat), steatorrhea exists and various disorders must be ruled out.[21] In the child, a loss of fecal fat greater than 5 percent of the ingested fat constitutes steatorrhea.[22]

Metabolism of Fat

Once chylomicrons reach the liver they are metabolized or are converted to alpha- and beta-lipoproteins which are used for energy, if needed, or stored in adipose tissue.

Fat storage is an active process. *Lipogenesis* (synthesis and deposition of fat) and *lipolysis* (mobilization and oxidation of fat) are ongoing processes. Fatty acids and glycerol are the end products of these reactions. The hydrolysis of triglycerides to glycerol and fatty acid is one of the first steps in fat synthesis and deposition. Fatty acids are further broken down during oxidation into two carbon units and acetyl CoA. Thereafter, fat follows the same oxidative pathway as carbohydrate (the Krebs cycle; see Chap. 9).

Incomplete oxidation of fat such as occurs during states of fasting or uncontrolled diabetes mellitus, leads to the formation of ketone bodies (acetoacetic acid, beta-hydroxybutyric acid and acetone) and accumulation in the blood (ketonemia) with subsequent excretion in the urine (ketonuria). This state is known as ketosis. Under this condition, the brain, which normally uses glucose for energy, utilizes ketone bodies. To a limited extent, other tissues of the body also utilize ketones in lieu of glucose.

Since glycerol cannot be oxidized by most tissues of the body, it is transported to the liver

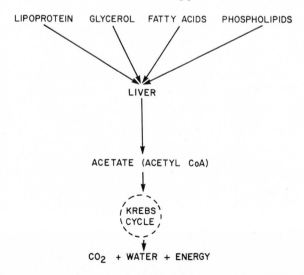

Figure 5-4
The metabolism of fat.

where it combines with fatty acids to form triglycerides, and is then transported to the cells. The liver plays an important role in fat metabolism; its functions are summarized as follows:

1 Synthesis of triglycerides from carbohydrate
2 Synthesis of cholesterol from triglycerides
3 Synthesis of phospholipid and lipoprotein from protein
4 Clearance of phospholipid, cholesterol, and lipoprotein from the plasma

In addition to the liver, hormones also affect fat metabolism, causing fat to be mobilized, synthesized, utilized, or released from tissue stores. Table 5-5 summarizes the effect of the body's hormones on fat metabolism.

Deposition of Fat

When fat has been metabolized and energy requirements have been met, excess fat is stored or deposited in certain anatomical sites, which include subcutaneous tissue, the peritoneal cavity, and intramuscular tissue.

The storage or deposition of excessive fat results in obesity. Normally fat comprises 15 to 18 percent of the body weight. This stored fat can supply the body with enough energy to meet an individual's requirements for a 4-week period,[23] enabling survival during a period of famine or starvation. During these periods fat is transported from the storage depots to the actively metabolizing tissue requiring energy. Those depots found under the skin respond first to dietary deprivation.

Types of Fat Deposition

Both age and diet affect the deposition and the composition of body fat. For example, the composition of adipose tissue of a newborn differs markedly from that of an elderly individual. In the newborn period, only 40 percent of adipose tissue is composed of lipid (the other 60 percent is mostly water with some nitrogen); however, in the elderly, adipose tissue contains approximately 75 percent lipid. Also, with age there is an tendency for more fat to be deposited since activity patterns usually decrease, and there may not be a concomitant decrease in food intake.

The fact that diet affects the type of body fat deposition has been demonstrated by animal studies. In animals fed on diets high in saturated fatty acids, the depot of animal fat was also high in saturated fatty acids. A comparable phenomenon was observed with diets high in unsaturated fatty acid. Humans consuming a high polyunsaturated diet have lower serum cholesterol levels and adipose tissue that is higher in unsaturated fatty acids than are found in individuals maintained on high saturated fatty acid diet.[24]

The extrapolation of this information to animal husbandry may provide a new therapeutic tool in the prevention of heart disease, whereby a change in animal feeds that alters the adipose tissue of animals might produce an effect on the type of fat in the human diet. A

TABLE 5-5 HORMONES AFFECTING FAT METABOLISM

Hormone	Effect on fat
↓ Insulin	↓ Fat synthesis ↑ Fat mobilization
↑ Insulin	↑ Fat synthesis ↓ Fat mobilization
↑ Growth hormone	↑ Release of FFA (free fatty acids) from adipose tissue
↑ Thyroxine	↑ Mobilization of fat by energy metabolism
↑ ACTH (adrenocorticotropic hormone)	↑ Mobilization of fat by energy metabolism
↑ Glucocorticoids	↑ Fat mobilization
↑ Epinephrine	↑ Fat mobilization
↑ Glucagon	↑ Fat mobilization ↓ Fat synthesis

reduction in the amount of fat produced in animals is already quite evident from the difference between corn-fed and grass-fed animals, with the latter having fewer fat stores.

DIETARY SIGNIFICANCE AND REQUIREMENTS OF FAT

In the United States, evidence of the effect of dietary fat composition on blood lipid levels has changed the research, production, and sales of fats and fatty acids. Since the early 1960s, there has been a profound increase in the consumption of salad and cooking oils. Presently, 40 percent of the fat consumed in the diet is in the form of meat, 20 percent is from dairy products, and 40 percent is from hidden fats.[25]

With the introduction of tub-type margarines and more stick-type margarines with higher levels of unsaturation, there has been a marked increase in the polyunsaturates/saturates ratio (P/S ratio) of the visible fat portion of the diet. The P/S ratio indicates the quantitative relationship between the polyunsaturated and the saturated fatty acids in the diet. Of interest is the increase in the P/S ratio, which was 0.5 to 1 in 1959 and grew to 1 to 1 in 1971.[26] Some questions have been raised as to whether the amounts of highly unsaturated fatty acids should be increased much above present levels and whether or not polyunsaturated fatty acids are benign compounds imposing risk with large consumption. Although these issues are unresolved, present information indicates that a P/S ratio of 1 to 1.5 is desirable.[27] This is achieved by placing dietary emphasis on vegetable oils and margarines (safflower, corn, soybean, sunflower, and sesame oils) and reducing the saturated fat content of the diet, thereby limiting animal meats and dairy products, with fish and fowl used as substitutes.

The total fat content of the diet has no specific requirement other than to provide

TABLE 5-6 THE FAT COMPOSITION OF SELECTED FOODS

Food	Household measure	Fat, g
Milk (whole)	8 oz	12.0
Milk (skim)	8 oz	0.2
Beef (ground lean)	3 oz	9.1
Chicken (breast)	3 oz	5.1
Fish (halibut)	3 oz	6.0
Margarine (stick type)	1 tsp	3.8
Butter (stick type)	1 tsp	3.8
Corn oil	1 tbsp	13.6
Peanut butter	1 tbsp	8.1
Salad dressing	1 tbsp	11.2

* Source "Nutritive Value of American Foods," *Agriculture Handbook No. 456*, Agriculture Research Service, USDA, 1975.

enough to supply the essential fatty acids and the fat-soluble vitamins. It is estimated that a diet containing between 15 and 25 g of appropriate food fat should provide the dietary requirement for fat.[28] (See Table 5-6.)

During infancy, clinical experience indicates that 30 to 55 percent of the calories should be provided from fat. Diets deviating from this range upwardly tax the infant's digestive and excretory capabilities.[29] With lower fat intakes, the carbohydrate and protein content of the diet increases. An increase in carbohydrate causes an increase in disaccharides in the intestinal lumen which may exceed the existing disaccharidase activity and cause diarrhea. An increase in protein may present an excessive renal solute load to the immature kidney. It is interesting to note that 50 percent of the calories in human milk are derived from fat, and therefore most commercial formulas which are produced to simulate human milk provide between 35 and 50 percent of the calories as fat.

Since fat has been associated as a risk factor in coronary heart disease, the American Heart Association now recommends that the fat content of the diet should represent no more than 35 percent of the total energy (see Chap. 17).

Another growing concern with our present fat consumption is the relationship between dietary fat and the incidence of cancer of the colon. In epidemiological surveys high-fat diets (also high in animal protein) have been identified as risk factors in countries with a high incidence of bowel cancer.[30]

Clinical Application

There are many conditions which affect lipid metabolism, as reflected in altered levels of lipid in blood plasma (see Tables 5-7 and 5-8). Some of these conditions will require regulation of dietary fat. For the most part, those conditions requiring fat modification or reduction are malabsorption syndromes, gallbladder disease, coronary heart disease, diabetes mellitus, fatty liver, cystic fibrosis, and obesity. Other conditions require fat additions; for example, the underweight individual or the use of fat to induce ketosis in seizure patients. (See Chap. 22.)

Dietary fat is regulated by changing the total amount of fat in the diet, by changing the type of fat in the diet, or by changing both. In order to be effective in helping the patient to modify the dietary fat intake, the student will need to understand the differences between saturated fatty acids, polyunsaturated fatty acids, cholesterol, and medium-chain triglycerides and to know their functions in the human body.

Dietary fat is becoming a significant risk factor in coronary heart disease and a possible risk factor in cancer of the colon and breast. Therefore, the control of fat is an important tenet of preventive nutrition. In addition, our population, for the most part sedentary, does not require the extra energy from fat.

A prudent, fat-controlled diet should be initiated during the early years of life. There are many risk factors to our health in our environment, such as noise and pollution, that cannot be easily controlled; however, fat can be controlled, and you as a future health profes-

sional, through nutrition education, can help our population to adopt the prudent diet and elicit the control of fat necessary to foster health (see Chap. 2).

TABLE 5-7 AVERAGE VALUES OF LIPID CONTENT OF BLOOD PLASMA*

Type	Age, y	Value, mg/100 ml
Cholesterol† (total)	Birth	40–90
	1–19	120–230
	20–29	120–240
	30–39	140–270
	40–49	150–310
	50–59	160–330
Cholesterol esters		Determined by 60–75% of the total cholesterol values
Triglycerides	1–19	10–140
	20–29	10–140
	30–39	10–150
	40–49	10–160
	50–59	10–190
Phospholipids		60–350
Vitamin A		65–275 IU 20µg/100 ml
Vitamin E (tocopherol)		>0.5 mg/100 ml
Carotene		100–300 IU
Vitamin D		0.7–3.3 IU/ml (Procedure not generally available.) Indirect estimate by serum alkaline phosphatase, calcium, and phosphorus

* Normal values vary depending on the individual laboratory and the method used.

† Total serum cholesterol as measured in the laboratory represents the sum total of cholesterol contained in high-density lipoprotein (HDL), low-density lipoprotein (LDL), very-low-density lipoprotein (VLDL), and the chylomicrons.

STUDY QUESTIONS

1 Explain the difference between a polyunsaturated fat and a saturated fat.

2 What unsaturated fatty acids have been identified as essential to the body and why are they called "essential"?

TABLE 5-8 CONDITIONS ALTERING LIPID CONTENT OF BLOOD PLASMA

Blood lipid	Condition	Increased in	Decreased in
Triglycerides	Familial hyperlipidemia	×	
	Liver diseases	×	
	Nephrotic syndrome	×	
	Diabetes mellitus	×	
	(higher values correlate with hyperglycemia and poorer control of diabetes; reduced by insulin therapy)		
	Pancreatitis	×	
	Von Gierke's disease	×	
	Acute myocardial infarction	×	
	(rise to peak in 3 wk; increase may persist for 1 year)		
	Malnutrition		×
	Congenital a-beta-lipoproteinemia		×
	(rare disease characterized by acanthocytes, absence of serum low-density lipoproteins, very low serum triglyceride values—i.e., less than 6 mg/100 ml)		
Cholesterol	Idiopathic hypercholesterolemia	×	
	Biliary obstruction	×	
	(stone, carcinoma etc. of duct; cholangiolitic cirrhosis)		
	Von Gierke's disease	×	
	Hypothyroidism	×	
	Nephrosis	×	
	(due to chronic nephritis, renal vein thrombosis, amyloidosis, systemic lupus erythematosus, periarteritis, diabetic glomerulosclerosis)		
	Pancreatic disease	×	
	Diabetes mellitus	×	
	Total pancreatectomy	×	
	Chronic pancreatitis (some cases)	×	
	Pregnancy	×	
	Severe liver damage		×
	(due to chemicals, drugs, hepatitis)		
	Hyperthyroidism		×
	Malnutrition		×
	(e.g., starvation, terminal neoplasm, uremia, malabsorption in steatorrhea)		
	Chronic anemia		×
	Pernicious anemia (in relapse)		×
	Hemolytic anemias		×
	Marked hypochromic anemia		×
	Cortisone and ACTH therapy		×
	A-beta-lipoproteinemia		×
	Tangier disease		
Carotenoids	Excessive intake	×	
	(especially carrots)		
	Postprandial hyperlipemia	×	
	Hyperlipemia (e.g., essential hyperlipemia)	×	
	Diabetes mellitus	×	
	Hypothyroidism	×	

TABLE 5-8 (continued)

Blood lipid	Condition	Increased in	Decreased in
	Carotenoid-poor diet (blood level falls within 1 wk, while vitamin A level is unaffected by dietary change for 6 months because of much larger body stores)		×
	Malabsorption syndrome (a very useful screening test for malabsorption)		×
	Liver disease		×
	High fever		×
Lipoproteins	Alterations in familial lipoprotein abnormalities* Tangier disease [marked decrease (heterozygous) or absence (homozygous) of high-density lipoprotein; pre-beta-lipoprotein is absent] A-beta-lipoproteinemia (low-density beta-lipoproteins are absent; high-density lipoproteins are normal; patients also have acanthotic RBCs and low serum carotene levels)		

* See Chap. 17.

Source: Jacques Wallach, *Interpretation of Diagnostic Tests: A Handbook Synopsis of Laboratory Medicine,* 2d ed., Little, Brown Company, Boston, 1974.

CASE STUDY 5-1

A 3-month-old girl was brought to the clinic because of irritability and marked failure to thrive. The past history revealed that at 3 weeks of age, the infant had been changed to a skim milk formula in attempts to control diarrhea.

On physical examination, the infant was found to be growing 2 standard deviations from the mean, with a height of 56.3 cm and a weight of 5.2 kg. Noted were scaly dermatitis on the forehead, the medial ends of the eyebrows, the points of the shoulders, and the scalp; multiple subcutaneous hemorrhages; and sparse hair. Present diet includes eight 6-oz bottles of skim milk, 3 oz of orange juice, and 4 teaspoons of rice cereal, providing a total of 537 kcal (2255 kJ) or 100 kcal per day (420 kJ). The infant was receiving supplemental vitamins A, C, and D.

Laboratory analysis revealed a triene/tetraene ratio of 0.85, a serum cholesterol level of 115 mg/100 ml, a total serum lipid level of 200 mg/100 ml, a hemoglobin level of 9.8 g/100 ml, a hematocrit of 31 percent, and a platelet count of 4.5×10^{-5} mm^3.

Case Study Questions

1 From the biochemical profile and clinical state, what deficiency state would you identify?

2 Based on your diagnosis, what recommendations would you make?

3 How would you relate the symptoms exhibited in this patient to the role of the missing nutrient?

3 What is the role of cholesterol in the body?

4 The mode of absorption of fat differs according to chain length. What is the clinical significance?

5 Excessive storage of fat results in obesity. What is the mechanism of fat deposition and in what areas of the body is fat stored?

REFERENCES

1 A. Keys, "Blood Lipids in Man: A Brief Review," *Journal of American Dietetic Association,* **51**:508, 1967.

2 H. B. Brown, "Food Patterns That Lower Blood Lipids in Man," *Journal of American Dietetic Association,* **58**:303, 1971.

3 J. F. Mead, "The Metabolism of Polyunsaturated Fatty Acids," in R. T. Folman (ed.), *Progress in Chemistry of Fats and Other Lipids,* vol. 9, Pergamon Press, Inc., New York, 1968, pp. 159–192.

4 B. Samuelson, "Biosynthesis of Prostaglandins," *Federation Proceedings,* **31**:1442, 1972.

5 Z. Friedman, A. Daron, M. Stahlman, and J. Oates, "Rapid Onset of EFA Deficiency in the Newborn," *Pediatrics,* **58**(5):640–648, November 1976.

6 W. F. Cuthbertson, "Essential Fatty Acid Requirements in Infancy," *American Journal of Clinical Nutrition,* **29**:559–568, May 1976.

7 M. Caldwell, H. Jonsson, and H. B. Othersen, Jr., "Essential Fatty Acid Deficiency in an Infant Receiving Prolonged Parental Alimentation," *Journal of Pediatrics,* **81**:894, 1972.

8 A. E. Hansen, M. E. Haggard, A. H. Boelsche, D. Adam, and H. F. Wiese, "Essential Fatty Acid in Infant Nutrition, Clinical Manifestations of Linoleic Acid Deficiency," *Journal of Nutrition,* **66**:565, 1958.

9 Food and Nutrition Board, National Research Council, *Recommended Dietary Allowances,* 8th ed. 1974.

10 Cuthbertson, op. cit., p. 565.

11 Brown, op. cit., p. 303.

12 R. Goodhart and M. Shils, *Modern Nutrition in Health and Disease,* Lea & Febiger, Philadelphia, 1973, chap. 4, p. 132.

13 B. T. Burton, *Handbook of Nutrition,* McGraw-Hill Book Company, New York, 1976, p. 71.

14 Montgomery et al., *Biochemistry: A Case Oriented Approach,* C. V. Mosby Co., St. Louis, 1974, chap. 8, p. 306.

15 D. S. Goodman "Cholesterol Ester Metabolism," *Physiological Reviews,* **45**:747–839, 1965.

16 L. Swell, E. C. Trout, J. R. Hooper, H. Field, C. R. Treadwell, "The Mechanism of Cholesterol Absorption," *Annals of New York Academy of Science,* **72**:813, 1959.

17 A. C. Guyton, *Textbook of Medical Physiology,* 4th ed., W. B. Saunders Co., Philadelphia, 1971, p. 808.

18 R. Pike and M. Brown, *Nutrition: An Integrated Approach,* 2d ed., John Wiley & Sons, New York, 1975, p. 46.

19 W. E. Nelson, *Textbook of Pediatrics,* 8th ed., W. B. Saunders Company, Philadelphia, 1964, pp. 1190–1191.

20 S. Williams, *Nutrition & Diet Therapy,* 2d ed., C. V. Mosby Co., St. Louis, 1973, chap. 3, p. 33.

21 J. Wallach, *Interpretation of Diagnostic Tests,* 2d ed., Little, Brown, Boston, 1974, p. 170.

22 Nelson, op. cit., p. 721.

23 F. P. Anitia, *Clinical Dietetics and Nutrition,* Oxford University Press, New York, 1973, p. 42.

24 Ibid., p. 42.

25 F. Wynder, "Diet and Cancer of the Colon," *Symposium on Nutrition and Cancer,* New York, November 1976.

26 American Medical Association, *Nutrients in Processed Foods,* vol. 3, *Fats & Carbohydrates,* Publishing Sciences Group, Inc., Acton, Mass., 1975, p. 8.

27 American Heart Association, *Diet and Coronary Heart Disease: A Statement for Physicians and Other Health Professionals by the Committee on Nutrition,* 1973.

28 Food and Nutrition Board, National Research Council, op. cit., p. 35.

29 S. J. Foman, *Infant Nutrition,* W. B. Saunders Co., Philadelphia, 1974, p. 164.

30 J. Berg, "Nutrition and Cancer," *Seminars in Oncology,* **3**:21, 1976.

CHAPTER 6

VITAMINS

Patricia A. Kreutler

KEY WORDS
Fat-soluble Vitamins
Water-soluble Vitamins
Provitamin A
β-Carotene
Retinol
Rickets
Tocopherol
Scurvy
Beri-beri
Pellagra
Cheilosis
Glossitis
Intrinsic Factor
Pernicious Anemia

INTRODUCTION

The vitamin story has had many exciting chapters. The current popular and scientific interest in nutrition, coupled with concerns about vitamin deficiencies and supplementation, promises to maintain the momentum in the efforts to unravel their mechanism of action.

The word *vitamine* was proposed by Casimir Funk in 1911 to describe a new "food factor" found to be necessary for health and life, but chemically different from the essential nutrients known at that time, namely, carbohydrates, fats, and proteins. As more and more of these factors were discovered, it was found that they were not amines, but a variety of chemical compounds; and the general name was changed to *vitamin*.

Vitamins are organic compounds that are required by the body in trace amounts to perform specific cellular functions. They are considered essential because they cannot be synthesized in sufficient amounts by the body, and the human body relies on an exogenous source for their supply. Vitamins differ in their chemistry, function, and distribution in foods.

Much of what we know about vitamins has resulted from the so-called deficiency diseases. Recognition of what happens when an essential substance is missing very often leads to definition of its particular and important function, and this has certainly been true in the study of vitamins. These essential compounds act as cofactors in reactions involving the transport and metabolism of other chemicals we call nutrients, and may perform structural functions as well.

Vitamins are generally divided into groups on the basis of their solubility. Vitamins A, D, E, and K are soluble in fat and fat solvents. This property is reflected in their distribution in foods, storage in the body, and mechanism of excretion. Because our bodies can store them, they do not have to be consumed every day, and there is also the danger of vitamin toxicity.

Vitamin C and the B complex vitamins are water-soluble, and because amounts in excess of what our bodies need are readily excreted, they must be provided in the diet regularly.

Because no one food contains all the vitamins our body needs, it is important to consume a variety of foods to ensure an adequate intake.

A vitamin deficiency can be classified as either primary or secondary. Primary deficiency is caused by consuming an inadequate intake; in secondary deficiency, the recommended allowance may be ingested, but because of disease, medication, or physiological states such as pregnancy, lactation, and growth, the actual individual requirement is increased. Regardless of the etiology of the deficiency, insufficient vitamins will be reflected in a decrease in the serum level of the vitamin, followed by or coincident with a decrease in the biochemical function for which it is required, and finally the manifestations of a clinical deficiency disease will appear.

FAT-SOLUBLE VITAMINS

Vitamin A

History and Discovery
Shortly after Funk proposed the vitamin theory, two independent groups of researchers reported the existence of a fat-soluble substance that affected growth and reproduction in rats, and might be a candidate for the newly designated vitamin category. In 1912 Osborne and Mendel, working at Yale, noted that rats demonstrated growth failure when milk fat was removed from their diet, and eye lesions also were apparent. Reintroduction of milk fat abated the symptoms. At about the same time, McCollum and Davis from the University of Wisconsin fed rats purified diets with the fat provided by lard. These rats failed to grow after several months, and also developed eye disease. If the rats were then provided with butterfat or egg yolk, the symptoms were reversed. The unidentified fat-soluble substance was named *vitamin A*. The next step in the understanding of this new growth factor was the work of Steenbock, who identified a yellow pigment, carotene, from yellow vegetables; this pigment also demonstrated growth-promoting properties, and was further identified as a precursor of the vitamin found in animal products.

In 1937 a fat-soluble substance with the physiological properties of vitamin A was isolated from cod liver oil, and in 1946 the vitamin was synthesized. It is colorless and heat-stable, but labile to oxygen and ultraviolet light.

Chemistry
Preformed vitamin A exists in three forms, retinol (an alcohol), retinal (an aldehyde), and retinoic acid. All of these are biologically active, although there is some specificity of function among the various forms. Fig. 6-1 demonstrates the chemical relationship between the three forms. Most of the vitamin A we ingest from food exists in the alcohol form, which can be reversibly oxidized to the aldehyde form. It is the latter which is functional in the response of vision in dim light. Further oxidation produces the acid form, which is no longer useful in the visual cycle, but retains the growth-promoting properties of the vitamin.

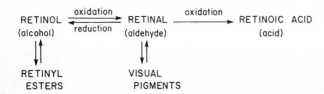

Figure 6-1
Chemical relationship between the three forms of preformed vitamin A—retinol, retinal, and retinoic acid.

Metabolism

Preformed vitamin A usually occurs in foods as a retinol ester. Ingestion of the vitamin is followed by its hydrolysis by pancreatic or intestinal enzymes to yield retinol and the fatty acid. Because vitamin A is a fat-soluble substance, those factors which enhance fat absorption also increase the absorption of the vitamin. After uptake of retinol into the mucosal cell, it is rapidly reesterified, primarily with palmitate, and is packaged into chylomicrons for transport via the lymph to the general circulation.

Provitamin A, carotenoid precursors, and α-, γ-, and especially β-carotene are converted to vitamin A, primarily in the intestinal mucosa. Theoretically, one molecule of β-carotene will produce two molecules of retinol, but because of decreased conversion efficiency, the cleavage enzyme is only about 50 percent effective; in addition, only one-third of the β-carotene which exists in food is biologically available. The net result is that β-carotene is approximately one-sixth as effective as the same amount of preformed vitamin A. This fact is reflected in the recommended dietary allowance (RDA) for vitamin A.

After absorption, vitamin A is transported to the liver, where it is stored as the alcohol ester. When vitamin A is needed by the body, it is mobilized from the liver and transported to the tissues by a special transport protein, retinol-binding protein (RBP). The protein forms a complex with prealbumin, which serves to protect against excessive loss of the vitamin and RBP from the kidney and therefore in the urine. The release of the binding protein appears to be dependent on the presence of vitamin A in the liver. Also, protein deficiency affects vitamin A status, probably by decreasing the synthesis of RBP. After dietary rehabilitation of malnourished patients, serum levels of both RBP and vitamin A increase.[1] The role of zinc in vitamin A metabolism is unclear.[2,3] Several other clinical conditions have been implicated in vitamin A metabolism. Liver disease will decrease serum levels of the vitamin and its binding protein, whereas in renal disease an increase is observed.[4] Several drugs have been shown to influence vitamin A status as well. Oral contraceptives increase serum vitamin A levels, probably by inducing the synthesis of RBP; cholestyramine (a drug used to lower blood cholesterol) and mineral oil interfere with its absorption.

Function

The only physiological function of vitamin A that has been worked out in detail is its role in the so-called visual cycle. In 1967 George Wald from Harvard earned a Nobel Prize for this discovery. Night blindness results from vitamin A deficiency, because the vitamin is required to regenerate the chemical which allows us to see in dim light. Rhodopsin is the complex of opsin (a protein present in the rods of the eye) and the retinal form of vitamin A. A simplified scheme of the process is shown in Fig. 6-2. Because some retinal is degraded in the process of rhodopsin degradation caused by bright light, we need a supply of vitamin A to regenerate the complex. Thus, normal vision cannot be attained quickly after rhodopsin bleaching by bright light, such as that from an oncoming car, unless there is an ample supply of vitamin A.

While only retinol and retinal can be used for maintenance of the visual cycle, all three forms function in maintaining growth. Rats fed retinoic acid will maintain their growth rate, but will soon develop eye lesions. Some research suggests that vitamin A allows the

Figure 6-2
Function of vitamin A in the visual cycle.

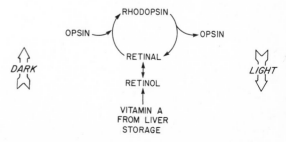

maturation of osteoblasts to osteoclasts, a conversion necessary for the remodeling and therefore continued growth of bone.

Vitamin A is also required for the maintenance of epithelial tissue; that is, of the cells which are found in the outer layers of the skin as well as lining the gastrointestinal, respiratory, and urogenital tracts. Likewise, in tooth development vitamin A is necessary for the normal differentiation and function of the ameloblasts, cells of ectodermal origin which are responsible for the formation of dental enamel.

Vitamin A deficiency results in a transformation of epithelial cells from soft, moist tissue to cells which are hard and dry, or keratinized. This effect has been related to the protective effect of vitamin A in maintaining the integrity of epithelial tissue against infective organisms, particularly of the respiratory tract. The biochemical effect of vitamin A in this function is not clear; it may exert a direct effect on the synthesis of mucopolysaccharides and protein.

Dietary Allowances and Sources

The 1974 recommended dietary allowances are expressed in both international units (IU) and retinol equivalents (RE). The latter term was introduced to take into account the presence of both preformed vitamin A and its provitamin carotene in foodstuffs, and the relative efficiency of carotene utilization. Allowances related to age and sex can be found in the RDA table (see Appendix, Table A-1). Retinol equivalents can be calculated by using the following information:

$$1 \text{ RE} = 1 \ \mu g \text{ retinol}$$
$$= 6 \ \mu g \ \beta\text{-carotene}$$
$$= 12 \ \mu g \text{ other carotenes}$$
$$= 3.33 \text{ IU activity from retinol}$$
$$= 10.0 \text{ IU activity from } \beta\text{-carotene}$$
$$= 20.0 \text{ IU activity from other carotenes}$$
$$1 \text{ IU} = 0.3 \ \mu g \text{ retinol}$$
$$= 0.6 \ \mu g \ \beta\text{-carotene}$$
$$= 1.2 \ \mu g \text{ other carotene}$$

Food sources of preformed vitamin A are liver, kidney, whole milk, eggs, and butter. Skim milk and margarine may be fortified with vitamin A. Major sources of provitamin A are yellow and green leafy vegetables, such as carrots, squash, kale, spinach, pumpkin, and red or green peppers. The deeper the green or yellow color, the higher the carotene content will be.

Processing and cooking cause little loss of vitamin A. Because the vitamin is insoluble in water, there is no loss in cooking. Some processing, in fact, such as mashing, cutting, or pureeing, may increase the availability of carotenes in plant products by rupturing cell walls and making the provitamin more available.

Clinical Deficiency

Less than an optimal supply of vitamin A results in some classic deficiency symptoms, which are night blindness, growth retardation, reproductive failure (in laboratory animals), and an increased susceptibility to infections, particularly those affecting the respiratory tract. The most serious public health problem associated with vitamin A deficiency is blindness due to changes in the eye tissue, leading to irreversible corneal damage. In xerophthalmia, keratinization of epithelial cells leads to a decrease in the protective secretions of the eye. The eye becomes dry and the cornea eventually loses its sensitivity. Continuation of the deficiency results in a lesion known as a Bitot's spot, and if unchecked, causes keratomalacia, when severe visual impairment and even blindness may result. These severe signs of deficiency are widespread in India, South and East Asia, Africa, and Latin America. It is no coincidence that these areas are also those which have a high prevalence of protein-calorie malnutrition. Preventive programs of vitamin A administration are effective in reducing the incidence and prevalence of xerophthalmia and keratomalacia.[5]

Toxicity Symptoms

Because vitamin A is fat-soluble, it is capable of being stored in the body, and the potential for toxicity exists. Hypervitaminosis A is a condition that includes symptoms of nausea, headache, peeling and flaking of skin, dizziness, and pain in the long bones. Progression to a chronic state may lead to growth failure and hair loss. Vitamin A toxicity symptoms have been reported on intakes of 10,000 to 75,000 IU per day. Causes of toxicity in children usually can be traced to overzealous parents who believe that if some is good, more is better. Symptoms generally disappear when the vitamin is discontinued, although some residual effects have been noted in children. Increased intake of provitamin A results in pigmentation of the skin as a result of carotenemia.

Large doses of vitamin A may be prescribed for the treatment of acne. The compound is irritating to the skin, causing peeling, and may favor the treatment of this condition; however, in some instances it has led to toxicity.

Vitamin D

History and Discovery

Vitamin D has been known as the "sunshine vitamin" or the "rickets-preventive factor," names which are related to the confusing history of the vitamin and to its role in preventing a debilitating bone disease. Cod liver oil had been used for centuries as a cure for rickets, a disease in which bone calcification is hampered, leading to bowed legs and knock-knees. It was not until the early part of this century that Mellanby presented evidence of a fat-soluble substance in the oil that could cure rickets in dogs. In 1924 Steenbock and Hess discovered independently that ultraviolet light would give antirachitic properties to certain foods. These findings began to resolve the long debate that involved the etiology of rickets. Because the disease existed in children living in crowded, smoky industrial cities, many thought that it was an infectious disease of bacterial origin. It was also noted that dark-skinned people who moved to England

from the tropics were susceptible to the bone deformity. We now know, from much research, that both food and sunlight have antirachitic properties. A new period of vitamin D research has been occurring recently. Within the past 10 years, it has been recognized that the vitamin is converted in the body to an active form which exerts a physiological effect on calcium metabolism.

Chemistry and Properties

As with vitamin A, there is a provitamin-vitamin relationship with vitamin D. Plant substances contain a sterol called ergosterol which, when activated by ultraviolet light, is converted to ergocalciferol, or vitamin D_2. In animal tissues, including the human body, the presence of 7-dehydrocholesterol in skin allows ultraviolet light (sunshine) to convert this provitamin to cholecalciferol, or vitamin D_3. These are fat-soluble substances which are remarkably stable to heat, light, and storage.

Measurement

Vitamin D activity is based on international units, where 1 IU equals 0.025 μg of pure crystalline vitamin D_3, also equivalent to 1 USP (United States Pharmacopoeia) unit. Bioassay techniques for the vitamin include the standardized line test, in which rats are treated with graded doses of vitamin D after rickets has been produced. Histological examination of the rats' long bones demonstrates areas of calcification (noted by a line that becomes visible after the bone is stained with silver nitrate) which are proportional to the amount of vitamin D administered. Because this is a time-consuming and expensive method of assay, newer techniques are being developed.

Metabolism

Vitamin D is absorbed from the small intestine in the presence of bile and is transported into the circulation via the lymph in chylomicrons, in much the same way as vitamin A. Again, factors which increase or interfere with fat absorption will influence the rate at which vitamin D is absorbed. The vitamin is removed from the circulation into the liver, where it is stored, although not to as great an extent as is vitamin A.

An exciting chapter in the history of vitamin D unfolded when it was discovered that the liver contains an enzyme which hydroxylates cholecalciferol to 25-hydroxycholecalciferol (25-HCC), which is a more potent form of the vitamin. Some evidence suggests that 25-HCC regulates its own synthesis, but other research has not been able to demonstrate this.[6,7] A specific transport protein carries 25-HCC from the liver to the kidney, where another hydroxylation takes place to produce 1,25-dihydroxycholecalciferol (1,25-DHCC), thus far identified as the most active form of the vitamin. This hydroxylation appears to be under the control of parathyroid hormone, the net effect of which is to raise plasma calcium and phosphate levels. It appears that DHCC is the form which influences calcium absorption (see p. 120).

Reserves of vitamin D are found in liver, bone, brain, and skin; some vitamin D metabolites are excreted in the bile.

Function

The primary role of vitamin D is to increase the absorption of dietary calcium. It is thought that vitamin D acts to induce the synthesis of a specific calcium-binding protein that binds to dietary calcium and increases its absorption. Phosphorus absorption is also increased by vitamin D.

Another site of vitamin D action is bone. Bone acts as a reserve to maintain the tightly controlled level of calcium in the blood. When serum calcium falls, vitamin D, in conjunction with parathyroid hormone and possibly magnesium, increases the release of calcium from bone to increase serum levels of the mineral. Vitamin D also has a positive, direct effect on bone mineralization, although the mechanism is not clear. Thus, in vitamin D deficiency, bone mineralization is impaired, resulting in osteomalacia in adults and rickets in children.

Phosphate reabsorption by the kidney is also increased by vitamin D.

Thus, vitamin D functions, in conjunction with parathyroid hormone, to provide the optimal amounts of calcium and phosphorus that are needed for bone mineralization by increasing their availability through increased absorption and, in the case of phosphorus, by preventing its loss in urine.

Clinical Implications

With the recognition that vitamin D is converted to active forms within the body, the use of its metabolites (25-HCC and 1,25-DHCC) to correct bone diseases associated with vitamin D-resistant rickets is being investigated. In kidney and liver disease, bone disease sometimes occurs, and this is understandable if we consider that reduced hydroxylation of cholecalciferol may result from the primary disease. The possibility also exists that an inborn error of metabolism, resulting from a genetic defect in production of the kidney enzyme hydroxylase, can cause vitamin D-resistant rickets as well. Patients often do not respond to massive doses of either vitamin D_2, D_3, or HCC, whereas much smaller doses of DHCC appear to correct the situation.

Certain drugs are known to antagonize the effects of vitamin D. Corticosteroids have a negative effect on vitamin D and calcium metabolism; patients with Cushing's disease (overproduction of hydrocortisone) and those undergoing cortisone therapy may develop osteoporosis. Thus, the requirement for D_3 increases in these conditions. Barbiturates and anticonvulsant drugs decrease the amount of 25-HCC, either by decreasing its synthesis by nonspecific hydroxylation, or by increasing its turnover. Cholestyramine, a drug used in cardiovascular disease, decreases the amount of bile, which is necessary for the absorption of the vitamin.

Dietary Allowances and Sources

Naturally occurring vitamin D is found only in small and insignificant amounts in common foods, such as cream, butter, eggs, and liver. Therefore, we rely on fortified foods or fish liver oil for our vitamin D requirements. Because children are highly susceptible to rickets, milk has been chosen as the vehicle for vitamin D fortification at a level of 400 IU/qt, equivalent to 10 μg of the vitamin.

Sunlight is the major nonfood source of the vitamin. In skin, 7-dehydrocholesterol is converted to cholecalciferol by ultraviolet light and absorbed into the circulation. For many of us, our requirement for the vitamin can be suitably obtained by this means. However, geography and climate modify the amount of sunlight, cultural customs and city living may diminish the amount of exposure, and infants and elderly people often do not get enough sunlight. Ultraviolet light cannot penetrate ordinary window glass, smog, or clouds; in addition, dark-skinned people living in temperate zones may not get enough exposure. Thus, certain population groups need an exogenous source of vitamin D, and this is generally provided by fortified milk. Because human milk is a poor source of the vitamin, breast-fed infants rely on supplementation.

The dietary requirement for vitamin D has been difficult to determine, since a substantial part of the necessary amount is supplied by sunlight. The Food and Nutrition Board recommended a daily intake of 400 IU from birth through 22 years of age, on the basis of observations of calcium absorption, bone mineralization, and satisfactory growth rate. The adult requirement is not known, but presumably most adults receive enough vitamin D by exposure to the sun. Pregnant and lactating women should receive 400 IU per day.

Clinical Deficiency

Rickets, formerly quite prevalent in infants and children, and identified as early as 1645, is characterized by bone malformation caused by insufficient deposition of calcium and phosphorus. Long bones are affected, so that bowed legs and knock-knees are generally found; ribs, skull, and pelvic bones often exhibit changes as well. Because mineralization is diminished, a tendency toward a thickening of wrists and ankles also exists. Poorly calcified and late-erupting teeth are often found in children with rickets.

The counterpart of the disease in adults is osteomalacia, characterized by a decalcification of bone shafts, increasing the tendency for fractures. Administration of vitamin D will ameliorate this condition.

Toxicity

Hypervitaminosis D can occur when excess vitamin D is provided in the diet, generally as supplements of cod liver oil. Symptoms produced by the condition are generally related to those produced by hypercalcemia and include nausea, weight loss, anorexia, calcification of bones and soft tissues, head pain, and in children a reduction in growth rate.[8] Certain infants may develop hypercalcemia on vitamin D intakes of 1800 to 2000 IU per day, and symptoms have been documented in adults receiving more than 100,000 IU per day. However, much lower levels of vitamin D (1000 to 3000 IU per day) may result in hypercalcemia. As with vitamin A, total intake must be monitored: pediatricians and mothers should be aware of the importance of vitamin D, but also that overuse of the vitamin produces pathological changes.

A recent report suggests that exceedingly large doses of the vitamin may also contribute to the development of atherosclerosis.[9] A symposium on vitamin D metabolism and function has recently been published.[10]

Vitamin E

History and Discovery

The presence of a dietary factor necessary for reproduction in the rat was recognized in 1922 by Evans and Bishop; 2 years later, Sure named it the "antisterility vitamin" or vitamin E. In the 1930s the substance was isolated from wheat germ oil and named *tocopherol,* from the Greek "to bear offspring."

Since that time, many investigators have sought to define its role in human nutrition. Many of the clinical signs apparent in vitamin E-deficient animals have not been documented in humans, and the role of the vitamin is not completely understood at the present time.

Chemistry and Properties

Tocopherols are oily yellow liquids, water-insoluble, but soluble in fat and fat solvents. Of the four naturally occurring tocopherols, the alpha form is the most active. They are heat-stable, but deteriorate upon exposure to light and on contact with iron and lead. Because the tocopherols are readily oxidized, they are said to have antioxidant properties and are therefore preferentially oxidized, thus preventing the oxidative breakdown of other substances, notably vitamin A and polyunsaturated fatty acids (PUFA).

Measurement

One milligram of *dl*-alpha-tocopheryl acetate, either natural or synthetic, is designated as 1 IU. Adjustments to this figure are made on the basis of the form of the vitamin contained in food or supplements. Dietary allowances are based on the alpha-tocopherol content of food.

Metabolism

Vitamin E is absorbed as are other fats and fat-soluble substances: it requires the presence of bile, and once absorbed into the mucosal cell, the vitamin is carried on chylomicrons to enter the general circulation via the lymph. The efficiency of absorption is relatively low and is further decreased by mineral oil and by conditions which affect fat absorption in general. Vitamin E is stored in liver and muscle, with significant amounts present in adipose tissue. Fat mobilization also releases vitamin E into the circulation. Metabolites of the vitamin are excreted in urine and feces.

Function

Until recently, the vitamin has been "in search of a disease." Since the function of most nu-trients has not been elucidated until deficiency symptoms have been produced, the lack of definite clinical signs has hampered the search for a physiological function of the tocopherols. However, several roles have been postulated. There is some evidence that the vitamin acts as a cofactor in the cytochrome system of the electron transport chain. There are also some studies that suggest a role for the vitamin in heme synthesis: in experimental vitamin E deficiency, two enzymes associated with the synthesis of the compound are decreased. Other heme-containing compounds are also decreased in vitamin E deficiency. Varying results have been reported in the use of vitamin E for the treatment of anemia associated with protein-calorie malnutrition.

Although the mechanism of action is not known, vitamin E increases the stability of cellular and intracellular structures, presumably related to its antioxidant properties. As such it may react with free radicals, thus sparing polyunsaturated fats, vitamin A, sulfur-containing enzymes, and cell wall constituents, including those of red blood cells, from damage. Vitamin E deficiency has also been associated with the aging process, perhaps "naturally" caused by cell destruction through lipid peroxidation. This kind of observation has led food faddists to advocate very large doses of vitamin E to prevent aging. Caution must be maintained in drawing this conclusion. Scientists do not really know what contributes to the aging process and to say that (1) aging is caused by lipid peroxidation and subsequent tissue damage, (2) vitamin E decreases lipid peroxidation, and therefore (3) vitamin E will retard aging, offers false security to many middle-aged and elderly people who can ill afford to spend their money on unnecessary vitamin supplements.

An interesting relationship between the mineral selenium and vitamin E has been observed. Selenium can replace some of the vitamin E needed for certain functions, thus reinforcing the idea that the primary role of the vitamin is as an antioxidant. Selenium is a necessary cofactor for the enzyme glutathione peroxidase, the function of which is to prevent peroxidation within the cytoplasm.

The controversy over and search for the molecular role of vitamin E will undoubtedly continue.

Dietary Allowances and Sources

For the first time, in 1968, the Food and Nutrition Board set a recommended dietary allowance for vitamin E. The figures were adjusted in its 1974 revision to 15 IU for males and 12 IU for females, on the basis of the vitamin E content of the average American diet; intakes have been assumed to be adequate since no biochemical or clinical evidence is available to indicate a deficiency state in most of the population. The requirement for infants is based on the vitamin content of human milk, 2 to 5 IU/l. Most investigators agree that the requirement for vitamin E increases with the content of polyunsaturated fat in the diet. When subjects are placed on a high polyunsaturated fatty acid diet with low vitamin E intake, increased in vitro red blood cell hemolysis has been noted.

The major sources of vitamin E in the American diet are fats and oils, particularly the unsaturated fat products. This is fortunate, since the vitamin requirement apparently increases with the polyunsaturated fatty acid intake. Animal foods are generally poor sources of the vitamin, although liver and egg contain moderate amounts. Vegetables, particularly green leafy ones, are also moderate sources. Vitamin E is the most widely available of the vitamins in common foodstuffs.

Clinical Deficiency

Until recently, deficiency symptoms had not been identified, and clinical evidence of deficiency is almost entirely restricted to premature infants. Newborn infants in general tend to have low plasma levels of vitamin E, and the levels normally rise (particularly in breast-fed infants) by about 1 month of age. Several reports have cited cases in which premature infants showed signs of irritability and edema,[11,12] accompanied by a hemolytic anemia. The deficiency was traced to their drinking a commercial formula which was low in vitamin E.

Normally, vitamin E deficiency is difficult to produce, since so many of our foods contain it. In the only long-term study thus far, adult men who consumed diets low in the vitamin for 3 years showed no symptoms, even though their plasma tocopherol fell to low levels. A slight decrease in red blood cell stability was apparent, but there were no clinical signs of anemia.[13]

Groups at risk of developing a vitamin E deficiency include premature infants and individuals who have a defect in the ability to absorb dietary fat, including patients with cystic fibrosis.

There is no substantial experimental evidence to suggest that vitamin E will prevent or cure muscular dystrophy, the aging process, cancer, ulcers, infertility, or sexual impotence, or that it will increase athletic performance,[14] for which the use of vitamin E in pharmacological amounts has been advocated.

Clinical Toxicity

Symptoms of toxicity have been produced in chicks, characterized by depression of growth and bone calcification. Some recent studies[15,16] have revealed a relationship between vitamin E status and blood clotting time. Large doses of the vitamin increase the time required for blood to clot; this may have clinical significance for women taking oral contraceptives who are at risk of developing thrombosis, and may, on the other hand, increase the requirement for vitamin K.

Vitamin K

History and Discovery

In 1935 Henrik Dam, a Danish scientist, identified a severe hemorrhagic disease in newly hatched chicks fed a ration adequate in all known essential nutrients. Analysis of blood showed a decrease in the amount of prothrombin, a factor involved in the normal blood clotting mechanism. Addition of hog liver fat or alfalfa to the ration improved and prevented the condition. The antihemorrhagic factor was named *vitamin K* for *k*oagulation vitamin.

Chemistry and Properties

Vitamin K is a fat-soluble yellowish crystalline compound that is stable to heat, air, and moisture. It is destroyed upon exposure to strong acids, alkalis, and light. There are several forms of the vitamin, all belonging to a family of chemical compounds called quinones. Vitamin K_1 (phylloquinone) occurs naturally in green plants; vitamin K_2 (menaquinone) is a product of bacterial synthesis in the intestine.

Measurement

No present system of standardization exists. The vitamin can be measured in micrograms of a pure synthetic compound, and a bioassay based on coagulation time in chicks has been used to quantify the vitamin.

Metabolism

Vitamin K is absorbed, with the aid of bile, in the upper part of the small intestine. Since it follows the same absorptive pattern as dietary fat, any interference with fat absorption will affect the absorption of vitamin K. Effective water-soluble preparations exist for patients with fat malabsorption syndromes.

After absorption, chylomicrons carry the vitamin to the liver, where much of the vitamin is transferred to β-lipoproteins. Liver concentrates the vitamin for a short period of time, and small amounts appear in heart, skin, muscle, and kidney. Storage of the vitamin in the human body is not extensive. Metabolites of vitamin K are excreted in bile and urine.

Function

The only known function of vitamin K is in the blood clotting mechanism, a process which depends on the presence of many protein factors. Prothrombin (factor II) is essential for the mechanism, and is directly affected by vitamin K. It is also known that the synthesis or activation of three other blood clotting factors (factors VII, IX, and X) are responsive to the vitamin. (It should be noted that vitamin K offers no therapeutic value to patients with hemophilia.) Knowledge of the molecular role of vitamin K in the blood clotting process has been studied largely during the last 10 years. Most investigation supports the hypothesis that a precursor protein in the liver is converted, probably by carboxylation, to prothrombin only in the presence of vitamin K.[17,18] A deficiency of the vitamin, or its antagonism by anticoagulants such as coumarins (warfarin and dicumarol) and salicylates (aspirin), will prevent prothrombin synthesis and consequently impair blood coagulation. Vitamin E may be metabolized to a vitamin K antagonist.[19]

Dietary Allowance and Sources

No allowance has been set for vitamin K by the Food and Nutrition Board. A significant portion of the vitamin found in liver stores arises from intestinal bacterial synthesis, and the vitamin is contained in a wide enough variety of foods that there is little danger of inadequate intake under normal conditions.

Newborn infants present a special circumstance, however, because placental transport of the vitamin is limited, and because the normal intestinal flora does not establish itself until some time after birth. Thus, it has been suggested that 1 mg of vitamin K_1 be administered to newborn infants to prevent hemorrhagic disease.

In addition to the extensive bacterial synthesis of the vitamin, only part of which may be available depending on the site of synthesis (if it is synthesized too far down in the gastrointestinal tract, it will not be absorbed), vitamin K is found in cabbage, cauliflower, spinach, alfalfa, and other leafy vegetables. Egg yolk and pork liver also provide moderate amounts. Human milk contains little of the vitamin.

Clinical Deficiency

Under normal conditions, vitamin K deficiency is unlikely. Interference with fat absorption; the presence of liver disease; the use of sulfonamides and tetracycline (which will depress bacterial synthesis); and the administration of anticoagulants, which antagonize the effects of vitamin K, and of some anticonvulsants, which increase its turnover, may precipitate deficiency symptoms, the only one of which thus far identified is a decrease in blood coagulation.

Toxicity

If given in large doses over a prolonged period of time, vitamin K may produce hemolytic anemia and jaundice in the infant.[20] Vitamin K_3, a synthetic form of the vitamin also known as menadione, has been removed from the list of over-the-counter drug preparations because of its toxic effect on membranes of red blood cells.

WATER-SOLUBLE VITAMINS

Ascorbic Acid

History and Discovery

Scurvy is one of the oldest deficiency diseases recognized by man, having been reported as early as 1500 B.C. It was a seasonal disease, and ruined many sailing and exploring expeditions, causing widespread morbidity and mortality. In a now classic nutrition experiment, James Lind in 1735 demonstrated that sailors provided with two oranges and lemons daily were cured of their disease; as citrus fruits were added to the rations of British sailors, the men were known as "limeys."

In 1907, Holst and Frölich produced scurvy in guinea pigs, one of the species which cannot synthesize the vitamin. Man, monkeys, and other more obscure animal species also cannot synthesize the compound; it must be provided in the diet.

In the 1930s, crystalline vitamin C had been isolated, and it was officially named *ascorbic acid* (a contraction of *antiscorbutic*, meaning "without scurvy").

Chemistry and Properties

Ascorbic acid is a white, crystalline material that is water-soluble and stable in dry form. In solution it is easily oxidized, particularly when heated and exposed to alkali. It is the most unstable of all the vitamins, and precautions must be taken to prevent its loss during the preparation of food.

Ascorbic acid has a structure closely related to monosaccharides, and exists in two biologically active forms. L-Ascorbic acid can be oxidized to L-dehydroascorbic acid, which has approximately 80 percent of the activity of the reduced form. Further oxidation, by an irreversible reaction, to diketogulonic acid produces a form which has no antiscorbutic activity.

Metabolism

Ascorbic acid is readily absorbed from the small intestine; the mode of transport is controversial, and may depend upon whether vitamin C is a required vitamin for the particular species studied. It is transported to the liver via the portal vein, and from the liver it is distributed to all tissues. There is a moderate amount of storage in liver and spleen, with a high concentration found in the adrenal gland, an observation which has led to much speculation on its relationship to steroid synthesis. Body stores generally amount to about 1500 mg. Tissue levels in kidney, liver, spleen, and adrenal appear to be in equilibrium with serum, and there is a limited amount of storage in the leukocytes, or white blood cells. Leukocytes take up the vitamin when tissue demands have been met, and white blood cell levels have been used to evaluate vitamin C status in man.

Metabolites of vitamin C are excreted primarily in the urine, as ascorbic acid and oxalic acid; some is expired as carbon dioxide. Approximately 3 percent of the body pool is excreted daily.

Several drugs have been shown to affect the metabolism of vitamin C. Among those which increase the urinary excretion of the vitamin are adrenal steroids, sulfonamides, tetracycline, and salicylates. Leukocyte and plasma levels are decreased by salicylates, tetracycline, and indomethacin. The effect of oral contraceptives on vitamin C metabolism is ambiguous. Horwitt et al.[21] demonstrated essentially no effect on blood levels of ascorbic acid in women taking contraceptive preparations, whereas Rivers showed a decrease in plasma and leukocyte content of the vitamin.[22] Cigarette smokers generally have lower plasma vitamin C levels than do nonsmokers, although results to the contrary have appeared in the literature.[23]

Function

Unlike the other water-soluble vitamins, ascorbic acid has not been positively identified as a catalyst or coenzyme in any metabolic system. Its biochemical mode of action has not been determined; some investigators feel that its reducing powers may account for its function, but this is a relatively nonspecific effect. However, some specific roles of the vitamin, again based on studies of deficiency states, have been identified.

The most basic function of vitamin C thus far identified is its role in collagen formation. Collagen is a protein which makes up connective tissue found in skin, bones, teeth, and muscle. Ascorbic acid appears to exert a posttranslational effect in the hydroxylation of proline and lysine to form hydroxyproline and hydroxylysine, substances present exclusively in collagen. The exact mechanism for the vitamin's role in this reaction has not been determined; it may be that it acts as a reducing agent and converts an inactive hydroxylase enzyme to an active form.[24]

The function of vitamin C in wound healing was recognized years ago. Ascorbic acid migrates to the site of the wound and presumably plays a role in the collagen formation required for such healing. It is for this reason

that many physicians recommend vitamin C treatment in postsurgical and burn patients. Vitamin C also has a positive effect on bone and dentin formation. Other sites of vitamin C action are related to neurotransmitter synthesis. Tyrosine and tryptophan hydroxylation require ascorbic acid, as does the conversion of dopa (3,4-dihydroxyphenylalanine) to norepinephrine.

Ascorbic acid enhances iron absorption by reducing the ferric form generally found in foods to the more readily absorbed ferrous form. Iron supplements frequently contain ascorbic acid to promote absorption of the mineral. Ascorbic acid may also influence the distribution of iron stores.

An interesting role for ascorbic acid in cholesterol metabolism, and thus its role in atherosclerosis, is a subject of controversy. Spittle[25] reported that daily doses of 1 g of ascorbic acid reduced the serum cholesterol level in young adults, but had no effect on older adults. However, Peterson et al. gave nine hypercholesterolemic patients 4 g of ascorbic acid per day for 2 months and noted no change in serum cholesterol levels.[26] It has been postulated that any cholesterol-lowering effect of the vitamin is mediated by a metabolite, ascorbic acid sulfate. More research needs to be done in this area.

Another interesting observation, which has fascinating implications, is that vitamin C is capable of converting hormone-sensitive lipase, found in adipose tissue, from an active to inactive form.[27] Whether this is a normal physiological function of ascorbic acid, or whether it is a pharmacological effect, remains to be resolved.

The much-heralded use of vitamin C for the prevention and cure of the common cold has not been strongly documented. Linus Pauling recommended that 0.5 to 5 g per day would prevent and reduce the symptoms of a cold. One of the best controlled studies was done by Anderson et al. in Canada. Using 800 subjects in a double-blind study, they demonstrated a positive effect of ascorbic acid on the frequency and severity of colds, but cautioned that it was a pharmacological rather than a nutritional effect.[28] Large doses of vitamin C may have an antihistaminelike effect, and thus ameliorate some of the symptoms of a cold. A recent study by Coulehan et al. involving 868 schoolchildren showed no effect of vitamin C supplementation. Of the children receiving ascorbic acid, 133 were ill with 166 cold episodes, and the mean duration of illness was 5.5 days. Among the control children who received placebos, 129 suffered 159 colds, with a mean duration of 5.8 days. The differences between these figures are not statistically significant.[29] Undoubtedly, the controversy will remain unresolved until more definite criteria for "colds" and their symptoms can be determined.

A recent report suggests that pharmacological doses of ascorbic acid may be helpful in chemically dissolving gallstones.[30]

Dietary Allowances and Sources

Although 10 mg of ascorbic acid per day will prevent scurvy, the level required for maintenance of health is considerably higher. The Food and Nutrition Board has currently set 45 mg as the recommended allowance for adults, with increases to 60 and 80 mg for pregnant and lactating women, respectively. Because of the body's limited storage capacity, a daily intake of the vitamin is recommended. An extensive monograph on the requirements of vitamin C has appeared.[31]

Commonly available fruits and vegetables are the richest sources of the vitamin. Fruits and vegetables provide 94 percent of our vitamin C intake, with broccoli, cantaloupe, and strawberries being excellent sources, in addition to the citrus fruits. The amount of vitamin C in products varies according to the variety, time of harvesting, processing procedures, and even the part of the plant. Because vitamin C is so easily destroyed, care must be taken to preserve its content. Frozen vegetables should be plunged into already boiling water, baking soda should never be added to cooking water,

and there should be a minimum of chopping and cutting of foods before cooking. Vitamin C will leach out into the cooking water and, in addition to its loss in discarded water, is destroyed by the heat and air exposure.

Less well known sources of vitamin C are the acerola (or West Indian cherry), rose hips, papaya, guava, and black currants. While potatoes do not have a high concentration of the vitamin, the quantity in which they are eaten in some population groups makes them a valuable source of the vitamin, if they are properly prepared.

Clinical Deficiency

Scurvy, a classic deficiency disease, is characterized by general weakness and lassitude, swollen joints, spongy and bleeding gums and loose teeth, and delayed wound healing. Muscle cramps, aching bones, and dry, rough skin are also symptoms. Infantile scurvy, because of the effect of vitamin C on bone formation, is manifested by a characteristic "frog's leg" position, and the child shows anorexia, lip tenderness, and extremely sensitive arms and legs—a generally irritable child. Scurvy is rare in breast-fed infants, unless of course their mothers are deficient. Bottle-fed infants may require supplementation, depending on the formula used. Scurvy is relatively rare in this country, although occasional epidemics are found. These are generally related to custom, ignorance, and poverty, but in two cases were due to technology. Blacks in the South were accustomed to consuming "pot likker," the liquid in which vegetables were cooked. When social changes led them to abandon this practice, children developed scurvy. Early in this century, pasteurization of milk, which destroyed the ascorbic acid, led to a scurvy outbreak. Fortunately, scurvy has been all but eradicated as a nutritional disease.

Toxicity

Because vitamin C is a water-soluble vitamin and little is stored, toxicity symptoms are unexpected. However, with many advocating the ingestion of very large doses to prevent the common cold, several effects have been noted. One report suggests the induction of kidney stones,[32] and another reports the inactivation of vitamin B_{12},[33] although this latter finding has been challenged recently.[34] Another adverse effect of a large vitamin C intake has been the false-positive results found in oral glucose tolerance tests, due to the cross-reactivity of urinary ascorbic acid and glucose. Some physicians have warned that large ascorbic acid intakes during pregnancy may create a "vitamin C-dependent" fetus whose requirements after birth may exceed the normal level. Clearly, further study is required to assess the risk-benefit ratio in prescribing high doses of ascorbic acid.

Thiamine (Vitamin B₁)

History and Discovery

Beriberi is a nutritional deficiency disease which was recognized as early as 2600 B.C. by the Chinese. It takes its name from the Oriental words which mean "I cannot," which appropriately describes the clinical state. In 1855 a Japanese naval officer named Takaki cured the disease by feeding milk and meat to his men. In 1897 a Dutch physician, Eijkman, who was working in Java, noted that the chickens in the yard of the prison hospital had symptoms similar to those of his patients with beriberi. Replacement of polished rice by brown rice in the poultry rations reversed their condition. Studies in later years demonstrated that an "accessory food factor" was present in the outer husk of rice. It was named vitamin B; subsequent investigators showed that there was more than one accessory food factor, and the antiberiberi factor was renamed vitamin B_1. Thiamine was isolated in 1926, and in 1936 R. R. Williams succeeded in synthesizing the vitamin.

Chemistry and Properties

The name *thiamine* was given to this substance because it contains a sulfur molecule (a thio

group) and an amine. It is available commercially as thiamine hydrochloride. It is a crystalline yellowish-white compound that is water-soluble and has a nutlike taste and odor. In the dry form, it is heat- and oxygen-stable. In solution, it becomes heat- and alkali-labile. In acid solution, it is a bit more stable to heat. For these reasons, addition of baking soda to preserve color in vegetables is not advised and, since the vitamin is water-soluble, minimal amounts of water should be used when cooking. In addition, antacids, because of their alkaline nature, will inactivate thiamine.

Metabolism

Dietary thiamine is absorbed from the upper part of the small intestine. In large amounts, it is passively absorbed. In smaller amounts, the absorptive process is an active one, requiring energy and sodium. Evidence suggests that thiamine is phosphorylated within the mucosal cell and is transported via the portal vein and then into the general circulation. Although bacteria in the gastrointestinal tract do synthesize thiamine, the product of their metabolism is thiamine pyrophosphate, which cannot be absorbed and is therefore unavailable. Alcohol and barbiturates decrease thiamine absorption, and oil from garlic and onions may enhance it.

Limited reserves of thiamine are found in the human body; of the 30 mg stored, 50 percent is found in muscle tissue. Amounts in excess of what the cells can use are excreted in the urine, either as intact thiamine or as the pyrimidine and thiazole moieties. Mercurial diuretics increase urinary loss of the vitamin.

Function

Thiamine, as thiamine pyrophosphate (TPP), functions as an important coenzyme in energy metabolism. Thiamine pyrophosphate is required for the oxidative decarboxylation of alpha-keto acids such as pyruvate and alpha-keto-glutarate, and the keto analogues of the branched-chain amino acids. It is also required for the transketolase reactions of the hexose monophosphate shunt (pentose phosphate pathway), and therefore plays an indirect role in nucleic acid metabolism. Thiamine is needed for the metabolism of carbohydrates, proteins, and fats.

In addition to its coenzyme role, thiamine pyrophosphate may have a specific role in neurophysiology, which may explain the devastating effects of thiamine deficiency on the nervous system. Itokawa and Cooper[35] have suggested that thiamine pyrophosphate (or thiamine triphosphate) is a component of the nerve cell membrane, and is part of the mechanism required for propagation of an electrical potential along the axon. However, other research does not support this hypothesis,[36] and the mechanism of thiamine deficiency in the production of neurological symptoms remains unresolved.

Biochemical Assessment

Several tests have been developed to evaluate thiamine status in man. Measurement of the vitamin in blood and urine, and blood levels of pyruvate and alpha-ketoglutarate, have been used to estimate the adequacy of thiamine stores. A load test has also been used. In this test, a standardized dose of thiamine (5 mg) is administered, and the urinary content of thiamine 4 h later is measured. An acceptable concentration, indicating adequate status, is more than 80 μg; a deficient subject will have less than 20 μg in a 4-h urine sample.

In recent years, a functional test to evaluate thiamine status has been developed.[37,38] Erythrocyte transketolase activity is measured; this may be a more reliable index of a subclinical deficiency state than blood or urine levels of the vitamin. The activity of this thiamine-dependent enzyme decreases in times of vitamin deficiency, and is stimulated in vitro by addition of thiamine pyrophosphate. When thiamine status is adequate, stimulation will not occur or will be only slight, while in deficient subjects there will be at least a 25 percent increase in enzyme activity following addition of the cofactor.

Dietary Allowance and Sources

A high intake of carbohydrate increases the need for thiamine, whereas protein and fat appear to act as thiamine sparers. The present recommended dietary allowance, based on excretion of thiamine and its metabolites, the effects of graded doses on signs of clinical deficiency, and the effect on the level of erythrocyte transketolase activity, is 0.5 mg/1000 kcal per day (0.5 mg/4200 kJ per day).

Thiamine is found in a wide variety of animal and plant foods, but occurs in large amounts in only a few. Pork and wheat germ are excellent sources. Whole grains and enriched grain products are the best daily sources, because of the quantity in which they are eaten. Milk and milk products are generally not good sources of the vitamin, but do make a contribution to the daily intake. In general, fruits and vegetables should not be relied upon to provide a significant source of thiamine.

Clinical Deficiency

The classic symptoms of beriberi affect the nervous, cardiovascular, and gastrointestinal systems. Infantile beriberi is a disease of rapid onset, striking infants whose mothers are in poor thiamine status. Cyanosis, tachycardia, vomiting, convulsions, and death follow if treatment is not instituted promptly.

In adults, the decrease manifests itself in one of two ways, each, however, characterized by irritability, disorderly thinking, and nausea. "Dry" beriberi is a wasting disease, with nervous manifestations and paralysis of the lower extremities. In "wet" beriberi the edema associated with heart failure is the predominant sign, with noticeable swelling of the limbs, feet, and heart.

In addition to deficiency symptoms produced by inadequate intake of the vitamin, antivitamins can alter thiamine status. Thiaminase, a heat-labile enzyme present in uncooked shellfish and some types of freshwater fish, causes hydrolysis of the vitamin. A heat-stable factor found in certain plants is related to caffeic and tannic acids, both components of tea; this also has antithiamine effects.

Chronic alcoholics may also become thiamine-deficient, for several reasons. Low thiamine intake, impaired intestinal absorption, a phosphorylating defect, and apotransketolase deficiency have been implicated in their condition.

Patients with simple deficiency can be treated with physiological doses of thiamine. Thiamine has been used in pharmacological doses to treat patients with several inborn errors of metabolism, such as lactic acidosis due to low activity of liver pyruvate carboxylase, and branched-chain ketoaciduria due to decreased activity of keto acid dehydrogenase.[39]

Beriberi has been eradicated in the United States, largely because of the enrichment of grain products. In areas of the world where enrichment is not a standard processing procedure, and people subsist on a diet of polished rice, beriberi remains a public health problem.

Riboflavin (Vitamin B$_2$)

History and Discovery

In the 1920s it was recognized that there is more than one B vitamin, since some growth-promoting properties were retained after heat treatment had destroyed the antiberiberi properties of certain foods. In 1933 a yellow-green pigment was isolated from milk, and was found also in liver and eggs. The compound was identified as part of "Warburg's yellow enzyme," and in 1935 vitamin B$_2$ was synthesized.

Chemistry and Properties

Vitamin B$_2$ is a member of the chemical family called *flavins,* which are fluorescent compounds. Attached to the flavin moiety is a five-carbon sugar, ribose; the newly identified vitamin was therefore christened *riboflavin.* It is stable to heat, acid, and oxidation, but is unstable in alkaline solution and is readily destroyed by light. Less of the vitamin is lost by

normal cooking procedures than is thiamine. The relatively high riboflavin content in milk requires that milk be packaged in an opaque container to prevent decomposition by light.

Metabolism

Riboflavin is absorbed from the small intestine; it must be phosphorylated, and there appears to be a specific transport system required for its absorption. It is transported to the liver by albumin, where it is further phosphorylated. Absorption of the vitamin increases with age, and riboflavin is apparently better absorbed when eaten with a meal than when ingested separately. Although liver and kidney have moderate amounts of riboflavin, very little of the vitamin is stored and it must therefore be supplied regularly. Excess riboflavin is excreted in the urine.

Several drugs affect the metabolism of this vitamin. Tetracycline and the thiazide diuretics increase urinary excretion, as does probenecid (used in the treatment of gout). The latter drug also causes a decrease in absorption. Sulfonamides, the antimicrobial agents, depress bacterial synthesis of the vitamin, but to what extent bacteria normally serve as a source of riboflavin is questionable. Some oral contraceptive preparations have been associated with a reduction in serum levels of the vitamin, although no deficiency symptoms have been noted.

Function

Riboflavin functions in conjunction with phosphoric acid as two coenzymes which are necessary for the release of energy from carbohydrates, fats, and proteins. Flavin mononucleotide (FMN) and flavin adenine dinucleotide (FAD) are important coenzymes which catalyze oxidation-reduction reactions, notably in the electron transport system, where cellular adenosine triphosphate (ATP) and water are produced. The coenzymes also function in the tricarboxylic acid cycle in dehydrogenase reactions, and in fatty acid oxidation. Oxidative deamination of amino acids requires the vitamin as FMN. The vitamin may also play a role in corticosteroid synthesis and in the production of red blood cells in the bone marrow.

Biochemical Assessment

Urinary levels of riboflavin have been used to evaluate vitamin status, but these primarily reflect immediate past intake, and are easily influenced by temperature, stress, and exercise. Therefore, other methods have been sought. A functional test similar to that described for thiamine has been developed and shows promise as an indicator. Riboflavin is bound to the enzyme glutathione reductase, an erythrocyte enzyme required to maintain the levels of reduced glutathione, necessary for the maintenance of red blood cell membranes. Results are usually expressed in terms of *activity coefficients,* determined by the in vitro addition of FAD to the assay mixture. The coefficient is 1.0 to 1.2 if adequate riboflavin is present, and increases to greater than 1.4 if the subject is at high risk of developing a riboflavin deficiency.[40]

Dietary Allowance and Sources

The 1974 recommendations for riboflavin are based on energy intake, being set at 0.6 mg/1000 kcal (0.6 mg/4200 kJ). Thus, for adult men and women, daily intakes should be 1.6 and 1.2 mg, respectively. Pregnancy and lactation require additions of 0.3 and 0.5 mg per day, making the daily allowances 1.5 and 1.7 mg, respectively.

Riboflavin is widely distributed in food, but, like thiamine, only in small amounts in most commonly eaten foods. Milk and milk products, organ meats, and green leafy vegetables provide a substantial part of our daily intake. Although cereals and breads enriched with the vitamin do not contain large amounts, they too contribute significant amounts of riboflavin to our food supply. Strict vegetarians may have a marginal intake of the vitamin, since riboflavin consumption is apt to be low if milk is not part of the menu plan.[41]

Clinical Deficiency

Riboflavin deficiency generally occurs in concert with other B vitamin deficiencies, and the specific clinical signs associated with riboflavin are less dramatic than those seen in beriberi and pellagra (niacin deficiency). Vitamin deficiency results in growth retardation and several abnormalities of the mouth and eyes. Cracks at the corners of the mouth (cheilosis) appear, and the tongue becomes smooth and purplish (glossitis). Dry and scaly skin is also apparent. The eyes may itch, become sensitive to light, and be susceptible to strain and fatigue.

There is no known toxicity from the vitamin.

Pyridoxine (Vitamin B₆)

History and Discovery

Another of the water-soluble vitamins, sought after because none of the known B vitamins could cure a specific type of dermatitis in rats, was isolated in 1938, synthesized in 1939, and named *pyridoxine.*

Chemistry and Properties

Vitamin B_6 is a complex of closely related compounds, all of which are interconvertible and biologically active. The parent compound is a pyridine with either an alcohol (pyridoxine), aldehyde (pyridoxal), or amine (pyridoxamine) group attached to the pyridine nucleus. The complex is a white, crystalline, and odorless compound which is both water- and alcohol-soluble. It is heat-stable in acid solution, and is relatively heat-labile in an alkaline medium and upon exposure to light.

Metabolism

The absorption of pyridoxine from the upper segment of the small intestine is unremarkable, except perhaps in children with acute celiac disease,[42] chronic alcoholics[43] (synthetic pyridoxine preparations appear to be better absorbed by the latter group), and persons who have had a jejunoileal bypass for the treatment of obesity.[44] There is only limited storage of the vitamin in human tissue, occurring mostly in muscle. The primary metabolite is pyridoxic acid, which is excreted in the urine.

Function

Pyridoxine functions as a coenzyme, pyridoxal phosphate, in protein, carbohydrate, and perhaps fatty acid metabolism. By far the most extensive function of the vitamin is its role in protein and amino acid metabolism. It functions as a coenzyme in several types of reactions: transamination and deamination (gluconeogenesis and the synthesis of nonessential amino acids), decarboxylation (serotonin, norepinephrine, and histamine synthesis), and desulfuration (conversion of serine to cysteine). Pyridoxal phosphate is required for the formation of a heme precursor, delta-aminolevulinic acid. It appears to stabilize phosphorylase, which functions to release glucose-1-phosphate from liver and muscle glycogen. It may also be involved in the conversion of linoleic to arachidonic acid. An important function of the vitamin is its role in the conversion of tryptophan to niacin, and deficiency therefore may be manifested to some extent as niacin deficiency. In fact, a limited intake of pyridoxine may play a contributory role in the pathogenesis of pellagra.

Biochemical Assessment

The traditional method of evaluating pyridoxine status has been the tryptophan load test. In a B_6-deficiency state, administration of a large dose of tryptophan results in an abnormally high urinary excretion of xanthurenic acid, an intermediary product in the conversion of the amino acid to niacin. Urinary excretion of the vitamin or of pyridoxic acid has also been used to determine adequacy. More recently, a functional test has been developed, in which erythrocyte levels of glutamic acid–oxaloacetate transaminase activity (EGOT) or glutamic acid–pyruvate transaminase activity

(EGPT) are measured. In vitro simulation with pyridoxal phosphate is used as a measure of in vivo pyridoxine deficiency.

Dietary Allowance and Sources

As a result of the close association between protein metabolism and vitamin B_6, it is not surprising that the requirement for pyridoxine is increased with increasing intakes of protein. Although vitamin B_6 is present in a wide variety of foodstuffs, concern about requirements has arisen because the vitamin is easily depleted by a number of physiological and pathological conditions. The Food and Nutrition Board first established a dietary requirement in 1968, and set the allowance at 2 mg per day for adults, with an increase to 2.5 mg for pregnant and lactating women. Current research suggests that the allowance for pregnant and lactating women should be reevaluated: 4 or 5 mg per day may be required to maintain maternal serum pyridoxine levels and an adequate content of the vitamin in human milk.[45,46] Of concern also is the fact that women taking oral contraceptive agents demonstrate abnormal tryptophan metabolism which can be normalized by large doses of pyridoxine. Many investigations have been carried out to determine the clinical significance of this finding. Most researchers now feel that pharmacological pyridoxine supplementation is probably unnecessary for most women, although some benefit has been seen in women who show signs of mental depression. This finding has been related to the role of pyridoxine in serotonin synthesis.

Pyridoxine has at times been used to prevent morning sickness in pregnancy; its effectiveness is not widely accepted, and questions of its potential harmful effects have been raised. Although it does not seem to be teratogenic, Rose has cautioned that large doses of the vitamin might cause a detrimental decrease in plasma amino acid levels, because of the induction of amino acid catabolizing enzymes by estrogen and their potentiation by pyridoxine.[47]

Requirements for infants (0.3 to 0.4 mg per day) are largely based on studies which followed an incident about 20 years ago when, through overprocessing, vitamin B_6 was accidentally destroyed in a commercial infant formula, and the lack resulted in irritability and convulsions in infants.

Very little is known about nutritional requirements in general for the elderly. Since this age group is becoming a proportionally larger segment of our population, it behooves nutritional researchers to look into this important question. Some evidence suggests that vitamin B_6 requirements may increase with age.[48]

Several medical conditions requiring drug therapy have been shown to affect pyridoxine status, and therefore to affect the requirement for the vitamin. Antitubercular drugs, such as cycloserine and isoniazid (INH), bind with the vitamin and if used without adjuvant B_6 therapy result in serious neurological symptoms. Therefore, pyridoxine supplementation accompanies administration of these drugs. The use of the antibiotic chloramphenicol also produces neuritis, and this untoward effect can be prevented by simultaneous administration of large amounts of pyridoxine. Hydralazine (an antihypertensive agent) and certain diuretics also cause increased urinary loss of vitamin B_6. Penicillamine, which binds copper and is used in the treatment of Wilson's disease, also increases the requirement for pyridoxine. Finally, levodopa (L-dopa), used in the treatment of Parkinson's disease, can cause a polyneuropathy related to pyridoxine depletion. Unfortunately, increasing the intake of pyridoxine decreases the effectiveness of L-dopa; the use of carbidopa (which enhances the effects of L-dopa) and B_6 with L-dopa therapy is recommended. Pyridoxine therapy may be warranted in uremic patients undergoing hemodialysis.[49]

The best dietary sources of pyridoxine are pork, wheat germ, organ meats, whole grain cereals, legumes, and bananas. Milk and eggs provide only small amounts.

Clinical Deficiency

Rats deficient in pyridoxine develop a characteristic dermatitis and growth failure, weakness, and mental changes, which cannot be counteracted with niacin. Adults given a pyridoxine antagonist (deoxypyridoxine) develop nausea, depression, neuritis, and dermatitis. The most extreme symptom of severe pyridoxine deficiency involves the central nervous system, as demonstrated by the incident with the overprocessed infant formula and by the effects of certain medications.

Vitamin B_6 has been used therapeutically in certain inborn errors of amino acid metabolism. Some success in ameliorating the formation of oxalate kidney stones has been reported. Although pyridoxine supplementation increased the serum levels of the vitamin in patients with rheumatoid arthritis, there was no improvement in their clinical condition.

Niacin (Nicotinic Acid)

History and Discovery

In the early part of this century, thousands of Americans, mostly poor Southerners, were suffering from a debilitating disease that resulted in many of them being confined to mental institutions. It was a disease that had been described by Casal of Spain in 1735 and also was rampant in Italy, where it received its name, pellagra (rough skin). Although many theories were proposed for its existence, Goldberger clearly and gallantly determined that it was a dietary deficiency disease, although he was unable to identify the pellagra-preventive factor. Diets based on cornmeal appeared to precipitate the symptoms, and high-quality protein diets prevented or cured them. It was not until 1937, when Elvehjem demonstrated that nicotinic acid cured blacktongue in dogs, the counterpart of human pellagra, that nicotinic acid, or niacin, was recognized as a dietary essential. Further research elucidated the reason why high-protein diets abated the symptoms, when it was recognized that tryptophan is a precursor from which the body can synthesize niacin.

Chemistry and Properties

Niacin (nicotinic acid) is a white crystalline powder that is remarkably stable to light, heat, acid, and alkali, but because it is water-soluble, may be lost in cooking water. It is readily converted to nicotinamide, the active form of the vitamin.

Metabolism

Niacin is rapidly absorbed in the upper part of the small intestine, probably by passive diffusion. Limited storage exists in the body and the vitamin is excreted in the urine as N-methylnicotinamide or 2-pyridone.

We cannot discuss niacin metabolism without mentioning its synthesis from tryptophan. Investigators have concluded that roughly 60 mg of the amino acid are converted to 1 mg of niacin, although this approximation may not apply to certain conditions such as pregnancy. The synthesis of niacin requires pyridoxine, riboflavin, and thiamine; deficiencies of these vitamins may also be implicated in the etiology of pellagra.

Function

Niacin and its active form nicotinamide are intimately related to energy release from fat, carbohydrate, and protein. The vitamin functions as a part of two important coenzymes, NAD (nicotinamide adenine dinucleotide) and NADP (nicotinamide adenine dinucleotide phosphate), which are involved with hydrogen transfer in metabolic reactions, in both their oxidized and reduced forms (NADH and NADPH). The coenzymes are utilized in the glycolytic and tricarboxylic acid pathways, and in the synthesis and breakdown of fatty acids. Transfer of hydrogen from NADH to the riboflavin-containing coenzymes occurs in the electron transport system, by which ATP and water are formed. NADP is utilized in the pentose phosphate pathway, in which ribose is synthesized. Thus, a variety of important

metabolic pathways are influenced by the availability of niacin.

Biochemical Assessment

Dietary surveys do not provide a good index of niacin status, as there is a question about the availability of niacin in foods. Biochemical methods of estimation are more meaningful, although present methods are not particularly suitable or accurate. Measurement of niacin metabolites in urine, and recently the ratio of 2-pyridone to N-methylnicotinamide, have been used. Measurement of NAD levels in blood has been disappointing; there are no satisfactory and reliable differences between pellagrins and normals. Clearly, more research is needed, particularly to identify subclinical cases of pellagra.

Dietary Allowance and Sources

The allowance for niacin is based on niacin equivalents, to take into account its in vivo synthesis from tryptophan. Requirements for niacin are based on caloric intake, 6.6 mg/1000 kcal (6.6 mg/4200 kJ), with the recommendation that a minimum of 13 mg per day be ingested, even at energy intakes of less than 2000 kcal (8400 kJ). Note that the requirement for this vitamin is considerably higher than that recommended for any of the other water-soluble vitamins. Pregnancy increases the daily requirement by 2 mg, and lactation by 4 mg. Patients with Hartnup's disease (a rare familial disorder in which there is decreased intestinal absorption and renal reabsorption of the neutral amino acids, including tryptophan) often develop pellagralike symptoms which are responsive to niacin treatment.

Meat, poultry, and fish are better sources than are plant products, on the basis not only of preformed niacin content, but also of their tryptophan content. Enrichment procedures have also made enriched bread and bread products good sources of the vitamin, primarily because of the quantity in which they are eaten, although our weight-conscious society often shuns these products. Peanut butter can be an important source of the vitamin. Fruits and vegetables are generally poor sources; milk and eggs have little preformed niacin, but are good sources of tryptophan.

Clinical Deficiency

Pellagra is the classic disease associated with niacin deficiency and is characterized by the "three D's": *dermatitis, diarrhea,* and *dementia* (a fourth "D," *death,* is often added). The observed dermatitis is interesting in that the rash generally shows a symmetrical pattern and is accentuated by exposure to sun or heat. *Casal's necklace* describes the rash apparent in the neck area of affected persons. Mouth, tongue, and intestinal tissues become inflamed in niacin deficiency. Mental confusion, anxiety, and depression are manifestations of the effects of the disease on the central nervous system. Many of the symptoms are reminiscent of riboflavin and thiamine deficiencies; recent work suggests that pellagra is a mixed deficiency and that riboflavin and thiamine (and perhaps also pyridoxine) nutriture are important factors in its development. In addition, millet (sorghum)-based diets may be responsible for the onset of pellagra in some cases. This grain contains high concentrations of available niacin and is not low in tryptophan, but it is high in leucine content; this branched-chain amino acid may interfere with the conversion of tryptophan to niacin.

Fortunately, most pellagra has disappeared in the United States. It is still found, however, in the corn-eating countries of Europe. Of interest is the fact that the people of Latin and Central America have not been prone to pellagra, even though their dietary staple is corn. This is probably related to the fact that the corn is treated with lime salts, which may release bound forms of niacin and make the vitamin available for absorption.

Toxicity and Pharmacological Effects

Large doses of nicotinic acid (but not nicotinamide) have a vasodilating effect, causing transient tingling and flushing of the skin.

Pharmacological doses of niacin (3 g or more daily) have been used to lower serum cholesterol and lipoprotein levels; this caused a short-lived hope for the control of coronary diseases. The Coronary Drug Project Research Group recently released a statement concerning the safety and efficacy of this form of treatment:

[There is] no evidence that niacin influences mortality of survivors of myocardial infarction; this medication may be slightly beneficial in protecting persons to some degree against recurrent nonfatal myocardial infarctions. However, because of the excess incidence of arrhythmias, gastrointestinal problems, and abnormal chemistry findings in the niacin group, great care and caution must be exercised if this drug is to be used for treatment of persons with coronary heart disease.[50]

Another highly touted use of niacin has been in the treatment of schizophrenia. In addition to questionable effects on the mental disorder, massive doses of the vitamin may cause liver toxicity. Diabetes and activation of peptic ulcers may also be long-term consequences of niacin therapy. Niacin is not, therefore, a totally harmless water-soluble vitamin.

Pantothenic Acid

History and Discovery

This B vitamin gets its name from the Greek *pantos,* meaning "everywhere"; its unbiquitous presence in all plants and animals led to its nomenclature. The vitamin was recognized as essential for several species, including humans, and was isolated in 1938 and synthesized in 1940.

Chemistry and Properties

Pantothenic acid (composed of pantoic acid and β-alanine) is a water-soluble white crystalline compound, available as calcium pantothenate. It is easily decomposed by alkali, acid, and dry heat; it is more stable in solution than in the dry state.

Metabolism

Little is known about the absorption of pantothenic acid. Storage sites, although limited, are liver, adrenal, brain, kidney, and heart. Its excretion has not been extensively studied.

Function

The essentiality of pantothenic acid was recognized when it was determined that it was part of the coenzyme A molecule, a very important compound in intermediary metabolism. Coenzyme A forms thioesters with carboxylic acids, and is intimately involved in the metabolism of carbohydrate, protein, and fat. Acetyl CoA, the entry point for many compounds into the tricarboxylic acid cycle, is also involved in fatty acid and sterol synthesis. It provides acetyl groups for acetylcholine, a neurotransmitter, and is also required for the synthesis of porphyrin, the pigment portion of the hemoglobin molecule.

Another function of pantothenic acid is its role in the structure of acyl carrier protein (ACP), necessary for the transport of acetyl CoA from mitochondria to cytoplasm for use in fatty acid synthesis. ACP is required in all subsequent steps of fatty acid synthesis.

Dietary Allowance and Sources

Lack of adequate evidence about the actual requirement for pantothenic acid has led the Food and Nutrition Board to merely suggest a daily intake of 5 to 10 mg of the vitamin. The upper level is suggested for pregnant and lactating women. It has been estimated that the average American diet contains 10 to 20 mg per day, therefore making a deficiency unlikely.

Although pantothenic acid is present in all foods, eggs, liver, yeast, salmon, and heart are the best-known sources. Mushrooms, cauliflower, molasses, and peanuts are also good sources. Fruits generally are relatively poor sources of the vitamin. Grains are an important source of pantothenic acid; however, approximately 50 percent is lost in the milling process.

Clinical Deficiency

One of the reasons that the Food and Nutrition Board has not been able to set a recommended dietary allowance is that no spontaneous deficiencies of pantothenic acid have been shown to occur in man. In fact, experimentally induced deficiencies, either by use of purified diets or pantothenic acid antagonists, have not been "successful" either, in that they, too, are difficult to produce. In one study, subjects on a deficient diet experienced insomnia, leg cramps, and paresthesias of hands and feet. Addition of an antagonist produced burning feet, insulin sensitivity, and mental depression.

Lower species do show specific signs of deficiency: chicks develop ocular dermatitis and spinal cord degeneration, and rats develop red whiskers, growth failure, alopecia, and graying of hair. Contrary to the claims of vitamin advocates, pantothenic acid will not prevent the appearance of gray hair in humans.

In some patients treated with streptomycin, a polyneuropathy may develop which is responsive to pantothenic acid. A recent report suggests that in patients with chronic ulcerative and granulomatous colitis a block in the conversion of pantothenic acid to coenzyme A occurs within the intestine.[51]

The vitamin has been used clinically after surgery to stimulate gastrointestinal motility, but large doses will cause diarrhea and should be avoided.

Biotin

History and Discovery

Variably known as vitamin H and coenzyme R, biotin was recognized as a growth factor for microorganisms in 1924. It was synthesized in 1943 and recognized as a compound which protected rats against "egg white injury," caused by the feeding of raw egg whites. Symptoms which appeared included dermatitis, paralysis of the hind legs, and a characteristic alopecia around the eye, appropriately called "spectacle eye." Cooked egg white did not produce these signs. It is now known that raw egg white contains a heat-labile protein, avidin, which binds dietary biotin and makes it unavailable for absorption.

Chemistry and Properties

Biotin is a sulfur-containing monocarboxylic acid which is water- and alcohol-soluble, and stable to heat but destroyed by oxidation, alkali, and strong acids.

Metabolism

Except for its being made unavailable for absorption by avidin, the absorption of biotin from the gastrointestinal tract is unremarkable. In addition, synthesis of the vitamin by bacteria is extensive and probably largely available to man. Little is known about its storage, and most of it appears to be excreted intact in the urine.

Function

Biotin acts as a coenzyme in many important biochemical reactions. It is involved in amino acid metabolism (in some deamination reactions) and may be involved with protein synthesis. Carbohydrate metabolism (glycolysis and gluconeogenesis) also requires biotin as a coenzyme. Some possible functions include a role in niacin synthesis from tryptophan, formation of antibodies, and the synthesis of pancreatic amylase; further investigation of these proposed roles must be undertaken. It appears to be closely related to the functions of vitamin B_{12} and folic acid.

Dietary Allowance and Sources

No requirement has been stated by the Food and Nutrition Board for biotin, although they recommend a daily intake of 150 to 300 μg. Most American diets contain at least this much, and intestinal production by the microflora seems to provide a substantial amount.

Although many foods have not been analyzed for biotin content, it is present in milk, liver, egg yolk, mushrooms, and legumes.

Clinical Deficiency

Biotin deficiency in humans has not been documented, although a biotin deficiency has been produced in animals by dietary means. Experimental deficiency has been induced by feeding large amounts of raw egg white, and produced dermatitis, anorexia, lassitude, muscle pain, and nausea. The symptoms have been reversed by giving a biotin concentrate.

Consumption of an occasional raw egg, as in an eggnog, will not precipitate deficiency symptoms. It is only large amounts, estimated to be more than 20 eggs per day, that cause the deficiency. This equivalent is highly unlikely in the typical American diet.

Folic Acid

History and Discovery

In 1930 Wills reported an often fatal macrocytic anemia among the pregnant women of India, and suggested that it might be a symptom of a dietary deficiency disease. Further investigation with animals led to the conclusion that the substance was identical to a bacterial growth factor isolated from spinach leaves. Folic acid (from the Latin *folium,* meaning "leaf") was subsequently isolated and synthesized in 1948.

Chemistry and Properties

The folacin group of water-soluble crystalline yellow compounds contains several forms of the vitamin which are biologically active. The parent compound is known as *folic acid* or *pteroylglutamic acid* (PGA), the latter describing its chemical nature: pteroic acid (of which para-aminobenzoic acid, once thought to be an essential vitamin for man, is a part) and one or more molecules of glutamic acid. Folacin is a heat-labile compound in acid solution and unstable to sunlight in the dry form. Considerable loss of the vitamin occurs in high-temperature processing and during storage.

Metabolism

The primary site of folate absorption is the upper part of the small intestine, where both active and passive transport contribute to its entry into mucosal cells. Before the folate in foods, in which it occurs primarily as polyglutamates, can be absorbed, excess glutamates must be enzymatically removed by conjugase, a hydrolytic enzyme present in intestinal tissue or secretions. The rate of absorption of dietary folate may be inversely related to the length of the polyglutamate chain, and current research is attempting to determine the availability of the various forms of folate. Chronic alcoholics are unable to absorb dietary folate; synthetic forms of the vitamin are apparently better utilized.

Liver stores contain about half of the vitamin found in the body, although folate is found in all cells. It is bound to a protein for transport and storage. Small amounts are found in the urine, as a folate metabolite.

The metabolism of folate may be influenced at several points by interactions with pharmaceutical agents. Among those which cause a decrease in its absorption are alcohol, the antitubercular drugs aminosalicylic acid and cycloserine, and some anticonvulsants. The antimalarial drugs trimethoprim and pyrimethamine inactivate folate; methotrexate is a powerful folate antagonist used in antitumor treatment. A growing literature describes the effects of oral contraceptive agents on serum folate levels, a marked decrease being observed. In some women taking these preparations, the histology of the cervical epithelium may be abnormal; the changes are responsive to folate therapy.[52]

Function

A discussion of the function of folic acid requires discussion of its own metabolism. Folic acid is reduced to tetrahydrofolic acid (THFA) in the presence of NADPH (a niacin coenzyme). Addition of a one-carbon fragment to one or two of the nitrogen molecules in pteroic acid completes the synthesis of the active coenzyme form of folic acid. As the coenzyme, folate participates in the transfer of single carbon units (formyl, methyl) to intermediates in the biosynthesis of purine and pyrimidine (precursors for the nucleic acids), and in several amino acid interconversions. The latter reactions include the methylation of homocysteine to methionine, and the conversion of histidine to glutamic acid.

Folacin is required for heme synthesis, and is necessary for the formation of blood cells in the bone marrow, and for their maturation.

Biochemical Assessment

Serum folate levels of less than 3 ng/ml are indicative of a folic acid deficiency. Another widely used assessment method is the histidine load. Histidine requires folate for its metabolism and when the vitamin is not available, an intermediary metabolite, formiminoglutamic acid (FIGLU), accumulates and is excreted in the urine. After a 20-g histidine load, more than 50 mg of FIGLU in a 12-h urine sample is considered abnormal and suggestive of a folic acid deficiency.

Dietary Allowance and Sources

The recommended dietary allowance for adults is 400 μg per day. Because requirements are substantially increased during periods of extensive cell multiplication (owing to the role of folic acid in nucleic acid synthesis), the requirements for pregnancy and lactation are 800 and 600 μg per day, respectively. Infants require 50 μg. If they are fed either human or cow's milk their folic acid intake should be sufficient, but goat's milk is low in this essential nutrient.

Folic acid is found in green leafy vegetables, liver, fish, meat and poultry, legumes, and whole grains. Chemical determinations of folate vary widely; newer and more accurate analyses are being developed.

Clinical Deficiency

In man, folate deficiency results in megaloblastic anemia, gastrointestinal disturbances, glossitis, and growth retardation. Because of the close relationship between folic acid and vitamin B_{12} metabolism, several of the same clinical signs appear when either of these is deficient. It should be stressed that folate will cure the anemia due to B_{12} deficiency, but will not alleviate the more serious neurological symptoms that accompany the anemia in B_{12} deficiency. For this reason, over-the-counter vitamin preparations cannot contain more than 0.1 mg of folic acid, the rationale for this law being that supplementation with folic acid might mask a potentially lethal vitamin B_{12} deficiency.

Vitamin B_{12} (Cobalamin)

History and Discovery
In 1926 pernicious anemia was a fatal disease of unknown origin, characterized by neurological damage and a megaloblastic anemia. Castle postulated the existence of an *intrinsic factor,* which he believed to be present in gastric secretions, and an *extrinsic factor,* both at the time unidentified, which were involved in the etiology of the disease. When physicians in Boston demonstrated that raw liver cured patients with pernicious anemia, the search for the so-called extrinsic factor began. In 1948, the isolation of vitamin B_{12} from liver proved to be a turning point in the understanding of the disease.

Chemistry and Properties
Vitamin B_{12} is a complicated molecule which was not synthesized in the laboratory until 1973. It contains the mineral cobalt and is an extremely potent compound. It is a water-soluble reddish molecule and is sensitive to acid, alkali, and oxidizing agents.

Metabolism
The unfolding of the B_{12} mystery was a challenge to biochemists. The vitamin, presumably because of its large size, is poorly absorbed without the presence of intrinsic factor, a large

mucopolysaccharide found in gastric juice. Vitamin B_{12} is released from food and combines with intrinsic factor in the stomach. The complex is bound to a receptor in the intestinal wall; this attachment is calcium-dependent. The vitamin is released from the mucopolysaccharide and transported through intestinal cells into the bloodstream, where it is carried by transcobalamin, a transport protein, to the tissues. Storage occurs in the liver, and in contrast to other water-soluble vitamins, the extent to which this vitamin is conserved, relative to its utilization, is substantial. Excess vitamin B_{12} is excreted in the urine.

Absorption of vitamin B_{12} appears to decrease with age, and in iron and pyridoxine deficiency. Diminished absorption occurs in patients with gastritis and those with congenital intrinsic factor deficiency. Pregnancy enhances the absorption of the vitamin.

Function
Vitamin B_{12} functions as a coenzyme in cellular reactions. The synthesis of nucleic acids is dependent upon vitamin B_{12}, and this is probably related to its interactions with folate metabolism. The metabolism of odd-chain fatty acids is also B_{12}-dependent, as is the conversion of homocysteine to methionine.

Biochemical Assessment
Evaluation of nutritional status can be done by measuring serum levels of B_{12}, and by determining the amount of methylmalonic acid (MMA) in the urine. MMA requires B_{12} for its conversion to succinic acid, and in the absence of the vitamin, urinary excretion is increased, which is diagnostic of a vitamin B_{12} deficiency.

Dietary Allowance and Sources
The present recommendation for vitamin B_{12} intake is 3 μg per day for adults, increasing to 4 μg during pregnancy and lactation. In patients whose liver stores have been depleted, 15 μg per day is recommended.

The only sources of the vitamin are animal products such as seafood, meat, eggs, and milk. Foods of vegetable origin contain no vitamin B_{12} unless it is added by fortification.

Clinical Deficiency

Signs of vitamin B_{12} deficiency are manifested by both blood and nervous system disorders. The megaloblastic anemia is presumably due to the effect that the vitamin has on maturation of immature red blood cells; nervous system disorders may be due to defective myelin synthesis and fatty acid metabolism.[53] Pernicious anemia is classically due to the congenital absence of intrinsic factor, in which case milligram doses of vitamin B_{12} must be administered parenterally on a daily basis. Iatrogenic (physician-induced) deficiency is produced by gastrectomy or surgical removal of the ileum. Malabsorptive states may induce a deficiency. In some populations, infestation of the gastrointestinal tract with a particular fish tapeworm, which dissociates the B_{12}–intrinsic factor complex, may precipitate a deficiency state. A recent report cites evidence that in patients undergoing maintenance dialysis for renal failure, serum levels of vitamin B_{12} are decreased and are associated with slow nerve-conduction velocities. The patients in the study responded to parenteral administration of the vitamin.[54]

Of increasing concern to nutritionists is the effect of a strict vegetarian diet on vitamin B_{12} status. Adults who choose this type of diet generally have enough of the vitamin stored in their liver to last for 5 or 6 years before deficiency symptoms set in. However, children consuming a vegetarian diet have not accumulated stores of the vitamin and are at higher risk of developing a deficiency. Parents are urged to include at least some animal products (milk and eggs) in their children's diets. If that is unacceptable, a vitamin preparation containing cobalamin is necessary.

VITAMINLIKE FACTORS

There are several compounds which at one time or another have been considered as vitamins. As we learn more about their metabolism and function, a decision will be made as to their inclusion in the vitamin category.

Choline

Choline is a bitter-tasting, water-soluble compound that is widely distributed in plant and animal tissues. It can be synthesized by the human body in the presence of sufficient serine, methionine, folate, and vitamin B_{12}, but probably not in amounts adequate for the maintenance of health. Choline is used as a source of labile methyl groups needed for synthetic processes, and is a structural component of phospholipids, lecithin, and sphingomyelin, in addition to being a precursor of acetylcholine. Along with methionine, choline is known as a *lipotropic factor*, that is, "fat-attracting," and is necessary for the prevention of fatty liver. Fatty liver is observed in kwashiorkor and alcoholism; choline has been used to treat the condition. Under normal circumstances, choline deficiency does not occur in man; sources of this compound include egg yolk, organ meats, legumes, and wheat germ. Dietary requirements are not known; the average American diet provides 800 mg per day, and this appears to be sufficient.

Inositol

Inositol is a colorless water-soluble compound and is structurally related to glucose. In animal tissues it occurs as a component of phospholipids in muscle, and this is its primary function in man; phytic acid, an inositol-phosphate complex, is found in plants and is known to decrease the absorption of calcium and iron. Besides its occurrence in large amounts in common foods, the body appears to be able to synthesize adequate amounts; most researchers no longer include it as a vitamin.

Ubiquinone

Ubiquinone or coenzyme Q, chemically related to vitamin K, is present in mitochondria and plays a major role in the operation of the electron transport system. Adequate in vivo synthesis takes place in man, and its inclusion as a vitamin is not warranted.

Lipoic Acid

Another substance that serves as a coenzyme in intermediary metabolism is also synthesized in sufficient amounts by the human body. Lipoic acid is a sulfur-containing fat-soluble compound that functions in conjunction with thiamine pyrophosphate in decarboxylation reactions, particularly the conversion of pyruvate to acetyl CoA.

SUMMARY

Although the classic signs of vitamin deficiency are seldom manifest in our population, certain altered physiological states and diseases can place individuals at nutritional risk. Since these deficiencies evolve in a gradual continuum and in clusters, the diagnosis must be based on medical and diet histories, and on physical, laboratory, and anthropometric data. Medical and surgical patients, by virtue of their conditions, are at particular risk and should be monitored accordingly. However, given the wrong circumstances, anyone can be at risk of developing vitamin deficiencies, especially the poor, the ignorant, and the elderly. It is the astute health professional who looks for the obscure signs of vitamin deficiencies rather than the classic manifestations, and who counsels against the indiscriminate use of vitamin supplements.

STUDY QUESTIONS

1 What are the similarities and differences between the fat-soluble and water-soluble vitamins?

CASE STUDY 6-1

A 53-year-old woman went to her physician complaining of achy bones and distressed that her skin had recently turned yellow. She prided herself on her "health IQ"; she had always had annual physicals and knew that vitamin pills were unnecessary if you ate balanced meals. Further discussion revealed that she had stopped menstruating 8 years previously, and was recently divorced and had reentered the work force. Because she wanted to lose weight, and influenced by the young people she worked with who are vegetarians, she adopted vegetarianism 8 months ago. She reduced her daily intake to 1200 kcal (500 kJ), and had learned to combine vegetable proteins to ensure an adequate amino acid intake. She ate no eggs or dairy products. She liked carrots and had recently begun con-

suming a package a day. Her physician performed a physical examination, noting dry scaly skin around the corners of her nose and mouth. Because of the physical findings the doctor ordered a vitamin profile in addition to usual laboratory tests. The results showed elevated serum carotene and alkaline phosphatase levels, and low levels of riboflavin.

Case Study Questions
1 *Relate this woman's physical symptoms and blood chemistry to her dietary pattern.*
2 *What recommendations would you make?*
3 *What occurs when there is an inadequate intake of vitamin D or calcium?*

2 What are the chief symptoms of vitamin A deficiency? Vitamin D? Vitamin E? Vitamin K?

3 Explain three specific types of information you might use to determine nutritional status with regard to the vitamins. Of what value is this information in nutrition education?

4 Why are the requirements for thiamine and riboflavin related to energy intake? Why is pyridoxine related to protein intake?

5 Name the criteria which are used to designate a nutrient as a vitamin. Why are carbohydrates, fats, proteins, and minerals not considered to be vitamins?

REFERENCES

1 F. R. Smith, R. Suskind, O. Thanangkul, C. Leitzmann, D. S. Goodman, and R. E. Olson, "Plasma Vitamin A, Retinol-binding Protein and Prealbumin Concentrations in Protein-Calorie Malnutrition. III. Response to Varying Dietary Treatments," *American Journal of Clinical Nutrition,* 28:732–738, 1975.

2 J. E. Smith, E. D. Brown, and J. C. Smith, Jr., "The Effect of Zinc Deficiency on the Metabolism of Retinol-binding in the Rat," *Journal of Laboratory and Clinical Medicine,* 84:692, 1974.

3 S. M. Carney, B. A. Underwood, and J. D. Loerch, "Effects of Zinc and Vitamin A Deficient Diets on the Hepatic Mobilization and Urinary Excretion of Vitamin A in Rats," *Journal of Nutrition,* 106:1773–1781, 1976.

4 F. R. Smith and D. S. Goodman, "The Effects of Diseases of the Liver, Thyroid and Kidneys on the Transport of Vitamin A in Human Plasma," *Journal of Clinical Investigation,* 50:2426–2436, 1971.

5 D. P. Sinha and F. B. Bang, "The Effect of Massive Doses of Vitamin A on the Signs of Vitamin A Deficiency in Preschool Children," *American Journal of Clinical Nutrition,* 29:110–115, 1976.

6 M. H. Bhattacharyya and H. F. DeLuca, "The Regulation of Rat Liver Calciferol-25-Hydroxylase," *Journal of Biological Chemistry,* 248:2969–2973, 1973.

7 G. Tucker III, R. E. Gagnon, and M. R. Haussler, "Vitamin D_3-25-Hydroxylase: Tissue Occurrence and Apparent Lack of Regulation," *Archives of Biochemistry and Biophysics,* 155:47–57, 1973.

8 "Hazards of the Overuse of Vitamin D," *Nutrition Reviews,* 33:61, 1975.

9 F. A. Kummerow, B. H. Semon Cho, W. Y.-T. Huang, H. Imai, A. Kamio, M. J. Deutsch, and W. M. Hooper, "Additive Risk Factors in Atherosclerosis," *American Journal of Clinical Nutrition,* 29:579–584, 1976.

10 "Symposium on Vitamin D," *American Journal of Clinical Nutrition,* 29:1253–1329, 1976.

11 J. H. Ritchie, M. B. Fish, V. McMasters, and M. Grossman. "Edema and Hemolytic Anemia in Premature Infants. A Vitamin E Deficiency Syndrome," *New England Journal of Medicine,* 279:1185–1190, 1968.

12 F. A. Oski and L. A. Barness, "Vitamin E Deficiency: A Previously Unrecognized Cause of Hemolytic Anemia in Premature Infants," *Journal of Pediatrics,* 70:211–220, 1967.

13 M. K. Horwitt, "Vitamin E and Lipid Metabolism in Man," *American Journal of Clinical Nutrition,* 8:451–461, 1960.

14 J. D. Lawrence, R. C. Bower, W. P. Riehl, and J. L. Smith, "Effects of Alpha-Tocopherol Acetate on the Swimming Endurance of Trained Swimmers," *American Journal of Clinical Nutrition,* 28:205–208, 1975.

15 J. J. Coorigan and F. I. Marcuss, "Coagulopathy Associated with Vitamin E Ingestion," *Journal of the American Medical Association,* 230:1300–1301, 1974.

16 M. K. Horwitt, "Vitamin E: A Reexamination," *American Journal of Clinical Nutrition,* 29:569–578, 1976.

17 G. L. Nelsestuen, T. H. Zykovicz, and J. B. Howard, "The Mode of Action of Vitamin K. Identification of *Gamma-Carboxylglutamic Acid as a Component of Prothrombin,*" *Journal of Biological Chemistry,* 249:6347–6350, 1974.

18 C. T. Esmon, J. A. Sadowski, and J. W. Suttie, "A New Carboxylation Reaction. The Vitamin K-dependent Incorporation of $H^{14}CO_3$ into Prothrombin," *Journal of Biological Chemistry,* 250:4744–4748, 1975.

19 M. K. Horwitt, op. cit., *American Journal of Clinical Nutrition,* 29:569–578, 1976.

20 V. M. Crosse, T. C. Meyer, and J. W. Gerrard, "Kernicterus and Prematurity," *Archives of Diseases in Childhood,* 30:501–508, 1955.

21 M. K. Horwitt, C. C. Harvey, and C. H. Dahm, Jr., "Relationship between Levels of Blood Lipids, Vitamins C, A, and E, Serum Copper Compounds, and Urinary Excretions of Tryptophan Metabolites in Women Taking Oral Contraceptive Therapy," *American Journal of Clinical Nutrition,* 28:403–413, 1975.

22 J. M. Rivers, "Oral Contraceptives and Ascorbic

Acid," *American Journal of Clinical Nutrition,* **28:**550–554, 1975.

23 D. L. Yeung, "Relationships between Cigarette Smoking, Oral Contraceptives, and Plasma Vitamins A, E, C, and Plasma Triglyceride and Cholesterol," *American Journal of Clinical Nutrition,* **29:**1216–1221, 1976.

24 "Activation of Prolyl Hydroxylase by Ascorbic Acid," *Nutrition Reviews,* **31:**255–256, 1973.

25 C. R. Spittle, "Atherosclerosis and Vitamin C," *Lancet,* **2:**1280–1281, 1971.

26 V. E. Peterson, P. A. Crapo, J. Weininger, H. Ginsberg, and J. Olefsky, "Quantification of Plasma Cholesterol and Triglyceride Levels in Hypercholesterolemic Subjects Receiving Ascorbic Acid Supplements," *American Journal of Clinical Nutrition,* **28:**584–587, 1975.

27 S. C. Tsai, H. M. Fales, and M. Vaughan, "Inactivation of Hormone-sensitive Lipase from Adipose Tissue with Adenosine Triphosphate, Magnesium and Ascorbic Acid," *Journal of Biological Chemistry,* **248:**5278–5281, 1973.

28 T. W. Anderson, R. B. W. Reid, and G. H. Beaton, "Vitamin C and the Common Cold: A Double Blind Trial," *Canadian Medical Association Journal,* **107:**503–508, 1972.

29 J. L. Coulehan, S. Eberhard, L. Kapner, F. Taylor, K. Rogers, and P. Gary, "Vitamin C and Acute Illness in Navajo Schoolchildren," *New England Journal of Medicine,* **295:**973–976, 1976.

30 E. Ginter, "Chenodeoxycholic Acid, Gallstones and Vitamin C," *New England Journal of Medicine,* **295:**1260–1261, 1976.

31 M. I. Irwin and B. K. Hutchins, A Conspectus of Research on Vitamin C Requirements of Man," *Journal of Nutrition,* **106:**823–879, 1976.

32 M. P. Lamden, "Dangers of Massive Vitamin C Intake," *New England Journal of Medicine,* **284:**336–337, 1971.

33 V. Herbert and E. Jacob, "Destruction of Vitamin B_{12} by Ascorbic Acid," *Journal of the American Medical Association,* **230:**241–242, 1974.

34 H. L. Newmark, J. Scheiner, M. Marcus, and M. Prabhudesai, "Stability of Vitamin B_{12} in Presence of Ascorbic Acid," *American Journal of Clinical Nutrition,* **29:**645–649, 1976.

35 Y. Itokawa and J. R. Cooper, "Ion Movements and Thiamin. II. The Release of the Vitamin from Membrane Fragments," *Biochimica et Biophysica Acta,* **196:**274–284, 1970.

36 K. Berman and R. A. Fishman, "Thiamin Phosphate Metabolism and Possible Independent Functions of Thiamin in Brain," *Journal of Neurochemistry,* **24:**457–465, 1975.

37 M., Brin, "Erythrocyte Transketolase Activity in Early Thiamine Deficiency," *Annals of the New York Academy of Sciences,* **98:**528–541, 1962.

38 Y. H. Chong and G. S. Ho, "Erythrocyte Transketolase Activity," *American Journal of Clinical Nutrition,* **23:**261–266, 1970.

39 C. R. Scriver, "Vitamin-responsive Inborn Errors of Metabolism," *Metabolism,* **22:**1319–1344, 1973.

40 H. E. Sauberlich, J. H. Judd, G. E. Nichoalds, H. P. Broquist, and W. J. Darby, "Application of the Erythrocyte Glutathione Reductase Assay in Evaluating Riboflavin Status in a High School Student Population," *American Journal of Clinical Nutrition,* **25:**756, 1972.

41 P. T. Brown and J. G. Bergan, "Dietary Status of 'New' Vegetarians," *Journal of the American Dietetic Association,* **67:**455–459, 1975.

42 L. Reinken, H. Zieglauer, and H. Berger, "Vitamin B_6 Nutriture of Children with Acute Celiac Disease, Celiac Disease in Remission, and of Children with Normal Duodenal Mucosa," *American Journal of Clinical Nutrition,* **29:**750–753, 1976.

43 H. Baker, O. Frank, R. K. Zetterman, K. S. Rajan, W. ten Hove, and C. M. Leevy, "Inability of Chronic Alcoholics with Liver Disease to Use Food as a Source of Folates, Thiamin and Vitamin B_6," *American Journal of Clinical Nutrition,* **28:**1377–1380, 1975.

44 L. Howard, M. Oldendorf, and R. Chu, "Pyridoxine Deficiency: Another Potential Sequel of the Jejunal-Ileal Bypass Procedure," *New England Journal of Medicine,* **295:**733, 1976.

45 L. Lumeng, R. E. Cleary, R. Wagner, P-L Yu, and T-K Li, "Adequacy of Vitamin B_6 Supplementation during Pregnancy: A Prospective Study," *American Journal of Clinical Nutrition,* **29:**1376–1383, 1976.

46 K. D. West and A. Kirskey, "Influence of Vitamin B_6 Intake on the Content of the Vitamin in Human Milk," *American Journal of Clinical Nutrition,* **29:**961–969, 1976.

47 D. P. Rose, J. E. Leklem, R. R. Brown, and C. Potera, "Effect of Oral Contraceptives and Vitamin B_6 Supplements on Alanine and Glycine Metabolism," *American Journal of Clinical Nutrition,* **29:**956–960, 1976.

48 C. S. Rose, P. Gyorgy, M. Butler, R. Andres, A. H. Norris, N. W. Shock, J. Tobin, M. Brin, and H. Spiegel, "Age Differences in Vitamin B_6 Status of 617 Men," *American Journal of Clinical Nutrition,* **29:**847–853, 1976.

49 W. J. Stone, L. G. Warnock, and C. Wagner, "Vitamin B_6 Deficiency in Uremia," *American Journal of Clinical Nutrition,* **28:**950, 1975.

50 "The Coronary Drug Project Research Group: Clofibrate and Niacin in Coronary Heart Disease," *Journal of the American Medical Association,* **321:**360–381, 1975.

51 J. J. Ellestad-Sayed, R. A. Nelson, M. A. Adson, W. M. Palmer, and E. H. Soule, "Pantothenic Acid, Coenzyme A, and Human Chronic Ulcerative and Granu-

lomatous Colitis," *American Journal of Clinical Nutrition,* **29:**1333–1338, 1976.

52 J. Lindenbaum, N. Whitehead, and F. Reyner, "Oral Contraceptive Hormones, Folate Metabolism and the Cervical Epithelium," *American Journal of Clinical Nutrition,* **28:**346–353, 1975.

53 E. P. Frenkel, "Abnormal Fatty Acid Metabolism in Peripheral Nerves of Patients with Pernicious Anemia," *Journal of Clinical Investigation,* **52:**1237–1245, 1973.

54 S. G. Rostand, "Vitamin B_{12} Levels and Nerve Conduction Velocities in Patients Undergoing Maintenance Dialysis," *American Journal of Clinical Nutrition,* **29:**691–697, 1976.

CHAPTER 7

MINERALS

*Jean Hine**

KEY WORDS
Macrominerals
Microminerals
Calcium/Phosphorus Ratio
Tetany
Osteoporosis
Iron Deficiency Anemia
Ferritin
Goiter

INTRODUCTION

Our food supply provides us with the inorganic elements, or minerals, of which many are essential to the body's metabolic processes. The mineral content of food varies with local soil and water conditions. The total mineral content of a food is determined by burning a specific amount of the food and weighing the remaining ash, which is then analyzed for the individual minerals that are present.

Of the 103 known elements (Fig. 7-1, periodic table), 11 constitute the bulk of living matter, while the remainder are present in much smaller or trace amounts. Minerals can be viewed as falling into two categories: those required in amounts at or above 100 mg per day (*macrominerals*) and those needed in amounts no higher than a few milligrams per day (*microminerals*) (Table 7-1). Calcium, chloride, magnesium, phosphorus, potassium, sodium, and sulfur are classified as macrominerals and have well-documented roles in human nutrition. Essential minerals needed in microquantities are cobalt, copper, iodine, iron, manganese, molybdenum, and zinc. Chromium, fluoride, and selenium appear to be essential for most species, including humans.[1] Roles for nickel, silicon, tin, and vanadium have been identified in some laboratory animals and they may have some essential functions in humans as well (Table 7-2).

Within the body, minerals serve a variety of functions: as essential activators for a number of enzyme-catalyzed reactions (namely, zinc, molybdenum, and manganese), as components of skeletal structure (calcium and phosphorus), in hemoglobin synthesis and red blood cell formation (iron, cobalt, copper), and as part of thyroid hormone (iodine). In addition, they control the water and electrolyte balance (sodium, potassium, calcium, phosphorus, chlorine) and are necessary for nerve cell function (calcium, magnesium).

* Supported by UAF federal grant Project MCT-3000-915-080.

H																	He
Li 2.2	Be 36											B 48	*C*	*N*	*O*	F 3300	Ne
Na	*Mg*											Al 100	**Si** 1100	*P*	*S*	*Cl*	Ar
K	*Ca*	Sc	Ti 9	**V** 10	**Cr** 3	**Mn** 14	Fe 4500	Co 1.3	Ni 8	Cu 87	**Zn** 2000	Ga	Ge 20	As 14	**Se** 21	Br 200	Kr
Rb 320	Sr 340	Y	Zr 340	Nb 120	**Mo** 13	Tc	Ru	Rh	Pd	Ag 0.8	Cd 34	In	**Sn** 42	Sb 6	Te 7	**I** 15	Xe
Cs 1.4	Ba 22	La	Hf	Ta	W	Re	Os	Ir	Pt	Au	Hg 13	Tl 7	Pb 122	Bi 0.2	Po	At	Rn
Fr	Ra	Ac															

Figure 7-1

The Periodic Table. The **bold** *chemical symbols represent the trace elements present and essential in the human body. The italic chemical symbols represent trace minerals present in the human body which at this time are not known to be essential. The numbers represent the amount in milligrams of trace elements present in the human body.* (Adapted from Periodic Table prepared by Maria Linder for Perinatal Physiology, Plenum Press, 1977.)

The Food and Nutrition Board of the National Academy of Sciences has established recommended dietary allowances for calcium, phosphorus, iodine, magnesium, and zinc. The allowances for other essential minerals have yet to be established and much research is under way. Investigations have been stimulated by the increasing concern over the pollution of our environment and its possible effect on the mineral content of food. The inclusion of a wide variety of foods in the diet formerly assured an adequate intake of most minerals; however, due to negative ecological trends, modern food processing, and changing food habits, this assertion may be somewhat questionable. However, it is still a generally accepted notion that when a diet provides sufficient amounts of calcium, iron, and iodine, the intake of other minerals will be adequate to meet body needs.

Mineral absorption is influenced by both endogenous and exogenous factors. Once in the blood, the minerals are bound to protein, act as free ions, or are assigned to a specific transport carrier. They are then utilized, stored in the liver, skin, skeleton and possibly in fat tissue, or excreted in the urine, feces, sweat, and bile.

In human physiology, the minerals are interrelated; they do not function with circumscribed roles but work in concert. However, for the sake of discussion, this chapter will examine each mineral separately: calcium, phosphorus, sulfur, magnesium, iron, iodine, fluorine, chromium, manganese, cobalt, zinc, selenium, molybdenum and copper. (Sodium, potassium and chloride will be discussed in Chap. 8.) This chapter will elucidate the importance of these minerals in human nutrition

TABLE 7-1 MACROMINERALS AND MICROMINERALS

Macrominerals	*Microminerals*
Calcium	Chromium
Chloride	Cobalt
Magnesium	Copper
Phosphorus	Fluorine
Potassium	Iodine
Sodium	Iron
Sulfur	Manganese
	Molybdenum
	Selenium
	Zinc

and emphasize the effects of clinical disturbances on mineral metabolism.

MACROMINERALS

Calcium

A 70-kg adult's body contains approximately 1200 g of calcium, 99 percent of which is found in the skeleton. In the bones, calcium is present in the form of deposits of calcium phosphates in a soft, fibrous, organic matrix.[2] The unique structure of the matrix is required for normal calcification. The principal inorganic compound of bone is a form of calcium phosphate which is similar to the mineral hydroxyapatite:

$$CA_{10}(PO_4)_6(OH)_2$$

The precise chemical nature of bone is unknown because of transitional forms which are present as the bone matures and because of ion exchange and substitution that can take place in the crystalline structure. It is known that calcium in the bone is precipitated initially as an amorphous material which is changed to a crystalline precipitate and subsequently converted to the final crystal.[3] In adult bone, approximately 40 percent of the total calcium is present in the form of a non-apatite material; in younger persons, the amorphous material predominates. Sodium and small amounts of carbonate and magnesium are also present in bone.

Function

Bone formation Bone is constantly being formed and resorbed. In adults, the skeleton is completely replaced every 10 to 12 years. However, in children the renewal process takes only 1 to 2 years.[4] The formation of bone and the control mechanisms which influence formation and dissolution are incompletely understood.[5] Bone is formed by *osteoblasts*, which form new bone crystals in the matrix by the deposition of calcium phosphate, and *osteoclasts* balance this process by resorbing or phago-

cytizing and digesting the minute bone crystals. Physical stress stimulates osteoblastic deposition of bone and bone is deposited in proportion to the load that the bone must carry. For example, bones are heavier in athletes than in nonathletes; and when an individual is in a cast and continues to walk on one leg, the bone of the disabled leg becomes thin and decalcified while the bone in the opposite leg remains thick and calcified.

Calcium in the skeletal framework is in a dynamic state of equilibrium with body tissues and fluids, and balance mechanisms work to maintain the level of calcium in the plasma within its narrow normal range. In fact, the rate of exchange between the plasma and bone calcium is greater than the rate of original deposition of new bone. The calcium stored in the trabeculae at the ends of bones is most readily mobilized and responds to the increasing demands during pregnancy, lactation, and periods of malnutrition. The calcium contained in the dentin and enamel of teeth is more stable. This fact negates the old wives' tale that for every baby, the mother loses a tooth.

In teeth, the crystalline salts are similar to those of bone and are composed basically of the hydroxyapatite with absorbed carbonates and varying cations bound together as a hard crystalline substance. As in bone, new salts are constantly being deposited, while old salts are being resorbed from the teeth. This deposition and resorption occurs mainly in the cementum with some activity in the dentin and minimal occurrence in the enamel (see Chap. 23).

Circulating calcium The small but significant quantity of circulating calcium plays an important role in the maintenance of normal body function. Levels of calcium range from 8.5 to 10.5 mg/100 ml (somewhat higher in children) with no more than a 10 percent variation.[6] The level of circulating calcium is independent of the dietary calcium intake.

Calcium is present in the serum mostly in a soluble ionized form; the remainder occurs in a protein-bound form (mainly bound to al-

TABLE 7-2   THE CONTENT, ABSORPTION AND DISTRIBUTION OF TRACE ELEMENTS IN THE NORMAL ADULT HUMAN*

Element (*essential)	Content in adult body, mg	Ease of absorption from diet, %	Blood distribution and plasma binding (*most in red cells)	Blood concentration µg/100 ml	Main organ of accumulation or storage (*airborne source)	Main route of excretion
*Iron (Fe)	4000–5000	5–15	*Transferrin	50,000	Liver	Bile
*Fluorine (F)	2600–4000	40–100	Mostly free (like Cl⁻)	10–20	Bone	Urine
*Zinc (Zn)	1600–2300	31–51	*α_2 globulin, also α_1 globulin albumin	100	Skin, bone	Pancreatic secretions, bile
*Silicon (Si)	(1100)†	(1–4)	Monosilicic acid	500	Skin	
Zirconium (Zr)	250–420	0.01	Like V?		Fat? (*lungs)	Bile
Strontium (Sr)	340	20	½ loosely bound to protein ½ small chelates		Bone	
Rubidium (Rb)	320	90	*Free (like K⁺)		None	
Bromine (Br)	200	99	Free (like Cl⁻)	300	None	
Lead (Pb)	122	5	*Protein bound (?)	15–40	Bone	Bile
Aluminum (Al)	50–150	0.1	?	13–17	(*lung)	Urine
Copper (Cu)	72–100	30–60	Ceruloplasmin, also albumin	100	Liver	Bile
Boron (B)	48	99	?		Bone	Urine
*Tin (Sn)	(42)‡	2	?		Lung? Liver?	Urine
Cadmium (Cd)	30–38	25	Protein bound (like Ca^{++}, Zn^{++}?)	0.5–0.7	Kidney	Urine
Barium (Ba)	22	1–15	?	2–10	Skin?	Urine
*Selenium (Se)	21	35–85	Firmly to 2 proteins, loosely to others	10–30	Kidney?	Urine (bile, exhalation)
Germanium (Ge)	(20)	easy	?		Spleen	
*Iodine (I)	10–20	100	Almost all protein bound (as thyroid hormone)	2–4	Thyroid	Urine

Arsenic (As)	8–20	(5)	*	10–64	Skin? Hair?	Urine (organic), bile (inorganic)
*Manganese (Mn)	12–16	3–4	Transferrin (?)§	1–2	Liver, bone	Bile
*Molybdenum (M)	9–16	40–100	Protein bound	1	Liver	Urine (bile?)
Mercury (Hg)	13	5–10	As natural complex absorbed from diet	0.5–1	Kidney	
Vanadium (V)	10	0.1–1	Almost all in plasma	0.5–23	Fat?	Urine
Titanium (Ti)	9	1–2	Like Zr?		(*lung)	Urine
*Nickel (Ni)	5–10	3–6	Most albumin bound; some free	2–4	Skin, liver, muscle	Urine
Tellurium (Te)	7	20–50	Like Se?		Bone	
Antimony (Sb)	6	poor	Like As?		Spleen, liver, kidney	
*Chromium (Cr)	1–5	1	Transferrin,§ also globulins	1–6	Spleen, heart	Urine
*Cobalt (Co)	1.1–1.5	63–97	Albumin (little as vitamin B_{12})	0.007–6	Liver, fat	Urine

Source: Maria Linder, *Perinatal Physiology*, Plenum Press, 1977.

* This table is based on information from many sources extrapolated to the 70-kg adult, notably Underwood (1971), Schroder (1973), Schwarz (1974), Nielson and Ollerich (1974), Hopkins and Mohr (1974), Linder and Munro (1973), and Tipton and Cook (1963). Values in parentheses are tentative or controversial.

† Based on concentrations found for blood (7%), skin (10%), and other tissues (70% of body weight).

‡ Based on an overall concentration of 0.6 µg/g.

§ Cueather et al. (1974).

bumin and globulins), with very small quantities complexed with organic acids. In the blood, calcium functions in the following roles:

1 *Transmission of nerve impulses* Calcium is necessary for the release of neurotransmitters such as acetylcholine, serotonin, and norepinephrine from nerve endings.

2 *Muscle contraction* Muscle is composed of many long cells or fibers, formed by many longitudinally arranged fibrils containing hundreds of protein myofilaments composed of myosin and actin. Beside the myofilaments is the sarcoplasmic reticulum, a system of fine tubes which contain sacs stored with calcium ions. These calcium ions are essential for the actin, myosin, and adenosine triphosphate (ATP, a high-energy phosphate compound) to function in muscle contraction. The contraction of muscle or the sliding of filaments involves a reaction between actin and myosin in which actomyosin is formed and a large amount of energy is released from the cell. Contraction is initiated when the nerve signal reaches the muscle fiber, calcium is released from the reticulum sacs into the fluid surrounding the filaments where it is bound to the calcium-receptive protein of muscle (troponin), and the contraction is activated. The calcium immediately returns to the storage vesicles in the sarcoplasmic reticulum and the muscle relaxes. Magnesium is also a mineral essential to this process, since it is required for the release of energy from the cell. Without a source of energy or a loss of ATP, necessary to cause a separation of the actin and myosin filaments, muscles remain stiff, accounting for the rigor mortis that develops in muscle after death. With low levels of circulating calcium, *tetany* occurs. Tetany is a symptom complex characterized by increased neuromuscular excitability. It is a state in which the nerve fibers beome so excitable that they discharge spontaneously, initiating nerve impulses that pass to peripheral skel-

etal muscles, where they elicit tetanic contractions which may lead to cardiac and respiratory failure. Usually, tetany occurs when the blood concentration of the calcium falls below 8 mg/100 ml, which is 30 percent below the normal calcium concentration.

3 *Blood coagulation* Calcium is required for the conversion of prothrombin to thrombin during formation of the fibrin clot (see Chap. 6). Since blood clotting is normal in hypocalcemic tetany, it can be inferred that only minute quantities of calcium are required for prothrombin activation.

4 *Enzyme activation* Calcium is necessary for the activation of certain enzymes, including pancreatic lipase, plasma lipoprotein lipase, phospholipase, and phosphorylase kinase.

5 *Cell membrane permeability* Calcium regulates the transport of ions across cell membranes.

6 *Maintenance of the integrity of the intracellular cement substances and of various membranes.*

7 *Enhancement of normal cardiac function* Fluctuations in calcium blood levels affect cardiac function.

Abosrption and Utilization

Calcium for the most part is absorbed in the proximal end of the small intestine (the duodenal area).[7] Only 20 to 30 percent of dietary calcium is absorbed and the remainder is excreted in the feces, urine, and sweat. The amount of calcium absorbed is controlled by the following factors:

1 *Body need* With a small dietary supply or an increased need, the body becomes more efficient in absorption. A state of increased need is found during growth, pregnancy, stress, and calcium depletion. Under usual conditions, calcium absorption is not increased proportionately with an increased intake.

2 *Intestinal pH* An acid pH enhances calcium absorption, since calcium salts, namely

phosphates and carbonates, are soluble in acid solutions and relatively insoluble in an alkaline medium; thus, the normal gastric hydrochloric acid is necessary to facilitate efficient absorption.

3 *Food components* Substances in food that exert an influence over calcium absorption can be grouped into three categories: those exerting a positive, a negative, or a questionable effect.

- *Vitamin D* The major regulator of calcium absorption is 1,25-dihydroxycholecalciferol, a vitamin D metabolite produced by the kidney. When the plasma calcium level goes down, production of the metabolite is stimulated; when the plasma calcium goes up, lesser amounts of the metabolite are produced.

- *Calcium/phosphorus ratio* The optimum dietary calcium/phosphorus ratio for absorption of both elements has been considered to be about 2 to 1. The explanation is that an excessively high ratio of calcium causes a decrease in the absorption of phosphorus, and excessive phosphorus in relation to calcium in the intestine results in the formation of calcium phosphate, which makes the calcium unavailable for absorption. However, newer research indicates that under usual conditions a high calcium/phosphorus ratio may have little effect if the vitamin D intake is adequate.

- *Lactose* Lactose, the disaccharide found in milk, may promote calcium absorption. Two mechanisms have been suggested to explain this effect. Lactose is absorbed slowly and it is possible that a free sugar in the ileum could change the flora, thereby lowering the pH. An acid pH enhances calcium absorption. Others have suggested that lactose may combine with calcium to form a chelate which could protect it from precipitation and consequently promote absorption.[8]

- *Protein* A diet adequate in protein, particularly the amino acids lysine, arginine, and serine, has been viewed as exerting a positive effect on calcium absorption.

- *Oxalic acid and phytic acid* High levels of oxalic acid (found in spinach, chocolate, greens, rhubarb) and phytic acid (found in the outer husk of cereal grain) form insoluble salts which lower the concentration of ionizable calcium in the gut, with the net result of increasing the level of fecal calcium. This is not considered to be a problem when the dietary level of calcium is sufficiently liberal. Also, in research studies, subjects who were fed high-phytate diets adapted to the diets and, after a short period of negative balance, absorbed normal amounts of calcium. This same effect is observed in vegetarians in some parts of the world, who theoretically consume sufficient phytate to precipitate all of the calcium in the diet.[9]

4 *Quantity of bile salts present* Fats must be properly digested and absorbed or calcium absorption can be inhibited. When fats are not absorbed either because they are not hydrolyzed by lipases or because the absorption of fatty acids is impaired, fatty acids combine with free calcium and form insoluble calcium soaps, which are excreted. Also, the fat-soluble vitamin D is not absorbed, promoting a deficiency state (calcium deficiency can occur in prolonged obstructive jaundice, pancreative insufficiency, celiac disease, and sprue).

5 *Serum level of inorganic phosphorus* The metabolism of calcium is closely related to that of phosphorus, and a serum calcium/phosphorus ratio must be maintained (serum calcium level, 8.5 to 10.5 mg/100 ml; serum phosphorus level, 2.0 to 4.5 mg/100 ml).[10] A change in the serum calcium/phosphorus ratio, such as is seen in kidney disease, interferes with calcium absorption.

6 *Hormonal influences* Both the parathyroid and thyroid glands are active in influencing calcium homeostasis. When circulating plasma calcium drops, the parathyroid gland releases parathyroid hormone, which acts to (*a*) liberate calcium from the bone and (*b*) increase intestinal absorption. The liberated calcium is reabsorbed by the renal tubules, producing a rise in the serum calcium. At the same time, the parathyroid hormone causes phosphorus excretion, thus maintaining the calcium-phosphorus ratio. Calcitonin, a hormone formed by the thyroid gland, is secreted when plasma calcium levels are elevated. Calcitonin acts to decrease plasma calcium and phosphorus by (*a*) enhancing resorption of these minerals by bone and (*b*) decreasing loss of minerals from bone.

Excretion

Homeostatic mechanisms regulate the amount of calcium retained from food so that it does not exceed the amount needed by the body, thereby producing calcium equilibrium. Of the calcium ingested, 70 to 80 percent is excreted. When serum calcium is depressed or dietary intake is low, calcium absorption is more efficient, and thus excretion is less. High levels of serum calcium cause loss of calcium via the urine. Calcium excreted in the stool is mostly unabsorbed calcium from food. In persons with steatorrhea, substantial amounts of calcium can be lost in the stool. Calcium is also lost via bile and digestive secretions, and in sweat.

Calcium losses	
Fecal	100 to 200 mg/day
Urine	150 mg/day
Bile and digestive secretions	500 mg/day
Sweat	Depends on temperature; may be as high as 1 mg/day

Dietary Allowances

Evidence regarding human calcium needs has been derived from balance studies, in which calcium intake and excretion are measured. In a normal adult, it is assumed that the requirement for calcium will be equal to the excretion and that individuals can accommodate to different levels of calcium intake. Since it is difficult to establish a baseline of need, there has been much discussion concerning the levels of calcium requirements.

The 1974 edition of the National Academy of Sciences *Recommended Dietary Allowances* recommends a dietary intake level of 800 mg per day for both children and adults.[11] However, the committee does acknowledge the growth needs of children and the fact that adults are capable of maintaining a positive balance on lower intakes. The WHO Food and Agriculture Organization suggests an adult intake of 400 to 500 mg per day. The recommended intake for calcium is therefore probably somewhere between 500 and 800 mg per day.[12] During states of increased need, such as pregnancy, lactation, and adolescence, 1200 mg is recommended.

Dietary Sources

Milk and milk products are the richest food sources of calcium. Without the use of milk products, which provide 85 percent of the dietary calcium, it is very difficult to meet the recommended levels of intake. Foods containing smaller amounts of calcium are grains, fruits, nuts, vegetables, shellfish such as clams and oysters, fish (sardines and salmon), eggs, and molasses. In certain areas of the country, the drinking water may contain absorbable calcium. Table 7-3 compares the calcium content of selected foods (see also Appendix, Table A-9).

Supplementation

When calcium supplements are necessary calcium lactate and calcium gluconate are the therapeutic agents of choice. Approximately 30 to 50 percent of the available calcium is absorbed. Calcium lactate is often prescribed because it is less expensive than calcium gluconate. Calcium gluconate, however, may be preferred because of its better taste.

TABLE 7-3 CALCIUM CONTENT OF SELECTED FOODS

Type	Household measure	Weight, g	Calcium content, mg
Milk, whole*	1 cup	244	288
Milk, skim*	1 cup	244	296
Yogurt (made from whole milk)	8 oz	226	251
Cheddar cheese	1 oz	28	213
Cottage cheese (creamed)	1 oz	28	27
Ice cream (10% fat)	1 cup	133	194
Vanilla pudding (made with milk)	1 cup	255	298
Blackstrap molasses	1 tbsp	20	137

* Cow's milk contains approximately 4 times the amount of calcium in an equal volume of human milk.

Source: USDA Handbook 456, 1975.

Children who are allergic to cow's milk or who have another condition that precludes its use in the diet will need a milk substitute, such as a soy formula, or a calcium supplement to meet their needs. Other individuals, under no therapeutic restriction but eating diets that are minimal in calcium, can increase their dietary intake through the addition of fluid milk or milk solids to soups, gravies, casseroles, or baked goods.

Clinical Application

There are many disease conditions that cause clinical disturbances of calcium metabolism which are reflected in abnormalities of serum calcium or of the skeletal framework. Tables 7-4, 7-5, and 7-6 summarize those conditions that alter calcium metabolism as reflected in serum levels, urinary excretion, and fecal excretion. Although the conditions causing these alterations will be discussed in detail in later chapters, it is important to acknowledge the interrelationship between calcium and the disease state.

Osteoporosis is a metabolic disorder that causes a decrease in the amount of bone (deossification) without any change in its chemical composition or histological structure. Osteoporosis is most prevalent in postmenopausal women and in men over the age of 50. It is more common in females than in males. A decrease in estrogen production as well as unknown factors associated with the aging process cause the diminished bone formation. Other factors associated with deossification are malnutrition, especially protein malnutrition, conditions associated with protein breakdown

TABLE 7-4 CONDITIONS ALTERING SERUM CALCIUM LEVELS

Condition	Serum calcium level	
	Increased	Decreased
Primary hyperparathyroidism	×	
Secondary hyperparathyroidism	×	
Hypervitaminosis D	×	
Neoplastic disease of bone	×	
Hypophosphatasia	×	
Milk-alkali syndrome	×	
Hypoparathyroidism		×
Vitamin D deficiency (rickets, osteomalacia)		×
Steatorrhea		×
Nephrosis		×
Nephritis		×
Maternal tetany		×
Neonatal tetany		×

Source: Adapted from J. Wallach, Interpretation of Diagnostic Tests, 2d ed., Little, Brown, Boston, 1974.

TABLE 7-5 CONDITIONS ALTERING URINE CALCIUM LEVELS

	Urine calcium level	
Condition	Increased	Decreased
High calcium diet	×	
Hyperparathyroidism	×	
Hyperthyroidism	×	
Immobilization (especially children)	×	
Hypervitaminosis D	×	
Hypoparathyroidism		×
Hypothryoidism		×
Renal failure		×
Vitamin D deficiency		×

Source: Adapted from J. Wallach, *Interpretation of Diagnostic Tests*, 2d ed., Little, Brown, Boston, 1974.

(e.g., Cushing's syndrome), acromegaly, hyperthyroidism, lack of exercise, and prolonged immobilization. It can also occur following a prolonged course of corticosteroid therapy.

Osteoporosis per se causes no disability, except that it increases the likelihood of broken bones. However, there are several clinical symptoms of osteoporosis. Hypercalciuria may develop initially, especially when prolonged immobilization is a factor and renal calculi form. Besides bone fractures, other symptoms of osteoporosis include weakness, anorexia, hip and back pain, muscle tenderness, and cramping. Stooped posture and a loss of height result from a shrinking spine.

The best prophylaxis for middle-aged persons is to remain physically active. Cyclic administration of estrogen has been used in the treatment of osteoporosis. It frequently relieves pain and has been suggested to be the only long-term treatment which prevents additional fractures. Androgens and other anabolic steroids were formerly used but are now used infrequently because of their virilizing effects on women.[13] The use of fluoride for treatment of osteoporosis is under investigation (see "Fluoride," below).

Because osteoporotic bones have already lost both calcium and phosphate it would seem reasonable to conclude that diets low in these minerals might accelerate the process. However, there is no firm evidence to support this contention. A 1972 investigation found no significant correlation between the calcium intake and the bone density of middle-aged subjects.[14]

Phosphorus

After calcium, phosphorus is the most abundant mineral in the body. There are approximately 12 g of phosphorus per kilogram of fat-free body tissue. Although most phosphorus (85 percent) is present in the skeleton, smaller amounts are found in the red blood cells and plasma. The plasma inorganic phosphate level in adults is usually 3 to 4 mg/100 ml. Children have slightly higher levels.[15]

Function

All body cells contain organic phosphates, which play a vital role in cellular functioning:

1 *Component of ribonucleic acid (RNA) and deoxyribonucleic acid (DNA)* The nucleic proteins involved in reproduction, cell division, and transmission of hereditary traits.

2 *Component of cellular membranes* Phospholipids which are present in cell membranes are major determinants of cell permeability.

TABLE 7-6 CONDITIONS ALTERING FECAL CALCIUM LEVELS

	Fecal calcium level	
Condition	Increased	Decreased
Rickets	×	
Osteomalacia	×	
Sprue	×	
Celiac disease	×	
Chronic nephrosis	×	

Source: Adapted from J. Wallach, *Interpretation of Diagnostic Tests*, 2d ed., Little, Brown, Boston, 1974.

3 *Phosphorylation in metabolic pathways* For example, the oxidation of carbohydrate, culminating in the formation of adenosine triphosphate (ATP), requires phosphorus because phosphorylation is a required step in the metabolism of monosaccharides.

4 *Component of high-energy phosphate compounds.* Phosphorus is a part of the structure of adenosine diphosphate (ADP) and ATP, which are compounds involved in processes related to the storage and release of energy.

5 *Component of B vitamin coenzymes.* Several B vitamins (e.g., niacin) are effective only in the coenzyme form, which contains phosphorus.

Absorption and Utilization

Approximately 70 percent of the phosphorus that is ingested is absorbed. There is minimal control over the absorption of phosphorus and body content is principally regulated by urinary excretion. Provided that vitamin D intake is adequate, wide variations in the intake ratio of calcium to phosphorus are tolerated. An acid pH in the upper intestine and normal motility of the gastrointestinal tract promote absorption of phosphorus.

Dietary Allowances

There is little direct information concerning the human requirement for phosphorus. In adults, the intake of phosphorus often exceeds that of calcium. The intake recommended by the National Academy of Sciences is the same as that for calcium, except in the infant. Current evidence supports a calcium/phosphorus ratio of 1.5 to 1 in early infancy. The calcium/phosphorus ratio of cow's milk is 1.2 to 1 while in human milk it is 2 to 1. Some investigators have suggested that a phosphorus intake such as that provided by cow's milk could contribute to the occurrence of neonatal tetany.[16] Infants on formulas derived from soybeans or other vegetable sources may not get sufficient posphorus because some of it is in the form of phytate and consequently not readily available for absorption.[17]

Dietary Sources

Because phosphorus is present in nearly all foods, there is no indication that human intake of the mineral is ever low enough to interfere with vital body processes. Diets which provide adequate levels of protein and calcium can be inferred to contain a sufficient amount of phosphorus as well. Foods rich in phosphorus include milk and milk products, nuts, legumes, cereals, meat, fish, poultry, and eggs. Cow's milk has a greater phosphorus content than human milk. Food manufacturers use phosphorus as an additive in many processed foods.

Clinical Application

Depletion of body phosphorus can result from prolonged intake of high doses of nonabsorbable antacids. Clinical signs of depletion are weakness, anorexia, malaise, bone pain, and bone demineralization, coupled with a marked increase in urinary calcium excretion. Treatment involves discontinuing the use of antacids and ingestion of a diet high in phosphorus. Metabolism of phosphorus can be disturbed in many disease states, especially in kidney and bone disorders (see Chaps. 19 and 20).

Sulfur

Sulfur is found in all body cells and is essential to life. It is principally found as a part of the protein structure of the living cell. Sulfur-containing compounds play several important roles in the body. Sulfur and nitrogen metabolism are closely related.

Function

1 *Part of the structure of amino acids* Sulfur is a component of the chemical structure of methionine, cysteine, and cystine (the double form of cysteine). Keratin, the protein of hair, is rich in sulfur.

2 *Component of two known vitamins* Thiamine and biotin contain sulfur.

3 *Required for many oxidation-reduction reactions and coenzymes* Enzyme systems containing coenzyme A and glutathione depend on free sulfhydryl (SH) groups for their activity. SH groups are important in tissue respiration. Other organic compounds of sulfur include heparin, lipoic acid, ergothioneine, taurocholic acid, and chondroitin sulfate.

4 *Contained in blood and other tissues*   Small amounts of inorganic sulfates, along with sodium and potassium, are present in blood and other tissues.

5 *Active in detoxification mechanisms*   Sulfur-containing compounds such as sulfuric acid combine with other components to detoxify compounds which would otherwise be harmful to the body.

6 *Contained in polysaccharides.*   Sulfur is a part of polysaccharides found in cartilage, tendons, bones, and skin.

No conclusive studies of sulfur intake and output have been reported in the literature. This can probably be attributed to the difficulty in estimating small amounts of sulfur. An adult normally excretes between 1 and 2 g of sulfur daily. Some effects of protein deficiency may be due to inadequate synthesis of sulfur-containing enzymes or polysaccharides.

Dietary Allowances and Dietary Sources

No specific recommendation for sulfur intake has been established. The primary sources of sulfur in the diet are the sulfur-containing amino acids. A mixed diet providing 100 g of protein will provide a range of 0.6 to 1.6 g of sulfur.[18]

Magnesium

A 70-kg human contains 20 to 28 g of magnesium.[19] Magnesium is found principally in bone and muscle tissue. Approximately half of the body's magnesium content is not freely exchangeable.[20] The normal range of magnesium in the serum is 1.8 to 3.0 mg/100 ml.[21]

Function

1 *Essential for the mobilization of calcium from bone.*

2 *Ranks after potassium as the most important cation in living cells.*

3 *A part of many enzyme systems.*   It is essential for cellular respiration; specifically, in the oxidative phosphorylation process leading to the formation of adenine triphosphate. It is critical to all phosphate transfer systems. It functions as an activator for many of the enzymes of the glycolytic systems.

4 *Plays a role in protein synthesis.*   Magnesium binds messenger RNA. It is also important in the synthesis and degradation of DNA.

5 *May also influence parathyroid hormone secretion.*[22]

6 *Plays a possible role in the prevention of cardiovascular disease.*[23]

Absorption and Excretion

There is great variability in the levels of magnesium intake. Approximately 30 to 40 percent of the magnesium that is ingested is absorbed and utilized by the body. Several factors influence the absorption of magnesium; among these are the amounts of calcium, phosphate, and lactose in the diet; intestinal transit time; and the rate of water absorption from the gastrointestinal tract.

Maintenance of a normal range of magnesium in the blood depends on a balance between absorption and renal excretion of sodium. There is no known hormonal regulatory mechanism.

Magnesium is lost via both urine and feces. Gastric juice is relatively high in magnesium content, so that significant amounts can be lost during prolonged episodes of vomiting or diarrhea.

Dietary Allowances

A magnesium intake of 350 mg for men and 300 mg for women has been suggested. Human milk contains 4 mg/100 ml, and recommendations for infants have been formulated in relation to that level. Recommendations for childhood and adolescence are estimates, designed to allow for rapid growth. To date, there is little information concerning needs during pregnancy and lactation.[24]

Dietary Sources

The mineral is widely distributed in foods, particularly in vegetables, which contain chlorophyll, a magnesium porphyrin. The typical diet in Western countries provides about 5 mg of magnesium/kg of body weight per day. Oriental persons typically ingest a diet rich in magnesium and their intake has been found to be approximately 6 to 10 mg/kg of body weight per day.

Clinical Application

Acute deficiency in humans is manifested by tremors, tetany, repetitive involuntary movements, seizures, mental disorientation, and tachycardia. Magnesium deficiency affects calcium, phosphorus, and sodium metabolism.

Several clinical conditions can predispose the individual to magnesium deficiency. Among these are malabsorption syndromes, loss of gastrointestinal fluids, chronic diarrhea, and ulcerative colitis. Severe protein depletion such as that which occurs in protein-calorie malnutrition can increase the risk of magnesium depletion. Increased renal excretion of magnesium can result from the use of diuretics and can occur in severe alcoholism. Prolonged parenteral feeding using solutions which contain little or no magnesium can lead to deficiency. Patients on hemodialysis should be carefully observed for signs of hypomagnesemia. Conditions that elevate or decrease serum magnesium levels are summarized in Table 7-7.

MICROMINERALS

Iron

Function

The body of a 7-kg adult contains between 4 and 5 g of iron. Of this, 70 percent may be classified as functional or essential iron and 30 percent as storage iron. Because of its presence

TABLE 7-7 CONDITIONS ALTERING SERUM MAGNESIUM LEVELS

Condition	Serum magnesium level	
	Increased	Decreased
Renal failure	×	
Diabetic coma	×	
Hypothyroidism	×	
Addison's disease and after adrenalectomy	×	
Controlled diabetes mellitus in older age groups	×	
Administration of magnesium-containing antacids	×	
Malabsorption and abnormal loss of gastrointestinal fluids*		×
Acute alcoholism or alcoholic cirrhosis		×
Insulin treatment of diabetic coma		×
Hyperthyroidism		×
Aldosteronism		×
Hyperparathyroidism	×	
Hypoparathyroidism		×
Lytic tumors of bone		×
Renal disease		×
Excessive lactation		×

* E.g., nontropical sprue, small bowel resection, biliary and intestinal fistulas, abdominal irradiation, prolonged aspiration of intestinal contents; celiac disease and other causes of steatorrhea.

Source: Adapted from J. Wallach, *Interpretation of Diagnostic Tests,* Little, Brown, Boston, 1974.

in the hemoprotein enzymes and in the cytochromes, iron is vitally involved in the oxidative mechanisms of all living cells.[25] It is complexed with a variety of protein molecules which determine its function. When the iron-containing pigment heme combines with the colorless protein globin, the resultant molecule is hemoglobin. Iron is also combined in other enzymes such as catalase, peroxidase, and Warburg's respiratory enzyme which perform their electron transport in tissue respiration by virtue of their iron content.

As part of hemoglobin, four atoms of iron are combined with two alpha- and two beta-polypeptide chains and four protoporphyrin molecules. The hemeglobin molecule is 4 percent heme and 96 percent globin. The ability of hemoglobin to carry oxygen from the lungs to the tissues and to carry carbon dioxide back relates to the presence of iron in the heme molecule. Without iron, the oxygen supply to tissues is diminished and hypoxia of blood and tissues results.

Absorption

Iron absorption is affected by the body's iron status, the state of health, age, and gastrointestinal conditions. Absorption is also influenced by the amount and form of iron ingested as well as the amounts of various other substances in the diet. Iron absorption is an active process and iron is absorbed only in the ferrous state. Under usual conditions, only 5 to 10 percent of the iron ingested is absorbed by the body; however, in those who are iron-deficient, the amount absorbed can range from 10 to 20 percent, as the ability to absorb iron increases in states of deficiency. Infants and children absorb a greater proportion of ingested iron than adults do because of their increased growth needs.

The primary absorption site for iron is in the upper small intestine (duodenum and jejunum), although a limited amount is absorbed in the stomach. Ascorbic acid and other reducing substances, such as cysteine, facilitate the absorption of iron through reducing the ferric form (FE^{3+}) to the ferrous form (FE^{2+}), while phytates and cellulose diminish the absorption of iron. Geophagia (the practice of eating clay) also interferes with absorption.

There are great differences in the availability of different forms of iron for absorption.[26] Most available is ferrous sulfate; other organic complexes or chelates of iron are also easily absorbed. The availability of reduced metallic iron is moderate and is probably related to the particle size of the preparation. Iron phosphates and carbonates are poorly absorbed.[27]

Absorption is sometimes impaired in persons who have had total or subtotal gastrectomies and in those who have had portions of the small intestine removed.

Absorption of iron is an active process. Mucosal cells of the duodenum and jejunum send part of the iron directly to the bloodstream where most of it is bound as *apoferritin.* This protein combines with iron to form *ferritin.* Ferritin is the major storage form of iron in the tissues and the serum ferritin concentration is in direct equilibrium with the total body iron content. Immunoassays of serum ferritin are increasingly being used to identify minor dietary deficiencies of iron before a frank clinical deficiency state develops. *Hemosiderin* is another storage form of iron.

Excretion

Under usual circumstances, little iron is absorbed and the amounts excreted in the urine are small. Iron is also lost in feces and sweat and, in women, as a result of blood losses during menstruation and pregnancy. Menstrual losses of iron can vary widely.[28] The average amount of iron lost during each menstrual period is 30 mg. Because of the small percentage of iron absorbed, and the amount lost monthly, females have a higher iron requirement than males.

There is no physiological mechanism which allows the body to excrete excess iron effectively. Therefore, control of absorption is the first line of defense in preventing the accumulation of iron in toxic amounts in body tissues.

Dietary Allowances

During the life cycle, there appear to be three periods when iron intake may be inadequate: (1) infancy, especially for infants born of women with low stores and from low socioeconomic families; (2) the years of menstruation; and (3) pregnancy and childbirth. The increased need during pregnancy is due to increased blood volume, necessitating an increased production of red blood cells to maintain a near-normal hematocrit. Also, an average of 270 mg of iron is transferred to the fetus and another 240 mg is lost at delivery. Iron stores in the normal infant born at term are exhausted in 3 to 6 months if not replaced.

Consequently, recommendations for infants and women are generous. The recommended allowance in infancy is based on an average need of 1.5 mg/kg of body weight per day.[29] Recommended daily allowances are 10 mg for infants and 15 mg for children. The allowance for women of child-bearing age is 18 mg per day, which allows for the needs imposed by menstruation, pregnancy, and lactation. A woman on an adequate diet, ingesting calories at the recommended levels, will only derive 9 to 12 mg of iron per day from dietary sources. It can be particularly difficult to ingest adequate amounts if the woman is a vegetarian. During pregnancy, a supplementary intake of 30 to 60 mg of iron per day is recommended. For postmenopausal women and for men, an intake of 10 mg per day is recommended.

Dietary Sources

Organ meats are excellent sources of dietary iron. Red meats are also rich in iron. Other good sources include fortified cereals, cooked dried beans, peas, spinach, dried fruits, enriched breads and cereals, and molasses. Milk and milk products are poor sources. Table 7-8 provides a comparison of the iron content of selected foods.

Clinical Application

The primary consequence of iron deficiency is anemia. The causes of iron-deficiency anemia are given in Table 7-9. They can be summarized under four categories:

1 Iron-poor diet
2 Increased iron losses
3 Malabsorption of iron
4 Increased iron requirements

Iron-deficiency anemia is characterized as microcytic hypochromic anemia because the red cells are small (microcytic) and pale (hypochromic). As anemia develops, there is a nat-

TABLE 7-8 IRON CONTENT OF SELECTED FOODS

Type	Amount of food	Iron content, mg
Beef liver (fried)	1 slice (85 g)	7.5
Chicken liver (chopped)	½ cup (70 g)	6.0
Braunschweiger (liver sausage)	1 slice (18 g)	1.1
Roast beef (chuck roast)	1 piece (85 g)	2.9
Hamburger	4 oz patty (113 g)	3.5
Kidney beans	1 cup (185 g)	12.8
Peas	1 cup (160 g)	2.9
Dried apricots	½ cup (50 g)	2.7
Raisins	½ cup (67 g)	2.3
Whole-wheat bread	1 slice (25 g)	0.8
Enriched white bread	1 slice (28 g)	0.7
Molasses (blackstrap)	1 tbsp (20 g)	3.2
Fortified instant-cooking wheat cereal	½ cup (122 g)	1.1
Infant rice cereal (dry)	3 tbsp (7 g)	6.6
Strained beef	3½ oz jar (100 g)	2.0
Strained beef with vegetables	4½ oz jar (128 g)	1.5
Strained vegetables with beef	4½ oz jar (128 g)	1.0

Source: USDA Handbook 456, 1975.

ural sequence of compensatory mechanisms. Initially, as iron stores become depleted, the body becomes more efficient in iron absorption. Then the serum level of iron decreases and the iron-binding capacity of serum transferrin increases.[30] The percent of transferrin saturation is indicative of the amount of iron available to the erythroid marrow for red blood cell formation (average values: serum iron, 80 to 160 μg/100 ml in males, 60 to 135 μg/100 ml in females; iron-binding capacity, 250 to 350 μg/100 ml; percent saturation, 20 to 55 percent; transferrin, 300 to 359 mg/100 ml).[31]

As time progresses, the red cell pattern emerges. If the anemia is untreated, characteristic tissue changes may appear, including

TABLE 7-9 CAUSES OF IRON DEFICIENCY

I   Iron-poor diet
II   Increased iron loss
    A   Excessive menstruation
    B   Chronic blood loss
       1   Peptic ulcer
       2   Lesions of gastrointestinal tract
       3   Lesions of genitourinary tract
    C   Chronic hemoglobinuria
    D   Parasitic infections (e.g., hookworm)
    E   Blood loss due to other causes (surgery, trauma)
III   Malabsorption of iron
    A   Postgastrectomy
    B   Small-bowel disease
IV   Increased iron requirements
    A   Pregnancy
    B   Infancy

Source: J. A. Koepke, "Iron Deficiency Anemia," *Postgraduate Medicine,* 163:163, 1972.

spoon nails, cheilosis, glossitis, and, on rare occasions, a membranous obstruction of the upper esophagus.

Clinical signs of mild iron-deficiency anemia are weakness, lassitude, and fatigue. Pagophagia (ice eating) has been observed in some iron-deficient persons. Some investigators have suggested that in utero or during the first 2 years of life an infant can sustain permanent damage through effects on the cerebral oxidative metabolism, neurotransmitter synthesis, or brain cell mitosis.[32] Others have demonstrated disruptive behavior in anemic adolescents and have observed apathetic and irritable behavior, along with short attention span, in anemic preschool youngsters.[33] These behaviors were observed in children with hemoglobins in the 8.5 to 10 g range. The incidence iron deficiency may be as high as 20 percent among certain pediatric populations.

The hematocrit and the hemoglobin level are used as routine screening measures of populations. These measures must be interpreted according to age and physiological state, since variations in total blood volume affect the definition of anemia. (See Table 7-10.)

In the treatment of iron-deficiency anemia, the use of iron medication should be teamed with nutritional education centered on the importance of consuming a diet that is adequate in iron and also in vitamin C, which aids in absorption. Parents of young children may be given additional counseling help concerning introducing new foods and weaning from the bottle. Within 7 days after initiation of oral iron therapy, the hemoglobin begins to rise. Within 4 to 8 weeks, hemoglobin values approach normal levels; however, therapy should be continued for 6 to 12 months if stores are to be repleted.

Oral administration of ferrous salts (sulfate, gluconate, or fumarate) provides therapy. The therapeutic dose is calculated in terms of elemental iron present, and varies with the type of iron used. Ferrous sulfate yields 20 percent elemental iron. A total daily dose of 4.5 to 6 mg/kg of body weight is divided into three doses, which is considered optimal for bone marrow utilization. Iron should be given

TABLE 7-10 NORMAL VALUES BY AGE

Age	Hemoglobin, g	Hematocrit, %
6–23 months	10	31
2–5 years	11	34
6–14 years	12	37
15 years + (male)	13	40
15 years + ∓female)	12	37
15 years + (pregnant female)	11	34

Source: Center for Disease Control, Department of Health, Education, and Welfare.

HOW IRON DEFICIENCY EVOLVES:

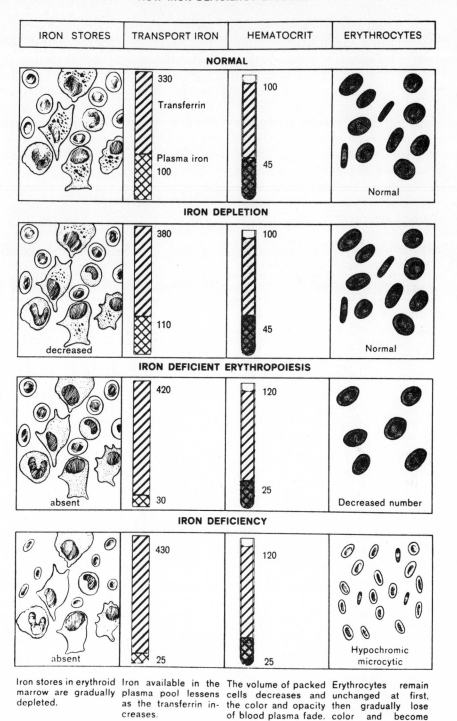

IRON STORES	TRANSPORT IRON	HEMATOCRIT	ERYTHROCYTES

NORMAL

330
Transferrin

Plasma iron
100

100

45

Normal

IRON DEPLETION

380

110

100

45

Normal

decreased

IRON DEFICIENT ERYTHROPOIESIS

420

30

120

25

absent

Decreased number

IRON DEFICIENCY

430

25

120

25

absent

Hypochromic
microcytic

Iron stores in erythroid marrow are gradually depleted.

Iron available in the plasma pool lessens as the transferrin increases.

The volume of packed cells decreases and the color and opacity of blood plasma fade.

Erythrocytes remain unchanged at first, then gradually lose color and become smaller.

Figure 7-2

The progression of iron-deficiency anemia. (From Clement Finch, "Iron Metabolism," Nutrition Today, Summer 1969, p. 6.)

between meals to avoid interference with absorption from chelating agents contained in foods. Ingestion of milk interferes with absorption, and medication should not be placed in an infant's bottle.

Hemochromatosis is a genetic disorder of iron metabolism which is characterized by a large accumulation of iron, as hemosiderin, in the tissues. Hepatic, pancreatic, and cardiac problems are common. Pigmentation, diabetes mellitus, and hepatic cirrhosis are classic signs of the disorder. The excessive accumulation of iron is the result of long-term elevated absorption of iron.[34]

In the treatment of hemochromatosis, the objective is to remove excess iron from the body. Usually, phlebotomy (incision of a vein and removal of blood) is the method used to achieve mobilization of parenchymal iron stores. However, in anemic persons deferoxamine (a chelating agent) has been used to promote iron excretion.[35]

Besides hemochromatosis, there are several other conditions which may result in markedly increased levels of iron. Among these are repeated transfusions, excessive administration of intravenous iron, and excessive intake of dietary or supplementary iron, causing an increased storage of iron or hemosiderosis.

Iodine

The adult body contains approximately 10 to 20 mg of iodine. Most iodine is concentrated in the thyroid gland and deficiency states cause an enlargement of the gland, producing a swelling in the front part of the neck (goiter).

Function

The sole function of iodine is to serve as a component of the thyroid hormones thyroxine and triiodothyronine, and of other compounds produced by the thyroid gland.

Absorption and Excretion

Dietary iodine is converted to iodide in the gastrointestinal tract; iodide is efficiently ab-

sorbed. The thyroid gland is the only tissue that has a capability for utilizing iodide, which it does in the synthesis of the two thyroid hormones, thyroxine and triiodothyronine. The activity of the thyroid gland is regulated by thyrotropic hormone, which is secreted by the pituitary gland. There is no mechanism which allows for the conservation of iodine in the face of dietary deficiency. Iodine is excreted via the urine.

Dietary Allowances

The dietary need for iodine is probably different in different regions of the country. In general, it is recommended that an intake of 100 μg daily will provide a sufficient amount of iodine, providing that intake of goitrogens (substances that have antithyroid activity) is limited. Goitrin is a goitrogen and is found in turnips, rutabagas, and other members of the cabbage family. It is unlikely that goiter will develop solely as the result of ingesting large amounts of these foods. Some medicines, such as the thiocarbamides, are also known for their antithyroid activity.

Dietary Sources

Seafood is the only naturally occurring major source of iodine. The iodine content of a particular agricultural food can vary greatly depending on local variations in soil and fertilizers. Generally, land nearer the sea has a better natural iodine content than the mountainous regions of the midwest. Iodized salt provides a primary source of iodine for many persons. Also, milk and bread made with iodate dough conditioners can be considered as contributors to dietary iodine.

Clinical Application

Iodine deficiency, manifested as simple goiter, can occur in areas where the soil is low in iodine and dietary intake of iodine-rich substances such as seafoods and iodized salt is inadequate to meet body needs. Endemic goiter (see Chap. 20) occurs principally in two areas of the United States: the Great Lakes and the Rocky Mountain regions. Treatment involves administration of iodine-containing preparations, ingestion of a diet rich in iodine, and use of iodized salt. Originally, iodine deficiency was considered to be the cause of all cases of goiter. However, iodine replacement therapy alone has not always been effective in eliminating goiter. Consequently, those treating goiter have carefully monitored the efficacy of iodine replacement therapy.

During fetal or neonatal periods, thyroid deficiency results in cretinism, a syndrome of infancy and early childhood (see Chap. 20). The etiology can be identified as an abnormal development of the thyroid gland, an inborn error of thyroid hormone metabolism, or, in endemic goiter regions a dietary iodine deficiency.

Clinical signs of cretinism are thick, dry skin, thick lips, and a broad face. Infants with cretinism usually are lethargic and show mild to severe mental retardation; hypotonia and constipation are also noted.

Treatment involves administration of desiccated thyroid until a euthyroid (normal) state is achieved. Adequate dietary intake of iodine is stressed and use of iodized salt is recommended.

Fluoride

Fluoride is widely distributed in soils and water as well as in plant and animal life. Traces of this mineral are present in teeth, bones, skin, and the thyroid gland.

Function

Fluoride provides protection against dental caries (see Chap. 23). It has been suggested that fluoride may strengthen the structure of the tooth and limit the solubility of tooth minerals.[36] Although its anticariogenic action is especially important during the growth years, it persists throughout adult life.

Fluoride is an inhibitor of some enzyme systems, such as enolase, the enzyme in the process that converts glyceric to pyruvic acid during glycolysis. Inhibition of the citric acid cycle has also been described. Excess intake of fluoride can therefore have potential effects on metabolism.

Dietary Allowances and Sources

There are no specific dietary recommendations relating to fluoride intake. Dietary intake has been observed to range from 0.3 mg per day in low-fluoride areas to 3.1 mg per day in high-fluoride areas.[37]

Drinking water can provide a major source of fluoride. Many areas have fluoridated their water supplies to a standard level of 1 ppm (part per million), which equals 1 mg of fluoride per liter of water. Seafood and tea are considered to be good dietary sources of the mineral.

Clinical Application

Some researchers have studied the use of fluoride in the treatment of osteoporosis and Paget's disease of bone. To date, results are inconclusive, although some patients with osteoporosis have been reported to be improved through administration of sodium fluoride.

Fluoride can be poisonous if consumed in large amounts. Toxicity has been identified in industrial workers handling fluoride-containing substances such as cryolite. One of the initial signs of fluoride excess (fluorosis) is mottling of tooth enamel. Toxic signs include anorexia and sclerosis of the spine. (see Chap. 23.) Dietary deficiency may result in serious problems with dental caries.

Copper

Copper is an essential mineral for most animal species. The highest concentrations of copper in the body are found in the plasma and red blood cells. The normal plasma level ranges from 65 to 170 μg/100 ml.[38] Copper is also present in muscle, liver, brain, heart, and kidney tissues.

Function

The mineral is a constituent of several enzymes or is essential in their activity; these include cytochrome, cytochrome oxidase, catalase, tryo-sinase, monoamine oxidase, and ascorbic acid oxidase. Together with iron, copper is required for the synthesis of hemoglobin. The copper-binding protein in plasma is ceruloplasmin, which may act in the oxidation of plasma iron to allow formation of transferrin-bound iron. Cerebrocuprein is a copper protein which has been isolated from brain tissue.

The role of copper in human nutrition is incompletely understood; some have suggested that it may be involved in bone formation, in maintenance of myelin in the nervous system, and in gastrointestinal function.

Absorption and Excretion

Copper is absorbed from the stomach and upper small intestine (duodenum). It is excreted via the bile, urine, feces, sweat, and menstrual fluid. Only about 5 percent of the copper ingested is retained by the body.

Dietary Allowances and Sources

Copper intakes ranging from 1.3 to 2 mg per day seem to be adequate for adolescents and adults. For children, an intake of 0.08 mg/kg of body weight per day appears adequate. In general, most individuals' copper intake is in excess of requirements.[39]

Fish, poultry, liver, oysters, kidney, chocolate, nuts, green vegetables, dried fruits, legumes, and whole grains are good dietary sources of copper.

Clinical Application

Copper deficiency, as manifested by hypocupremia, has been observed in individuals with protein-calorie malnutrition, sprue, cystic fibrosis, or kidney disease, and in those undergoing prolonged parenteral nutrition. Infants who were maintained for extended periods of time on diets consisting only of milk manifested symptoms similar to those seen in copper-deficient animals.[40,41] These symptoms include hypoproteinemia, hypocupremia, ane-

mia, poor growth, neutropenia (a decrease in neutrophilic leukocytes in the blood), and low ceruloplasmin levels. These symptoms are reversed by the administration of iron and copper.[42]

Menke's kinky hair syndrome in infants is a genetically determined disorder of copper metabolism which manifests itself in kinky hair (due to lack of keratinization), mental retardation, hypothermia, low plasma copper, skeletal changes, and degenerative changes in heart tissue. With copper therapy, children with the disease are surviving longer than before such intervention was attempted.

Wilson's disease is a rare autosomal recessive disease which is characterized by degeneration of brain tissue and cirrhosis of the liver. Large amounts of copper are deposited in the tissues. The serum copper and copper content of ceruloplasmin are low. Large amounts of copper are excreted in the urine. Kidney problems are also common. Therapy for this disorder involves use of a chelating agent which promotes copper excretion. A low-copper diet has been viewed as an effective therapeutic adjunct. If diagnosed early and treated throughout life, prognosis is fairly good for those who have the disorder.

Table 7-11 presents a summarization of disorders which can affect serum copper.

Recently it has been postulated that a metabolic zinc-copper imbalance may be a major factor in the etiology of coronary heart disease.[43] This imbalance, a relative or absolute deficiency of copper with a high ratio of zinc to copper, may result in hypercholesterolemia and an increased mortality due to coronary heart disease.

Zinc

The human body contains 2 to 3 g of zinc. Although the need for zinc in animals has been recognized for several decades, clinical signs of human zinc deficiency were initially described in 1961 in males. Ten years later, similar symptoms were documented in females.

TABLE 7-11 CONDITIONS CAUSING AN INCREASE OR DECREASE IN SERUM COPPER

Increased in

Anemia

Pernicious anemia

Megaloblastic anemia of pregnancy

Iron-deficiency anemia

Aplastic anemia

Leukemia

Infection

Malignant lymphoma

Hemochromatosis

Collagen diseases

Hyperthyroidism, hypothroidism

Oral contraceptive users

Decreased in

Nephrosis

Wilson's disease

Acute leukemia in remission

Some iron-deficiency anemias of childhood requiring both copper and iron therapy

Protein-calorie malnutrition

Function

Zinc is an essential constituent for the activity of a number of metalloenzymes such as carbonic anhydrase, carboxypeptidase, alkaline phosphatase, aspartate transcarbamylase, mannisodase, aminopeptidase, dehydrogenases dipeptidase, superoxide, dismutase, DNA polymerase, and aldolase. Zinc is a component of insulin and has a role in taste, auditory, and olfactory acuity. It is required for normal growth and sexual maturation. Zinc has been identified as important in the wound healing process.[44]

Absorption and Excretion

Approximately 20 to 30 percent of dietary zinc is absorbed.[45] The site and mechanism of absorption are not clearly understood. Presence of phytates in the diet can compromise the absorption of zinc. These phytates tend to form insoluble zinc-phytate complexes. High levels of calcium can further decrease zinc availability by forming a zinc-calcium-phytate complex. Geophagia (clay eating) has also been noted to interfere with absorption of zinc.

Excretion of the mineral is via gastrointestinal and pancreatic secretions. Body reserves of zinc are not easily mobilized, and consequently there is a need for a regular intake of the mineral, particularly during periods of growth and stress.

Dietary Allowances and Sources

The 1974 edition of the National Academy of Sciences *Recommended Dietary Allowances* suggests a zinc intake of 15 mg per day for the adult, with an additional 5 mg per day during pregnancy and 10 mg during lactation. Recommendations for infants and children range from 3 mg for infants up to 6 months of age, to 10 mg for early childhood.

Though zinc is widely distributed in foods, perhaps the best source is red meats. Seafood and oysters are also relatively high in zinc content. The zinc content of foods is subject to wide variation, related to a net loss of zinc in the soil due to natural leaching, erosion, and constant removal of crops without repletion.

Clinical Application

One study of 35 persons with zinc deficiency noted hypogeusia (diminished taste sensation), anorexia, weight loss, and psychological problems.[46] Another noted poor growth and impaired taste acuity in school-aged children. Growth retardation, sexual immaturity, and skin lesions have been observed in other zinc-deficient subjects. Some have suggested that zinc deficiency impedes wound healing through allowing lipid peroxidation of cellular membranes. Administration of supplementary zinc allows stabilization of the cell membranes through decreasing lipid peroxidation of these structures. Various teratogenic effects of zinc deficiency have been noted in rats and chicks.

Zinc poisoning can occur as a result of eating foods stored in galvanized containers. Toxic signs are gastrointestinal distress, vomiting, diarrhea, and fever.

Several conditions known to lower serum zinc levels are pregnancy, upper respiratory infections, kidney disease, sickle cell anemia, myocardial infarction, and malignant neoplasms. Oral contraceptives may also lower serum zinc. Zinc levels are decreased in pernicious anemia; however, this is reversed by vitamin B_{12} therapy. The metabolism of zinc is significantly altered in persons with alcoholic cirrhosis of the liver, since a key step in the metabolism of alcohol requires an enzyme containing zinc (liver alcohol dehydrogenase).

Manganese

Despite the fact that manganese deficiency has not been described in human subjects, it has been postulated that the mineral plays a role in human lipid metabolism. The largest concentrations of manganese are found in the bone, liver, pancreas, and pituitary. The adult human body contains approximately 16 to 20 mg of manganese.

Function, Absorption, and Excretion

Manganese is important in bone formation, brain function, and reproduction. It is a component of several enzyme systems.

Manganese is absorbed rather poorly from the gastrointestinal tract. About 40 percent of the 2.5 to 7 mg typically ingested by adults is absorbed from the small intestine. High levels of calcium and phosphorus in the diet are known to diminish absorption. Excretion of manganese is through the bile and pancreatic juice.

Dietary Allowances and Sources

No formal recommendations for manganese intake have been established. Since no cases of overt deficiency have been described in humans, it seems reasonable to assume that the average daily intake of 2.5 to 7 mg meets the requirement.

Nuts, seeds, and whole grains are good sources of manganese; fruits and vegetables provide moderate amounts.

Cobalt

Cobalt is a component of vitamin B_{12} (see Chap. 6). The bacterial synthesis of vitamin B_{12} requires the mineral. Cobalt has been used in the treatment of anemia in children. Aside from this, no metabolic role for the mineral has been discovered.

Selenium

The body contains approximately 21 mg of selenium. There is evidence that selenium is an essential component of the enzyme glutathione peroxidase. It is known that glutathione protects red blood cells through destruction of hydrogen peroxide and fatty acid hydroperoxides through reactions catalyzed by glutathione peroxidase. This role for selenium clarifies the relationship between vitamin E and selenium in the prevention of lipid peroxidation.

Both selenium deficiency and excess are important diseases in animals in some locales. Although suboptimal selenium nutriture has been observed in severely malnourished persons, neither overt deficiency nor excess has been reported. To date, no recommended dietary allowance has been set. The average American diet provides about 1 μg per day. High-protein foods such as meats and seafoods have been found to be the best sources of selenium. Although grains can provide a reasonable source, their content varies depending on the soil in which they are grown.

Chromium

Chromium probably acts as a cofactor for insulin. In some individuals with diabetes an improvement of glucose tolerance has been observed following the administration of chromium. Also, research has demonstrated improvement in glucose tolerance of malnourished children as a result of chromium administration.

The mean daily chromium intake of subjects consuming institutional diets has been reported as 52 to 78 μg daily.[47] Approximately 10 to 25 percent of chromium from foods is absorbed. Sources of chromium include most animal proteins (except fish), whole grains, and brewers' yeast. Refinement of cereal products can markedly lower the chromium content and this loss is not replaced by current fortification. Several investigators have suggested that marginal chromium deficiencies may occur among elderly persons, pregnant women, and those suffering from protein-calorie malnutrition. There is no basis upon which to establish a firm recommendation for chromium intake.

Molybdenum

Molybdenum is an essential component of xanthine oxidase, the enzyme responsible for the conversion of xanthine to uric acid. The estimated average intake of the mineral in the United States is between 45 and 500 μg per day. No dietary recommendations have been established. Beef kidney, some cereals, and legumes are considered to be good sources.

Other Minerals

Nickel, tin, vanadium, and silicon have been found to be essential for some animal species, thereby raising speculation that they might be required for humans as well. To date, their implications for human nutrition have not been adequately explored.

STUDY QUESTIONS

1 Differentiate between macrominerals and microminerals.

CASE STUDY

Past History

Jeremy, aged 19 months, was brought by his parents to the clinic pediatrician with the chief complaints of listlessness, irritability, and constipation. The past history was unremarkable. Initially, he fed well on a standard infant formula (not fortified with iron) and accepted all baby foods well. At 6 months of age, when junior foods were introduced, food refusals became pronounced, and Jeremy developed very specific preferences which excluded meat and vegetables.

Present History

Physical examination revealed a pale child whose height was at the 25th percentile for his age and whose weight was between the 50th and 75th percentiles. Laboratory analysis revealed the following: hemoglobin 9.6 g/100 ml, hematocrit 31 percent, serum iron 59 μg/100 ml, iron-binding capacity 365 μg/100 ml, and saturation of transferrin less than 16 percent.

Present food intake consists of 40 oz of milk, 8 oz of fruit juice, presweetened cereal, white toast, canned vegetable soup, ice cream, and canned spaghetti. Although drinking from a cup, Jeremy continues to take a bottle at nap and bedtime. Intake of iron was estimated to be 4.5 mg.

Case Study Questions

1 *Based on laboratory and clinical findings and dietary intake, what condition would you diagnose?*

2 *Why is the serum iron-binding capacity value high when the hemoglobin value is low?*

3 *What are your recommendations for treatment?*

2 Describe the interrelating role of calcium and phosphorus in the human body.

3 Cite the factors which influence calcium absorption.

4 Describe the progression of iron-deficiency anemia in the human body. What clinical and laboratory symptoms would you expect to find?

5 What predisposing factors lead to magnesium deficiency?

REFERENCES

1 R. L. Pike and M. L. Brown, *Nutrition: An Integrated Approach,* 2d ed., John Wiley & Sons, Inc., New York, 1975, chap. 5, p. 181.

2 *Recommended Dietary Allowances,* 8th ed., National Academy of Sciences, Washington, D.C., 1974, p. 82.

3 A. S. Posner, "Crystal Chemistry of Bone Mineral," *Physiology Review,* **49:**766, 1969.

4 S. Davidson, R. Passmore, J. Brock, and A. Truswell, *Human Nutrition and Dietetics,* 6th ed., Churchill and Livingstone, London, 1975, chap. 9, p. 108.

5 R. Goodhart and M. Shils, *Modern Nutrition in Health and Disease,* 5th ed., Lea & Febiger, Philadelphia, 1973, chap. 6, p. 269.

6 J. Wallach, *Interpretation of Diagnostic Tests,* 2d ed., Little, Brown, and Company, Boston, 1974, chap. 1, p. 8.

7 W. F. Ganong (ed.), *Medical Physiology,* 7th ed., Lange Medical Publications, Los Altos, Calif., 1975, p. 291.

8 Goodhart and Shils, op. cit., p. 274.

9 *Recommended Dietary Allowances,* op. cit., p. 83.

10 Wallach, op. cit., p. 10.

11 *Recommended Dietary Allowances,* op. cit., p. 89.

12 FAO/WHO (Food and Agriculture Organization/World Health Organization). "Calcium Requirements," *WHO Technical Report* 230, 1962, p. 54.

13 D. N. Holvey (ed.), *The Merck Manual of Diagnosis and Therapy,* 12th ed., Merck, Sharp and Dohme Research Laboratories, Rahway, N.J., 1972, chap. 10, p. 1237.

14 S. Garn, "The Course of Bone Gain and Phases of Bone Loss," *Orthopedic Clinics of North America,* **3:**503, 1972.

15 Ganong, op. cit., p. 208.

16 A. Mizrhai, R. D. London, and D. Gribetz, "Neonatal Hypocalcemia: Its Causes and Treatment," *New England Journal of Medicine,* **278:** p. 1163, 1968.

17 S. J. Fomon, *Infant Nutrition,* 2d ed., W. B. Saunders Company, Philadelphia, 1974, chap. 11, p. 271.

18 Davidson, Passmore, et al., op. cit., p. 121.

19 Goodhart and Shils, op. cit., p. 287.

20 *Recommended Dietary Allowances,* op. cit., p. 87.

21 Wallach, op. cit., p. 9.

22 P. K. Bondy and L. E. Rosenberg (eds.), *Duncan's Diseases of Metabolism,* 7th ed., W. B. Saunders Co., Philadelphia, 1974, chap. 20, p. 1318.

23 R. Masironi, *Trace Elements in the Etiology of Cardiovascular Disease,* WHO Technical Report 5, Geneva, 1974, p. 628.

24 *Recommended Dietary Allowances,* op. cit. p. 89.

25 E. Underwood, *Trace Elements in Human and Animal Nutrition,* Academic Press, New York, 1971, chap. 2, p. 16.

26 J. D. Cook and E. R. Monson, "Food Iron, I: Use of a Semi-Synthetic Diet to Study Absorption of Nonheme Iron," *American Journal of Clinical Nutrition,* **28:**1289, 1975.

27 J. Fritz, *Measures to Increase Iron in Foods and Diets,* Food and Nutrition Board, National Research Council, National Academy of Sciences, Washington, D.C., 1970, p. 633.

28 A. Jacobs and E. Butler, "Menstrual Blood Lost in Iron Deficiency Anemia," *Lancet,* **2:**407, 1965.

29 *Recommended Dietary Allowances,* op. cit., p. 94.

30 Committee on Nutrition of the American Academy of Pediatrics, "Iron Balance and Requirements in Infancy," *Pediatrics,* **43:**134, 1969.

31 Wallach, op. cit., p. 15.

32 Pollet and Leibel, "Iron Deficiency and Behavior," *Journal of Pediatrics,* **88:**372, 1976.

33 M. S. Read, "Anemia and Behavior," *Moderne Probleme der Paediatrie,* **14:**189, 1975.

34 J. Stanbury, J. Wyngaarden, and D. Frederickson, *The Metabolic Basis of Inherited Disease,* 3d ed., McGraw-Hill, New York, 1972, chap. 44, p. 1051.

35 Holvey, op. cit., p. 1093.

36 C. L. Comar and F. Bronner (eds.), *Mineral Metabolism,* Academic Press, New York, 1964, p. 672.

37 J. C. Muhler, *Fluorine and Human Health,* World Health Organization, Geneva, 1970, sec. II, "The Supply of Fluorine to Man," pp. 32–40.

38 Wallach, op. cit., p. 8.

39 Fomon, op. cit., p. 326.

40 A. J. Cordano, J. M. Baertl, and G. G. Graham, "Copper Deficiency in Infancy," *Pediatrics,* **34:**324–366, 1964.

41 Underwood, op. cit., p. 25.

42 R. S. Goodhart and M. E. Shils, op. cit., p. 381.

43 Klevay, L. M., "Cornary Heart Disease: The Zinc/Copper Hypothesis," *American Journal of Clinical Nutrition,* **28:**764, 1975.

44 R. E. Burch, H. Hahn, and J. F. Sullivan, "Newer Aspects of the Roles of Zinc, Maganese, and Copper in Human Nutrition," *Clinical Chemistry,* **21:**502, 1975.

45 H. H. Sandstead, "Zinc Nutrition in the United States," *American Journal of Clinical Nutrition* **26:** 1215, 1973.

46 R. I. Henkin, P. Schecter, R. Hoye, and C. Mattern, "Idiopathic Hypogeusia with Dysgeusia, Hyposonia, Dysomia: A New Syndrome," *Journal American Medical Association,* **217:**434, 1971.

47 O. A. Levander, "Selenium and Chromium in Human Nutrition," Journal American Dietetic Association, **66:**338, 1975.

CHAPTER 8

WATER AND ELECTROLYTES

Grace Shen

KEY WORDS
Electrolytes
Ions
Osmotic Pressure
Sodium
Potassium
Chloride
Dehydration
Acidosis
Alkalosis

INTRODUCTION

The fundamental unit of life in all organisms is the cell. Each cell of the human body is bathed in a tissue fluid of water and certain electrolytes (sodium, potassium, calcium, magnesium, chloride, phosphophate, and sulfate) and is regulated by the integration of many physiological processes.

Illness, trauma, or surgery can cause an alteration in the amount and composition of tissue fluids, which may have profound effects (dehydration, shock, death) if not corrected by the administration of suitable replacement fluids. Successful fluid and electrolyte therapy is based on the fundamental concepts governing water and electrolytes, which this chapter presents.

BODY WATER

Function

All biological functions require a suitable concentration of water as the solvent for inorganic electrolytes and other substances. Thus, water is an essential nutrient. As the most important body solvent, it provides a normal constant internal environment for body function. It serves as the vehicle to deliver oxygen and nutrients to tissues and cells. It excretes wastes from the body. It is essential for metabolism. In periods of growth, it also expands different fluid compartments. Water is the largest single component of the body, and a loss of even 10 percent can cause metabolic disorders.

Body Water Distribution

Two-thirds of the total body weight consists of water. It is distributed throughout the body in all cells, in the extracellular fluids, and in the solid supporting structures of the body. However, there are three designated functional fluid compartments: the intracellular compartment (the cellular fluid), which contains the

TABLE 8-1 BODY FLUID COMPARTMENTS IN THE ADULT MALE

Compartment	Volume in man, ml	Percentage of body weight
Plasma	3,500	5
Interstitial fluid	10,500	15
Total extracellular fluid	14,000	20
Intracellular compartment	28,000	40
Total	42,000	60

Source: Adapted from J. H. Bland, *Clinical Metabolism of Body Water and Electrolytes*, W. B. Saunders Company, Philadelphia, 1963, p. 36.

largest percentage of water, the extracellular (intravascular) compartment (the plasma); and the extravascular compartment (the interstitial fluid). (See Table 8-1.)

Total body water as a percentage of body weight changes with age from 78 percent of body weight at birth to 60 percent by adulthood. This is related to a changing body surface area and metabolic activity, both of which are high in infancy. Also, body water tends to decrease as body fat increases, since fat is essentially water-free; the leaner and more muscular a person is, the higher the body content of water. Thus, while the total body water is 60 percent of the body weight for a normal person, it is 50 percent for an obese person and 70 percent for a lean person.

Water Balance

Normally there is a maintenance or balance between the *intake* and *output* of water, and an osmotic equilibrium between the different body fluid compartments.

Water intake is controlled by the thirst center in the hypothalamus, which is stimulated by a rise in the tonicity of the extracellular fluid, or by the generalized dehydration of all tissues. Water output is controlled by the antidiuretic hormone of the posterior pituitary gland. This hormone is secreted in response to an increase in the osmotic pressure of the blood plasma.

Water intake has two routes, *ingestion* and *metabolism.* The chief sources of fluid intake in health are (1) liquids and (2) water derived from solid foods, which can contain considerable amounts of water. For example, bread contains 38 percent moisture; potato 60 percent, and cooked meat 50 percent. In a normal diet, 350 ml of the daily water intake may be derived from solid food.

Metabolic water is water obtained from chemical oxidation of foodstuffs; carbohydrate, protein, and fat in the body must therefore be considered as part of the fluid intake. Thus, 1 g of food protein provides 0.41 g of water; 1 g of food carbohydrate provides 0.61 g of water; and 1 g of food fat provides 1.07 of water. Under abnormal conditions, imposed by disease states or starvation, the catabolism of body tissue also yields water. One kilogram (2.2 lb.) of oxidized body fat will yield 1 l or 1000 ml of water.

Water output or elimination is largely through secretion of urine by the kidneys. Part of the urine is obligatory water, obligated to excrete the end products of metabolism, and the rest is facultative water, varying with conditions (diet, temperature). Normally an adult has to excrete a minimum of 500 ml of urine as obligatory water in order to eliminate approximately 25 g of urea produced in the average daily metabolism of protein and other metabolic waste products. Total urine output, including facultative losses, for an adult male is between 1000 ml and 1500 ml per day. Other water losses are:

TABLE 8-2   WATER INTAKE AND OUTPUT IN ADULTS

Mode of intake	Amount	Mode of output	Amount
Water and other beverage	1250 ml	Insensible perspiration	
Water of solid foods	1000 ml	Skin	600 ml
Metabolically produced	350 ml	Lungs	400 ml
		Sweat	50 ml
		Feces	100 ml
		Urine	1450 ml
Total	2600 ml		2600 ml

Source: Adapted from *Recommended Dietary Allowances*, 8th ed., National Academy of Sciences, Washington, D.C., 1974.

100 ml in feces

600 to 700 ml as insensible perspiration or evaporation through the skin

400 to 500 ml in air expired through breathing

Both expiration and insensible perspiration (not sweating) are electrolyte-free water. The amount of water lost by sweating under conditions of moderate temperature and humidity is small and fairly constant. Under these conditions, the electrolyte losses are also small. However, with elevated temperature or vigorous exercise water and electrolyte losses can be excessive (e.g., an athlete can lose up to 5 lb during marathon running or a tennis match). In a lactating woman, water is also lost in the breast milk.

For the most part, the amount of water taken in each day approximates the amount of water lost. (See Table 8–2.)

The daily minimum fluid intake should cover the total amount of water lost per day through the lungs, skin, feces, and urine. Water requirements are based on body size and determined per kilogram of body weight (see Table 8-3). If based on recommended energy intake, it is suggested that the daily intake be 1 ml of fluid/kcal (4.2 ml/kJ) for adults and 1.5 ml of fluid/kcal (4.2 ml/kJ) for infants.

INFLUENCES ON BODY WATER DISTRIBUTION

The influences that control the body water distribution are (1) the solutes present in the body water and (2) membrane or osmotic pressure. A solute is a substance which can be dissolved in a solvent to make a solution. There are three types of solutes governing changes in the body fluids—*electrolytes* (e.g., sodium chloride), *nonelectrolytes* (e.g., glucose, urea, creatinine), and *large molecules* (e.g., plasma protein).

TABLE 8-3   WATER REQUIREMENT

(Milliliters per kilogram body weight)*

	Age, years	Water, ml per kg body weight
Infants	Birth–1	120–100
Children	1–10	60–80
Adolescents	11–18	41–55
Adults	19–51 +	20–30

* The daily maintenance requirement is based on body surface area, at 1500 to 2000 ml/m² of surface area per 24 h.

Source: Adapted from G. H. Bell, *Textbook of Physiology and Biochemistry,* 6th ed., Williams and Wilkins Company, Baltimore, 1965, p. 166; and W. Waring and L. Jeansonne, *Practical Manual of Pediatrics,* The C. V. Mosby Company, St. Louis, 1975, p. 217.

Solutes

Electrolytes are electrically charged particles when they are dissociated in aqueous solutions.

Ions are the dissociated particles of electrolytes in solution which carry the electrical charges. A positively charged ion is a *cation,* while a negatively charged ion is an *anion.*

The main cations in the body fluids are sodium (Na^+), potassium (K^+), calcium (Ca^{2+}), and magnesium (Mg^{2+}). The main anions in the body fluids are chloride (Cl^-), bicarbonate (HCO_3^-), phosphate (HPO_4^{2-}), and ions of organic acids such as lactate, pyruvate aceto-acetate, and many proteinates.

Electrolytes are essential for forming and retaining water in the extracellular and intra-cellular compartments and are evenly distrib-uted between the compartments (see Table 8-4). The even distribution of such positive and negative charges is known as electroneu-trality. This ionic equilibrium within the body fluid compartments maintains the homeostasis within the body. Homeostasis is affected by both electrolyte concentration—the number of particles per unit volume, expressed as *milli-moles* (mmol); and the electrolyte activity—the number of charges present, expressed as *milli-equivalents* (meq).

The conversion formulas are:

$$mmol/l = \frac{mg/100 \text{ ml} \times 10}{molecular \ wt}$$

$$meq = \frac{mg/100 \text{ ml} \times valence}{atomic \ wt}$$

In the case of ions containing one electrical charge (such as sodium, potassium, and chlo-ride), the numerical values for millimoles and milliequivalents are the same. However, with ions carrying two charges or having a valency of two, such as calcium or magnesium, the val-ues for milliequivalents and millimoles are dif-ferent in the solution; since there are more charges present in the solution once the com-pound with the higher valence is dissolved.

For example, 1 liter in which 24 mg of mag-nesium is dissolved contains only 1 mmol of magnesium but 2 meq of magnesium.

Role of Membranes in Fluid and Electrolyte Distribution

Since all biological membranes which separate extracellular and intracellular fluids are com-pletely permeable to water, the total solute concentrations in both extracellular fluid and

TABLE 8-4   IONIC CONCENTRATION IN EXTRACELLULAR FLUID (ECF) AND INTRACELLULAR FLUID (ICF)

Cation	Anion	Extracellular fluid		Intracellular fluid	
		Cation, meq/l	Anion meq/l	Cation, meq/kg intracellular water	Anion, meq/kg intracellular water
Na^+		142		11	
K^+		5		164	
Ca^{2+}		5		2	
Mg^{2+}		3		28	
	Cl^-		103		
	HCO_3^-		27		10
	HPO_4^{2-}		2		105
	SO_4^{2-}		1		20
	Protein		16		65
	Organic acids		6		5
Total		155	155	205	205

Source: Adapted from D. Black, *Essentials of Fluid Balance,* 4th ed., Blackwell Scientific Publications, Oxford, 1969, p. 9.

intracellular fluid are approximately equal. Water molecules will move from the extracellular fluid to the intracellular fluid when the latter has a higher solute concentration. The reverse process occurs when the solute concentration of the extracellular fluid is higher—water then moves to it.

Membrane pressure exerts a significant influence on body water distribution. A living cell membrane is the site of continuous activity; molecules of solute and water are constantly being transported to and fro across the cell membrane, which is semipermeable, producing a membrane barrier. Each molecule of solute added to a solution occupies an element of volume formerly occupied by water molecules. The more solute added, the greater the number of water molecules displaced and the greater the pressure against the membrane.

Osmotic pressure can be defined as the pressure exerted by a solute on a semipermeable membrane in order to attract water. Since the amount of pressure is proportional to the concentration of the solute or numbers of molecules or ions present, the measure of osmotic pressure is the number of particles present in a unit of volume. The unit of measurement of the osmotic activity is the *milliosmol* (mosmol), representing the amount of work that dissolved particles must do in order to draw fluid through a semipermeable membrane. It is a measure of the osmotic contribution of a solute to a solution. Since a solute ionizes in water, the osmotic pressure depends on the number of ions or particles present in solution rather than on the amount of solute present. For example, 1 mmol of calcium chloride produces 3 mosmol, while 1 mmol of sodium chloride produces 2 mosmol and 1 mmol of a nonelectrolyte such as glucose produces 1 mosmol.

There are several mechanisms by which water and solutes move across a semipermeable membrane; among these are osmosis, diffusion, filtration, active transport, and pinocytosis.

Osmosis   The net diffusion of water between two compartments separated by a semipermeable membrane is known as osmosis. This process occurs in the simple movement of water through a semipermeable membrane.

Diffusion   When the pressure on the two sides of a membrane is *equal,* the solute molecules move across the separating membrane from a region of higher concentration to a region of lower concentration. This process is known as diffusion.

Filtration   Water molecules are filtered through membranes when there is a difference in pressure on the two sides of the membrane.

Active transport (Energy-dependent)   When the solute molecules must cross a membrane against significant pressure, both energy (which comes from cell metabolism) and some vehicle of transport is required. This process is called active transport. For example, glucose is absorbed from the intestinal lumen and is actively transported across the intestinal wall by the *sodium pump.* Amino acids and fatty acids also enter and leave the cell by active transport (see Chapter 9).

Pinocytosis   Through the mechanism of pinocytosis, the cell membrane forms a pocket (*vesicle*) on the cell surface, engulfing molecules which are eventually released into the cell cytoplasm. Pinocytosis provides a major route for the entry of molecules into the cell. Proteins, fats, and various ions appear to increase the rate of vesicle formation in certain cells and use this mechanism as the mode of cell entry.

Role of the Kidneys in Regulation of Fluid and Electrolytes

In regulating the fluid and electrolyte balance, the kidneys, more than any other organ, control the volume, the osmolality, and the composition of the extracellular fluid compartment in accordance with the body's constantly changing needs.

Whenever there is a change in the extracellular fluid volume, the kidneys can vary the urinary volume to handle the water load. In response to hypovolemia (a decrease in the blood plasma volume) the renin-angiotensin system of the kidneys is activated, which stimulates the adrenal gland to release aldosterone and facilitates the reabsorption of sodium and water by the kidneys (see also "Sodium: Balance Mechanisms," below). This interaction between aldosterone and the kidneys can maintain the normal ratio of water to solute in the body at 3.3 ml of water to 1 mosmol of electrolyte.

Whenever there is a change in tonicity of the extracellular fluid, the kidneys can change the urine osmolarity from 50 mosmol/kg of water [giving urine a specific gravity (sp gr) of 1.001] to 1300 mosmol/kg of water (urine sp gr 1.040). The kidneys regulate the concentration of solutes in this way through interaction with the hypothalamus and the pituitary gland. The

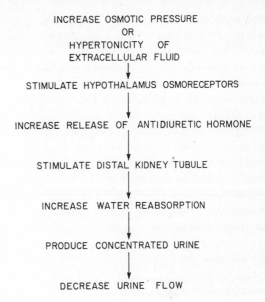

Figure 8-2

Interactions between the release of antidiuretic hormone by the hypothalamus and water reabsorption by the kidneys, serving to stabilize the osmotic pressure of the body fluids.

Figure 8-1

Interaction between the renin-angiotensin system of the kidney and the adrenal cortex, serving to stabilize the volume of body fluids.

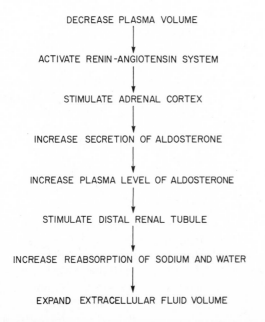

hypothalamus secretes an antidiuretic hormone (ADH) which is stored in the pituitary. The function of ADH is to promote an increase in water reabsorption by the kidneys. When the osmotic pressure of the blood plasma increases, that is, in response to hypertonicity of the extracellular fluid, the pituitary gland releases ADH, which stimulates the kidneys to reabsorb more water. In this way, the release of ADH helps in the production of concentrated urine and the restoration of a normal extracellular fluid volume. With hypotonicity of the extracellular fluid, no ADH is released and a diluted urine is excreted.

Role of the Gastrointestinal Tract in Regulation of Fluid and Electrolytes

Besides the kidneys, the gastrointestinal tract, the lungs, and the skin also play a role in regulating the fluid and electrolyte balance.

The exchange of water and electrolytes

between the extracellular compartment and the gastrointestinal tract is considerable, with a negligible loss of gastrointestinal secretions. However, persistent vomiting, diarrhea, or drainage from an intestinal fistula may quickly cause a serious contraction in volume of the extracellular fluid compartment, and a serious deficiency of potassium, chloride, and bicarbonates. In determining replacement needs, both the volume and the electrolyte composition of vomitus, diarrhea fluids, and drainage fluids must be considered. The approximate electrolyte content of these fluids is summarized in Table 8-5.

Role of Lungs and Skin in Regulation of Fluid and Electrolytes

Normal insensible water loss from the lungs and the skin is mainly electrolyte-free water, ranging in volume from 250 ml to 750 ml per day. It increases in cases of fever, hyperventilation, dyspnea, and burns, as well as in some trauma to the body, including surgery.

ELECTROLYTES

Sodium

Distribution in the Body
Sodium is the principal cation of the extracellular fluid, found in concentrations between

TABLE 8-5 ELECTROLYTE COMPOSITION OF FLUID LOSSES FROM VOMITING, DIARRHEA, AND FISTULA DRAINAGE

Type of fluid	Sodium, meq/l	Potassium, meq/l
Gastric (suction, vomiting)	75	15
Small bowel (suction, vomiting)	135	15
Diarrhea	50	40

Source: Adapted from W. Waring and L. Jeansonne, *Practical Manual of Pediatrics,* The C. V. Mosby Company, St. Louis, 1975, p. 220.

136 and 145 meq/l while only approximately 10 meq/l is found in the extracellular fluid. Of the exchangeable sodium, 90 percent is in the extracellular compartment; the remainder is in the intracellular fluid and in bone. The chief function of sodium is to maintain osmotic pressure in the extracellular fluid compartment.

Sodium in the body is in the form of sodium chloride—that is, the same as common table salt. Under normal conditions an individual consumes about 85 to 100 meq of salt per day (5 to 10 g per day). Ninety percent of the sodium intake is then excreted in the urine. Stool and sweat losses are less than 10 meq per day. In the adult, sodium intake and excretion are in equilibrium. For children, a positive sodium balance is necessary to expand the extracellular fluid compartment during growth.

The kidneys are the principal sodium excretory organ and regulate excretion closely. The body is very efficient in sodium conservation. In case of zero intake of sodium, the kidneys and sweat glands reduce the sodium output to zero. The body can maintain sodium balance with an intake of as little as 12 to 15 meq (0.2 to 0.3 g) of sodium per day and can tolerate an acute load of 400 meq (9.2 g) per day.

Balance Mechanisms
Sodium balance is controlled by the renin-angiotensin-aldosterone system. Angiotensinogen is a liver plasma protein, circulating in the blood. Renin is an enzyme secreted by the kidneys which catalyzes angiotensinogen to angiotensin. The angiotensin in turn stimulates the secretion of aldosterone by the adrenals. With sodium depletion, the secretion of renin by the kidneys is in inverse proportion to the amount of sodium present in the tubules of the kidneys. This increased production of renin by the kidneys is followed by the formation of angiotensin in the plasma. Angiotensin then stimulates the release of aldosterone from the adrenal cortex, which causes the kidneys to reabsorb sodium. In the complete absence of aldosterone, as occurs in Addison's disease, the

patient may excrete 25 g of salt per day, whereas excretion may be negligible when aldosterone is present in large quantities.

Daily Sodium Intake

Daily intake of sodium is regulated more by taste, custom, and habit than by need. The normal intake ranges from 100 to 300 meq, or 6 to 18 g of sodium chloride per day. The quantity of sodium in most infant formulas is around 3.3 meq/100 kcal (420 kJ) which means that a 3-month-old infant consuming 600 kcal (2520 kJ) per day would take 20 meq of sodium daily. Certain commercially prepared strained junior foods (e.g., meats, vegetables) provide more than 100 meq of sodium/100 kcal (420 kJ), which may be excessive. Salt is added to certain infant foods primarily to cater to the taste of the parents rather than to meet nutritional needs and has caused concern regarding the long-term effect on the incidence of cardiovascular disease, raising the question whether early introduction of salt into infants' food creates a "taste" for salt that leads to overuse later in life. Since 1970, the amount of sodium chloride added to baby foods has been decreased.

Clinical Application

Disorders arise when sodium intake or losses exceed the adaptive balance mechanisms. This can occur in conditions resulting from kidney or heart failure. In renal disease problems are due to the inability of the kidneys to excrete sodium normally, whereas in heart failure the problem is caused by increased levels of aldosterone, which promotes the retention of sodium. In such cases sodium intake may be restricted. In other conditions, such as the nephrotic salt-losing syndrome or adrenal insufficiency, there is sodium loss because of renal or adrenal cortical damage. Vomiting, diarrhea, drainage from an intestinal fistula, and other extrarenal losses of sodium may also cause a problem of excess losses. Without replacement therapy, the volume of water in the extracellular space or the sodium concen-tration in all extracellular water (including plasma) or both may fall, leading to dehydration, shock, and death.

Potassium

Distribution in the Body

Potassium is the chief cation in the intracellular compartment. There is approximately 164 meq of potassium/l of intracellular fluid. In the extracellular compartment, potassium is present in small amounts, 5 meq/l; however, the cation is very significant for maintenance of body process and survival. The body contains a total of 3200 meq of cellular potassium, and only 70 meq of potassium in the extracellular fluid. Since potassium is the predominant cation of cells, its distribution among the organs of the body is related to their cell number. Retention of this potassium is associated with an increase in the lean body mass, and the total-body counting of the naturally occurring radioactive isotope of potassium, ^{40}K, is an indirect measure of the total-body potassium.

Balance Mechanism

The minimum amount of potassium that the body can function with is approximately 30 meq, while the maximum load is approximately 400 meq per day. Normally, 90 percent of the potassium intake is excreted in the urine; stool and sweat losses are less than 10 meq per day. In the adult body, the potassium intake and output are in equilibrium. However, a positive balance is necessary for children, to increase their cellular growth and expand the intracellular fluid compartment. There is always an obligatory potassium loss even with negligible intake. In contrast to sodium ions, which are completely reabsorbed when the plasma sodium level is low, the reabsorption of potassium ions from renal tubules does not increase when the plasma potassium level is low. Normally, reabsorption of potassium from the glomerular filtrate takes place in the proximal tubules and some potassium is secreted into the urine in the distal part of the tubules. The average serum potassium levels are maintained between 3.5 and 5.5 meq/l.

The chief function of extracellular potassium is to control cardiac function and muscle and nerve irritability. The heart muscle is subject to injury if the serum potassium is outside the range of 3 to 7 mEq/l. Intracellular potassium is essential in many cellular enzymatic functions, such as glycogen synthesis and glucose degradation, and in amino acid uptake. In homeostasis, the total-body potassium and the extracellular potassium remain relatively constant. Since potassium can enter cells easily, the potassium of the liver, kidneys, lungs, gastrointestinal tract, and muscle is exchanged rapidly.

Potassium Intake and Dietary Sources

The dietary intake of potassium must be adequate to maintain electrolyte balance in the body. Potassium is widely distributed in milk, meats, fruits, and vegetables, and the usual intake is somewhere between 50 and 150 meq (1.9 to 5.8 g) per day. It is estimated that adults need approximately 64.1 meq (2.5 g) per day of potassium and children, according to their age, need between 25 and 100 meq (0.98 to 3.9 g) per day.

Potassium supplementation must be administered with care when potassium deficiency occurs. This can result from low potassium intake or from excessive losses due to diarrhea, diabetic acidosis, other disease states, or use of drugs such as diuretics, steroids, and purgatives.

Clinical Application

Potassium deficiency can cause structural and functional changes in the intestines, myocardium, kidney tubules, pancreas, and liver. Under abnormal conditions, causing cellular breakdown, such as hemolysis, acidosis, and starvation, potassium moves from the intracellular fluid compartment to the extracellular fluid compartment, and potassium losses can

result from renal as well as extrarenal origin. Renal losses can be exaggerated by diuresis, acidosis, renal tubular damage, or excessive secretion of adrenocortical hormone, as occurs in Cushing's syndrome. Extrarenal losses usually take the form of vomiting, diarrhea, and intestinal fistula drainage. Usually the loss of potassium from the upper gastrointestinal tract is insignificant. However, losses from the lower gastrointestinal tract may be considerable in abnormal conditions.

Chloride

Distribution in the Body

Chloride is the predominant anion in the extracellular fluid compartment, providing two-thirds of the anions in the plasma. It is almost entirely absent within cells and occurs mainly in combination with sodium. The extracellular fluid compartment normally contains about 80 percent of the body chloride. The plasma normally contains 100 to 110 meq/l and the red blood cells about 58 meq/l. The principle role of chloride is to regulate the osmotic pressure and water content of the body. It is also the predominant component in the gastric juice. The chloride anion acts as a coenzyme for digestive amylases. It helps to buffer the acid-base balance of blood by exchange of chloride from the plasma for bicarbonate from the red blood cells.

Balance Mechanism

The plasma chloride level is affected only slightly by the ingestion of chloride; it decreases about 2 meq/l at the height of gastric secretion because of the need to produce hydrochloric acid. Approximately twice the quanity of chloride present in the plasma is secreted daily in the gastric juice and is reabsorbed again.

In healthy adults the chloride intake and output are in equilibrium. Normally more than 90 percent of the body chloride is excreted in the urine, the remainder mostly in the feces and sweat. But a positive balance is necessary for children in order to expand the extracellular fluid compartment. The rate of urinary chloride excretion depends on the chloride intake and the water balance. The retention of chloride occurs readily during periods of fluid retention (edema).

Chloride Intake and Dietary Sources

Most dietary chloride is derived from dairy products and meat with some from vegetables and fruit. The chloride content of foods is roughly proportional to the sodium content and inversely proportional to the potassium content. The daily intake is about 60 to 100 meq (2.1 to 3.5 g).

Clinical Application

Starvation, fever, vomiting, diarrhea, and excessive sweating will lower the urinary chloride output. When the plasma chloride is low, the urinary excretion of chloride is markedly decreased except in adrenal cortical insufficiency. Deficit of adrenocortical hormone increases the chloride output by interfering with tubular reabsorption of chloride. In abnormal conditions such as starvation, fever, diarrhea, excessive vomiting, and excessive sweating there is a decrease in the plasma chloride. As with the marked loss of potassium, the marked loss of chloride can result in hypokalemic alkalosis for the following reasons: If there is a decrease in the chloride concentration in the extracellular fluid, there is a concomitant increase in the bicarbonate concentration, which leads to the state of alkalosis. Since the availability of chloride ions as anions to accompany sodium is limited, the reabsorption of sodium is diminished. However, there is a mechanism for the reabsorption of sodium without chloride, known as the *exchange mechanism,* whereby there is an accelerated excretion of potassium in the urine in exchange for sodium reabsorption without chloride ions. Therefore, in replacement therapy, if potassium is supplied without chloride, hypokalemic alkalosis may persist. Chloride supplementation in addition to the potassium is needed to correct hypokalemic alkalosis (see below).

Acid-Base Balance

Water and electrolytes act together within the body to maintain the acid-base balance.

The acidity or alkalinity of a substance or a solution is determined by the concentration of hydrogen ions. The more hydrogen ions present, the more a solution is acid; a decrease in hydrogen ions makes the solution more alkaline or basic. The degree of acidity is expressed by the symbol *pH.* The pH of a solution is defined as the negative logarithm of the hydrogen ion concentration. The definition is based on the fact that the quantity of hydrogen ions present in a solution is best expressed mathematically as a negative logarithm, since the weight of hydrogen in water is about one ten millionth of a gram per liter (0.0000001 or 10^{-7}g). Therefore, a hydrogen ion concentration of 0.0000001 g/l equals 10^{-7} g/l or a pH of 7.

A solution with a *pH of 7* is at the neutral point between an acid and a base because at that concentration the number of hydrogen ions (H^+) is in equilibrium with the number of basic or hydroxyl ions (OH^-). Because of the use of a negative "log," an acid solution has a pH below 7 and a basic solution has a pH greater than 7.

Buffer Systems

The body, through a buffer system (see Figure 8-3), maintains the extracellular fluid within a narrow pH range of 7.35 to 7.45. The buffer system involves certain combinations of chemicals in the extracellular fluid which can act as buffers or protectors against changes in the hydrogen ion concentration. The importance of this system lies in the fact that the chemical processes of living cells are exceedingly sensitive to changes in pH.

A *buffer* is a substance capable of maintaining the relative concentrations of hydrogen

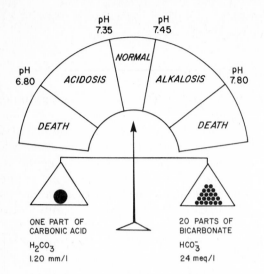

Figure 8-3
The buffer system of the body, which maintains a ratio of 1 part carbonic acid to 20 parts bicarbonate (1:20). (Adapted from Fluid and Electrolytes; Some Practical Guides to Clinical Use, Abbott Laboratories, (North Chicago, Ill., May 1969, p. 23.)

and hydroxyl ions in a solution by neutralizing within limits and offsetting rapid changes. It is a mixture of acidic and alkaline components which are protective against either added acid or base. When a strong acid is added to a buffered solution, the base component of the acid-base buffer combines with the added acid to form a weaker acid. Similarly, when a strong base is added to the buffered solution, the acid component of the acid-base buffer donates ionized hydrogen to form a weaker base and restore the pH.

Although there are several buffer systems in the human body, the most important one in the extracellular fluid is the *carbonic acid-sodium bicarbonate system* (H_2CO_3-$NaHCO_3$). Under normal conditions a ratio of 1 part carbonic acid to 20 parts bicarbonate is present (1:20).

When the extracellular environment becomes more acid, the buffer system activates. The bicarbonate ions alkalize, since they have an affinity for hydrogen ions, binding them,

removing them from solution, and thereby neutralizing or buffering the effect of the acid. This is observed in the following reaction:

$$H^+Cl^- + Na^+HCO_3^- \longrightarrow Na^+Cl^- + H_2CO_3$$

| Hydro-chloric acid | Sodium bicarbonate | Salt | Carbonic acid |

These events cause the bicarbonate carbonic acid ratio to become altered, giving an acid pH. The carbonic acid formed is excreted via the lungs as carbon dioxide—the depth and rate of breathing increases to exhale more carbon dioxide and control the level of carbonic acid in the blood.

$$H_2CO_3 \xrightarrow{\text{carbonic anhydrase}} CO_2 + H_2O$$

This increased exhalation of carbon dioxide decreases the raw material for carbonic acid production, while the decreased level of sodium bicarbonate signals the renal tubules to reabsorb sodium. Both of these mechanisms serve to restore the 1:20 ratio of the buffer system; i.e., 1 part carbonic acid to 20 parts bicarbonate.

Disturbances in Acid-Base Balance

Disturbances of the acid-base balance consist of major shifts in the electrolyte patterns related to failure of the compensatory responses of the buffer system, the lungs, or the kidneys. The resulting conditions are referred to clinically as *acidosis*, in which an increase in hydrogen ion concentration causes a shift in pH to an acidic medium, or *alkalosis*, the opposite state, in which the hydrogen ion concentration is below normal, causing a shift in Ph to a basic medium.

The disturbances of the acid-base balance of the body are characterized according to their origin: imbalances caused by failure of the lungs are either respiratory acidosis or respiratory alkalosis; imbalances caused by failure of the renal system are either metabolic acidosis or metabolic alkalosis.

Acid-base disturbances are differentiated

by determining three components of the blood: (1) the respiratory component, plasma carbon dioxide pressure or P_{CO_2} (normal range 35 to 45 mmHg); (2) the metabolic component, plasma bicarbonate or HCO_3 (normal range 22 to 26 meq/l); and (3) the blood pH, (normal 7.40; normal range 7.35 to 7.45).

Acidosis and Alkalosis

Respiratory Acidosis

Respiratory acidosis is due to disturbances in regulatory mechanisms in the respiratory center, or to disorders of muscles involved in respiration, or to diseases of the lungs such as emphysema. These conditions cause a retention of carbon dioxide (CO_2), with an increase in the partial pressure of CO_2 (P_{CO_2}) and carbonic acid (H_2CO_3) and a decrease in pH.

Respiratory Alkalosis

Respiratory alkalosis is due to hyperventilation, which causes a decreased arterial P_{CO_2} and an elevated pH. It is associated with many stressful conditions. Hyperventilation also results from many hypermetabolic states. It is common in gram-negative sepsis and peritonitis, salicylate poisoning, and encephalitis.

Metabolic Acidosis

Metabolic acidosis is due to a loss of base resulting from disorders of either the kidney or the gastrointestinal tract. Causes include the accumulation of acidic compounds in the extracellular fluid, such as occurs in lactic acid acidosis of diabetes; and renal failure involving retention of phosphates, sulfates, and organic acid anions as a result of the kidney's inability to regenerate bicarbonate. Metabolic acidosis also occurs with improper use of parenteral hyperalimentation solutions, in other diseases causing loss of bicarbonates from extracellular fluids and in renal tubular acidosis, which causes abnormal loss of bicarbonate from renal tubules. Loss of small intestinal secretions from fistulas, vomiting, and diarrhea may also induce metabolic acidosis.

Metabolic Alkalosis

Metabolic alkalosis is due to a loss of acid by either the renal or the gastrointestinal route. Examples of diseases due to gastrointestinal loss are pyloric obstruction and loss of hydrochloric acid from the stomach via a gastric tube. Metabolic alkalosis of renal origin is usually caused by loss of potassium from the kidney. Diuretics, which are used in many different diseases, are likely to cause this problem.

CLINICAL APPLICATIONS

Principles of Electrolyte Therapy

When the normal oral route is insufficient to replace fluid and electrolyte substances as a result of surgery, dehydration, or severe burns, parenteral fluid therapy must be instituted. This therapy is based on the principles of providing the body with optimal amounts of water and a suitable mixture of electrolytes in order to either maintain water and electrolyte balance or replace frank losses. The principles discussed above under the sections on body water distribution, electrolyte composition of fluid compartments, and acid-base balance become operational in considering replacement therapy.

Each patient requires a special therapeutic formulation to meet specific needs, which must be closely monitored and reevaluated on a daily basis. The average daily maintenance requirements of sodium, water, potassium, and glucose per square meter of body surface area must be considered for parenteral therapy (see Table 8-6).

The normally functioning kidney is selectively able to retain or excrete ions as needed and thereby maintain water and electrolyte balance. However, in illness states requiring replacement therapy, the osmolarity of the pa-

TABLE 8-6 AVERAGE DAILY MAINTENANCE REQUIREMENT FOR ELECTROLYTE THERAPY

Nutrient	Amount required per m² in 24h
Water	2000 ml
Sodium	40 meq
Potassium	30 meq
Glucose	100 g

m² = square meter of body surface area.

Source: Adapted from W. Waring, and L. Jeansonne, *Practical Manual of Pediatrics,* The C. V. Mosby Company, St. Louis, 1975, p. 218.

tient's serum, the urine volume, and the fluid and electrolyte intake must be carefully monitored. A 24-h flow sheet (input-output) is recommended for this purpose.

Dehydration

Dehydration is a consequence of deficits of either water or electrolytes or both water and electrolytes. Two conditions may result: *hypotonic dehydration* or hypertonic dehydration. When there is a loss of electrolytes in excess of water, the result is hypotonic dehydration. It is seen in patients with diarrhea whose fluid losses have been replaced with excessive amounts of carbohydrates in water solutions without added electrolytes. When there is a loss of water in excess of electrolytes, the result is hypertonic dehydration.

Infants are particularly sensitive to shifts in fluid and electrolyte balance and are prone to hypertonic dehydration because of their large body surface area and relatively greater evaporative losses. For example, a 1-year-old child weighing 10 kg has a body surface area of 0.50 m², whereas an adult weighing 68 kg has a body surface area of 1.8 m², which is not proportionately higher. (See Appendix for nomogram to determine body surface area.)

Another factor making the infant particularly vulnerable to hypertonic dehydration is that the infant kidney is immature in its ability to concentrate urine. (Infants can concentrate urine only to 553 mosmol/l whereas adults concentrate urine to 1200 mosmol/l.) Also, the fact that infants are totally dependent on others for their fluid intake places them at further risk. This dependency for water is also true for debilitated, elderly, or handicapped patients, all of whom should be closely monitored for signs of dehydration (dry parched lips, scant and thick saliva, reduced urine output), especially during states of fever or illness.

STUDY QUESTIONS

1 What is the role of water within the human body?
2 How is water distributed within the body and what are the influences on the pattern of distribution?
3 Does water intake equal water losses on a daily basis? Describe.
4 What are the rules of the kidney, lungs, skin, and gastrointestinal tract in regulating the body's fluid and electrolyte balance?
5 How does the body maintain the extracellular fluid within a narrow pH range of 7.35 to 7.45?

CASE STUDY 8-1

A 7-month-old male infant with moderate dehydration and lethargy was brought to the emergency ward for therapy. The parents reported that on the advice of their physician, they had

been treating a 7-day bout of infantile diarrhea with boiled skim milk, which they had been giving the infant for 2 days.

On physical examination the infant was

found to be lethargic and semicomatose, with dry mouth and parched lips. Admission weight was 6.3 kg, which represented a weight loss of 0.7 kg, or 10 percent of body weight. Laboratory analysis revealed the following:

blood urea nitrogen	*40 ml/100 ml (average, 8 to 18 mg/100 ml)*
serum sodium	*159 meq/l (average, 134 to 145 meq/l)*
serum potassium	*5.5 meq/l (average, 3.5 to 5 meq/l)*
serum chloride	*110 meq/l (average, 98 to 100 meq/l)*
serum bicarbonate	*15 meq/l (average, 25 meq/l)*
urinary specific gravity, with collection by catheter	*1.027 (average, 1.018)*

Case Study Questions

1 *List those factors involved in precipitating hypertonic dehydration.*

2 *How does the body respond to hypertonic dehydration?*

3 *How would you monitor the effectiveness of the fluid and electrolyte therapy?*

BIBLIOGRAPHY

Black, D. A. K.: *Essentials of Fluid Balance,* 4th ed., 2d printing, Blackwell Scientific Publications, Oxford, 1969.

Bland, John, H., ed.: *Clinical Metabolism of Body Water and Electrolytes,* W. B. Saunders., Philadelphia, 1963.

Christensen, Halvor, N.: *Diagnostic Biochemistry,* Oxford University Press, New York, 1959.

Gamble, James L.: *Chemical Anatomy, Physiology and Pathology of Extracellular Fluid,* 6th ed., Harvard University Press, Cambridge, Mass., 1967.

Goldberger, Emanuel: *A Primer of Water, Electrolyte and Acid-Base Syndromes,* 5th ed., Lea & Febiger, Philadelphia, 1975.

Loeb, John N.: "Current Concepts: The Hyperosmolar State," *New England Journal of Medicine,* **290:** 1184, 1974.

Snively, William D. and Michael J. Sweeney: *Fluid Balance Handbook for Practitioners,* Charles C Thomas Publisher, Springfield, Ill., 1956.

Talbot, Nathan B., Richie H. Robert, and Crawford D. John: *Metabolic Homeostatis,* Harvard University Press, Cambridge, Mass., 1959.

Waring, William W. and Louis Jeansonne: *Practical Manual, of Pediatrics,* The C. V. Mosby, St. Louis, 1975.

Welt, Louis G.: *Clinical Disorders of Hydration and Acid-Base Equilibrium,* Little, Brown and Company, Boston, 1959.

CHAPTER 9

THE BODY'S USE OF FOOD AND NUTRIENTS

Christine Adamow Murray

KEY WORDS
Absorption
Anabolism
Basal Metabolic Rate
Calorie
Catabolism
Digestion
Krebs Cycle
Embden-Meyerhof Glycolytic Pathway
Glycolysis
Gluconeogenesis
Glycogenolysis
Joule
Metabolism

INTRODUCTION

The body's utilization of food is one of the most impressive and important human functions. The nutrients, when allowed to follow an uninterrupted course through the ten feet of the small intestine and onward to the colon, provide for the building, upkeep, and operation of the body.

Having previously considered the nutrients on an individual basis, we will now examine their interrelationships within the gastrointestinal system.

In this chapter the process of nutrient utilization will be considered on the basis of the specific contribution made by each of the various gastrointestinal organs in successive order, so as to help the student follow the common pathway of food from digestion to excretion. It is important for the student who will become a health professional to recognize the significant contributions of each gastrointestinal organ to the biochemical breakdown and final utilization of food.

This chapter will enable the health professional to understand the processes of digestion, absorption, and metabolism as a whole, as the consequences of food digestion and energy metabolism are discussed and related to body composition. It is with this understanding, namely, that of an integrated gastrointestinal system, that the health professional can conceptually integrate nutrients into the human system and thereby forward the practice of nutrition-centered health care.

INGESTION

The process of digestion begins with the intake of food into the alimentary tract. There are many factors contributing to the individual's selection of foods that ultimately affect the body's nutritional status. Food availability, eye appeal, cultural preferences, and taste—all influence the daily nutrient intake.

Four primary groups of taste buds, located

on the papillae of the tongue (Fig. 9-2), enable an individual to perceive the tastes of sweet, sour, salty, and bitter. With these four basic tastes an individual is able to perceive hundreds of taste combinations. The number of taste buds increases slightly during childhood to become representative of a variety of tastes, and declines after the age of 45. During the adult years there are over 10,000 taste receptors located along the entire surface of the tongue.

Mouth

The primary mechanical action occurring in the oral cavity is the mastication of ingested food. Through the grinding bilateral motion of the teeth, food particles are broken into smaller units and mixed with saliva. The

process of digestion begins at this point because saliva contains the starch-splitting enzyme, salivary amylase. This enzyme is secreted in response to the presence of food as an unconditioned reflex. It has been shown that the conscious act of thinking about food can also trigger its secretions as a conditioned response. Salivary amylase acts on starch molecules to produce units of maltose, a simple sugar, in the presence of the optimal oral pH of 6.9. However, as with all enzyme-catalysed reactions, the length of time that the enzyme is in contact with the substrate will significantly affect the degree of starch breakdown that occurs in the oral cavity. Therefore, the longer the mastication time, the greater the degree of starch degradation in the mouth.

However, the amount of time that food is actually chewed depends on a multitude of variables. The nature of the food, the amount of conversation, individual habit, and early training all contribute to the mastication time and eventually to the extent of starch breakdown in the oral cavity.

Following mastication, involuntary reflex actions close the passages going from the pharynx to the nose and trachea, allowing the swallowing reflex to initiate the passage of food to the esophagus. Swallowing can be started at will or by the stimulation of a number of areas in the mouth and pharynx.

The preformed food mixture is now able

Figure 9-1

The gastrointestinal system.

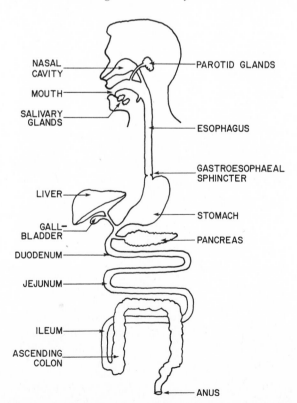

Figure 9-2

Primary sets of taste buds.

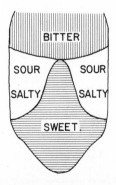

to proceed towards the antrum of the stomach via the esophagus. The esophagus utilizes strong muscular contractions to propel the food mass through its length to the stomach. At the lower end of the esophagus the muscle is slightly hypertrophied to form the gastro-esophageal constriction. This muscle allows for passage of the swallowed food into the stomach and prevents reflux of the stomach contents into the upper esophagus where the acid gastric secretions could damage the esophageal mucosa.

DIGESTION

Stomach

The gastric mucosa resembles the foothills of a large mountain range. The stomach's interior is heaped in folds and ridges which contribute significantly to the process of digestion. Closer examination of the mucosa reveals column-shaped cells, called *columnar epithelial cells.* A microscopic view of these cells reveals the presence of tiny pores leading to the gastric glands from which the gastric secretions that are responsible for aiding digestion arise. These secretions are the products of the parietal, chief, and mucous gastric cells (see Fig. 9-3). Each of these cells is specific for its contribution to digestion.

Figure 9-3
Gastric gland showing cells responsible for gastric secretions. (Adapted from A. C. Guyton, Textbook of Medical Physiology, W. B. Saunders, Philadelphia, 1976.)

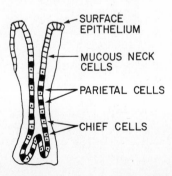

Parietal cells   The parietal cells rising from the glandular mucosal lining of the stomach are the production sites of hydrochloric acid. The normal stomach contains sufficient hydrochloric acid to produce a pH of 1 or an acid medium many times more acidic than lemon juice. The production of this acid, a complicated process, is stimulated by the gastrointestinal hormone, gastrin, upon distention of the stomach by food. Davenport reported that the body uses 324 kcal (1360.8 kJ) to produce the normal hydrochloric acid content found in the stomach at 1 h after a meal.[1] Hydrochloric acid is fundamental in the digestive process by acting to:

1   Partially break off some glucose molecules from starch
2   Slightly alter the condition of fats and proteins in preparation for further action by other digestive enzymes
3   Activate the transformation of pepsinogen to active pepsin, a protein-digesting enzyme

Chief cells   The gastric mucosa also produces enzymes that digest protein and certain fats. Pepsin is the major protein-digesting (proteolytic) enzyme and is manufactured in the chief cells of the gastric mucosa. Pepsin breaks down large protein molecules to form peptides (see Chap. 3). This enzyme relies on the acid medium of the stomach for its proteolytic action. In the absence of the hydrochloric acid, pepsin is relatively inactive and very little protein digestion will occur.

Besides producing pepsin, the lining of the stomach secretes gastric lipase. This enzyme acts principally on fats containing short- and medium-chain fatty acids (see Chap. 5), yielding smaller units of short-chain or free fatty acids. The stomach contains no enzymes specific for carbohydrate digestion. However, a negligible amount of starch digestion can occur in the stomach from swallowed salivary amylase or regurgitated pancreatic amylase.

Mucous cells   The mucous cells of the stomach produce another important gastric product, mucus. Mucus creates the slimy, slippery appearance of the gastric lining and seems to be a protective element. It is believed to lubricate the mucosal surface of the stomach and to protect the stomach from harmful irritants.

Gastric digestion relies not only on biochemical reactions, but also on various mechanical actions of the stomach wall. Immediately upon entry of food particles into the stomach cavity, tonus or mixing waves move along the stomach wall to help the gastric secretions combine with the stomach's contents. Besides these mixing waves, strong peristaltic movements occur in the gastric musculature which squeeze the partially digested food particles toward the body of the stomach. Once the food has become mixed with the gastric secretions it is called *chyme*. Chyme has a murky, milky color and a semifluid consistency.

Stomach emptying is aided by peristaltic waves moving from the stomach to the duodenum. Opposition to passage of the food is created by the pylorus. However, the creation of a pressure gradient and certain tonic contractions allow for emptying of the chyme from the stomach cavity into the duodenum.

Gastric emptying is regulated by neural and hormonal controls as well as by the physical properties of the chyme. Additional factors affecting the rate of emptying are:

Particle size
Viscosity of the chyme
Osmotic pressure
Gastric acidity
Gastric volume

Monosaccharides tend to pass through the stomach quickly in proportion to their duodenal osmolarity, while complex carbohydrates such as cellulose (a polysaccharide providing bulk in the normal diet) pass through the gut most rapidly because of the body's inability to break down the molecule's organic bond. There is no enzyme that is specific for the breakdown of cellulose to a smaller carbohydrate unit. In contrast, protein molecules in-

crease the release of the hormones gastrin and cholecystokinin, which tends to inhibit gastric motility. However, fatty meals tend to empty from the stomach most slowly because they stimulate mucosal production of enterogastrone. This hormone is absorbed into the blood and within minutes inhibits gastric motility, thereby slowing the stomach's emptying time and prolonging the digestion time of fats in the small intestine. It is for this reason that meals high in fat are said to have a high satiety value.

Pancreas, Liver, Gallbladder, and Small Intestine

The digestive process proceeds toward the small intestine, where the pancreatic duct supplies the duodenum with enzymes for protein, fat, and carbohydrate breakdown. The pancreas is stimulated by the hormones secretin, cholecystokinin, and pancreozymin to produce several important digestive enzymes. These enzymes act on the partially digested nutrients to prepare them for the absorption process in the small bowel.

Two pancreatic enzymes, hydrolase and cholesterol esterase, which act on the esters of glycerol and cholesterol respectively, depend on bile salts for their action. The liver is weakly stimulated by the hormone secretin to secrete bile. Cholecystokinin stimulates the gallbladder to contract and allow the flow of bile to mix with the contents of the duodenum. These hormones are synthesized by the intestine and are released when the contents of the stomach pass to the duodenum. In the duodenum, bile acts as an emulsifying agent, improving the solubility of fat molecules and thus aiding the process of fat absorption. The major components of bile are conjugated bile acids, bile salts, pigments, and cholesterol. Bile salts act as detergents that contain both fat- and water-attracting regions. Their action in fat and cholesterol digestion is to allow these nutrients to form a complex called a *micelle*. This micellar complex allows the otherwise insoluble fat and cholesterol molecules to enter into aqueous so-

TABLE 9-1 DIGESTIVE ENZYMES AND SECRETIONS RESPONSIBLE FOR THE BIOCHEMICAL DEGRADATION OF PROTEIN, FAT, AND CARBOHYDRATE

Site	Secretion	Substrate	Product
Oral cavity	Salivary amalse (ptylin)	Starch	Maltose
Stomach	Hydrochloric acid	Pepsinogen	Pepsin
	Pepsin	Protein	Peptides
	Gastric lipase	Fat	Medium-chain triglycerides & short-chain fatty acids
Pancreas	Trypsin	Protein, polypeptides	Smaller polypeptides
	Chymotrypsin	Protein, polypeptides	Smaller polypeptides
	Carboxypeptidases	Polypeptides	Lower peptides & amino acids
	Amylase	Starch	Dextrins
	Lipase	Fats	Monoacylglycerols, fatty acids, & glycerols
	Cholesterase	Cholesterol	Cholesterol esters with fatty acids
Gallbladder, liver	Bile	Unemulsified fats	Miscelle

lution, thereby facilitating their uptake by cells of the intestinal wall.

Gastrointestinal Flora

Normally, there are approximately 10^{14} living bacterial cells in the gut.[2] The effect of the gastrointestinal flora in the digestion-absorption process is often overlooked.

The most commonly found enteric bacteria are anaerobic streptococci, gram-positive bacilli, gram-negative cocci, and gram-negative bacilli. These bacteria inhabit the lower small intestine of humans and are found embedded in the mucus attached to the intestinal mucosa. However, they are found in significant numbers only in the large intestine.

The gastrointestinal tract is sterile at birth but becomes inhabited by bacteria via the oral route within the first few days of life. The diet is the principal determinant of the type of bacteria that will inhabit the gastrointestinal tract. All surfaces of the human body are covered with a normal flora population which has been shown to be stable in composition. Relatively little is known concerning the control of this population on the body's surface, including the gastrointestinal colonies.

Moore and Holdeman have reported the presence of 400 to 500 different kinds of bacteria in the feces of the population studied.[3] Their study indicated the existence of a strong interaction between the microenvironment and mechanisms by which one bacterial population controls the growth of others.

Intestinal bacteria are responsible for the production of several enzymes involved in the digestive and absorptive process. Many members of the body's normal bacterial flora produce fatty acids and carbon dioxide and are responsible for the formation of flatus in the gut and lower gastrointestinal tract. The gastrointestinal flora also serves as a catalyst in the production of bile acids and in the intermediate stages of carbohydrate and fat digestion.

Colonic bacteria are capable of producing vitamin K and several of the B complex vitamins. *Staphylococcus aureus*, a common gastrointestinal inhabitant, is responsible for the synthesis of vitamin K. Vitamin K injections are necessary for newborn infants because they lack an intestinal flora at birth and therefore lack vitamin K, which is needed to prevent hemorrhages.

The presence of bacteria has also been shown to alter the mucosal structure of the intestinal wall. In animals raised in a sterile environment, the intestinal wall appears thinner and lighter in composition when compared to the thicker mucosal structure of the bacteria-inhabited gastrointestinal tract of ordinary animals. Nutritional and environmental factors affect the normal intestinal flora and can affect the resulting function of the inhabited gastrointestinal structure. One of the frequent side effects of antibiotic therapy is sterilization of the bowel. Research is underway to determine the level of antibiotic ingestion that is necessary to effect a change in the gastrointestinal population resulting from the action of these drugs on the gastrointestinal flora. At present, there are few data citing the limits of antibiotic usage that will result in decreasing the bacterial colonization of the lower gastrointestinal tract.

Shapiro has cited evidence that a yogurt diet supplement containing *Lactobacillus bulgarius* and *staphylococcus thermophilus* can aid in restoring the physiological balance and bacterial colonization of the small bowel after extensive antibiotic therapy in some disease states.[4] The implications of extensive antibiotic use and its effect on the intestinal bacterial flora remain of paramount concern in long-term antibiotic therapy.

Neurohormonal Control of Digestion

Until now, digestion has been viewed in this chapter as a chemical and mechanical process utilizing the secretions and muscular actions of the pancreas, liver, gallbladder, and stomach.

Four hormones have been identified as the initiators of enzyme secretions—gastrin, cholecystokinin, pancreozymin, and secretin. It is also important to understand the significant neurohormonal control that is exerted on the digestive process.

The complex interconnections between the cerebral cortex, hypothalamus, and vagus nerve have been propounded by Go and Summerskill.[5] The homeostasis of the digestive process is shown to be coordinated by both local and central mechanisms while being modified by neural, hormonal, and metabolic relationships.

The process of digestion becomes an integrated process by virtue of impulses transmitted via the vagus nerve which regulate the gastrointestinal secretions that are ultimately responsible for the digestive process. These impulses arise from the ventral medial center of the hypothalamus (believed to be the center of satiety) in response to blood sugar levels, initiating a feeling of hunger when the blood sugar level is below normal. In response to the hypoglycemia, secretion of insulin and glucagon are regulated by the pancreas, and gastrointestinal secretions begin urging the initiation of eating.

The presence of food in the gut as well as vagal stimulation initiates the secretion of the hormones gastrin from the gastric mucosa and secretin, cholecystokinin, and pancreozymin from the intestinal mucosa. The central nervous system and gastrointestinal system influence each other by vagal efferent and afferent pathways, resulting in the secretion of these gastrointestinal hormones.

These hormones in turn are responsible for stimulation of the stomach, intestine, liver, gallbladder, and pancreas to produce the specific enzymes that are necessary to further the breakdown of nutrients in the gut. Thus the integrated mechanisms of hunger, ingestion, and digestion are regulated.

Bearing in mind the relationship between the neural cortical centers and hormone secretions, it becomes clear that digestion can be

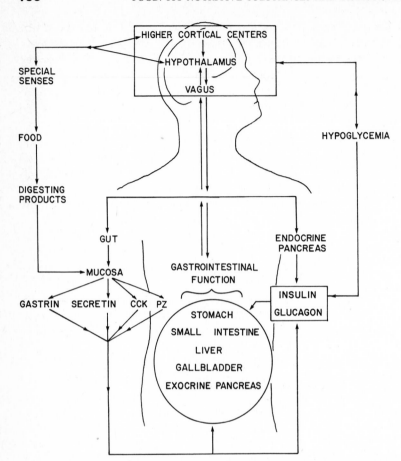

Figure 9-4
Neural-hormonal relationships in digestion. (Cholecystokinin is abbreviated as CCK; pancreozymin as PZ). (Adapted from V. L. W. Go, and W. H. J. Summerskill, American Journal of Clinical Nutrition, 1971, p. 160.)

significantly affected by a disturbance in the delicate neural biochemistry. Stress, anxiety, fatigue, and illness can alter vagal control of the gastrointestinal secretion and may thereby interrupt the dynamics of the digestive process. Therefore, in order to understand how the digestive process contributes to a homeostatic milieu, the role of the brain in relation to the process of food utilization must not be overlooked.

ABSORPTION

Stomach

Very little absorption takes place in the stomach. It functions rather as an organ of prepara-

tion for the digestion and absorption that are carried out in the gut.

Small Intestine

The small bowel is the primary site of nutrient absorption. It is approximately 300 cm (10 ft) long; however, its absorbing surface is larger than one-third of a football field. The large absorptive surface of the small bowel is due mainly to its mucosal structure. The exterior, or serosal, surface of the small intestine appears smooth. However, the inside luminal or mucosal surface is heaped in folds. On microscopic examination of this irregular mucosal surface, fingerlike projections known as *villi* are evident. When these villi are examined more closely with high-power electron microscopy, the epithelial cells covering these villi are seen to be covered themselves with bristlelike projections known as the *microvilli*. This luminal surface housing the microvilli is known as the *brush border*. The presence of the villi and the microvilli enlarges the potential absorptive surface of the small intestine to an area as much as 600 times greater than the outside serosal area.

The mucosal lining of the small intestine consists of a single layer of columnar epithelial cells that rests on a layer of supporting connective tissue, the *lamina propria*. Fig. 9-5 illustrates the structure of the jejunal mucosa, showing the columnar epithelial cells, nuclei, and villi. Note the contribution of the villi to the increased absorptive capacity of the small bowel.

Mucosal Function

The primary function of the small intestine is to absorb the end products of digestion. Once inside the mucosal cell, the nutrients traverse the membrane and are carried through the

Figure 9-5

Photomicrograph of human jejunal mucosa. Note the tall, finger-like villi and short crypts (ratio, approximately 4 to 1). The cells lining the villi are columnar, with basally oriented nuclei and an even surface layer. Lamina propria and supporting elements show normal cellularity. (Original magnification × 125. Photo courtesy of Dr. Richard J. Grand.)

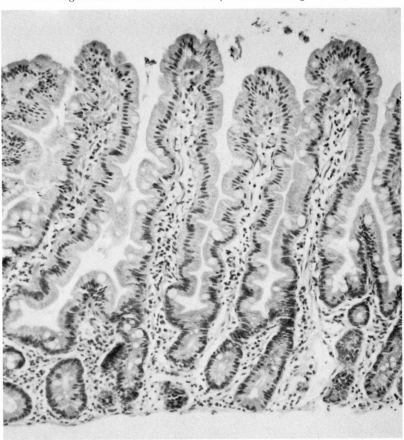

serosal layer and eventually enter the intestinal fluid. From here, the nutrients are able to pass through the vascular or lymphatic capillary network for transport to the sites of metabolism.

Mucosal Transport

A knowledge of the various means of molecular transport is important in understanding the passage of nutrient molecules to their sites of absorption and metabolism. The mucosal cells require special transport systems to accommodate the cellular absorption of nutrient molecules. These transport systems are known as:

Passive diffusion
Bulk flow
Solvent drag
Carrier-mediated diffusion
Active transport
Sodium pump

Passive diffusion   Absorption from the duodenum usually occurs by *passive diffusion*. Passive diffusion, or osmotic pressure, allows substances that are small enough in size to pass from one side of a membrane to the other, from an area of greater concentration to one of lesser concentration. Monosaccharides, fat-soluble vitamins, and several water-soluble vitamins pass across the intestinal mucosa via passive diffusion.

Bulk flow   In bulk flow negatively charged ions such as chloride move from an area of higher concentration to an area of lesser concentration in an attempt to equalize the osmotic pressure.

Solvent drag   Some molecules may be small enough to pass through the intestinal mucosal pores, thus utilizing the transport process known as *solvent drag*.

Carrier-mediated diffusion   Following a meal, when the contents of the intestinal lumen are high in digested carbohydrates and proteins, a means for ferrying these molecules into the blood from the gut is needed. The intestinal epithelium contains a large quantity of carriers that act as ferries to transport these water-soluble complexes through the lipoprotein membrane. Passive diffusion of this type is known as *carrier-mediated diffusion*.

Active transport   Transporting a substance against an electrochemical gradient or other forces is known as *active transport*. It differs from passive transport in that more energy is required to transport materials against a gradient to permit a homeostatic equilibrium of concentration. Although there is much disagreement over which substances rely on active transport, the major nutrients believed to enlist this mechanism include sodium, calcium, iron, glucose, galactose, many amino acids, and vitamin B_{12}.

Sodium pump   The final transport phenomenon to be considered is the *sodium pump*. Possibly this mechanism is the most crucial of all. This system has the ability to extract sodium ions from isotonic or even hypotonic salt solutions in the intestinal lumen, in order to move sodium into, through, and out of the intestinal epithelial cell and into the vessels draining the area. The movement of this positively charged ion produces an electrical gradient which allows negatively charged ions to follow. Thus, an osmotic pressure is created and water molecules move in response to the pressure gradient.

Large Intestine

Most of the ingested water and electrolytes are absorbed in the colon. Sodium and chloride ions are actively absorbed in the proximal half of the colon, creating an osmotic gradient. This osmotic gradient between the intestinal lumen and the plasma is the major determinant of water absorption. The normal colon absorbs approximately 1400 ml of water daily, with the movement of the water molecules

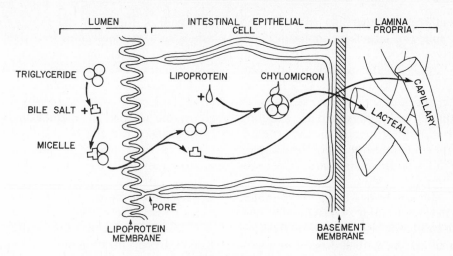

Figure 9-6
Cellular absorption. (Adapted from F. J. Ingelfinger, Nutrition Today, 2:3, 1967.)

closely paralleling movement of the sodium ions that are present.

A few bacteria in the colon are capable of digesting small amounts of cellulose. However, the major portion of ingested cellulose, hemicellulose, and other roughage is excreted as the principal component of the feces.

The rectum plays a small part in water and sodium absorption, and is most involved with the process of elimination.

Protein Absorption

The intestinal mucosa allows for a small, nutritionally insignificant, amount of large, intact protein molecules to pass into the epithelial cells. Gastric, pancreatic, and intestinal enzymes break large protein molecules into the smaller amino acids. Through active transport, amino acids are absorbed into the intestinal mucosa. Several factors affect macromolecular transport:

1 *Presence of localized antibodies* Local antibody deficiency may increase the number of large protein molecules that are absorbed. An example can be found in the fish-protein–sensitive individual. When

fish protein is ingested by an individual who has developed an antibody to the protein, an allergic reaction to the protein molecule occurs at the site of the antibody, thus blocking the protein molecule and ultimately affecting its absorption.

2 *Anatomy of the intestinal mucosa* Alterations in the mucosal barrier, such as ulceration, inflammation, or mucosal surface changes, will affect the receptor sites for nutrient absorption and hinder the transport of the large protein molecule.

3 *Physiology of lysosomes* Lysosomal dysfunction can interfere with the intracellular digestion process and affect the transport of large molecules also.

4 *Gastric acidity* Finally, low gastric acidity, pancreatic insufficiency, and other factors can alter the ability of the gut to absorb large nutrient molecules and thus can interfere with the absorption of proteins.

Lipid Absorption

(See also Chap. 5.) Fat absorption is a process involving several interdependent steps. Fat is most often ingested as triglycerides. In the upper small bowel, pancreatic enzymes and secretions split the larger fat molecules into smaller fatty acid units. Bile salts help to emulsify these fatty acids and put them into solution, forming a unit known as a *micelle* for continuation in the absorption process. Once in solution, the fat molecules which are traveling as a micellar complex are able to reach the microvilli of the small intestine. Here the complex splits, the bile salts traveling down to be reabsorbed in the distal ileum and the free fatty acids and monoglycerides being reassembled to form a new triglyceride. To enable the passage of this newly formed triglyceride through the intestinal lumen, a small droplet of a protein called a beta-lipoprotein surrounds the fat molecule. The new compound, called a *chylomicron,* is the form that can penetrate the epithelium of the lamina propria, or basement membrane, of the small intestine. The chylomicron enters the lymphatic system via the lamina propria and travels through the portal blood system, completing the process of fat absorption.

Cholesterol absorption (see also Chap. 5) is poorly understood. Cholesterol is usually ingested with fat and requires the pancreatic enzyme cholesterol esterase to emulsify the compound and make it available for absorption via the intestinal lumen. Cholesterol is also synthesized in the intestinal mucosa, which makes absorption studies difficult to execute. There is evidence that cholesterol absorption occurs at a steady rate when dietary intake is moderate but seems to increase with the ingestion of a diet high in fats.

Carbohydrate Absorption

(See also Chap. 4.) Carbohydrate is most often ingested as a disaccharide or polysaccharide. Salivary and pancreatic enzymes break the complex molecules into disaccharides which are then passed on to the intestinal lumen. Because of their still large molecular structure, the partially digested disaccharides are acted on by a variety of disaccharides found in the

microvilli of the intestinal lumen. These enzymes split the molecules into their constituent simple sugars, or monosaccharides—glucose, fructose, and galactose.

Glucose is water-soluble and, despite its large molecular size, is readily transported across the lipoprotein membrane. Other six-carbon sugars can also be absorbed readily because of their ability to pass through the narrow passages of the luminal pore system. Glucose can be absorbed actively or passively, depending on the degree of concentration in the gut. Because of the nature of this transport, glucose is capable of being absorbed even when the concentration of sugar in the blood is relatively high, as in diabetes mellitus.

Once absorbed, the monosaccharides enter the capillary network and circulate throughout the blood system.

Vitamin and Mineral Absorption

It is important to remember that ingestion of a meal will result in the intake of a variety of vitamins and minerals along with the basic nutrients. The small intestine is the site of absorption for these vitamins and minerals, the most active absorptive area being the lower part of the duodenum and the first part of the jejunum. (See Chaps. 6, 7, and 8.)

METABOLISM

The process of food ingestion, breakdown, and utilization involves a number of biochemical processes aided by enzyme-catalyzed reactions. It is important to understand that the major outcome of the digestion and absorption process is the production of energy.

In the living cell the nutrients work synergistically in cellular metabolism. Through this metabolic process energy is released and utilized for the synthesis of the cell's own biochemical composition and byproducts.

Metabolism is the sum total of all the chemical processes occurring in the body that result

TABLE 9-2 SITE OF ABSORPTION OF NUTRIENTS FROM THE GASTROINTESTINAL TRACT

Nutrient	Site of absorption
Glucose	Lower duodenum, upper jejunum
Sucrose	Lower jejunum, ileum
Lactose	Jejunum, upper ileum
Maltose	Jejunum, upper ileum
Amino acids	Lower duodenum, jejunum
Fats	Lower duodenum, upper jejunum
Cholesterol	Lumen of small intestine
Iron	Duodenum (limited absorption), jejunum
Calcium	Duodenum
Vitamin D	Ileum (disputed)
Vitamin A	Duodenum, jejunum
Vitamin E	Duodenum
Vitamin K	Duodenum
Folic acid	Upper duodenum
Pyridoxine	Jejunum
Riboflavin	Duodenum
Thiamine	Duodenum
Ascorbic acid	Jejunum
Water	Colon

in the utilization of ingested food. Energy production is a result of the body's ability to digest, absorb, and finally metabolize nutrients.

The Measurement of Energy

The body's ability to do work and operate its biochemical system is dependent on the production of energy. Energy can be measured in units of heat equivalents. A *calorie* is a unit of heat measurement. In nutritional and physiological studies the traditional unit of heat measurement has been the large calorie or *kilocalorie* (equal to 1000 small calories), which is defined as the amount of heat required to raise 1 kg of water 1°C. In practice, the terms calorie and kilocalorie are used interchangeably as a measure of food energy content.

In the metric system, the *joule* is the unit of energy; 1 calorie (1 kcal) equals 4.184 joules (4.184kJ). Caloric values of food may be con-

verted to the metric equivalent (joules) by multiplying the number of calories by 4.184. For example: 1 g of carbohydrate contains 4 kcal or approximately 17 kJ.

Through the use of an instrument known as a bomb calorimeter, energy values have been determined for a large variety of foodstuffs. A specific amount of food is placed in the inner center of the calorimeter and the instrument is submerged in water. In the presence of oxygen, the food is ignited and burned. The water surrounding the food chamber increases in temperature during the combustion process, signifying the number of calories obtained through the oxidation of the food.

With this process, the *fuel factor*, or average number of calories per gram of nutrient, has been established for each of the three energy-producing nutrients and for alcohol:

$$
\begin{aligned}
1 \text{ g of carbohydrate} &= 4 \text{ calories (kcal)} \\
&= 17 \text{ joules (kJ)} \\
1 \text{ g of protein} &= 4 \text{ kcal} \\
&= 17 \text{ kJ} \\
1 \text{ g of fat} &= 9 \text{ kcal} \\
&= 37.6 \text{ kJ} \\
1 \text{ g of alcohol} &= 7 \text{ kcal} \\
&= 29.3 \text{ kJ}
\end{aligned}
$$

CATABOLISM

Catabolism is the metabolic process involving the breakdown of molecules, resulting in the release of energy. Fig. 9-7 shows the interrelationships between carbohydrate, protein, and fat during the catabolic process.

These compounds are all processed eventually in the same cycle for the production of energy. The Krebs cycle produces about 90 percent of the body's energy requirements of adenosine triphosphate (ATP). ATP is a high-energy compound which provides the body with an easy source of energy in a stored form.

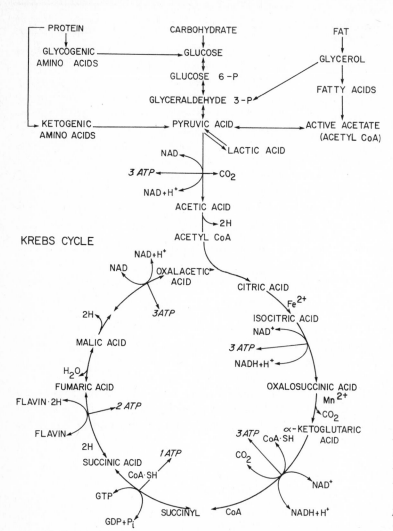

EMBDEN - MEYERHOF
GLYCOLYTIC PATHWAY

KREBS CYCLE

Figure 9-7

Interrelationships between the two energy-producing cycles—the Embden-Meyerhof glycolytic pathway and the Krebs cycle. A total of 38 molecules of ATP (adenosine triphosphate) are produced from the combination of these cycles for every 1 molecule of glucose.

Several vitamins are needed to catalyze certain reactions within the Krebs cycle:

Pantothenic acid

Niacin

Lipoic acid

Thiamine

Riboflavin

Nutrient catabolism yields 2 molecules of ATP from the Embden-Meyerhof glycolytic pathway and 36 ATP molecules from the electron transport chain for every glucose molecule catabolized. Thus, the body receives a constant supply of chemical energy to maintain its physiological and biochemical functions.

ATP is stored in a small metabolic pool for use as needed. However, because of the body's constant need for energy, there is a rapid turnover in this pool.

All products of endogenous or exogenous

metabolism have been shown to be in a state of active turnover. The concept of a metabolic pool was elaborated by Schoenheimer, who clearly demonstrated that all components of living matter are in a steady state of flux.[6] Thus, the metabolic pool is the quantity of a substance that is in a state of rapid turnover.

Carbohydrate Catabolism

(See also Chap. 4.) Glucose is converted through a series of biochemical reactions from a six-carbon sugar to pyruvic acid, allowing entry of this molecule into the energy-producing Krebs cycle. This sequence of catabolic reactions, referred to as *glycolysis,* results in the release of energy and the production of pyruvic acid. In this process of glycolysis, two molecules of the high-energy compound ATP are used and four are produced, with the net gain of two molecules available for immediate use. The pyruvic acid, under aerobic conditions (available oxygen), then enters the Krebs cycle. However, when there is insufficient oxygen or under anaerobic conditions such as during heavy exercise, the pyruvic acid is converted to lactic acid and does not enter the Krebs cycle. The lactic acid accumulates in the blood and can be converted back to glucose, mostly in the liver.

Protein Catabolism

(See also Chap. 3.) Early studies have led to the classification of amino acids into two categories according to the type of end products after degradation: those amino acids with glucose as an end product are known as *glycogenic,* whereas those amino acids producing ketone bodies are known as *ketogenic* amino acids (see Table 9-3).

Glycogenic amino acids are deaminated by coenzyme vitamin B_6 to form pyruvic acid in the Embden-Meyerhof glucolytic pathway. They may undergo decarboxylation to form acetic acid or they may go through the process of gluconeogenesis to form glucose and glycogen. Gluconeogenesis is the formation of

TABLE 9-3   CLASSIFICATION OF AMINO ACIDS FORMED BY CATABOLISM OF PROTEIN

Glycogenic	Ketogenic	Glycogenic & ketogenic
Alanine	Leucine	Isoleucine
Arginine		Lysine
Aspartic acid		Phenylalanine
Cystine		Tyrosine
Glutamic acid		
Glycine		
Histidine		
Hydroxyproline		
Proline		
Serine		
Threonine		
Tryptophan		
Valine		

glucose from noncarbohydrate sources. Ketogenic amino acids are processed as fatty acids and are eventually converted to acetyl coenzyme A (acetyl CoA).

Fat Catabolism

Fatty acids undergo a degradation process resulting in the formation of acetyl coenzyme A, allowing entry into the same pathway as carbohydrate.

ANABOLISM

Anabolism is the biochemical process of synthesizing large molecules from small molecules. This process is responsible for the maintenance of body tissue and ultimately for the synthesis of body components. Nutrients in excess of the energy needs of the cells are used for growth, development, and body maintenance.

Glucose is converted to glycogen by the liver and is stored in that organ when there is more glucose in the circulation than can be used by the cells for energy. Glycogen is also stored in muscle tissue and can be used for muscle function during periods of increased exercise or muscular stress that will require increased energy needs. Liver stores of glycogen can be mobilized and converted back to glucose by the process known as glycogenolysis. *Glycogenolysis* is the process resulting in the conversion of glycogen to glucose for eventual entry into the Krebs cycle. In starvation or with energy-deficient diets, liver and muscle stores are mobilized to provide glucose for energy and cellular functioning. (See also Chap. 4.) Fat stores are also mobilized for energy through the breakdown of lipid molecules. Resynthesis of these molecules to glucose supplies the body with energy when the exogenous supplies of energy are limited.

Glycerol, an intermediate metabolic product of lipid digestion, can enter the Krebs cycle or can be reconverted to glucose or glycogen. Glycogenic amino acids can provide energy through entry into the Krebs cycle or can be converted to glucose for either conversion to glycogen or the production of energy.

The process of *gluconeogensis* (glucose production from a noncarbohydrate source) provides a source of glucose for circulation or for storage or glycogen. However, since glucose production results from the degradation of protein, fats, and carbohydrates, it must be noted that ingesting these nutrients in amounts beyond normal energy demands can result in the increase of glucose in the system. Since all amino acids, carbohydrates, fatty acids, glycerol, and glucose eventually enter the Krebs cycle, the potential for increased lipid synthesis in response to increased nutrient intake is real. The energy that is produced as a result of these nutrients' entering the Krebs cycle will be converted to storage forms of glycogen or fat. Thus, the response to a nutrient intake that is greater than the energy need is the production of adipose tissue as a source of stored energy.

Besides carbon dioxide and water, energy is one of the major metabolic products derived from the utilization of ingested food (Table 9-4). A metabolic homeostasis, with energy input (nutrient intake) equaling energy output (catabolism), results in the maintenance of essential body functions.

BASAL METABOLIC RATE

Energy expenditure can be defined as the metabolic cost of a period of work. This cost can be calculated as gross kilocalories (kilojoules) or net kilocalories (kilojoules). However, the net kilocalories used by the body include two other factors that must be deducted from the net caloric expenditure during a period of work: (1) the basal metabolic rate and (2) the specific dynamic action of food.

The *basal metabolic rate* (BMR) is the energy expended by an awake individual at rest. The BMR requires the individual to be at physical, digestive, and emotional rest. The rate of oxygen consumption can be used as a measure of energy expenditure. Energy costs are most often expressed in kilocalories per minute but can be readily converted to kilocalories per 24h.

TABLE 9-4 FINAL PRODUCTS OF NUTRIENT DIGESTION, ANABOLISM, AND CATABOLISM

Nutrient	Digestion	Anabolism	Catabolism
Protein	Amino acids	Tissue, enzymes, hormones, fat	CO_2, energy, H_2O urea
Fat	Fatty acids & glycerol	fat	CO_2, energy, H_2O
Carbohydrate	monosaccharides	glycogen & fat	CO_2, energy, H_2O

The BMR can be measured by direct or indirect methods or determining oxygen consumption and carbon dioxide expiration per unit of specified time. The individual is required to observe a 12-h fast to ensure that the energy costs of digestion are excluded. With the individual awake and in a reclining position, the oxygen and carbon dioxide status are recorded.

The BMR is influenced by many factors:

Age

Body size

Temperature

Physical exercise

Fever

Specific dynamic action of food

Because of these variables it is difficult to predict the basal metabolic requirements of an individual. However, the BMR is commonly calculated by allowing 24 kcal kg body weight (101 kJ kg body weight) per day:

$$BMR = 24 \text{ kcal} \times \text{weight (kg) /day}$$
$$= 101 \text{ kJ} \times \text{weight (kg)/day}$$

Any condition that increases or decreases the body's expenditure of energy will inevitably reflect a proportionate change in the BMR. Some conditions that alter the BMR are listed in Table 9-5.

Age The basal oxygen consumption per kilogram of body weight decreases approximately 5 to 10 percent every 10 years after age 14. This decrease reflects a general decrease in cellular growth and activity and seems to be at the lowest levels in the elderly population over 65 years of age.

Body size The relationship between body size and metabolism is an inverse proportion. The smaller the animal the larger the BMR. In early studies done with animals of various sizes, it was found that an indirect relationship existed between metabolism and body weight. However, there seems to be a direct relationship between body surface area and BMR. That is, the larger the organism's surface area the greater the metabolic rate. This seems to be due to the processes of temperature regulation and heat loss, which are both related to surface area. Therefore, as surface area increases, the BMR increases the compensate for heat loss and to help control body temperature.

Environmental temperature Exposure to cold increases energy needs in response to the increased need for maintenance of body heat. Studies have shown that the metabolic rates of people living in the Arctic are 10 to 20 percent higher than those of people living in tropical areas. This increase reflects an adaptation of the thyroid gland, resulting in increased thyroid secretion in cold climates and decreased secretion in warm climates.

Physical exercise Physical activity increases the BMR in proportion to the type of exercise and the manner in which the activity is undertaken.

Fever Disease and physiological stress increase the BMR 7 percent for every 1°F above the norm. This is because every chemical reaction in vitro or in vivo increases its reaction 130 percent for every rise in temperature of 50°F (10°C). Therefore a body temperature of 105°F (40.5°C) represents a 90 percent increase in the metabolic rate.

Specific dynamic action of food Net Energy expenditure is a result of the energy required to maintain metabolic processes when the body is at rest, plus the energy produced after the ingestion of food. Energy is measured in units of heat, as previously mentioned. It has been reported that heat production increases during food ingestion. This effect of food on the production of heat is referred to as the *specific dynamic action* (SDA) of food. The SDA accounts for approximately 10 percent of the

TABLE 9-5 CONDITIONS ALTERING BASAL METABOLIC RATE

Condition	Increase	Possible increase	Decrease	Possible decrease
Increased physical activity	×			
Pregnancy	×			
Fever	×			
Endocrine disorders:				
Hyperthyroidism	×			
Hypersecretion of pituitary gland		×		
Cushing's syndrome		×		
Tumors of adrenal glands		×		
Blood diseases:				
Leukemia (most often)	×			
Pernicious anemia		×		
Essential hypertension		×		
Myocardial stress	×			
Diabetes insipidus		×		
Shock			×	
Malnutrition			×	
Anemia (Severe)				×
Chronic Arthritis				×
Peptic Ulcer				×
Nephrotic syndrome (lipid nephrosis)			×	
Endocrine disorders:				
Hypothyroidism			×	
Addison's disease				×
Hypopituitarism				×
Nervous system diseases:				
Schizophrenia				×
Psychoneurosis				×
Autonomic imbalance (vagotonia)				×

Source: Adapted from A. Cantarow and M. Trumperer, *Clinical Biochemistry*, W. B. Saunders Company, Philadelphia, 1975.

total energy intake but represents the energy value of the nutrient that is not available to the body for metabolism. Some of the ingested food is not absorbed by the body and is excreted as feces. These losses are due to the SDA and the excretion of the metabolic by-products creatinine, urea, and other organic components of the urine. The caloric values of foods as listed in diet tables are energy values for the food items after the SDA and other losses have been deducted.

ENERGY REQUIREMENTS

An individual's caloric or energy requirements are a function of his whole psychosocial-physiological state. Muscular activity influences the body's total energy needs perhaps more than any other environmental factor. In determining the average energy need of an individual, it is necessary to assess his activity level as related to his life style and add this increased need to his BMR. In very broad terms, a sedentary life style will require additional calories equal to 30 percent of the BMR. Moderate activity will increase the energy needs by 40 percent of the BMR, and a very active life style will increase the caloric needs by 50 percent of the BMR. For example, a 60-kg woman who leads a very active and full day would require 2160 kcal (9072 kJ) to accommodate her BMR and daily activity needs, as illustrated below.

$$BMR = 60 \text{ kg} \times 24 \text{ kcal/day}$$
$$= 1440 \text{ kcal/day} = 6048 \text{ kJ/day}$$
$$\text{Heavy activity} = 50\% \text{ BMR} = 50\% \times 1440$$
$$= 720 \text{ kcal/day} = 3024 \text{ kJ/day}$$

Total energy needs
$$= BMR + \text{calculated activity requirement}$$
Total energy needs per day = 1440 + 720
$$= 2160 \text{ kcal/day} = 9072 \text{ kJ/day}$$

This method for determining an individual's energy needs can be made more specific by determining his exact energy expenditure per day by activity. Table 9-6 lists specific activities and related energy expenditure in calories (joules) per minute of activity as elaborated by Passmore and Durin.[7]

Emotional stress, growth, muscle activity, health, and body size are key factors in determining the body's energy needs for energy balance. The Food and Nutrition Board of the National Academy of Sciences–National Research Council has established energy allowances for adults on the basis of age and sex (Table 9-7). These figures are to be used as a guideline in determining energy needs. It must be remembered that any deviation from the individual's normal psychosocial-physiological status will reflect an increase or decrease in these estimated energy needs, depending upon the nature of the change.

BODY COMPOSITION

Body composition can be defined as the chemical composition of the body's stores of:

Bone tissue
Connective tissue
Soft tissue
Adipose tissue

In vitro and in vivo studies have been utilized to determine the exact chemical composition of the body's tissues. Via chemical analysis there seems to be general agreement on body composition of vitamins, minerals, and other nutrients. Friis-Hansen has quantitated the

TABLE 9-6 CALORIC EXPENDITURE PER MINUTE OF SPECIFIED ACTIVITY FOR A REFERENCE 65-KG MAN

Activity	kcal/min	kJ/min
Sewing, 30 stitches/min	1.14	4.8
Sewing by machine	1.6	6.7
Sitting, playing cards	1.9	7.9
Brushing boots	2.2	9.2
Driving a car	2.8	11.7
Peeling potatoes	2.9	12.1
Stirring	3.0	12.5
Horseriding, walk	3.0	12.5
Kneading dough	3.3	13.8
Driving a motorcycle	3.4	14.2
Volleyball	3.5	14.6
Mopping	4.2	17.6
Ironing	4.2	17.6
Cycling, 5.5 mph	4.5	18.8
Golf	5.0	20.9
Dancing, waltz	5.7	23.8
Tennis	7.1	29.7
Grooming horses	8.3	34.7
Football association	8.9	37.2
Horseriding, galloping	10.0	41.8
Cross-country running	10.6	44.4
Skiing, moderate speed	10.8	45.2
Swimming, breast stroke	11.0	45.3
Cycling, 13.1 mph	11.1	46.4
Swimming, back crawl	11.5	48.1
Walking, on hard snow, 6 km/hr	11.9	49.8

Source: Adapted from R. Passmore and J. V. G. A. Durin, "Human Energy Expedition," *Physiological Reviews,* 35: 801–840, 1955.

TABLE 9-7   SUGGESTED WEIGHTS FOR HEIGHTS AND BASAL METABOLIC RATES (BMR) OF ADULTS

Height		Men				Women			
		Median weight		BMR		Median weight		BMR	
in	cm	lb	kg	kcal/day	kJ/day	lb	kg	kcal/day	kJ/day
60	152					109 ± 9	50 ± 4	1399	5853
62	158					115 ± 9	52 ± 4	1429	5979
64	163	133 ± 11	60 ± 5	1630	6820	122 ± 10	56 ± 5	1487	6222
66	168	142 ± 12	64 ± 5	1690	7071	129 ± 10	59 ± 5	1530	6402
68	173	151 ± 14	69 ± 6	1775	7427	136 ± 10	62 ± 5	1572	6577
70	178	159 ± 14	72 ± 6	1815	7594	144 ± 11	66 ± 5	1626	6803
72	183	167 ± 15	76 ± 7	1870	7824	152 ± 12	69 ± 5	1666	6971
74	188	175 ± 15	80 ± 7	1933	8088				
76	193	183 ± 16	83 ± 7	1983	8297				

To determine the daily energy need of an individual, allow for hours of sleep at 90 percent of BMR and for time periods engaged in various activities as indicated in Table 9–6.

Source: Recommended Dietary Allowances, National Research Council, Washington, D.C., 1974.

percentage of mineral, protein, and fat composition for the water-free body area as 6, 16, and 18 percent respectively.[8] In determining exact proportions of body nutrients, it has been estimated through chemical analysis that 25 to 50 percent of the body is water-free tissue.

The difficulties of studying the human body by direct chemical analysis plus the desirability of studying in vitro measurements has led to the development of indirect methods of determining body composition, namely:

Bone density
Fat fold measurements
Radiography
Anthropometric measurements

Anthropometric Measurements

Body measurements provide a good estimation of fat stores and thus give an indication of body composition. Traditionally, height and weight measurements have been utilized to relate physical size to an estimated set of standards established by the National Research Council. However, bone and muscle, as well as adipose tissue, cannot be quantitated accurately by these gross measurements. The use of skinfold calipers can aid in the estimation of body fat stores via measurement of skinfold thickness (see Chap. 12). Skinfold thickness standards have been established for measurement of the triceps muscle and abdominal and midthigh regions.

Body density, as demonstrated by Ingalls and by Baker and Newman, can provide an accurate measurement of lean body mass, defined as the whole body less the excess fat.[9,10] Submersion of the entire body in a tankful of water, and then recording the air volume in the lungs and measuring the rise in water volume, can provide statistics that yield the body density of the subject through mathematical equations. Body density is related to the physical activity of the individual, which increases metabolism and places extra stress on muscles and bones, thus affecting lean body mass.

Factors Affecting Body Composition

The study of body composition must take into account the functional, physiological, genetic, and nutritional factors that are significant determinants of body tissue structure.

Diet has an effect on body composition, perhaps most evident in the bone density and extent of adipose tissue. Bone density has been shown to vary up to 50 percent among individuals with similar stature. The amount of bone mineral seems to be greater in males than in females, greater in adults than in adolescents, and greater in individuals with higher calcium and phosphorus intakes.

According to Garn, subcutaneous fat deposits are greater in females than in males.[11] This may be due to the role of adipose tissue as insulation during childbearing.

Weight loss can significantly affect total body composition by decreasing adipose tissue stores. When increased exercise is coupled with a energy deficient diet, fat stores will be mobilized and converted to energy in order to accommodate for the increased energy expenditure caused by increased activity.

Body composition also reflects an individual's age and stage of development. Differences in electrolyte, mineral, protein, fat, and water content per kilogram of body weight between a full-term newborn infant and an adult male have been recorded by Brozek.[12] As the body approaches maturity, the electrolytes in the diet and the ratio of these electrolytes of dietary protein seem to influence body composition, reflected in an increase of these nutrients per kilogram of body weight.

STUDY QUESTIONS

1 Starting with the "port of entry," follow a meal progressively through the gastrointestinal system.
2 What are the neurohormonal control mechanisms that are operative in the process of digestion?
3 Describe the interrelationships between carbohydrate, protein, and fat metabolism in the body.
4 List those factors influencing the basal metabolic rate.
5 How would you go about calculating your own daily energy needs? Proceed to do so.

CASE STUDY 9-1

Past History
S. J. is a 35-year-old woman with obesity, elevated blood pressure, and increased triglyceride levels. Past history reveals a sedentary life style with an early diagnosis of obesity in childhood. At age 15, S. J. weighted 170 lb (77 kg) and was 5 ft 5 in (165 cm) tall. Past attempts to control weight gain were without success.

Present History
A physical examination reveals an adult woman in no apparent distress. Her height is 5 ft 7 in (170 cm) and her weight is 280 lb (127 kg). Blood pressure is recorded at 190/110. Other significant laboratory data include:

Serum cholesterol	*260 mg/100 ml*
Serum triglycerides	*200 mg/100 ml*
SGOT (serum	*30 units/ml*
glutamic oxalacetic transaminase)	
Alkaline phosphatase	*10 king-Armstrong units*
Serum glucose (after 2-h fast)	*70 mg/100 ml*

Present food intake is 3700 kcal/day (15481 kJ) (250 g protein, 400 g carbohydrates, 125 g fat).

Because of the increased stress to the cardiovascular system and the threat to S. J.'s general health, a jejunoileal bypass was performed. This is an extraordinary procedure reserved for extreme cases of intractable obesity.

The procedure creates a surgical bypass of the jejunal and ileal segments of the small intestine, resulting in direct passage of nutrients from the duodenum to the colon.

The postoperative course was complicated by diarrhea, steatorrhea, and electrolyte imbalance. Progressive weight loss followed.

Case Study Questions

1 *Describe the function of the jejunum and ileum in nutrient absorption. Relate this function to the problems of diarrhea and steatorrhea that S. J. encountered postoperatively.*

2 *List those nutrients most likely to be affected in a jejunoileal bypass. Why?*

3 *Determine the actual energy needs of this 35-year-old sedentary female.*

REFERENCES

1 H. W. Davenport, *Physiology of the Digestive Tract,* Year Book Medical Publishers, Inc., Chicago, 1961.

2 Williams, "Benefit and Mischief from Commensal Bacteria," *Journal of Clinical Pathology,* **26:** 811–818, 1973.

4 S. Shapiro, "Control of Antibiotic Induced Gastrointestinal Symptoms with Yogurt," *Clinical Medicine,* **7**(2): 295–301, 1960.

3 W. E. C. Moore, and L. V. Holdeman, "Human Fecal Flora: The Normal Flora of 20 Japanese-Hawaiians," *Applied Microbiology,* **27:**961, 1974.

5 V. L. W. Go, and W. H. J. Summerskill, "Digestion, Maldigestion, and the G. I. Hormones," *American Journal of Clinical Nutrition,* **24:**160–167, 1971.

6 R. Schoenheimer, *The Dynamic State of Body Constituents,* Harvard University Press, Cambridge, Mass., 1942.

7 R. Passmore, and J. V. G. A. Durin, "Human Energy Expenditure," *Physiologic Reviews,* **35:**801–840, 1955.

8 B. Friis-Hansen, "Body Composition During Growth," *Pediatrics,* vol. 47, pt. II, January 1971.

9 N. W. Ingalls, "Observations on Bone Weight," *American Journal of Anatomy,* **48:**45–97, 1931.

10 P. T. Baker, and R. W. Newman, "The Use of Bone Weights," *American Journal of Physical Anthropology,* **15:**601–618, 1957.

11 S. M. Garn, "Roentgenogrammetric Determinations of Body Composition," *Human Biology,* **29:**337, 1957.

12 Josef Brozek, *Human Body Composition Approaches and Application,* Pergamon Press, New York, 1955.

PART TWO

FOOD

AND THE HUMAN

ENVIRONMENT

The principles of nutrition do not operate in a vacuum but in the human environment, one which is dynamic and impinged on by many forces. This part will examine these forces, which are operative both within the individual—growth, development, psychosocial influences—and around the individual in the community in which we all live.

CHAPTER 10

THE PSYCHOLOGY OF DIET AND BEHAVIOR MODIFICATION

*Rosanne B. Howard
and Richard R. Schnell*

KEY WORDS
Food Symbol
Feeding Problem
Helping Relationship
Diet Counseling
Observational Learning
Stimulus-Response Learning
Operant Learning
Reinforcement
Extinction
Guiding Behavior
Self-Management

THE PSYCHOLOGY OF DIET*

Rosanne B. Howard

INTRODUCTION

Success in diet counseling depends on directives being followed. This can only be accomplished when health professionals involved in diet counseling look beyond the food that is eaten and consider all those factors influencing food behavior, a process implied in the word *psychodietetics*.[1] Psychodietetics describes the complex interaction between diet and behavior and the need to look beyond the diet to the emotional aspects of eating—the need to consider all that is going on "in between the food and the mouth." This means considering all the determinants of food intake—sensory, personal, social. It involves taking an interest in the patient—in his feelings and attitudes about food—and giving them careful consideration in the planning of a diet. To do so, the nutrition educator must establish a counseling relationship that is a helping relationship. This section on psychology of diet focuses on the determinants of food intake and the approach needed to influence the formation of positive food habits. We begin by reflecting on the meaning of food: the diversity of meanings and how food meanings are acquired.

THE MEANING OF FOOD

Food choices are influenced by a whole host of factors that include:

Cultural background
Religious beliefs
Psychological acceptance (pleasing to see, taste, smell, feel)

* The author of this section wishes to acknowledge the support of Dr. Alexandria Manning Kiniry.

General economic situation (inflation, depression, recession)
Family finances
Susceptibility to advertising media
Level of education
Emotions
Society

Both consciously and unconsciously, all individuals are influenced by these factors as they make their food choices. However, these factors impinge differently on each individual and, in their totality, are particular to that person, causing each individual to evolve his or her own unique food meaning or symbols.

Food is essential for both the body and spirit. It not only calls forth much of thinking and emotion, but food can also be endowed readily with meaning and attitudes that are indeed "the body and the soul" of the person who partakes or rejects the food available to him. The ability of the body and spirit to utilize food may change within any given person in the face of any stress (be it physical, societal, or emotional) that is of sufficient duration and of such timing as to influence the balance within which the organism was operating in the immediate past. . . .[2]

Symbolic Meanings of Food

A categorization of food symbolisms is a somewhat arbitrary task; however, it does provide a framework around which to organize those meanings that are primarily operative in any individual (see Table 10-1). For the most part, food meanings of consequence relate to security. These food meanings emanate from the residual emotions of infancy and make the individual secure, whether biologically, socially, or emotionally secure. It is through food and feeding that an individual learns trust in the environment. As a child is held, cuddled, and fed, biological as well as emotional needs are met. Thereafter, a full stomach is identified with the person who provides the satis-

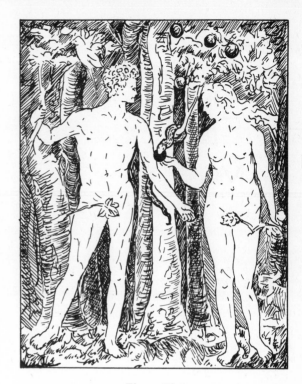

Figure 10-1
The apple—a universal food symbol of human weakness

faction and food becomes "love." Developmentally, many food problems may emanate from this basic perception, as the toddler and the adolescent refuse food in their struggle to establish their own ego identity (see Chap. 11).

Food Symbolism and Illness

Feelings regarding food are difficult to intellectualize. During stress and illness distortions of food behavior and a poor or fluctuating appetite are often the first signs of underlying pathology. In these periods, food can be used as an emotional crutch to gain security. For example, individuals may sublimate anxiety by eating continually or may seek attention in the same way. Often hospitalized patients may manipulate the staff through food rejections or impossible requests (e.g., wanting the breakfast egg cooked exactly 2½ minutes—no more, no less).

TABLE 10-1 SYMBOLIC MEANINGS OF FOOD

Food symbol	*Symbol formation*
Love Security Trust Gratification Sensory pleasure	Food from early feeding experiences imparts feelings of security, trust, love; as the infant suckles from breast or bottle, is cuddled closely, and is filled with warm milk, he feels sensory pleasure
Reward Punishment	Food can be used as a method of discipline, withheld to enforce behavior (a tool to provoke fear or hunger) or given as a reward for good behavior
Self-fulfillment	Food, so paramount to the infant's development, can become the focus of the parent-child relationship; and as such, the means through which parents achieve self-fulfillment. For example, the act of feeding becomes the act of nurturing and the fulfillment of parental esteem is heavily at stake in feeding the family.
Religion: Foods that derive a separate meaning only from religious rites on feast days, e.g., matzo Prestige: Foods whose major value is to demonstrate an ability to pay, e.g., gourmet or exotic foods such as caviar or quality foods such as brand-name products Taboo: Foods proscribed for irrational and nonscientific reasons, e.g., Hindu prohibition of beef Socialization: Food and eating that carry the perceptible symbolic undertone of sociability, e.g., a wedding banquet, testimonial dinner, holiday feast, coffee klatch, cocktail party Health: Foods purported to have magical properties, e.g., used to cure ailments, ward off old age, or function as aphrodisiacs	Food customs are part of our cultural heritage. From the beginning, societies developed patterns around the conduct of food activities. These standardized practices are unique to each society, having evolved from different environmental factors and having been incorporated into the society to maintain the viability of the group
Language: Meat, steak, potatoes — masculinity, aggression Vegetables, fruits — femininity Fruits — love, affection, sexuality ("bearing fruit," fruition) Olives — sophistication or adult taste Peanut butter — childhood	Foods communicate meanings that justify the simile of a language

Source: Adapted from H. B. Moore, "The Meaning of Food," *The American Journal of Clinical Nutrition,* 77–82, 1957.

Food also can be used as a vehicle by which stressed, handicapped, or debilitated individuals seek to exert control over their environment. In fact, one's relationship to food may be the last vestige of personal control as all else fails—eyes, motor ability, bladder and bowel control.

With illness and hospitalization, regression in feeding behavior and food preferences may occur. For example, an adult patient might show a preference for baby foods despite the patient's ability to masticate table food. The stress of hospitalization may cause a weaned child to seek his or her bottle and refuse food. The ability of the child to accommodate to stress and separation from parents depends on the child's age and stage of development. For the newborn to 6-month-old child, there is little separation anxiety. However, anxiety may be observed as the child approaches the 6th month and begins to develop a strong attachment to mother, so that adequate substitute mothering becomes difficult to provide. For all children under 4 years old, sudden prolonged separation can be overwhelming and food often becomes the vehicle through which the children vent their frustrations as they initiate the separation process, a process described by Robertson as progression from protest to despair to denial.[3]

In the protest phase, children cry a great deal and look for sights and sounds indicative of their parents. Next, children withdraw, as crying diminishes and apathy sets in. They make little attempt to alter their environment. With the onset of the denial phase, children demonstrate interest in their surroundings and acceptance of separation. They may appear to have forgotten their parents, even ignoring a parent's presence and allowing departure without complaint. An awareness of this process is important for health professionals who are working in a pediatric setting, when they attempt to interpret the cause of indifferent appetite or a regression in food behavior.

Feeding Problems

There are three main ways in which the function of eating is open to disturbance.[4]

1 *Organic feeding disturbances* Feeding problems related to severe physical illness, weakness, exhaustion, strain, or certain states of convalescence affecting the individual's drive to survive or the need for food

2 *Nonorganic feeding disturbances* Feeding problems related to an interference with the pleasurable character of eating such as occurs when a feeding schedule is imposed on a child with no allowance for individualization of frequency, quantity, or method of feeding (Feeding situations that lack a sense of synchrony between the food provider and the child, with little or no attention paid by the provider to the cues emanating from the child)

3 *Neurotic feeding disturbances* Feeding problems occurring when the function of eating is drawn deeply into the circle of the individual's emotional life (and is used as an outlet for libidinal or aggressive tendencies), causing extremes of appetite and aberrant food behavior which can be seen in the following conditions:
   - *Pica* The persistent ingestion of substances commonly considered unfit for food. Investigations support the concept that the interaction between the child and the mother is a critical factor in the development of pica which in part represents oral fixation serving as a relief of the child's anxiety in response to an absent or inadequately functioning mother.[5,6]
   - *Rumination* The regurgitation of previously swallowed food and the rechewing and reswallowing of the food. Findings suggest that the syndrome develops in response to a disordered relationship between parents and infant.[7]

- *Anorexia nervosa* A psychophysiologic disorder in which the ascetic pursuit of thinness is used as a tool in an individual's struggle for control—for a sense of identity and effectiveness.[8]

These major types of feeding disturbances are separated for the purpose of theoretical consideration; however, when observed clinically they are invariably intermixed and interrelated.

Organic feeding problems can lay the groundwork for the nonorganic type, as observed in the child with a tracheoesophageal fistula who, after the period of surgical repair, refuses food by mouth when it is first introduced, since the child's only knowledge of food and of the pleasure of feeling full had been by way of a gastrostomy tube.

Neurotic disturbances arise after the loss of pleasure in the function of eating. The child just described is at risk of developing a neurotic superstructure around feeding. Anticipatory guidance for the parents and the staff working with this child, along with considerate handling that allows some self-determination, can help the child reacquire pleasure in the function of eating.

Examples of neurotic feeding disturbances include those related to weight gain following some traumatic emotional experience or those in which obesity is interwoven with the whole development starting from birth. Feeding behavior is not innate, but rather is learned from birth. Learning is necessary for its organization into patterns.

Since feeding patterns are learned and not genetically determined they are subject to change. This change in food habits is a challenge to the nutrition educator who, because of concern with giving information rather than helping people, often fails to discover the relationship between food and behavior. Helping individuals to discover that there is more to learn about food than they have learned from their lifetime eating experiences is the goal of diet counseling.

DIET COUNSELING: AN INSTRUMENT OF CHANGE

Diet counseling is defined as "providing individualized professional guidance to assist a person in adjusting his daily food consumption to meet his health needs."[9] The definition does not imply how this is effectively done.

To be effective, information must be presented in such a way that the individual will discover personal meaning in it. The problem of helping people to learn is the problem of creating a closer meaningful relationship between the information and the self. This is the *basic principle of learning:* the closer the events are perceived to the self, the more likely it is that behavior will be affected.[10] This is vastly different from *knowing* the information which comes from acquiring information, a task at which most nutrition educators are proficient. Until patients do something with the information, it is unlikely to affect them in any important way. When patients are confronted with a prohibited food, they do not have time to decide what to do about it. They will naturally do those things that are most closely related to self and their past experiences. The importance of moving information into a closer and meaningful relationship to the self is thus evident and can be facilitated by establishing a helping relationship with the patient.

A Helping Relationship in Diet Counseling

Diet counseling begins with a patient interview, which all too often approximates an interrogation for the purposes of filling in a nutritional history form. This is unfortunate because it is during this initial interview that a rapport is developed between the patient and the nutrition educator which determines the success or failure in diet counseling. The ability to *engender trust* and *understanding* of the problem during this time may determine the patient's progress, and is essentially the basis of a helping relationship.

Carl Rogers, the noted psychologist, identified three characteristics necessary for effective helping: the counselor's *empathy, genuineness,* and *unconditional positive regard for his or her client.* He also once observed, in an article on the nature of the helping relationship, that it didn't seem to make much difference how the helper behaved so long as his intent was to be helpful.[11] There is no control implied. Since diet means food control, patients often tend to regard the nutrition educator as the controlling rather than the helping agent. Consequently, the walls are built between patient and nutrition educator before the process begins. The nutrition educator may also have walls already built, but of another variety—namely, those emanating from preconceived attitudes about certain cultural or economic backgrounds. Professional objectivity does not allow for any one value system to interfere with patient management. It is important for nutrition educators as helpers to understand themselves as they begin to interface with other human beings in a counseling relationship and to hold in respect the personal and societal values of patients.

A changing diet can be perceived as a detriment or a benefit, depending on one's value system. For example, an individual with the cultural tenets of poverty and a present-oriented, fatalistic outlook may find the concept of food planning completely alien. The same response may also be encountered with the directive to ghetto parents to remove candy from their children's diet (since candy may be the only attainable pleasure in a bleak inner-city environment). Another negative response may be encountered when instructions are given to wean a child when the cultural practices endorse a prolonged bottle- or breast-feeding period.

An important factor affecting the discovery of meaning and susceptibility to change is the threat to predetermined perceptions. Resistance to change is normal. The nutrition educator must help people to change perceptions, not cause them to defend those they already have. For example, some vegetarians may reject nutrition information that does not fit into their frame of reference on the premise that their practices are ecologically sound in terms of health and environment. The greater the degree of threat, the more tenaciously a person will hold to perceptions, ideals, or practices.

The Nutritional Interview

To understand the consequences of the diet prescription, a considerable knowledge of the patient is necessary. This can be gathered through the nutritional interview. Once the approach is decided upon, the objectives are to obtain reliable information in a manner that is both efficient and considerate of the patient. Helfer and Hess have identified 11 behaviors, 9 of them desirable and 2 undesirable, for evaluating the interviewing skills of medical students and physicians.[12] These can be applied to nutrition educators as well. They are as follows:

1 Observes social amenities
2 Invites expression of concern
3 Reassures, shows sympathy and warmth
4 Explains rationale
5 Inquires about the effect of illness
6 Clarifies prior statement or question
7 Makes non-leading inquiries
8 Makes leading inquiry
9 Uses common words
10 Ignores or shows misunderstanding; cuts off communication
11 Is impatient; shows lack of empathy

There are many different nutritional interview forms used to obtain information (see Appendix). However, there is no place on the forms to measure *feeling tones, incidental remarks,* and *body language* that give meaningful clues to the patient's attitudes and experiences, yet these are important in gathering knowledge which will aid the nutritional educator in helping patients to learn how to incorporate nutritional information into their way of life.

The Process of Learning as Part of Diet Counseling

During the course of the nutritional interview the nutrition educator must decide what change is needed in the diet, the individual's food habits, the feasibility of change, how best to go about making the necessary change, and how to plan for change. The key to planned change is motivation, which involves helping the individual to discover a *personal meaning* in the change. In every individual, self-concern is pervasive in deciding how to act.

To a healthy person, health does not serve as a motivational force to change eating patterns. Usually only when well-being is threatened will diet action be taken voluntarily, but even in these circumstances a person's perception of health is affected by age, and by biological and emotional factors. An example is the adolescent diabetic who is in poor control of his illness. Concerned with the here and now and with peer relations, this teenager will not be motivated by the threat of secondary diabetic complications. Other avenues must be sought to motivate diet change, such as social or academic incentives.

Besides considering the motivational forces that are operative within the individual, the nutritional educator must establish a receptive framework for learning. Conditions must allow flexibility and the freedom for verbal exchange. Responses from the patient could be encouraged. Psychological tension can be reduced by incorporating phrases like "let's think this through together."

The learning environment can be further enhanced by incorporating illustrative tools (food models, flip charts, videotapes, learning machines) into the educational session. Also the techniques of behavior modification can be utilized to help focus the attention of the patient on his or her own observable food behavior; these techniques will help to define the problem and to specify behaviors that must be increased, decreased, eliminated, or instituted in order to alleviate or solve the problem (see pp. 182–184).

Food habits are practiced and maintained by selective perception in which new nutritional information is evaluated. Nutrition education must be presented within the individual's framework of selective perceptions, the framework of self-needs and values. Krech et al. state that "the foods an individual chooses must not only satisfy his hunger but also be congruent with himself as a certain kind of person."[13] It is with this in mind, and with the attitude of developing a helping relationship, that the nutrition educator should commence counseling.

BEHAVIOR MODIFICATION*

Richard R. Schnell

INTRODUCTION

How can socially important maladaptive eating behaviors be changed? The procedures employed in changing or modifying any behavior often hinge upon the theoretical conceptions of personality and behavior that one holds. Traditionally, personality and subsequent behavior have been viewed as a consequence of psychic forces within the person, such as drives, needs, and motives. Problem behavior is seen as a symptom of dysfunction within the personality. To alter behavior requires that underlying aspects of the personality be uncovered. Another major position on ways of changing behavior, which has mushroomed in popularity during the past few years, is the so-called behavioral approach. This position

* Research upon which this section is based was supported in part through the U.S. Department of Health, Education, and Welfare: Maternal and Child Health Service (Project 928).

has its roots in the psychology of learning. The behavioral approach explains behavior as the product of external environmental, situational, and social determinants. Behaviors in the main are seen as learned and therefore as something that can be changed or modified through appropriate learning procedures. Problem behaviors are not seen as signs of a problem, but as the problem itself.

In day-to-day situations these two major approaches can, and often do, overlap to a great extent. Also, despite allegiance to either one of the positions it is obvious that aspects of the other approach might be useful in a particular circumstance to change behavior in a desired direction. There is no need to see the two viewpoints as incompatible or antagonistic to each other.

This section on behavior modification will focus on some of the basic issues in employing a behavioral approach and will present a case study to demonstrate the utility of the approach in clinical nutrition.

LEARNING AND BEHAVIOR

Current learning research has focused on three major approaches: observational learning, stimulus-response learning, and operant learning. In applying these different ways of changing behavior the distinctions between them become blurred and often different aspects of each approach may be used within the same situation. The operant approach will receive the most attention here because it appears to have the most flexibility for use in applied situations.

Observational Learning

Observational learning requires observation of the behavior of another person (model) to cause learning to take place. The observer need not overtly respond at the time but will later imitate the behavior. Parents can often be heard commenting on how the behavior of their child was close to perfect before the child went to school and was exposed to the behavior of many other children; with other children for models the child's behavior has taken a turn for the worse in the eyes of the parents. The qualities of the model exert an influence on the learning that takes place. When there are several models, when they are similar to the observer, and when they have high prestige and status, the observer is more likely to imitate the model.[14,15] The consequences associated with certain behaviors also influence whether the behaviors will be imitated. The importance of consequences will be discussed further in the operant learning section.

Stimulus-Response Learning

Stimulus-response learning or *conditioning* (also known as classic conditioning) was originally studied by Pavlov. In this type of learning, stimuli that produce a strong reflexive (unlearned) action, such as salivating to the taste of food, are paired with a neutral stimulus which does not elicit the response, such as the sound of a bell. This pairing of stimuli eventually results in the neutral stimulus (e.g., the bell alone) being able to elicit the response (e.g., salivating). In this type of learning an event can take on new powers in producing a behavior. The event must be paired with a stimulus that already elicits the behavior of interest and must precede the behavior to be able to produce the behavior without the original stimulus being present.

Desensitization is one of the widely used techniques of behavior modification which has evolved from the stimulus-response approach.[16] The technique has enjoyed good success when applied to specific anxieties and phobias. In using desensitization, stimuli that appear to elicit fear or anxiety are paired with an alternative and incompatible response to the fear such as relaxation. Desensitization breaks the stimulus-response association by developing an incompatible response to the same stimulus. Typically the person is exposed to the fear-eliciting stimuli in the order of their ability to arouse anxiety. Thus, the least anxiety-producing stimulus is used first and is coupled with the relaxation response. As the person is able to relax in its presence, the next level of anxiety-producing stimulus is introduced until the ability of this stimulus to produce anxiety is eliminated. Some researchers have claimed that desensitization is an effective technique in increasing food intake in people who have anorexia nervosa.[17]

Operant Learning

The history of operant learning, or *operant conditioning,* as it is most commonly called, begins with B. F. Skinner. Operant approaches focus on the learning that takes place as the result of the consequences of behavior. Positive consequences are systematically used to shape desired behaviors. In the case of operant learning the consequences determine how a stimulus influences the probability of a response's occurring and potentially the intensity, speed, and magnitude of the response.[18] It can easily be seen that much of our behavior might be affected by this approach, as most of us feel that the consequences of behavior have a direct influence on whether or not we perform certain behaviors. Operant learning, however, implies more, in that systematic procedures must be applied to gain control over the behavior. The following section will be an exposition of some of the most important components of operant learning.

PRINCIPLES OF OPERANT LEARNING

As in most theories of learning, the operant paradigm depends upon certain basic principles. The most basic, of course, is that behavior is controlled by the events or consequences that immediately follow it. Below are some of the essential ingredients necessary to an understanding of the operant approach.

Reinforcement

The behavior to be influenced is usually referred to as the *target behavior.* An event which immediately follows a target behavior and alters that behavior is called a *reinforcer.* Those reinforcers which follow a target behavior and which increase its frequency of occurrence are known as *positive reinforcers* or *rewards.* Those reinforcers which increase its frequency when *removed* after a target behavior are known as *negative reinforcers* or *aversive stimuli.*

When behavior is followed immediately by positive reinforcing consequences it will increase in strength. It should be noted that consequences that are rewarding for some people may not be for others, so that the best way to determine whether a consequence is reinforcing is to observe its effects upon behavior. If praising a child for eating a certain vegetable increases his consumption of that vegetable then the praise is reinforcing the behavior of eating that vegetable. Positive reinforcers can be divided into two categories, those which do not depend upon prior learning for their reinforcement value, e.g., water to a thirsty individual, and others which have been learned to be reinforcing by being paired with an unlearned reinforcer, e.g., money. Essentially unlearned reinforcers are called *primary reinforcers,* while learned reinforcers are referred to as *secondary reinforcers.*

An increase in target behavior is a sign of reinforcement, whether the reinforcing is positive or negative. A stimulus can only be negatively reinforcing if its removal causes the target behavior to increase. In negative reinforcement an aversive stimuli is presented to an individual before a response begins. The aversive stimulus is removed or moderated immediately after the appropriate response occurs. Negative reinforcement is not the same thing as punishment. Punishment is defined in operant terms as something that decreases the frequency of a response. Typically, in punishment an aversive stimulus is presented after a behavior is performed, which tends to decrease that behavior.

Punishment is often less effective than reinforcement and therefore is not as widely used in operant learning. Negative reinforcement is also used less often than positive reinforcement because positive reinforcement is usually as effective or more so, as well as being more socially acceptable. Negative reinforcement, however, can be useful in extreme situations in which positive reinforcement is difficult. Lovaas and his colleagues[19] have used it to develop more socially appropriate behavior in autistic children. Because other approaches had failed an electric shock was used as the negative reinforcer. When the autistic child began engaging in more socially acceptable behaviors such as moving toward or touching an adult the mild shock was terminated. Although the method is repugnant it did result in behavior change which could not be accomplished in any other known way. Whether that is adequate justification for its use remains a matter of dispute.

The frequency of the reinforcement that follows a desired behavior is an important variable. If reinforcement follows each occurrence of a desired behavior it is called continuous reinforcement. Continuous reinforcement is most effective in the acquisition of new behavior. Reinforcement that does not occur every time a target response is made is called intermittent reinforcement. Intermittent reinforcement is most effective in maintaining a behavior once it is established. Behavior is much more resistant to change if it is intermittently reinforced.

Extinction

Behaviors will decrease in frequency of occurrence if they are no longer reinforced. The process of stopping reinforcement of a behavior is called extinction. When a behavior is not reinforced the behavior is reduced or eliminated. Extinction should be clearly distinguished from punishment, in which an aversive stimulus follows a behavior and thus decreases its frequency. Extinction requires the total absence of reinforcement. Extinction can contribute to problem behavior, as well as help to change it. Positive behavior can be inadvertently extinguished by ignoring it. The child who always behaves well during mealtime may never be given any attention (extinction), while the disruptive child may be given a good deal of parental attention (reinforcement) for his misbehavior. Absence of reinforcement tends to weaken any behavior.

Guiding Behavior

If a desired behavior does not occur frequently or at all, it is difficult to reinforce it so that the behavior will increase in frequency. In this case a process called *shaping* can be used which reinforces closer and closer approximations to the desired behavior. Shaping uses behaviors which resemble the desired behavior and which the individual already frequently produces. These behaviors are initially reinforced and then reinforcement is altered so that the behavior must become more and more like that of the target behavior if it is to be reinforced. If one were trying to get an individual to eat half as much at mealtimes, it might prove difficult to reinforce that behavior because it might not readily occur. Systematically rewarding the person's eating somewhat less over a period of time until the person finally reached the appropriate amount would probably give better results.

Another procedure which facilitates the occurrence of a behavior which can be reinforced is called *prompting*. By helping an individual begin the behavior, faster approximations to the final behavior can be made. This can be accomplished by simple maneuvers like instructing the individual or even physically guiding him. For example, you might explain to an older child how to hold a knife to cut meat, while with a younger child you might help to guide the spoon from plate to mouth.

Self-Management

The principles already elaborated are most often used by someone to change the behavior of another. Usually the person who systematically attempts to alter the behavior of another is a professional in a discipline such as psychology, but others can be trained to apply behavioral techniques. Parents can serve as behavioral change agents for their children.[20] The greatest efficiency could be gained by educating individuals to exert control over their own behavior in problem situations according to the principles discussed previously. This would allow individuals to help themselves rather than becoming dependent upon others. Self-management techniques are being actively evaluated.[21,22]

In self-management procedures people are trained to control their own behavior by use of shaping and prompting, and by delivering reinforcement or punishment to themselves. They are required to monitor their own behavior. The most obvious merit of self-management techniques is also a potential problem. Since the individuals exert the control over the consequences of their behavior they may not choose to follow through on a behavioral program.

APPLICATION

Research

Over the years a great deal of research using both humans and animals has been devoted to developing behavior modification techniques. One of the results has been the application of these techniques to problems related to eating. Problems in eating behavior have become relatively important to our affluent society. Attention has been directed to those who eat too little or too much. In the case of those who significantly lose their appetite for food (anorexia nervosa) behavioral techniques have appeared to be helpful although they have as yet not been widely used.[23,24]

In the area of weight control for obesity, behavioral techniques have been used widely. Differing behavioral approaches have proved useful but a number of issues remain. It has been demonstrated that weight reduction can usually be accomplished with behavioral techniques but the reduction is often difficult to maintain.[25] Some investigators have approached the problem by examining how everyday eating habits are influenced by eating-related environmental cues while others have examined the influence of emotional states on eating habits.[26] Self-management techniques for weight loss have gained popularity, with self-reward strategies appearing to be more effective than other strategies.[28] In general, which techniques will be most useful for initiating and maintaining weight loss still depend upon the individual situation.

Common Concerns

In describing behavior modification it becomes evident that the principles are not necessarily new and in fact many of the techniques are practiced by, and on, all of us in a variety of situations. The principles and techniques of behavior modification are deeply woven into the fabric of major social institutions and human existence, in general, as evidenced by child rearing, education, business, government and law, and religion.[29] Although we can see aspects of behavior modification at work in components of our everyday life the important ingredients for using such techniques to change behavior is that they be *systematically* and *consistently* applied. If they are not so used their impact on behavior is not likely to be as great. Often these conditions do not obtain in our daily lives and it takes concern over a significant problem to mount a specific systematic and consistent program. With powerful enough consequences and systematic reinforcement, behavior change in most situations is possible.

Although the techniques of behavior modification are relatively simple their effects can be quite striking. It should be kept in mind that the techniques employed in modifying behavior are double-edged in that they can be used to promote socially relevant goals or they can be used in the service of less than ethical ends. In addition the techniques themselves can lead into problematic territory, as in the choosing of negative reinforcers or punishments. The use of aversive stimuli or consequences must be employed with great caution. Because the techniques are potentially so powerful a great deal of responsibility is placed on those who would use them. Careful consideration should always be given to ethical issues before behavior modification techniques are employed.

As you have seen, a knowledge of some of the principles of operant learning can help in structuring the environment so that desirable behaviors can be learned or, more precisely, the environment changes behavior, which, in turn, changes the environment.[29] There are certain procedures that need to be followed if a learning program is to be instituted. The behavior to be changed must be clearly described and observed. A baseline of present behavior is recorded for later use in ascertaining whether learning has taken place. Then the learning procedures are determined and begun. Typically an attempt is made to modify the behavior by rearranging the consequences which follow the behavior. The behavior is continuously recorded, often with the use of graphs, to give feedback on the effectiveness of the procedures. Often the procedures will be adjusted to promote maximum learning. If they are not working they can be rapidly disregarded. The behaviors at the end of the procedures can be compared with the initial baseline data to demonstrate how far behavior has changed.

STUDY QUESTIONS

1 List those factors that influence food choices.

2 What is the significance of food symbols?

3 What are the three ways in which the function of eating is open to disturbance?

4 How can a helping relationship be incorporated into diet counseling?

5 What is the goal of diet counseling?

6 Differentiate between observational learning, stimulus-response learning, and operant learning.

7 What is meant by reinforcement?

8 "Extinction should be clearly distinguished from punishment, in which an aversive stimulus follows a behavior and thus decreases its frequency." Explain this statement.

9 How can the techniques of behavior modification be used in nutrition practice.

CASE STUDY 10-1

This case will be devoted to a demonstration of how behavioral techniques were applied in a specific and complex situation to help Teddy, a child, modify his feeding behavior. The case will convey some of the complexities and problems in using a behavioral approach as well as demonstrating some of its advantages.

Past History
When we first met Teddy he was a 22-month-old boy with profound failure to thrive, cerebral palsy with generalized hypotonia, and phenotypic anomalies. Teddy had a striking physical appearance because of his small size, his hypotonia, and his unusual head, which had fine, dry hair, frontal bossing of the skull, and shallow ocular orbits which made his eyes prominent. Teddy lived at home with only his mother, who had lived in several cities during his 22 months.

Because he was unable to suck and swallow at birth he was begun on gavage feeding. Tube feeding continued because of persistent regurgi-

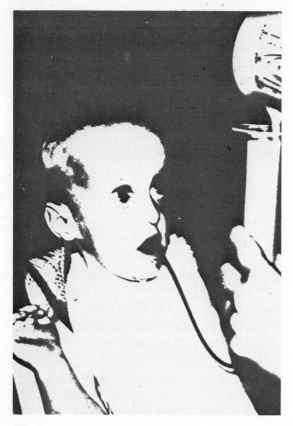

Figure 10-2
Weaning from the tube to the table. Teddy, a child literally tied to his tube feedings before a successful behavior modification allowed him to resume a normal feeding experience.

tation, poor sucking and swallowing reflexes, and choking. All attempts at oral feeding had failed. With the progression of time he became conditioned to his feeding tube and his response to oral feeding became further complicated by his lack of taste experience and his oral defensiveness. No physical abnormalities appeared to be present that required the use of the tube. He had had no major illnesses except for a brief bout of pneumonia for which he was hospitalized at 1 year of age. There was a history of recurrent urinary tract infections. His medical care had been erratic, with his mother receiving little help or encouragement. Developmentally, he had smiled at 2 to 3 months and rolled over at 1 year.

He had only a few bubbling sounds at 22 months of age, and was not yet walking.

Present History

At age 22 months he was admitted to Children's Hospital Medical Center for failure to thrive. He had a bone age of 9 months, with multiple growth-arrest lines, consistent with erratic food intake and malnutrition. His tube feeding had consisted of soy formula with an estimated caloric intake of 640 kcal (2688 kJ) per day. In the hospital, his tube feeding mixture was expanded to include all the basic food groups and was supplemented with multivitamins, vitamin K, B complex, folic acid, and iron. Upon discharge from the hospital he was enrolled in a physical therapy program and followed as an outpatient.

An outpatient program was introduced with the following goals:

1   Observation and documentation of Teddy's feeding behavior and his interaction with his mother
2   Weekly physical therapy sessions to develop better gross motor skills
3   Reduction of Teddy's oral sensitivity and introduction of foods orally
4   Monitoring of Teddy's growth, and his nutrient intake

Weekly sessions were held for Teddy and his mother with the nutritionist. At these times Teddy and his mother could be observed in a feeding situation and his feeding problems discussed. Teddy was encouraged to bring his hand to his mouth and to suck on his fingers. The nutritionist and mother would gently rub his gums with their fingers prior to feedings to decrease heightened oral sensitivity. A bottle and finger foods were presented along with the tube so that he would come to associate these with mealtime. This routine continued over a 6-month period, but he gained little in the way of actual food *acceptance. He did, however, come to explore objects with his mouth and he became less orally defensive.*

Teddy's mother tried oral feeding with him both at home and on her weekly visits to the hospital by attempting to get him to accept many different kinds of food. Many new foods with different shapes, colors, and tastes were presented, but without success. Teddy would not try any food orally and his mother found it difficult to persevere with any food once he had rejected it. After each refusal to eat orally he was always tube-fed, a practice that further conditioned him to the tube.

Because of the lack of success in getting him to eat orally a barium-swallow x-ray examination was performed. The result was a report of no coordinated muscle activity and no visible normal swallowing motions. However, we had observed how well Teddy swallowed his tube and

his ability to handle secretions was improving. Also, he had been known to drink water from a cup during episodes of throat inflammation. It was concluded that much of Teddy's inability to swallow was related to learned behavior and not due to physiological problems.

The physical therapy program had helped him to make some gains in motor development. During the 8 months since his discharge from the hospital, he had acquired sitting balance at the 5- to 6-month level, crawled with an alternate pattern at the 8-month level, and was cruising alone to tables at the 11- to 12-month level. Cognitively, he was functioning at the 15-month level on nonverbal tasks and his expressive language skills were at the 11-month level.

Teddy was still not showing significant catch-up growth on his tube feeding regimen. It was then decided that there would have to be a more concerted effort at oral feeding.

REFERENCES

1 M. D. Manning, "The Psychodynamics of Dietetic," *Nursing Outlook,* April 1965, p. 57.

2 C. G. Babcock, "Attitudes and the Use of Food," *Journal of the American Dietetic Association,* **38:**547, 1961.

3 J. Robertson, *Young Children in Hospitals, Tavistock Publications, London, 1958, pp. 20–23.*

4 Anna Freud, "The Psychoanalytic Study of Infantile Feeding Disturbances," in *The Psychoanalytic Study of the Child,* New York, 1947, pp. 119–132.

5 S. M. Pueschel, S. Cullen, R. Howard, and M. Cullinane, "Pica and Lead Poisoning," a study conducted in the Developmental Evaluation Clinic, Children's Hospital Medical Center, Boston, Mass. (to be published).

6 R. Lourie, E. Layman, and F. Millican, "Why Children Eat Things That Are Not Food?" *Children,* **10:**143–146, 1963.

7 J. B. Richmond, D. Eddy, and M. Green, "Rumination: A Psychosomatic Syndrome of Infancy," *Pediatrics,* **22:**49–55, 1958.

8 H. Bruch, *Eating Disorders, Obesity, Anorexia Nervosa and the Person Within,* Basic Books, Inc., Publishers, New York, 1973.

9 American Dietetic Association Position Paper on Diet Counseling, *Journal of the American Dietetic Association,* **66:**571, 1975.

10 A. Combs, D. Avila, and W. Purkey, *Helping Relationships,* Allyn and Bacon, Inc., Boston, 1976, p. 93.

11 C. R. Rogers, "The Characteristics of a Helping Relationship," *Personnel and Guidance Journal,* **37:**6–16, 1958.

12 R. D. Helfer and J. Hess, "An Experimental Model for Making Objective Measurements of Interviewing Skills," *Journal of Clinical Psychology,* **26:**327, 1970.

13 D. Krech, R. S. Crutchfield, and E. L. Ballachecy, *Individual in Society,* McGraw-Hill Book Company, New York, 1963, p. 83.

14 A. Bandura, "Psychotherapy based upon modeling principles," in A. E. Bergin and S. L. Garfield (eds.), *Handbook of Psychotherapy and Behavior Change: An Empirical Analysis,* John Wiley and Sons, Inc., New York, 1971.

15 S. Rachman, "Clinical Application of Observational Learning, Imitation, and Modeling," *Behavior Therapy,* **3:**379–397, 1972.

16 J. Wolpe, *Psychotherapy By Reciprocal Inhibition,* Stanford University Press, Stanford, Calif., 1958.

17 A. T. Schnurer, R. R. Rubin, and A. Roy, "System-

atic Desensitization of Anorexia Nervosa Seen As A Weight Problem," *Journal of Behavior Therapy and Experimental Psychiatry,* **4:**149–153, 1973.

18   A. E. Kazdin, *Behavior Modification In Applied Settings,* The Dorsey Press, Homewood, Ill., 1975.

19   O. I. Lovaas, B. Schoeffer, and J. Q. Simmons, "Building Social Behavior In Autistic Children By Use Of Electric Shock," *Journal of Experimental Research in Personality,* **1:**99–109, 1965.

20   B. P. Berkowitz and A. M. Graziana, "Training Parents As Behavior Therapists: A Review," *Behavioral Research and Therapy,* **10:**297–317, 1972.

21   M. R. Goddfried and M. Merbaum, *Behavior Change Through Self Control,* Holt, Rhinehart and Winston, Inc., New York, 1973.

22   M. J. Mahoney, "Research Issues In Behavior Management," *Behavior Therapy,* **3:**45–63, 1972.

23   F. J. Bianco, "Rapid Treatment Of Two Cases of Anorexia Nervosa," *Journal of Behavior Therapy and Experimental Psychiatry,* **3:**223–224, 1972.

24   A. Stunkard, "New Therapies For The Eating Disorders: Behavior Modification Of Obesity And Anorexia Nervosa," *Archives of General Psychiatry,* **26:**391–398, 1972.

25   R. B. Stuart and B. Davis, *Slim Chance In A Fat World,* Research Press, 2621 North Mattis Avenue, Champaign, Ill., 1972.

26   G. R. Leon and K. Chamberlain, "Comparison Of Daily Eating Habits And Emotional Status Of Overweight Persons Successful Or Unsuccessful In Maintaining A Weight Loss," *Journal of Consulting and Clinical Psychology,* **61:**108–115, 1973.

27   M. J. Mahoney, N. G. Moura, and T. E. Wade, "Relative Efficiency Of Self Reward, Self Punishment, and Self Monitoring Techniques For Weight Loss," *Journal of Consulting and Clinical Psychology,* **40:**404–407, 1973.

28   B. F. Skinner, *Science And Human Behavior,* The Free Press, New York, 1953.

29   A. Bandura, *Principles Of Behavior Modification,* Holt, Rhinehart and Winston, Inc., New York, 1969.

CHAPTER 11

DEVELOPMENTAL CONSIDERATIONS IN INFANT FEEDING

Robert W. Telzrow*

KEY WORDS
Interaction
Synchrony
Autonomy
Temperament

INTRODUCTION

Some of the most attractive and nutritionally balanced meals prepared for infants by both parents and dietitians go untouched. The solutions to this dilemma rarely lie in the foods themselves but in the fact that "eating does not occur as an isolated phenomenon but as part of a complex of interlocking social and biological conditions."[1] Nowhere, perhaps, is the old adage "You can lead a horse to water, but you can't make him drink" truer than in consideration of infant feeding. While this is obvious to most, it is surprising how often one needs to be reminded of it.

Some studies have been concerned with the effects of nutrition on growth and development while frequently showing little interest in other environmental effects. By contrast, other studies devoted to enhancing the cognitive and social environment of infants (stimulation programs) have given little consideration to food as a major factor in the infant's experience. Obviously, an awareness of the interaction between food and environment is necessary but often absent.

In this chapter we will present prenatal and postnatal environmental influences on nutrition and development, citing those periods in the child's early development when the interaction between feeding and important developmental variables can result in either excellent positive opportunities for both the parent and child or, as a consequence of these influences, can result in feeding problems for parents and health care professionals. The discussion will be supported with case examples which provide the health care professional with the background needed to identify stages of child development around which anticipatory guidance can be structured in order to help prevent feeding problems.

* This work was completed in part while the author was a fellow at the Child Development Unit, the Children's Hospital Medical Center, Boston, Mass., under a grant from the Robert Wood Johnson Foundation.

PRENATAL ENVIRONMENTAL INFLUENCES ON FEEDING BEHAVIOR

Malnutrition

Nutrition plays a major role in the outcome of the developing fetus. The notion of the fetus as an effective parasite, able to leech whatever nutrients it needs from its mother in order to develop, has found little scientific support.[2–5] Protein deprivation in the infant before and after birth does result in brain cell deficiency and mental impairment.[2] Intrauterine growth failure can occur following undernutrition in the mother. Animal studies have suggested that there may even be a multigenerational effect.[6] There appear to be critical periods, both pre- and postnatal, when organs such as the brain are especially vulnerable to events like undernutrition. Thus, the timing as well as the severity of malnutrition determines the effect on the developing brain.[2] The long-term effects of this process remain unclear.[24]

Placental Deficiencies

Intrauterine growth failure is also felt to occur from placental vascular insufficiency. However, in animal studies utilizing vascular clamping to reproduce placental vascular insufficiency, the effects differed from the effects of maternal malnutrition.[2] While there was a reduction of cell size in a number of organs such as the liver, the fetal brain appeared to be spared such a reduction.

An important consequence of both undernutrition and vascular insufficiency, however, is that they do affect the behavior of the newborn infant, as demonstrated in a study comparing full-term newborns of recently urbanized, impoverished Zambian families with middle-class American families.[7]

The Zambian mothers had had several pregnancies in rapid succession coupled with historical evidence of low protein intake before and during pregnancy. This uterine depletion

and undernutrition contributed to small-for-gestational-age (SGA) infants. The infants' muscle tone was poor, and they showed no attempt to mold or adjust themselves when being held (seeming rather like sacks of meal). They were also unable to relate to their social or inanimate environment (as shown by a poor response when being cuddled and a poor response to visual stimulation). By 10 days of age their responses had improved considerably. This was felt to be due to the combined effects of breast feeding with subsequent rehydration, and of the way they were carried, which encouraged alertness and required good motor tone on the infants' part.

A subsequent study comparing a group of ten American infants who were SGA (not felt to be on the basis of nutritional inadequacies) with appropriate-for-gestational-age (AGA) infants as controls demonstrated similar findings in the newborn period, but also suggested possible long-term behavioral differences.[8] These newborn SGA infants, like the children from the Zambian study, had a low activity level and showed poor responsiveness to socially important stimuli when alert. They usually did not become upset; however, when they did, they were difficult to console. Overall, their behavior appeared to signal to their environment that they were stressed, exhausted, and preferred to be left alone. By 10 days of age two of the infants had shown recovery from the initial dysfunctional patterns of behavior.

On a follow-up home visit, still within the newborn period, all ten infants remained quiet and hard to arouse. This "undemanding" nature was very noticeable and a concern to most parents. There was no intervention or further contact between parents and investigators until a subsequent follow-up at 9 months of age which demonstrated a dramatic change. All ten SGA infants were developmentally age-appropriate on the basis of the Denver Developmental Screening Test.[9] However, eight of the ten had become unpredictable in eating and sleeping patterns and were intense and highly reactive. They were described by their parents as difficult to live with. The two described as normal in every way were the two who had shown initial recovery. All of these studies point to the clear evidence of the consequences of intrauterine environment on the nutritional, behavioral, physical, and developmental capacities of the child.

POSTNATAL ENVIRONMENTAL INFLUENCES ON FEEDING BEHAVIOR

Age 0 to 2 Months

Infant Sucking Patterns

In a series of studies reported by Kaye,[16] newborn infants have been shown to have a natural, regular, rhythmic sucking pattern consisting of bursts of sucking followed by pauses. The length of the bursts appears to be dependent on milk flow (longer if the flow is rapid, shorter if flow is insufficient), whereas the length of the pauses appears to be related to interactions between the infant and its mother.

Contrary to popular belief and current practice, stimulation (jiggling the bottle, etc.) during the pauses reduces the likelihood of the infant's immediately returning to a burst pattern of sucking. In fact, pauses during which the infant is stimulated are longer than pauses during which the infant is not stimulated. Stopping the stimulation, on the other hand, does increase somewhat the infant's return to sucking. Kaye has shown that over the first 2 weeks, mothers changed the way in which they stimulated their infants during these pause periods. Instead of stimulating until the child began to suck again as they had done initially, the mothers would stimulate briefly and then wait for the infant to respond before stimulating again.

This resulted in shortening both the duration of the stimulation and the duration of the pauses, and suggests that the mothers, in responding to the tendency of the infant to re-

sume feeding when the stimulation stopped, had changed their responses during the pauses. This indicates early evidence of a synchrony (mutual awareness) between the partners.

An additional aspect of infant sucking is the role of maternal parity. Studies by Thoman et al.[14,15] suggest that the feeding behavior of the infant differs as a function of parity independent of the contribution of the mother. They observed that infants born to multiparous mothers had more feeding intervals (pauses in feeding) than those of primiparous mothers. This was shown by recording the feeding behavior of these newborns while being fed by an experienced nurse for their first feeding. In contrast, however, when given their babies, it was the primiparous mothers who used a greater number of feeding intervals and spent more time in nonfeeding activities. It appeared that multiparous mothers were more sensitive to the infant's cues

in the observation that infants of multiparous mothers sucked more during breast feeding and consumed more during bottle feedings, even though the primiparous mothers spent more time feeding their infants and stimulated them more to get them to suck.[14]

Thoman[14] suggested that the primiparous mothers, because of their relative inexperience and increased eagerness, might be more likely to miss the types of cues or observations that Kaye is describing and go on stimulating their infants, thus prolonging the feeding. The length of time that these differences persist is unknown. Kaye, in his report, makes no reference to differences in parity. Brody,[17] however, showed in an earlier report that for infants up to 7 months of age there still were more feeding intervals among primiparous mothers.

This is not a question of the primiparous mother's underfeeding her infant, and thus is not a pattern which demands intervention. Certainly, the known higher expectations of primiparous mothers, both of themselves and of their infants, raises the likelihood of dis-synchrony and subsequent feeding problems. If, however, as Kaye suggests, the changing burst-and-pause pattern shows evidence of synchrony and contains the elements of turn-taking (learning to give and take turns) and learning how to anticipate one another's behavior, then the apparent inefficiency in feeding suggested in the frequent "interventions" of the parent may in fact be serving a different purpose for the parent and child, namely, providing an opportunity for social exchange between the parent and the infant.

It would be wrong to place undue emphasis on efficiency in a feeding interaction at a time when a parent, especially a primiparous parent, is in the process of trying to find regularity in an interaction. That it might take a primiparous parent longer should not surprise anyone. There is no suggestion at this time that this relative inefficiency is in any way disorganizing to the infant, or in any way rendering the infant incapable of good social interactions during those prolonged pause periods.

Attachment

One of the most important tasks awaiting a newborn is the development of ties between himself and his parents, referred to as the *attachment process*. An important component of this attachment is the establishment of a communication system between the infant and its caregiver within the first few months. When functional, this system shows a high degree of synchrony between the participants. When it fails, a lack of synchrony is evident.

Because feeding and feeding-related interactions occupy much of the infant's awake time during the first months, it is not surprising that major opportunities for further development of this synchrony occur during feeding times. These episodes can be very informative windows through which to view the attachment process. In fact, a correlation has been shown between events occurring around

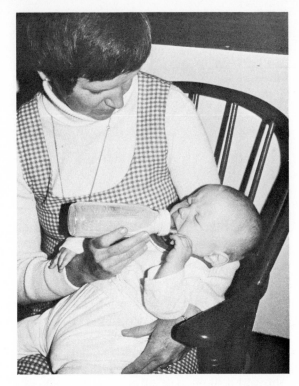

Figure 11-1
A lack of synchrony in feeding is evident between mother and child.

feedings in the first 3 months of life and the successful subsequent development of attachment between the infant and its mother.[10,11]

Since feeding problems often occur between some of the most apparently attached parents and their infants, it is necessary to differentiate between securely attached parent-infant pairs and anxiously attached pairs. The securely attached child at 1 year of age is able, for example, to use the parent as a secure base and shows a balance between using this base from which to explore the environment or to stay close to when stressed or needy. Following separation (e.g., having a baby-sitter for the afternoon) the infant shows positive behavior toward the parent when reunited (e.g., brightening, smiling, or cuddling). An anxiously attached child, on the other hand, at a similar age shows an imbalance between staying close and exploring. Following separation this child frequently shows a mixture of positive behavior and negative behavior (avoiding proximity, striking the parent, or even ignoring the parent).

Ainsworth and Bell[10] have shown that where synchrony has been achieved to a high degree in the first 3 months, as seen in the feeding interaction, subsequent attachment is strong. There are four points which they use to assess the degree of synchrony in a feeding situation. All have excellent clinical applicability.

1 The timing of the feeding—is it in response to a signal by the infant or determined primarily for the parent's convenience?

2 Who determines the amount of food ingested and the end of the feeding? Is it the infant or does the parent insist on a predetermined amount?

3 Is there tact in handling the infant's preferences when solid foods are introduced?

4 Who sets the pace or rate of intake? Is it in accordance with the baby's own rate or the caregiver's?

Securely attached infants had mothers who scored higher on these items and were felt to be more attuned to the infant's rhythm, signals, preferences, and pacing. This suggests a heightened awareness of the individuality of these infants and demonstrates the interaction between nutrition and other aspects of development (in this case, affective growth). Implications for counseling should center around promoting this awareness. This might best be done during the newborn period by fostering in parents an awareness of the unique qualities and individuality that newborns possess. Also helpful in some cases would be encouraging the parent and child to be alone for some of the feeding episodes where they will not be distracted by ongoing events in their household.

Disorganization Secondary to Organic Illness

There are a number of events that can occur to both parents and infants alike which have an

---

CASE STUDY 11-1

Timothy A. was a 2.95-kg infant born following a 38-week gestation. Pregnancy, labor, and delivery were benign. He was a slow eater during the first few days, but his mother persisted and he took up to 2 oz at most feedings. On the third day he was noticeably jaundiced and appeared sleepier than usual. His serum bilirubin level rose to 18.0 mg/dl, and fluorescent phototherapy was begun. He remained blindfolded and under the fluorescent lights for 3 days except for brief feeding periods. His mother had been discharged but was able to visit once a day to feed him.

Timothy's bilirubin responded to light treatment and he was discharged. However, when he arrived home he appeared to be overly sleepy, and to have many brief episodes of being irritable. If left alone, he would sleep 6 or 7 hours at a time. He would then become very hungry and have difficulty taking his bottle while so irritable. When his parents tried to wake him up sooner, he often fell asleep after taking only an ounce. This meant he was getting no more than 10 to 12 oz of formula in a day. His mother became more concerned and began to question her own ability to care for her child. In addition she also began to wonder whether Timothy was ill or abnormal.

effect on each one's ability to be attuned to these signals and rhythms and thus affect infant feeding.

Here is a case where an infant has become disorganized in areas of state control (a loss of control over normal rhythms like sleeping and waking cycles) following the stress of hyperbilirubinemia and the use of phototherapy. (Phototherapy is the process which takes advantage of the fact that bilirubin concentration can be reduced by exposure to visible light, primarily in the blue spectral range, which minimizes the need for exchange transfusion. Therapy is necessary when bilirubin concentration becomes elevated to levels which can cause brain damage.) Behavioral effects of jaundice and phototherapy have been shown to be manifested as altered state control and poor interactive qualities (responsiveness to social stimuli such as faces and voices).[12] These effects appear to persist for at least 1 week following phototherapy.

Jaundice and phototherapy are by no means the only disorganizing influences on the newborn. Medication during delivery, for example, can also have such effects if not used sparingly.[13] Other infants have poor state control for reasons we do not understand.

This information is important because we know that the infant's level of participation in the parent-child interaction is of such significance that it becomes a major determinant of parental caregiving responses. It is not uncommon for a disorganized child to elicit confusion and concern in parents. This brings into play the uncertainties and fears that all parents have, leading some to respond to their unpredictable child by being unpredictable themselves. Support by health care personnel during these episodes is necessary. Proper information about the child's transient disorganization and suggestions for intervention which might minimize this disorganization would be appropriate, including, where applicable, a feeding schedule.

For example, in Timothy's case, a suggestion on how to arouse a sleepy baby would be appropriate. If we were to arouse him indiscriminately, we might undermine any attempts on his part to organize his own sleep cycles. Waking him when he is in a light sleep state minimizes this disruption. Light sleep is easy to recognize: eye movements are noticeable under the eyelids, respiration is irregular, and body movements are frequent. Following arousal from light sleep the infant is more prone to respond to a feeding. Seeing this as the infant's problem, and recognizing that the parents can help him resolve it with proper information, will minimize the kinds of responses noted in the case example. Since there is some evidence of dehydration following phototherapy, which can certainly contribute to these observed behaviors, appropriate fluid intake can then be maintained.

Environmental and Emotional Stimulation

One of the more striking examples of the interaction between environment and nutrition is seen in the infant with failure to thrive. Powell et al.[18,19] described children of varying ages with signs of possible hypopituitarism (decreased ACTH reserve and diminished release of growth hormone) who were also noted to have very bizarre behaviors, ravenous appetites, failure to grow, and very stressed home lives. Restoration of their depressed growth hormone levels occurred following their removal from the stressed environment. Following this, growth was rapid unless they returned home, in which case they stopped growing and growth hormone levels diminished. Administration of growth hormone without altering their environment was less successful than changing their environment alone, suggesting an altered psychological response to growth hormone.[19,20]

These reports, along with others, have increased physicians' awareness of environmental (nonorganic) failure to thrive, to the point that the presence of an infant on a pediatric ward with a diagnosis of nonorganic failure to thrive has become almost routine. Such infants have a variety of histories, and only a very small number show the picture of possible hypopituitarism.

When first encountered, these infants have weights below the 3rd percentile. Some also show a fall-off in length and head circumference. They are pathetic, unhappy-looking babies with sunken, wary eyes. They frequently show very little motor activity. One striking observation is that if hospitalized and put on an optimal caloric intake they often do not begin to gain weight for up to 2 weeks. Some (about one-third) actually lose weight while in the hospital.

A recent study by Rosenn et al.[21] has defined the failure-to-thrive infant behaviorally and has chronicled the infant's behavior during the recovery period. It showed that the infant with nonorganic failure to thrive, when compared to those with organic failure to thrive or compared to controls, preferred distal to proximal social interactions. The child would show eye contact from a distance but would look away when approached. Such infants preferred objects to people. If handed a toy, they would use it to keep the observer away rather than to draw the observer into an interaction (social exchange) as the controls did. These and other behaviors were scored using an approach-withdrawal scale which

---

CASE STUDY 11-2

Amanda C. was a 2½-month-old baby admitted to the hospital because of failure to thrive. Her perinatal history was unremarkable. She had been born weighing 3.32 kg to a gravida 4, para 4, 24-year-old mother. While in the nursery she was an alert baby with no feeding difficulties. When seen at her 6-week follow-up visit she was still at just above her birth weight but overall appeared healthy. Her mother expressed minimal concern over this and felt that Amanda ate well. She described her as an easy baby. One month later, on follow-up, she was still not gaining weight (3.75 kg) and was admitted to the hospital.

Her physical examination showed her to be somewhat hypotonic, with poor head control and possibly some spasticity in her lower limbs. Neurological consultation raised the question of cerebral palsy. Behaviorally she showed evidence of neglect. She showed initial interest but no excitement when interacting with the nursing staff. There was no quick smile or the rhythmic churning of her arms and legs that one expects

from a 2- to 3-month-old. Instead she averted her gaze, her respirations became irregular, and her arms remained flexed with her hands held back on either side of her head. At times she showed mottling of her skin. Her behavior suggested that she was incapable of interacting without being easily overstimulated, as evidenced by changes in respiration and the vascular instability of mottling.

Mrs. C. was very depressed, and her history revealed that she had been so from the time she first learned she was pregnant with Amanda. Her marriage had been a disappointment. She lost many of her friends following the birth of her oldest son because she had to quit her job. She had been planning to return to work when she realized she was pregnant with Amanda. Seeing Mrs. C. sitting with Amanda lying on her lap in a limp, almost ragdoll, posture yet still staring at her mother's expressionless face, with Mrs. C. unable to look back at her daughter, told the whole story.

places infant behaviors on a continuum from extremely negative to extremely positive.

The study suggests that when weight gain begins to occur it follows by 24 to 48 hours a change in the infant's behavior profile from the above negative description seen in Amanda to a positive one similar to that of the controls.

Animal studies have also shown the interactive effect of nutrition and environment. Levitsky and Barnes[22] found that the adverse behavioral effects of early malnutrition in rats were exaggerated in a deprived environment and significantly reduced in an enriched environment.

They suggested two possible mechanisms:

Malnutrition may change the experience or perception of the environment during the period of early development by physiologically rendering the animal less capable of receiving, or integrating, or both, information about the environment. Another mechanism may be purely behavioral. Malnutrition may produce behaviors which themselves are incompatible with the incorporation of environmental information necessary for optimal cognitive growth.[22]

The converse would also appear to be true, in that environmental events such as neglect may alter children emotionally and physiologically to the extent that they make poor use of the nutrients they have been given.

When applied to our clinical experience we can easily see the child, apathetic and withdrawn because of malnutrition or the lack of appropriate social stimulation or frequently both, incapable of either processing information from the environment or interacting with it. It is remarkable how in the light of this affront children are able to recover when given an appropriate environment, including good nutrition.

In Amanda's case an intervention program was designed to provide her with a more appropriate social experience. This had to be done gradually because it was so easy to give her more stimulation than she could tolerate. Using a primary nursing approach that al-

lowed the nurse to develop a relationship with Amanda, at Amanda's own pace, was the first step. Often such children can only tolerate being stimulated for brief periods of time and through a single sensory modality. Amanda was cuddled when fed and only spoken to softly. She was not bounced or played with in any way which expected too much response from her. Following the first week she began to have eye contact with the nurse while being fed. This was the first sign of a trusting relationship. Continued efforts paid off and she soon began to gain weight, and with that her abnormal muscle tone and questionable neurological signs resolved.

Influences on Feeding Behavior Age 2 to 4 Months

Most feeding problems which arise in healthy children from this point on center around two issues. The first is the parent's concern (often unfounded) over inadequate intake, the second is concern over allowing the child to become the master of what he eats. In this section we will be discussing a number of developmental milestones, infants' differences in temperament, and parental concerns which have a bearing on how a child eats and how much he eats.

Quantity of Intake

Concern about whether a child is getting enough to eat is universal. The particular problems encountered by Jason's parents are common manifestations of this concern. Jason's fussiness always seemed to be less when he was sucking. This was interpreted to mean that he was hungry. We know now that a lot of sucking by infants is not related to hunger. Nonnutritive sucking appears to be a way in which infants quiet themselves. It helps them contain themselves in much the same way that adults do when they swaddle or hold a crying, fussy baby. The difference is that sucking is the baby's own attempt to accomplish this. Since

CASE STUDY 11-3

Jason Q. was an excellent eater. He was born weighing 3.868 kg following an uneventful pregnancy, labor, and delivery. His mother, aged 28, planned to nurse him as she had her two older children. Jason, however, never appeared to be satisfied. Unlike his two older siblings, Jason was a very intense, fussy baby. His parents found themselves supplementing his feedings with a bottle by the time he was 2 or 3 weeks of age. This satisfied him for a while but soon he was fussing

again. Cereal was added to his milk for a few weeks, and by 7 weeks of age he had been introduced to a number of solid foods. Most of it came back out as soon as it was into Jason's mouth. He occasionally gagged and even vomited. At other times when fed he would suck on his fingers. When he did this he did not have as much difficulty with eating. It seemed that the harder Jason's parents tried, the more he would gag and spit up.

offering the breast or bottle does quiet the baby, it reinforces the notion of hunger as the cause. In addition, it fails to allow the child an opportunity to begin to achieve competence in controlling some of his or her own frustration.

Extrusion Reflex

The second problem in this case grew out of the first. Solid foods were introduced in response to Jason's apparent hunger. Newborns do not have the ability to swallow voluntarily much before 10 or 12 weeks of age. They can swallow only if their sucking reflex is stimulated first. Even when voluntary swallowing does occur, the infant will still suck on its fingers while attempting to swallow. Although it did not happen in Jason's case, this hand-to-mouth behavior is frequently discouraged by parents who see it as interfering in their attempts to feed their child.

Influences on Feeding Behavior Age 4 to 9 Months

As a child develops, new skills and a broader awareness of the environment change the ways in which the child approaches a feeding.

Response to Breast Feeding

Sharon is an excellent example of three common feeding problems. The first is seen in her response to nursing. She would appear to be uninterested, and in fact Mrs. E. felt Sharon had begun to wean herself. What we are seeing is how individual temperament influences behavioral patterns. Sharon, while showing herself to be highly adaptable when she began to nurse and with the introduction of solids, is also showing that she is very easily distracted. Extraneous stimuli, such as another adult in the room or minor noises, are now capable of attracting her attention, making her curious, and interfering with her ongoing behavior.

This seems to be more common among breast-fed infants, perhaps because the nursing child's field of vision is more confined by this position. It can usually be handled by firmly coaxing the child back and by nursing in a quiet room with dim light at least once or twice a day (preferably morning and evening), when distractions are at a minimum. With minimal distractions the child is able to focus on the ongoing feeding process and is usually reinforced by the parent's more relaxed and focused response.

CASE STUDY 11-4

Sharon E. is a 6-month-old infant brought to the clinic because of a feeding problem. She had been a healthy infant whose only medical contact had been for well-child visits. Mrs. E. had been very successful in nursing Sharon. At 4 months of age solid foods were introduced with Sharon taking to them in her usual eager way.

Now, however, when her mother attempts to nurse her Sharon is continuously pushing away from the nipple after a few sucks. She will look around the room, return briefly to the breast, and look around again. If her mother is speaking to another person or if there is any activity or

noise in the room, the pushing away is more frequent. At other times she looks up at her mother and becomes interested in reaching for her mother's face and hair.

In addition, both parents report difficulties in giving her her solids. She frequently turns away as the spoon approaches, waving her arms wildly and occasionally sending the spoon flying. There are certain foods which she repeatedly spits out. Because of this her parents became concerned about her food intake and sought help. Her physical examination was entirely normal.

Acquisition of Reaching

The second development of significance is Sharon's acquisition of reaching. As with any new skill, it is immediately put to use to explore her environment. In Sharon's case, in combination with her distractibility she becomes interested in her mother's face and reaches out in gross sweeping movements. As her reach develops, she gets great pleasure in going after almost anything and putting it into her mouth. Almost simultaneous with this acquisition of reaching is the first evidence of autonomy.

Autonomy

We see in Sharon's case real evidence of preference and independence. Food preferences are not part of a child's genetic endowment but are acquired and thus individualized. Every household has a number of common foods missing from the dinner table because of the preference of the adult members. Why then are parents unaware or intolerant of food preferences in their children?

To a large extent it has to do with control, and represents the starting point for most of

the feeding problems encountered in the infant and preschooler. The development of autonomy and independence is every bit as important as the development of attachment. The participants in this process (too frequently a struggle) are the very people with whom the infant has just set up a dependent relationship. Most parents find the dependency needs of in-

Figure 11-2
Sarah, aged 7 months. Almost simultaneous with this acquisition of reaching is the first evidence of autonomy.

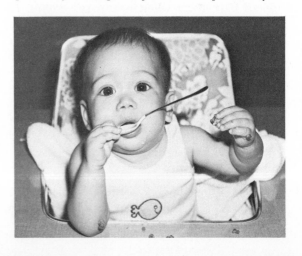

fants quite gratifying, so that when the child begins to separate from the parents and become autonomous they often feel a sense of loss. This is compounded by the child's vacillations between dependency and autonomy. Here is where allowing the child to be a more active participant in feeding should begin.

With the acquisition of an evolving pincer grasp using thumb and forefinger, children's reach will soon be developed to the point where they will be happily picking up pieces of food and stuffing themselves. They will also use these skills to explore their food. Finger foods allow this to happen. Usually parents still need to be actively involved in feeding at this point and frequently need ways to deal with the reaching and grabbing of the infant while the reach and pincer grasp is still inefficient. Giving the baby something to hold in each hand, like a breadstick or a spoon, eliminates the grabbing and provides something for the child to feed to himself. The spoon will in time facilitate imitative behavior when the child is ready to use it competently at about 15 or 16 months of age.

Spitting Up

Spitting up in infancy is common. There are a number of infants, however, who spit up regularly, sometimes 1 or 2 times per meal. An evaluation should be done on any infant who spits up this frequently. Some of these babies have chalasia (relaxation of a bodily opening such as the cardiac sphincter, a cause of vomiting in infants)[23] and are helped by being fed and kept upright in a chalasia chair for a period of time following their feeding. Other concerns, such as pyloric stenosis, also need to be considered during the newborn period.

A few of these infants, such as Daniel, who have no physical explanation for their failure to grow, end up being hospitalized. An understanding of the infant's temperament should be part of any evaluation. Among the children who make up "spitters" are a group like Daniel. They do not know the behaviors, described previously, of children with environmental failure to thrive. Almost in complete contrast, they are intense, easily excited infants who show good qualities of interaction and evi-

---

CASE STUDY 11-5

Daniel R. was hospitalized at 7 months of age because of failure to thrive. Mrs. R., aged 24, described a normal pregnancy, labor, and delivery. She reported that Daniel had been spitting up since birth. At age 2½ weeks, after he had been seen by his pediatrician, his milk was changed to a soy-based formula. This seemed to work for a few weeks, following which he began to spit up again. Subsequent formula changes also proved to be unsuccessful. At about 3 months of age cereals and fruits had been introduced with no change in his symptoms. Gradually he showed evidence of a decline in his growth curve. At birth he had weighed 3.26 kg and was 51 cm long. By his sixth month he was in the 3rd per-

centile for weight and was falling off in his length. A complete evaluation including a search for occult infection, malabsorption, chronic disease such as cystic fibrosis, evidence of central nervous system damage, and evidence of deprivation proved negative.

Daniel was described by his parents as a very intense child. When he cried, it was long and loud; when he was happy he was beside himself. His response to a new toy or new food was very positive. He always smiled at everyone he saw. He frequently was excited just prior to spitting up. These would often be times when he was playing with his mother or father.

dence of appropriate interpersonal experience. They frequently spit up when excited or in any way stressed.

This spitting up is often interpreted as overfeeding, and parents frequently try to deal with it by feeding the child less. At times this is done gradually and unknowingly, so that when such children are hospitalized they are being given less than adequate nutrition. The feeding experience usually becomes so negative and unrewarding that it affects the way in which the parents view their child. Almost universally the parents feel like failures.

When fed an adequate diet, while the parents receive support and reassurance, these infants gain weight even while continuing to spit up. Thus the notion that they fail to grow because of the food lost from spitting up is untrue. It is because they are underfed by their parents in response to their spitting up. This problem becomes much less frequent between 12 and 16 months of age. Interestingly, these infants remain intense children who in later years when stressed or excited (by birthdays, first day of school, etc.) often respond by vomiting.

Influences on Feeding Behavior
Age 9 to 16 Months

Independence

The list of important milestones during this period is significant—the infant will pull to stand, will cruise and probably walk; he or she will have developed a reach and pincer grasp and be able to manipulate and explore the environment; meaningful words will be uttered; a sense of spatial awareness, of the permanency of objects, of employing means to achieve ends, and of making causal connections will have developed. Throughout all of these accomplishments is a rapidly growing sense of competence and independence. By the end of this period children are quite capable of feeding themselves and will in fact insist on it.

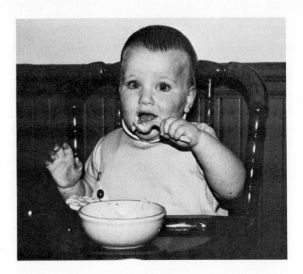

Figure 11-3
Tara, aged 12 months. Developing a facility with the spoon, she is becoming more independent, insisting on self-feeding.

By not encouraging independence parents frequently find themselves with a feeding problem. The two parental concerns (about enough to eat and about allowing autonomy) remain at the base of most feeding problems in healthy children at this age. An example of concern over the child's getting enough to eat is seen in the amount of food that children in this age group are given. Until the child is 8 or 9 months of age most parents are using commercially prepared baby foods which come in standardized volumes. Most parents mistakenly assume that the baby-food jar represents a desired, scientifically determined volume of food. This standard offers comfort and reassurance to parents. Once table foods are introduced, however, the parents' standard becomes whatever they determine it to be—usually a subjective percentage of an adult portion.

Once a standard has been set, an expectation has also been set. The child's own physiological response to food—an awareness of hunger or satiety—and attempts at autonomy have become challenged. The result is often food on the floor, an angry and frustrated parent, and a crying child. How much simpler it would be to put small amounts of food (chopped and cut table food) in front of children and to let them set their own pace and determine their own volume. It is wise to put out only small amounts at a time since children's temptation to play with and throw the food seems to increase with the amount in front of them.

At this point it is important to consider the adage cited at the beginning of this chapter in the light of what has been said in the preceding discussion about parental concerns over adequate volumes and the encouragement of autonomy in feeding. It is important to remember when bringing the horse to the trough that the objective is to satisfy the horse's thirst and not to drain the trough. Likewise, the goal to be set in feeding children should be to satisfy their hunger and caloric needs and not to get them to clean their plates. Further, optimal nutrition, a legitimate long-range goal, can be accomplished only by being aware of a child's total growth process. There clearly are times when meeting minimal daily requirements will appear as a challenge. It is felt that

an approach which appreciates the value of promoting the inherent sense of competence and mastery already present in children will minimize areas of conflict such as those described in this chapter. The end result will be a child who is not only well nourished physically but also well nourished cognitively and emotionally.

STUDY QUESTIONS

1 What are the prenatal influences that can affect infant feeding behavior?

2 Describe the postnatal influences on feeding behavior in the infant between the ages of birth and 2 months, 2 and 4 months, 4 and 9 months, 9 and 16 months.

3 How would you assess the degree of synchrony between a parent and child in a feeding situation?

4 Describe the behavioral characteristics of a child with nonorganic failure to thrive.

5 What are the major issues that surround feeding problems in the second year of life?

REFERENCES

1 H. N. Ricciuti, "Malnutrition, Learning, and Intellectual Development: Research and Remediation," in F. F. Korten, S. W. Cook, and J. I. Lacey (eds.), *Psychology and the Problems of Society,* American Psychological Association, Washington, D.C., 1970, pp. 237–253.

2 M. Winich, J. Brasel, E. Velasco, and P. Rosso, "Effect of Early Nutrition on Growth of the Central Nervous System," in D. Bergsma (ed.), *The Infant at Risk,* Birth Defects Original Article Series, vol. 10, National Foundation March of Dimes, Intercontinental Medical Books Corp., New York, 1974, pp. 29–36.

3 M. Winick and P. Rosso, "The Effect of Severe Early Malnutrition on Cellular Growth of Human Brain," *Pediatric Research,* **3**:181–184, 1969.

4 M. Winick, "Cellular Growth in Intrauterine Malnutrition," *Pediatric Clinics of North America,* **17**:69–78, 1970.

5 H. F. Eichenwald and P. C. Fry, "Nutrition and Learning," *Science,* **163**:644–648, 1969.

6 S. Zamenhof, E. Van Marthens, and L. Gravel, "DNA (Cell Number) in Neonatal Brain: Second Generation (F2) Alteration by Maternal (F0) Dietary Protein Restriction," *Science,* **172**:850–951, 1971.

7 E. Tronick, B. Koslowski, and T. B. Brazelton, "Neonatal Behavior among Urban Zambians and Americans," paper presented at the Society for Research in Child Development, Minneapolis, Minn., April 1971.

8 H. Als, E. Tronick, L. Adamson, and T. B. Brazelton, "The Behavior of the Full-Term yet Underweight Newborn Infant," 1975, unpublished report.

9 W. K. Frankenberg, J. B. Dodds, and A. W. Fandal, *Denver Developmental Screening Test,* University of Colorado Medical Center, 1970.

10 M. D. S. Ainsworth and S. M. Bell, "Some Contemporary Patterns of Mother-Infant Interaction in the

Feeding Situation," in A. Ambrose (ed.), *Stimulation in Early Infancy,* Academic Press, New York, 1969, pp. 133–170.

11 M. D. S. Ainsworth, S. M. Bell, and D. J. Stayton, "Individual Differences in Strange-Situation Behavior of One-Year-Olds," in H. R. Schaffer (ed.), *The Origins of Human Social Relations,* Academic Press, New York, 1971, pp. 17–52.

12 D. M. Snyder, R. W. Telzrow, E. Tronick, H. Als, and T. B. Brazelton, "The Effects of Phototherapy on Neonatal Behavior," *Proceedings of the Society of Pediatric Research,* April 1976.

13 E. Tronick, S. Wise, H. Als, L. Adamson, J. Scanlon, and T. B. Brazelton, "Regional Obstetric Anesthesia and Newborn Behavior: Effect over the First Ten Days of Life," *Pediatrics,* **58:**94–100, 1976.

14 E. B. Thoman, "Development of Synchrony in Mother-Infant Interaction in Feeding and Other Situations," paper presented at symposium of the American Institute of Nutrition, Federation of American Societies of Experimental Biology: Effects of Nutrition on Maternal-Infant Interaction, Atlantic City, N.J., April 9, 1974.

15 E. B. Thoman, C. R. Barnett, and P. H. Leiderman, "Feeding Behaviors of Newborn Infants as a Function of Parity of the Mother," *Child Development,* **42:**1471–1483, 1971.

16 K. Kaye, "Toward the Origin of Dialogue," paper prepared for the Loch Lomond Symposium, University of Strathelyde, September 1975.

17 S. Brody, *Patterns of Mothering,* International Universities Press, Inc., New York, 1966.

18 G. F. Powell, J. A. Brasel, and R. M. Blizzard, "Functional Deprivation and Growth Retardation Simulating Idiopathic Hypopituitarism. I Clinical Evaluation of the Syndrome," *New England Journal of Medicine,* **276:**1271–1278, 1967.

19 G. F. Powell, J. A. Brasel, S. Raiti, and R. M. Blizzard, "Emotional Deprivation and Growth Retardation Simulating Idiopathic Hypopituitarism. II Endocrinologic Evaluation of the Syndrome," *New England Journal of Medicine,* **276:**1279, 1967.

20 S. D. Frasier and M. L. Rallison, "Growth Retardation and Emotional Deprivation: Relative Resistance to Treatment with Human Growth Hormone," *Journal of Pediatrics,* **80:**603–609, 1972.

21 D. Rosenn, L. Stein, and M. Bates, "The Differentiation of Organic from Environmental Failure to Thrive," paper presented at the meetings of the American Pediatric Society and Society for Pediatric Research, April 1975.

22 D. A. Levitsky and R. H. Barnes, "Nutritional and Environmental Interactions in the Behavioral Development of the Rat: Long Term Effects," *Science,* **176:**68–71, 1972.

23 *Dorland's Illustrated Medical Dictionary,* 24th ed., W. B. Saunders Company, Philadelphia, 1965.

24 Z. Stein, M. Susser, G. Saenger, and F. Marolla: *Famine and Human Development: The Dutch Hunger Winter of 1944–45,* Oxford University Press, New York, 1975.

CHAPTER 12

GROWTH

AND NUTRITION

Christine E. Cronk
Rosanne B. Howard

KEY WORDS
Growth
Critical Periods
Growth Velocity
Cumulative Growth
Growth Assessment
Age Needs
Stage Needs

INTRODUCTION

Growth is the outward sign of a positive interaction between nutrition, genetics, and time. Nutrition operates within the confines of one's genetic background and environment to maximize growth potential. With a greater understanding of growth through the life cycle, as presented in pages 203 to 216, the student will readily appreciate nutrition through the life cycle, which is presented in pages 217 to 243 and continued in Chap. 13.

Although for the purposes of discussing nutrition in the life cycle chronological age is used as a point of demarcation to describe nutrient needs, it should be remembered that it is physiological age which is the true determinant. The spectrum of human variability is broad, and because a child is chronologically thirteen, she is not necessarily an adolescent, nor is a man at 65 always elderly. Within a single family, all ages and stages may be represented and the nutrient needs of everybody must be considered. As we look at the wheel of life, we can consider nutrition through the life cycle as a circular process. The influences of nutrition on the human body are continuous, with one generation passing the effect on to the next.

GROWTH THROUGH THE LIFE CYCLE

Christine E. Cronk

Definition

Growth, which is one measure of nutrient effectiveness in early life, is the increase in size attendant upon development of the organism from embryo to adult. It implies the physiological accretion of tissue, which in turn reflects the acquisition of protein and water.[1]

PROCESSES AND MECHANISMS UNDERLYING GROWTH

Growth takes place by way of three processes, (1) an increase in cell number, known as *hyper-*

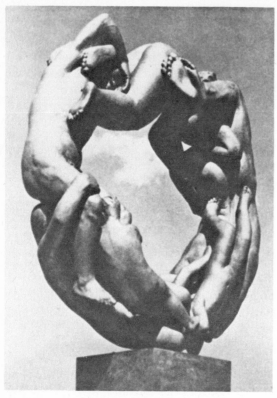

Figure 12-1
The wheel of life. (Gustav Vigeland, The Vigeland Sculpture Park, Oslo, Norway.)

plasia, (2) growth in cell size, or *hypertrophy,* and (3) an increase in the size of the intercellular matrix (material between cells). Hyperplasia characterizes very early embryonic growth, hypertrophy begins in the later fetal life, and growth of the intercellular matrix begins postnatally. While most tissues enlarge by way of a combination of hyperplasia and hypertrophy, some tissues grow largely by way of increases in cell size (muscle and fat, for example) and others, most importantly bone, get larger by way of an enlarging intercellular matrix.

Tissues are most vulnerable while their component cell numbers are increasing. When the cell division is disrupted because of deficient substrate, the basic cell population number may never be established; consequently,

nutritional deficiencies occurring during these periods are significant and may be irremediable. This fact underlies the concept of *critical phases* of growth. In contrast to this, disruptions or deficiencies that take place during the phases when cell enlargement predominates are more easily corrected.

The three growth processes are controlled by a number of internal and external factors, including genes, hormones (and related central nervous system factors), and environmental or extrinsic influences.

Genes

The understanding of the genetics of growth requires two different kinds of information: information concerning the relationship of genes to cell division and enlargement, and that concerning the inheritance of size. Within the nucleus of every cell are long strands of genetic material, deoxyribonucleic acid (DNA), which is organized in the shape of a double helix. During cell division, these long strands are coiled up into structures called *chromosomes.* The *genes* are segments of these long DNA double strands, and each gene is defined by a particular sequence of chemical bases. This sequence is a code or blueprint for how the cell should construct a particular protein from the raw materials (amino acids) that are available in the cell cytoplasm.

The code is carried from the nucleus into the cytoplasm by messenger ribonucleic acid (mRNA), which is single-stranded and is constructed at certain spots on the DNA strand. The mRNA moves into the cytoplasm and attaches itself to a spot called a ribosome. A second RNA, transfer RNA, also formed within the cell nucleus, collects the appropriate amino acids, brings them to the ribosomes to which their corresponding mRNA is attached, and hooks them onto the mRNA in the appropriate coded order. When the protein is completed it is released into the cytoplasm. This then is the link between the genes and their expression in the structure of the body.

Growth is one aspect of the realization of the genetic plan. In general, body size, weight, and head circumference are polygenically inherited; i.e., each involves more than one set of genes, in contrast to such traits as eye color or blood group (ABO), which depend on a single genic locus. This is not surprising since the combination of tissues and physiological processes on which growth depends are so various. From the standpoint of population genetics, an individual will tend to grow in the fashion and attain a size characteristic of his or her racial or ethnic group. This population variation simply reflects the "gene pool" created by restrictions of mating, whether determined geographically, socially, or otherwise. In turn, an individual's size will be closely related to that of his or her parents and siblings, the similarity arising from the even more restricted gene pool involved. Understanding this similarity is useful in growth assessment because it allows for a more accurate idea of how big an individual child "should" be.

Hormones

The hormones most important to growth are pituitary growth hormone, thyroxine, and insulin (see Chap. 20). At adolescence the sex hormones, including testosterone, estrogen, and the adrenal androgens, play a part in both the pubertal growth spurt and the subsequent completion of bone maturation.

Extrinsic Factors Influencing Growth

Nutrition

Several environmental factors are important in maintaining growth. First is adequate *nutrition*. At least a minimum intake of nutrients, vitamins, and minerals appropriate to body size is essential for support of normal growth. Severe and chronic malnutrition will lead to profound growth failure and wasting (as in kwashiorkor and marasmus). Less severe de-

ficiencies, however, may also affect growth. (See Chap. 16.)

Secular Trend, Immigration, and Socioeconomic Status

Three phenomena that are observable in growth differences among groups of people (rather than differences between individuals within a group) are related in part or in whole to a decline in the incidence of nutritional deficiency. *Secular trend* is a temporal phenomenon that has been evident in at least the last century, whereby European populations (and other populations where documentation has been provided) have appeared to mature earlier (i.e., reach final height sooner and grow bigger than earlier generations). This size increase is due to a differential increase in the size of long bones (as opposed to other tissues) and was most clearly demonstrated in Bowles's 1932 study of Harvard University fathers and sons.[2] Secular trend is partially due to improvements in diet, but may also be related to a host of other factors (e.g., improved health). The most recent United States growth data available[3] have demonstrated that the secular trend in this country has essentially ceased since 1955.

A phenomenon related to secular trend is the larger stature of second-generation immigrants to the United States. Again, nutritional and health factors account for this difference.

Larger average size characterizes higher *socioeconomic status*. This is clearest in third-world nations where differences in diet among the various socioeconomic classes are marked. Many studies of Guatemalan child growth, for example, establish the size advantage of the privileged Ladinos over the rural Guatemalan children.[4]

Health and Emotions

The *relative state of health* of the child influences growth. Ordinary illnesses like upper respiratory tract infections or chickenpox are usually not severe or prolonged enough to interfere with growth. Chronic, repeated, or severe illnesses, however, may conserve the body's resources for maintenance purposes, with few resources left for growth, so that growth arrest occurs. However, the arrested growth is often followed by a period of *catch-up growth*.[5] Catch-up growth is a phenomenon related to the fact that each individual is genetically programmed to be a certain size by the time growth ceases. If growth deficiency occurs, the body somehow recognizes this and makes up the deficit by growing faster than normal. In addition to recovery after illness, catch-up growth characterizes recovery from malnutrition, recovery from growth failure due to emotional deprivation, and recovery from some intrauterine growth retardation syndromes.

Emotions may also affect growth. While the mechanism for the growth failure observed in some neglected children is not understood in detail, it is presumed to be related to the close connection between neural centers for emotion and those controlling many other important physiological functions.

PERIODS OF BODY GROWTH

There are several distinct periods of growth, characterized by relatively accelerated periods and intervening steady periods of increase. While height and weight are closely interrelated, their individual schedules exhibit differences. Periods of accelerated growth are evident at *mid* and *later gestation, early infancy, and adolescence.* These periods are interspersed with times of slower growth that occur immediately post-conceptionally and during mid and late childhood. A less dramatic mid-childhood spurt of growth occurs in some children between 8 and 10 years of age (see Fig. 12-2 below).

Prenatal Growth

The very first part of growth, occurring from conception until 12 weeks after conception, is known as the *embryonic phase* and involves rela-

tively small increases in measurable size. After fertilization of the ovum, division of the first several generations of cells occurs simultaneously, with a consequent geometric increase in cell number. Soon the dividing times become staggered and the cells differentiate into those that will give rise to all of the important tissues and organs, in a process known as *morphogenesis*. At this point the cells are also increasing in size.

During the embryonic period the placenta transports and stores nutrients and synthesizes proteins and hormones. Important insults to the embryo such as infections, the introduction of harmful drugs or chemicals, or severe trauma may result in spontaneous abortion or in important anomalies. While the embryo is well protected during this time, inadequate nutrition may influence the integrity of its growth.

Beginning between 8 and 12 weeks after conception, the embryo becomes a *fetus,* a relatively more independent organism with primitive reflexes, a beating heart, and a functioning renal system. The fetal period is characterized by the most rapid increase in length (during the second trimester) and weight (during the final trimester) of the entire life cycle. In addition, the organ systems continue to differentiate and improve in function. Rapid growth occurs in all tissues and organ systems by expanding cell numbers. An increase in cell size occurs simultaneously in some tissues.

The integrity of fetal growth can be affected by smoking, high altitude, infection, toxemia of pregnancy, and the introduction of teratogenic agents. Although debate continues, some investigations demonstrate that pathophysiologic changes and compromise of growth occur in the fetus in the presence of maternal malnutrition.[6]

Birth Size

At birth, a child's size will reflect two factors: limitations imposed by the mechanics of birth (i.e., the size of the birth canal as it relates to the head size of the child) and those imposed by variations in the intrauterine environment. Birth size will be related more closely to these maternal factors than to a child's own genetic predisposition. Preterm babies will be smaller than those born at term (40 weeks). Because conceptional dates are often difficult to determine, distinguishing a child who is preterm from one who is small for reasons of inadequate intrauterine nutrient supply is often difficult. Charts are available as aids for such determinations.[7,8]

Postnatal Growth

Growth after birth can be roughly divided into three periods:

Infancy: birth to 2 years
Childhood: 2 to 10 or 11 years
Adolescence: 10 or 11 to maturity (16 to 21 years)

Reference to Fig. 12-2 provides a general idea of the shape of the cumulative curve for post-

Figure 12-2

Growth of the head and body from conception to 18 years. Head growth is most rapid prenatally and in the early postnatal months. It is nearly complete by age 1 year. Body growth is rapid in the late prenatal period and early postnatal years. However, final body size depends on a continued, steady rate of growth throughout childhood.

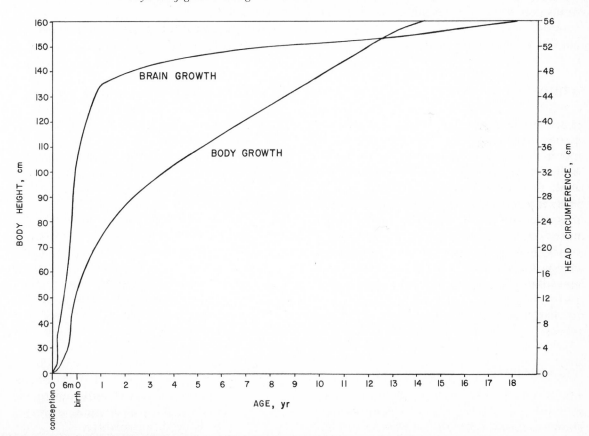

natal growth. (See "Growth Terminology" below for a discussion of the cumulative curve.)

Growth in *length* is most rapid in early life. A child has increased from birth length by 20 percent at 3 months, by 50 percent at 1 year, and by 75 percent at 2 years. Size at 2 to 2½ years is generally 50 percent of adult size. In the first 6 to 12 months of life children destined to be big grow faster and climb to higher percentile levels while smaller children grow more slowly, thus moving on to lower percentile levels. The percentile level established during this early infant growth is usually maintained at least until adolescence. Growth velocity decelerates steadily between birth and 4 to 5 years of age. Between age 5 years and just prior to adolescence, annual increments in length are about the same, although there may be seasonal variations in these gains (with peaks occurring between mid-April and mid-June).

Gains in length primarily reflect bone growth in three components: head, trunk (i.e., the spinal column), and legs. Since head height is 95 percent complete by 10 years of age, it comprises a greater percentage of the total length earlier in life than it does later. Growth in the first year of life occurs largely in the trunk, which gains 60 percent of its final adult size in this interval. Between 1 year and adolescence the most impressive relative growth takes place in the bones of the legs (about 66 percent of their total growth). The adolescent growth spurt is mainly due to increases in trunk length. Because of the differential growth rates of the components of stature, the body has a characteristic appearance at different ages.

Weight at birth is 3×10^6 times the weight of the ovum. The velocity of weight gain reaches its peak for the entire life cycle just after the early neonatal weight loss. Within the first few weeks after birth, weight gain proceeds very rapidly. Birth weight is doubled by 5 months, tripled by 1 year, and quadrupled by 3 years. As with length, increases in weight after the third or fourth year are steady, showing an unchanging annual velocity. Seasonal peaks also occur in weight, the winter months being characterized by the most rapid weight gains.

Weight gain is a composite of growth in all body tissues (muscle, bone, fat, and the organs). Its relation to length is expressed in the formula called the *ponderal index:* $100 \times weight/length^3$. The ponderal index is highest in infancy and early childhood (when weight is greatest relative to body surface area, $length^3$). It gradually falls toward the end of the adolescent growth spurt, after which it rises to the level it had attained at about age 8 or 9 years. The relation of bone weight to body weight is fairly constant throughout life. Skeletal muscle weight rises from 25 percent of body weight in infancy to 40 percent by adulthood. Changes in fat composition are discussed below.

Adolescence is the second postnatal period of rapid growth and a number of its features are important:

1 Changes at adolescence include:
   a Rapid growth in height and weight
   b Changes in body composition (primarily in proportions of fat, muscle, and bone) that are more marked in boys than in girls
   c Development of secondary sex characteristics
      (1) In girls these include breast development, appearance and elaboration of pubic and axillary hair, menarche, differential deposition of adipose tissue on hips, thighs, and buttocks, and characteristic changes of facial architecture.
      (2) In boys these include growth in the size of penis and testes, appearance and elaboration of pubic, axillary, body, and facial hair, increase in size of the larynx, broadening of the shoulder girdle, and increase in skeletal musculature.

2 In general, adolescent changes occur earlier in girls (between 9 and 16 years) than in boys (between 12 and 18 years).

3 Onset of pubertal development is controlled largely by circulating hormones. The mechanisms timing the release of these hormones are not well understood.

4 There is a wide variation in the times of onset and completion of the events of puberty, but the sequence of events is usually the same. Because of this variation, the use of growth charts and percentile levels is not reliable during adolescence.

Brain Growth

The schedule for brain growth differs from that for the body (see Fig. 12-2). In general the brain grows more rapidly and completes growth earlier than the rest of the body. Its growth is most rapid during last trimester of gestation and the first postnatal months. By 1½ years of age its growth is 90 percent completed and by 10 years of age it is 95 percent complete. No real adolescent growth spurt is evident in head circumference.

The growth schedule of different parts of the brain is important to the understanding of the potential effect of pre- and postnatal nutritional inadequacies. During the first 10 weeks of gestation the brain differentiates into its main parts. The cerebrum, which accounts for 85 percent of brain weight, increases in volume by means of an increase in the numbers of sulci (convolutions), which develop rapidly beginning at about 15 weeks of gestation. The rapid increase in volume of the cerebrum accounts for the largest part of the *first* growth spurt of the brain (occurring between 18 and 20 weeks postconception) and is largely due to neuronal hyperplasia. The number of cells established at this time will characterize the brain for life. During both the periods of differentiation and the periods of neuronal multiplication, the fetus is well protected by the intrauterine environment; as a consequence, maternal malnutrition at these times may have less impact on the growing brain than at later times. A second

spurt in growth is evident at 32 weeks of gestation. This second rapid period and much of the subsequent growth of the brain is attributable to the tremendous increase in dendritic complexity and synaptic interconnectivity of the neurons rather than to an actual increase in cell number. The cerebellum, a part of the brain located below the cerebrum and at the posterior end of the head, exhibits a different growth schedule. Its rapid cell multiplication begins during the last month of gestation and proceeds very rapidly during the first year of life. A particularly rapid phase in the cycle of cerebellar growth occurs at 5 months postnatally. The velocity of cerebellar growth is greater than that of the cerebrum. It begins later and is nearly completed by 18 months, at which time the cerebrum and other parts of the brain are only 60 percent of their final weight. Cerebellar growth takes place at a time when the growing fetus and then the infant is much more susceptible to the effects of malnutrition. Some investigators[9,10] have suggested that because of both the rate and the timing of its rapid increase, the cerebellum, which controls integration of motor activities, is most susceptible to the effects of malnutrition, particularly protein deprivation, during this period. The strongest evidence of this comes from animal research which demonstrates important limitations in cognitive functioning in all species subjected to nutritional deprivation during critical periods of postnatal brain growth.

In human research studies, malnourished children have demonstrated smaller head circumferences and, on postmortem analysis, reduced brain weight and protein content.[11] However, the distinction between the effects on intellectual functioning produced by nutritional limitation and effects which are due to other elements of environmental deprivation are difficult to disentangle.[12]

Adipose Tissue Growth

The dynamics of the growth of adipose tissue are of special interest because fat composition (as measured by skinfold thickness) is a useful means of assessing nutritional status. Table 12-1 shows body fat composition at various ages.

Girls are approximately 25 percent fatter than boys from birth onward. During the first part of intrauterine growth there is almost no adipose tissue. Fat begins to accumulate once the phase of increasing size is initiated in the second trimester, but is most rapid between the second fetal month and 6 months postnatally. During this time, fat acts to ensure energy stores for the rapidly growing body and to provide extra insulation for immature thermal regulation. Weight gain by the average infant is approximately 38 percent fat between birth and age 6 months but is only about 11 percent of the weight gained between 6 months and 1 year. A reverse relationship is evident between fat and protein composition of weight gain in that age interval. Between 1 year and 6 to 8 years of age there is a relatively lower percentage of body fat. The relative fat composition, increases again at 9 years as part of the adolescent growth phase. At the end of the growth spurt the fat/body size ratio again recedes to about that observed at birth. The prepubescent growth spurt in adipose tissue precedes

that of muscle and bone. Consequently, excess weight for height may be manifest at the onset of adolescence. It should be noted that this "fat phase" is transient and not predictive of adulthood obesity.

Though cell number continues to increase into early adulthood, an increase of cell size accounts for a larger percentage of the total gain in adipose tissue after infancy. Obese preadolescent children were demonstrated to have three to four times as many adipose cells as nonobese children by Hirsch, Knittle, and Salan.[13] These investigators suggest that proliferation of cell number in infancy is the important variable in determining their obesity.[14,15]

Measurement of fat composition can be accomplished fairly simply in a clinical setting by use of skinfold calipers, as discussed below, under "Measurement." Such measures are useful in assessment of obesity or malnutrition.

Growth Terminology

Three terms are essential in growth assessment: cumulative growth, growth velocity, and percentile levels. *Cumulative growth* is absolute growth, an individual's size at any point in time. The height and weight charts (see Fig. 12-5) provide a graph of cumulative growth. *Growth velocity* is the rate of growth during some interval of time (a year or six months, for example). It is obtained by subtracting an earlier measure from one taken later. Detection of abnormally fast or slow growth is accomplished by use of *percentile levels*. The National Center for Health Statistics (NCHS) charts (Fig. 12-5) show curves for the 5th through the 95th percentiles. Children at the 50th percentile will be average for their age while ones at the 5th or 95th percentiles will be respectively smaller and larger than their agemates. Because of the regular and predictable course of growth, a particular child will tend to stay within the same percentile level (beginning at about 6 to 12 months of age) throughout life. Maintenance of this percentile level depends on normal growth velocity. Deviations from the

TABLE 12-1 BODY FAT COMPOSITION AT VARIOUS STAGES OF DEVELOPMENT

Age	Bodyfat, % of total body weight
End of second trimester	0.5*
Birth (accrued in last 2 prenatal months)	12*
4 months	16*
6 months	26.3†
1 year	24†
4–6 years	22*
7–9 years	24*
10–12 years	28*
Adulthood	18*

* Source: Icie G. Macy and Harriet J. Kelly, *Chemical Anthropology: A New Approach to Growth in Children,* University of Chicago Press, Chicago, 1957, pp. 78–79.

† Source: Samuel Fomon, *Infant Nutrition,* 2d ed., W.B. Saunders Co., 1974, p. 74.

established percentile level will often indicate abnormal growth. These concepts will be important to the discussion of growth assessment below.

THE ASSESSMENT OF GROWTH

The assessment of growth has three components: information gathering, anthropometric measurement, and data analysis.

Information Gathering

The health professional, in looking at a child with a growth problem, is concerned with identifying both those problems directly attributable to dietary factors and those in which diet is a secondary but contributory factor. Because feeding difficulties and other aspects of diet are often synergistic with other phenomena related to poor growth, such determinations can be difficult. It is therefore essential to make a thorough documentation of all relevant information.

1 *Longitudinal data on growth* As many serial measurements as possible of height (or length), weight, head circumference, and chest circumference should be sought. These may be available in the child's hospital record, through the pediatrician or family physician, or in the baby book kept by the mother. In the case of very young children birth records (which will most often document birth length, weight, head circumference, and chest circumference) should be obtained. These data will be important in identifying whether the current measurements represent the beginning, continuation, or intensification of an abnormal growth pattern. It should also be clear that without some idea of when growth abnormalities began, the isolation of the cause is more difficult. Finally, when more data are available, a better documentation of growth pattern is possible. Growth

patterns, rather than single data points, are of the greatest use.

2 *Health history* Besides obtaining a diet history (see Chap. 15), a careful documentation of health status through life should be made.

   a Certain major disease entities have a known association with growth problems. These include diseases of the major organs, and inborn metabolic and endocrine disorders. Prenatally acquired infections (e.g., rubella) can seriously limit postnatal growth. Finally, surgery or prolonged hospitalization may slow growth. Some of these disease processes permanently impair growth. Others, including prenatal infections, may be followed by recovery (i.e., "catch-up" growth).

   b Sporadic or chronic minor illnesses, such as upper respiratory infections, may temporarily cause weight loss and slow the velocity of linear growth. Because ground lost during episodes of surgery, hospitalization, or illness will be regained, it is essential not to confuse these temporary setbacks with growth failure that requires intervention.

3 *Relevant background data* A child's growth pattern and size at any point in time will be related to the height and build of other family members, to racial or ethnic background, and to environmental circumstances. Data on each of these are necessary for accurate assessment. Documentation of the size of as many other immediate and extended family members as is feasible will give some idea about the propriety of a child's size in the family context. Data on socioeconomic background and the family's country of origin are important because of the clearly different expectations for growth often associated with these factors (see above discussion). It may be necessary to obtain standards appropriate for these variables, such as those presented by Knott on Puerto Rican children.[15]

Measurement

Four measurements—height (length), weight, head circumference, and skinfold thickness—are necessary for assessment of growth. It should be remembered that each of these is a composite or summary measure which represent, respectively, bony growth (i.e., spine and long bones along with the head), weight (all the tissues together), skinfolds (fat composition), and head circumference (brain growth).

Figure 12-3

Measurement of recumbent length. The infant's head must be held in place against the headboard. The infant's feet with toes pointing directly upward are held by a second person with gentle traction, as the movable footboard is brought to rest against the infant's heels. Three measurements taken in this position should be attempted. Differences in the three values should then be averaged.

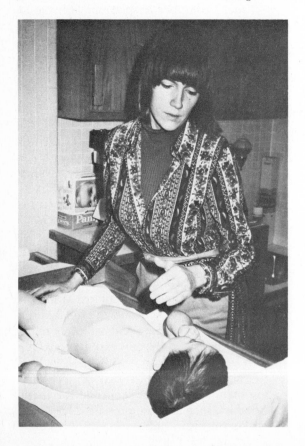

They are very general measures of the integrity of the biological operations of the individual being assessed.

Recumbent length (see Fig. 12-3) is the measure used for assessing size in young children. Some standards are based on recumbent length till age 2 years (NCHS charts for example) while others carry these standards to age 6. Because the recumbent length for a given child is about 2 cm greater than the child's standing height, the standards available will dictate which measurement is to be used.

Recumbent length is measured on a table with an immovable head piece and a movable foot piece. A measuring tape (preferably graduated in millimeters) runs along the table's length. The child is placed on his or her back with the head brought against the head piece and is held there with gentle pressure. The head, shoulders, hip and feet are oriented in a single line as they would be for a standing measurement. The knees are held flattened against the table and the toes point upward. The movable board is brought against the bottom of the feet with gentle pressure. Each measure should be repeated at least three times with any necessary adjustments in body orientation. Immediate accurate recording of each of the three measures is essential. The three measures should then be averaged.

Standing height is best measured by a fixed rather than a free-standing measuring device. The child is positioned with the back snugly against the measuring device. The feet should be close together and touching the device and the back should show as little curvature as possible. The whole body should be carefully centered, the head held erect with the gaze straight forward. The movable board should contact the top of the head midsagittally. Three repeated measurements should be taken and averaged.

Weight is best measured using a beam balance scales with nondetachable weights. As little clothing as possible should be worn. However, with serial measures the same amount of clothing should be worn at each measuring.

For infants, scales weighing to the nearest gram are desirable. The balance of the scale should be checked before each weighing. An infant should be either laid on the scale (if body size permits) or seated with the center of gravity at the exact center of the scale. On such sensitive scales, several different values should be tried to see which offers the best balance. An average of the best-balanced values should be taken.

Head circumference is taken with a measuring tape that is preferably made of fiberglass or steel rather than cloth. The tape is applied above the bony eminence slightly above the eyebrows and around the widest part of the back of the head. The largest point is sought, again with three averaged ascertainments.

Skinfold thickness: Skinfolds comprise the skin and a layer of subcutaneous fat pulled away from the underlying muscle (see Fig. 12-4). While there are a number of body sites where subcutaneous fat might be measured, two are easily used and have a reasonably high correlation with whole body fat composition. These are triceps and subscapular skinfolds.

Figure 12-4
Measurement of triceps skinfold thickness. (a) Location of the midpoint of the upper arm; (b) Application of the Lange calipers for measurement of triceps skinfold; (c) Representation of the tissues of the arm (bone, fat, and skin) and measurement of skinfold thickness.

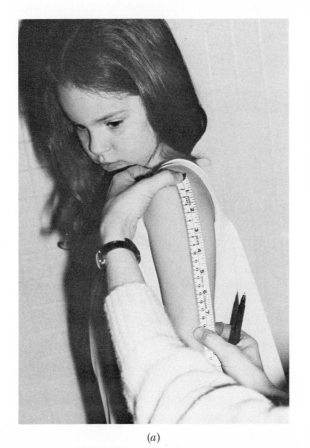

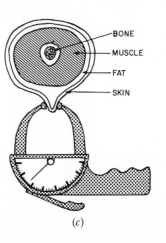

(b)

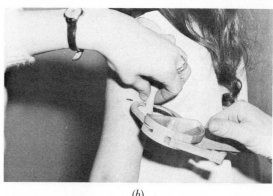

(a)

(c)

1 Triceps skinfolds are measured on one of the arms. The one measured should be that on which available standards are based. There are two instruments, the Lange and the Harpenden calipers, that may be used for the procedure. With a tape measure, the midpoint of the upper arm between the bony eminence at the shoulder (the acromion) and the olecranon (the lateral eminence at the elbow) is located. This midpoint is best marked with a felt-tip pen. The arm is held relaxed. The skinfold is grasped between the examiner's index finger and thumb at the back of the arm 1 cm above the marked midpoint.

2 Subscapular folds are taken at a point just below the lowest most lateral point of the shoulder blade in the line of the natural skin cleavage. Both triceps and subscapular readings are made to the nearest 0.5 mm at about 3 seconds after the application of the calipers. Again three readings with averaging are essential. (See appendix for skin fold standards.)

Data Analysis: Use of Growth Charts

The most commonly used tool for assessment of growth data are charts that plot the size of children by percentile level at consecutive ages (Fig. 12-5). The particular charts included here are selected for their high quality (in terms of sample size used and statistical rendering). Both past and current measures should be plotted. A number of observations should then be made concerning these data points and the following questions asked:

1 What is the child's current percentile level? If this is the only measurement available for this child, measures below the 3rd percentile or above the 97th percentile should arouse particular concern.

2 How does the current measure relate to the child's past measurement? Has the percentile level remained stable or has the child fallen or risen to a different percentile level?

3 How do the various measures interrelate?
   a Height/weight relations are best plotted on the newly generated height/weight grid. When these standards are unavailable separate graphs with height/weight plots more than 2 percentile levels apart are worthy of note.
   b Skinfold measures are best plotted by weight and age,[16,17] although age plots alone[18] are useful initially. Plots should be in line with percentile levels for weight.
   c The relation of head circumference to body size is not straightforward. In general a .25 correlation coefficient exists between stature and head circumference, indicating that it is not necessarily the case that big bodies and big heads (and vice versa) go together. There are certain characteristic relationships between head and body size during growth. At birth head circumference is larger than chest circumference but by age 1 year the opposite is true. Deviation from this relationship usually indicates deficits in body growth. One example of the cause for such a deviation is growth retardation due to emotional deprivation.

4 How do plots of other family members compare to that of the child? The reliability for predicting a child's size on this basis is limited. Two percentile levels of difference between a child and all the rest of his family is significant. More exacting standards can be used; for example, the Fels Parent Specific Standards for Height.[19]

5 At what ages have important illnesses, surgery, etc. occurred? These should be marked on the growth chart so that deviations from growth channels relative to them are evident.

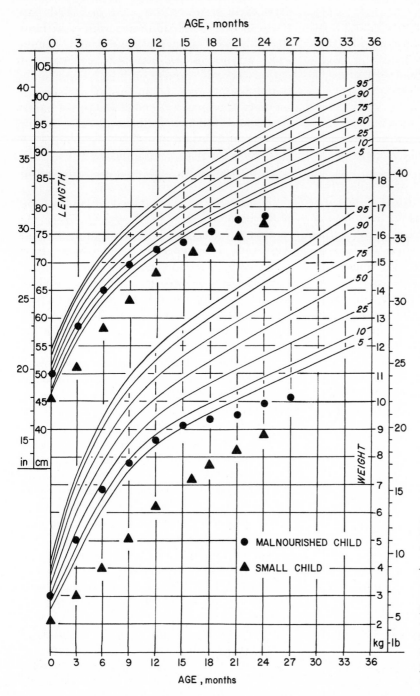

Figure 12-5

Serial measurements of length and weight of two children with abnormal growth patterns (see text for discussion). (Adapted from National Center for Health Statistics charts.) *The NCHS charts plot 5th through 95th percentiles. Normal children will generally fall within the upper and lower percentile limits and will maintain a particular percentile level throughout childhood.*

CASE APPLICATION: INTERPRETATION OF DEVIANT GROWTH

Growth charts plot data for a given child on a biologically normal curve. Consequently, patterns of growth that deviate from this curve can be easily seen. Two examples of unusual patterns in height and weight growth are given here.

Pattern #1 (Fig. 12-5) is the characteristic pattern of growth in height and weight for a chronically malnourished child. Weight drops precipitously at age 6 months and continues to move further below the 3d percentile, thus showing deficient velocity throughout the period plotted. Height begins to drop in percentiles (showing deficient velocity) somewhat after the weight falloff. The curve that is estimated through the points given is unlike the shapes of those on the normal chart.

Pattern #2 (Fig. 12-5) shows a child who was born at term but was small for gestational dates. At age 2 years, this child is continuing to grow at an essentially normal velocity but remains below the 3d percentile. Such a pattern indicates either a child whose nutriture in utero was inadequate enough to compromise growth recovery, or whose own internal biology is growth-limiting.

NUTRITION THROUGH THE EARLY YEARS

Rosanne B. Howard

Food is both the source of nutrients and the source of nurturance; it is the interpersonal matrix through which we learn about ourselves and our environment. In the process of nourishing, we feed more than food with its 50-odd known nutrients; we nurture and feed feelings as well.

Although the foods and the techniques (breast versus bottle) considered to be appropriate for infant and child feeding have varied over the centuries, the interpersonal aspects of feeding have prevailed. The colonial mother breast-fed by the clock, sometimes utilizing the services of a wet nurse, and prepared pap (flour or bread boiled in water with or without the addition of some milk) and panada (sometimes a synonym for pap; also, a mixture of various cereals, flours, or breads with some butter or milk cooked in broth)[20] as supplementary feedings.[21] A combination of ignorance and folklore influenced early infant feeding, and certain fruits and vegetables were forbidden for fear of infantile diarrhea.

Since that time, industrialization, urbanization, and the commercial activities of the formula industry have combined forces and the bottle became a new status symbol. Thus, the mother of today feeds her baby on demand with ready-to-feed formulas and baby foods or may choose to feed in the natural way—breast feeding and home-preparing baby foods—as these trends return to vogue. Whether baby is bottle or breast-fed, food and love become synonymous as the infant is held in the parent's comforting arms. As a "feeding couple," the needs of both parent and infant must be considered in deciding which mode of feeding is best, with breast feeding encouraged whenever possible.

From birth, feeding is a learned experience as the infant is placed at the breast or given a bottle, as soon as possible if in good physical condition. Usually 4 hours after birth, the normal, full-term infant is fed with 10 percent dextrose in water or plain water. Only after successful feeding is breast or formula feeding begun. (See Chap. 26, "Low-Birth-Weight, Premature Infants.") There is some evidence that nutritive sucking behavior in the newborn is affected by obstetric sedation, with the infants sucking at significantly lower rates and pressures and consuming less.[22] This lack of responsiveness is important for the nurse to recognize since this can interfere with nutrient intake and the developing mother-child relationship, as anxiety, tension, or frustration on the part of the mother can negatively reinforce the infant's early feeding experience.

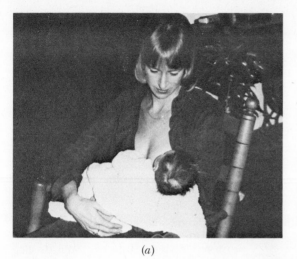 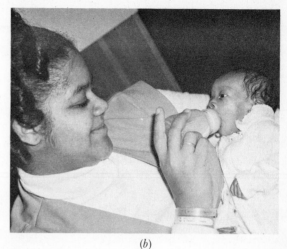

(a)   (b)

Figure 12-6
The mother and child, a "feeding couple." As a "feeding couple" the needs
of both must be considered in determining which mode of feeding is best.
(Photo courtesy of Jane McCotter O'Toole.)

INFANT

During the first year of life, the infant progresses from a totally dependent, somewhat passive, feeder to that of an active participant with a fair amount of independence. This transition follows the sequence of head, trunk, gross, and fine motor control as the infant's reflexive behavior now becomes voluntary. The infant will learn to chew and swallow rather than to suck solid foods, to drink from a cup, and to acquire all the manipulative skills that are necessary for independent feeding (see Table 12-2).

Growth is rapid and nutrient needs closely parallel growth. (See the first part of this chapter.) Energy needs approximate 117 kcal (466.2 kJ)/kg of body weight during the first 6 months and 108 kcal (453.6 kJ)/kg during the second half of the first year. For the most part breast milk or a sterilized formula with supplementary vitamins and iron can provide the needed nutrients for the first few months of life. Cow's milk or skim milk are not suitable for infant feeding. Proprietary formulas are processed to simulate human milk and are supplemented with vitamins and minerals [except for fluoride, which needs to be supplemented in areas without a fluoridated water supply (see p. 500)]. Special care is given to maintaining the calcium/phosphorus ratio, to monitoring the renal solute load, and to replacing trace elements. Iron is added to many proprietary formulas, the use of which is now advised by the American Academy of Pediatrics. Table 12-3 compares the composition of breast milk with that of a number of commercially available formulas.

The breast-fed infant requires supplementation of vitamin D (and fluoride in areas without water fluoridation), and mothers continue with prenatal vitamin supplements.

The sick, premature, or low-birth-weight infant will require special formula adaptations. (Table 12-4 summarizes some of these modifications.) Parents need to understand that their special infant may give clues to feeding needs that are weak, indistinct, or contradictory (see Chap. 11).

During this early period most healthy in-

TABLE 12-2 DEVELOPMENT OF FEEDING SKILLS

Age	Oral and neuromuscular development	Feeding behavior
Birth	Rooting reflex Sucking reflex	Turns mouth toward nipple or any object brushing cheek
	Swallowing reflex	Initial swallowing involves the posterior of the tongue; By 9–12 weeks anterior portion is increasingly involved which facilitates ingestion of semisolid food
	Extrusion reflex	Pushes food out when placed on tongue; strong the first 9 weeks
		By 6–10 weeks recognizes the position in which he is fed and begins mouthing and sucking when placed in this position
3–6 months	Beginning coordination between eyes and body movements	Explores world with eyes, fingers, hands, and mouth; starts reaching for objects at 4 months but overshoots; hands get in the way during feeding
	Learning to reach mouth with hands at 4 months	Finger sucking—by 6 months all objects go into the mouth
	Extrusion reflex present until 4 months	May continue to push out food placed on tongue
	Able to grasp objects voluntarily at 5 months	Grasps objects in mitten-like fashion
	Sucking reflex becomes voluntary and lateral motions of the jaw begin	Can approximate lips to the rim of cup by 5 months; chewing action begins; by 6 months begins drinking from cup
6–12 months	Eyes and hands working together	Brings hand to mouth; at 7 months able to feed self biscuit
	Sits erect with support at 6 months	Bangs cup and objects on table at 7months
	Sits erect without support at 9 months	
	Development of grasp (finger to thumb opposition)	Holds own bottle at 9–12 months Pincer approach to food Pokes at food with index finger at 10 months
	Relates to objects at 10 months	Reaches for food and utensils including those beyond reach; pushes plate around with spoon. Insists on holding spoon not to put in mouth but to return to plate or cup.
1–3 years	Development of manual dexterity	Increased desire to feed self *15 months*—begins to use spoon but turns it before reaching mouth; may hold cup, likely to tilt the cup rather than head, causing spilling *18 months*—eats with spoon, spills frequently, turns spoon in mouth; holds glass with both hands *2 years*–inserts spoon correctly, occasionally with one hand; holds glass; plays with food; distinguishes between food and inedible materials *2–3 years*—self-feeding complete with occasional spilling; uses fork; pours from pitcher; obtains drink of water from faucet

Source: Getchel and Howard, "Nutrition in Development," chap. 15, in Scipien et al., *Comprehensive Pediatric Nursing,* McGraw-Hill Book Company, New York, 1975, p. 220.

fants need between 6 and 8 feedings. As the child's stomach capacity (2 tablespoons at birth) increases, feedings are spaced farther apart with a large amount of individual variation. Parents of both the breast-fed and bottle-fed infant will need the assurance that appetite is the best indicator of the amount of formula the infant should take. (A rough way to estimate the amount per feeding is to take the infant's age and add 3 to get the total ounces per feeding). Parents should be helped to recognize the components of infant feeding (e.g., satiety; see Chap. 11). It is the failure to recognize infant cues such as satiety that has caused some pediatricians to blame the bottle for overfeeding and relate this to the cause of childhood obesity. It is postulated that since the bottle-fed infant relies on external cues emanating from the parent, the infant does not learn to rely on internal cues, thereby causing a functional deficit in hunger awareness with resultant weight gain.

Baby Foods

Around 3½ to 4 months of age, the infant's extrusion reflex (a thrusting movement of the tongue used to extract milk from the nipple) is diminishing, along with the birth stores of iron if the infant is not on an iron-fortified formula. Both these events indicate that baby food could be introduced, however, in attempts to prevent childhood obesity some nutritionists are encouraging the delay of food introductions until 6 months of age. In any event, there is no nutritional advantage to early introduction of baby foods, and in some instances it can be mutually frustrating to infant and parent alike as the infant pushes food back out with the tongue (because of the extrusion reflex) and the parent spoons it back in. Also, there is no evidence to support the claim that early introduction of food promotes night sleep. The achievement of an 8-h sleep interval is a developmental stage that can begin early in the second month[23] but on the average begins between 3 and 4 months of life.

Baby foods should be added one at a time and the child with a family history of allergy should be watched closely (see Chap. 25). Parents should understand that the infant's ability to eat solid food will improve with practice and that food pushed out of the mouth is not indicative of dislike or stubbornness but rather inexperience. Solids placed more to the center of the tongue with a slight downward pressure as the spoon is removed will facilitate the swallowing of the food. The sequence of food introduction will vary with cultural practice and pediatricians' preferences, with the usual sequence of cereal, then fruit, followed by vegetables and meats. Juice is added somewhere between 1 and 2 months of age, initially diluted to ensure tolerance (1 oz juice to 2 oz water). Fresh, frozen, and canned juices used for the family can also be used for the infant. Again, with an allergy history, a special alert is given to wheat cereal, orange juice, and whole egg, which is usually delayed to the end of the first year.

The selection of baby foods is important since replacement of formula with nutritionally inferior food can lead to a poor nutritional state; also, these foods have a high energy density which easily contributes to childhood obesity. Four categories of commercially prepared strained and junior foods—fruits, soups, dinners, desserts—account for 60 percent of baby food sales.[24] Unfortunately, three out of these four have distinct disadvantages. Soups and dinners with high water content have less protein when compared to plain baby meat (a better protein buy) and have modified food starches added, the effect of which has never been fully tested on infants. Desserts contain sugar, raising the concern toward early conditioning to sugar. (For the same reason, parents should be discouraged from adding sugar to cereal or to water bottles.) Both the sugar and salt added to baby foods has provoked consumer concern which has prompted the major baby food companies to reduce and in some products completely remove these additives (e.g., fruit processed without sugar). Table

TABLE 12-3 FORMULA COMPARISON CHART

Formula	Sources Carbohydrate	Sources Protein	Sources Fat	Per oz kcal	Per oz kJ	g/100 ml Protein	g/100 ml CHO
Breast milk	Lactose	Lactalbumin, casein	High in olein, lower in volatile fatty acids	22	92	1.1	6.8
Regular							
Enfamil [Mead Johnson (MJ)]	Lactose	Nonfat milk	Soy & coconut oils E/PUFA = 0.7:1	20	84	1.5	7.0
Modilac (Gerber)	Dextrins, maltose, glucose	Nonfat milk	Corn oil	20	84	2.2	8.0
Similac (Ross)	Lactose	Nonfat milk	Coconut, soy, & corn oils	20	84	1.5	7.1
Humanized							
Similac PM 60/40 (Ross)	Lactose	Nonfat milk, partially demineralized whey	Corn & coconut oils	20	84	1.6	7.6
SMA (Wyeth)	Lactose	Nonfat milk, demineralized whey	Oleo (destearinated beef fat), coconut, safflower, & soybean oils	20	84	1.5	7.2
Designed for Specialized Needs							
1 CHO-Intolerance CHO-Free (Syntex)		Soy protein isolate	Soy oil	20 with CHO added	84	1.8	6.4 (with CHO added)
2 Hypoallergenic Isomil (Ross)	Corn syrup, sucrose, modified corn starch	Soy protein isolate	Soy, coconut, & corn oils	20	84	2.0	6.8
Meat Base Formula (Gerber)	Cane sugar, starch, modified tapioca	Beef hearts	Sesame oil	17 (1:1.5 dilution)	71	2.9	4.2
Neo-Mull-Soy (Syntex)	Sucrose	Soy protein isolate	Soy oil	20	84	1.8	6.4
Nutramigen (MJ)	Sucrose, tapioca, starch	Hydrolyzed casein	Corn oil	20	84	2.2	8.6
ProSobee (MJ)	Sucrose, corn syrup solids	Soy protein isolate	Soy oil	20	84	2.5	6.8
3 Malabsorption Portagen (MJ)	Sucrose, maltodextrins	Casein	MCT, corn oil	20	84	2.3	7.7
Pregestimil (MJ)	Glucose	Hydrolyzed casein	MCT, corn oil	20	84	2.2	8.8
Probana (MJ)	Banana powder, glucose	Whole & skim milk curd (powdered), casein hydrolysate	Butter fat & corn oil	20	84	4.2	7.9
4 Inborn Errors of Metabolism Lofenalac (MJ)	Corn syrup solids	Casein hydrolysate (most phenylalemine removed. Fortified with tyrosine, tryptophan, histidine, methionine	Corn oil	20	84	1.9	8.7

Note: See page 222–223 for footnotes.

	mg/100 ml			meq/l			Osmolarity, mosmol/kg	Osmolality, mosmol/l	Estimated renal solute load, mosmol/l*
Fat	Calcium	Phosphorus	Iron	Na⁺	K⁺	Cl⁻			
4.5	34	14	0.05	7	13	11	273	300	75
3.7	54	46	0.14 (with iron 1.2)	11	19	12	262	300	102
2.8			0.05 (with iron 1.5)	16.9	27.1	18.4			152
3.6	60	44	trace (with iron 1.2)	10.9	19.2	16.6	262	300	109
3.5	35	18	0.26	6.9	14.9	12.9	275	300	97
3.6	44	32	1.2	6.5	14.4	10.4	272	300	91
3.5	88	68	0.83	15.8	22.6	9.4	†	355 (with glucose added)	120
3.6	73	52	1.2	12.6	18.2	14.9	28	232	126
3.3	102	68	1.5	7.9	9.9	7.3			141
3.5	†	†	†	16.1	23.1	9.5	245	273	124
2.6	63	47	1.2	13.6	26.7	23.4	416	484	155
3.4	78	52	1.2	18.1	18.7	11.8	225	258	149
3.2	70	55	1.2	18	26.7	16	203	236	154
2.8	94	73	1.2	18	24	22.9	539	627	153
2.2	114	88		26.3	30.7	20.8	549	639	250
2.7	63	47	1.2	20.3	26.7	22.9	393	457	146

(continued)

TABLE 12-3   (continued)

Formula	Sources			Per oz		g/100 ml	
	Carbohydrate	Protein	Fat	kcal	kJ	Protein	CHO
5 Adjusted Caloric Density‡							
Similac 13 (Ross)	Lactose	Nonfat milk	Coconut, soy, & corn oils	13	55	1.2	4.5
24	Lactose	Nonfat milk	Coconut, soy, & corn oils	24	101	2.2	8.3
27	Lactose	Nonfat milk	Coconut, soy, & corn oils	27	113	2.5	9.4
Skim Infant (Ross)	Lactose	Skim milk		10	42	3.5	4.9
Premature (MJ)	Lactose, sucrose	Nonfat milk	MCT, corn, coconut oils	24	101	2.2	9.2
6 Transition to Whole Milk							
Advance (Ross)	Sucrose	Nonfat milk and soy isolate	Corn oil	16.5	69	3.6	6.6
7 Water Electrolyte Maintenance							
Lytren (MJ)	Glucose			9	38		7.5
Pedialyte (Ross)	Glucose			6	25		5.0
5% glucose	Glucose			6	25		5.0
10% glucose	Glucose			12	50		10.0

* S. J. Fomon, *Infant Nutrition,* 24 ed., W. B. Saunders Co., Philadelphia, 1974. Using Fomon's simplified renal solute load calculation, 1 g of protein = 4 mosmol; each meq of Na^+, K^+, and Cl^- = 1 mosmol.

† Information not available.

12-5 lists the energy and protein content of some commercial baby foods.

Baby cereals are supplemented with calcium and phosphorus, and fortified with thiamine, riboflavin, niacin, and iron. The form of iron fortification (sodium iron pyrophosphate, electrolytic iron, or reduced iron) leaves open to question the actual availability of this iron to the infant since little is known about the efficiency of the human infant's absorption of these forms. Therefore, baby cereal cannot be considered a reliable source of iron.

Homemade vs. Commercially Prepared Baby Foods

Many parents are now preparing their own baby food mixtures with blenders or baby food mills or grinders instead of buying commercially prepared foods. At present there is no strong opinion favoring either practice, assuming that home cooking techniques are sanitary and that cost is not the factor in decision making.

In making baby foods, parents can control and even eliminate the amount of additives such as sugar, salt, and modified starch, yet some would argue that there is greater predictability of the vitamin content in manufactured foods because of rigid production control. However, with good techniques for food buying, handling, storing, and preparation, a more nutrient-concentrated baby food can be the final product with home preparation, since less water can be added during preparation.

With home-prepared baby food, the question of nitrite content has been raised. Plant nitrates commonly found in carrots, spinach, and beets can be converted under certain conditions to nitrites before consumption by the infant and with consumption can lead to methemoglobinemia. Cases have been reported

Fat	mg/100 ml			meq/l			Osmolarity, mosmol/kg	Osmolality, mosmol/l	Estimated renal solute load, mosmol/l*
	Calcium	Phosphorus	Iron	Na⁺	K⁺	Cl⁻			
2.3	45	35	trace (with iron 0.78)	10	15	11.3	155	†	84
4.3	83	64	1.5	13.5	26.2	21.4	310	†	149
4.9	94	73	trace	14.8	29.5	23.4	†	†	167
0.1	130	95	trace	†	†	†	†	†	†
4.1	125	62	1.77	14	23	19.4	358	407	144
1.6	100	30	1.8	17.4	28.2		230	251	†
				25	25	30	440	536	106
				30	20	30	405 (estimated)		116
							283	298	
							556	618	

‡ Mead Johnson also provides Enfamil 24 kcal/oz (100.2 kJ/oz) and skim milk 10 kcal/oz (42 kJ/oz).

Source: Courtesy of Nutrition Service, Dietary Department, Children's Hospital Medical Center, Boston, Mass.

Abbreviations used: CHO = carbohydrate; E/PUFA = Essential Fatty Acids/Polyunsaturated Fatty Acids; MCT = medium-chain triglycerides

from the consumption of home-prepared spinach soup, carrot soup, and carrot juice, whereas no cases of methemoglobinemia have been reported with commercially prepared foods because of the processing technique. Eliminating home-prepared beets, carrots, and spinach from the infant's diet can remove this potential health hazard.[25] Beets, whether home or commercially prepared, are not generally recommended for infant diets because of their high nitrate content.

Increasing Texture in the Infant's Diet

An infant does not need teeth before texture can be introduced into the diet; the baby can begin getting accustomed to the new feeling near the end of the fifth month with small amounts of soft mashed table foods (such as regular canned applesauce) mixed into baby food. Gradually less baby food and more table food can be added to the mixture as the child develops more tongue mobility and the lateral motions of the jaw commence (6 to 7 months), usually accompanied by the first appearance of the primary teeth (5 to 7 months). Failure to observe developmental readiness for texture makes the introduction increasingly difficult with the passage of time and the child is at risk of developing the "soft-solid syndrome."[26]

By 6 to 7 months, the child shows a readiness to begin munching. As children achieve sitting balance and eye-hand coordination, finger feeding can be encouraged. Hard toast, zwieback, and biscuits can initiate the feeding experience and help soothe gums that may be sore from teething. Thereafter, as they achieve motor control and sitting balance, foods with different textures, shapes, colors,

TABLE 12-4 MODIFICATIONS IN FORMULA COMPOSITION

Purpose	Available products	Indications for use	Rationale	Considerations
Humanize Milk *Casein—lactalbumin adjustment; addition of whey provides a 60:40 ratio. Whey is demineralized by electrophoresis.*	Similac PM 60/40 (Ross); SMA (Wyeth)	1 Infants predisposed to hypocalcemia; 2 Impaired renal function; 3 Decreased cardiovascular function; 4 Diabetes insipidus	Calcium/phosphorus ratio = 2:1; Protein & mineral content comparable to breast milk; lowered renal solute load. Sodium levels do not greatly exceed requirements; Decreased antidiuretic hormone, increased absorption of sodium	Not suitable for use with abnormal electrolyte losses (CF, salt-losing nephritis, hypokalemia from steroid therapy, adrenocortical insufficiency) Premature infants of less than 1500 g may require additional phosphorus and calcium with onset of rapid growth. Ross does not advocate PM 60/40 for use with premature infants because of: mineral needs for growth hyponatremia of premature concern for effects of electrophoresis process on trace mineral low protein level
Carbohydrate Adjustment *Elimination of carbohydrate (CHO)*	CHO-Free	1 Diarrhea assoc. with loss of disaccharidases. 2 CHO intolerance	CHO of choice can be added. Concentration can be controlled	Ketogenic without additional CHO *Note:* Should not be terminally sterilized
Elimination of lactose	Isomil (Ross); ProSobee (MJ); Meat Base (Gerber); Nutramigen (MJ)	1 Diarrhea assoc. with lactase deficiency; 2 Galactosemia	Lactase is first enzyme affected in GI disorders; Hydrolysis of lactose yields glucose and galactose	Pregestimil and Portagen also do not contain lactose but would not be formulas of choice except in fat malabsorption
Hypoallergenic *Altered protein source*	Isomil; ProSobee; Neo-Mull-Soy (Syntex); Meat Base	Sensitivity to cow's milk	Allergenicity reduced by heat & isolation of soybean protein. Strained meat generally well tolerated	
Hydrolyzed protein	Nutramigen	1 Sensitivity to intact protein; 2 Recovery stages of prolonged diarrhea	Provides high % of free amino acids; remainder is small polypeptides; Avoids possible GI absorption of intact protein	Metabolic acidosis has been known to occur in patients with long-term malabsorption or in premature infants given hydrolyzed casein. 2–3 meq sodium bicarbonate/kg per day reverses blood gas patterns to normal *Note:* Separates on standing. Shake before using. May be necessary to enlarge nipple holes
Elimination of corn	Neo-Mull-Soy	Sensitivity to corn	Elimination of corn syrup solids and corn-derived CHO	Corn syrup produced by hydrolysis of corn starch. Clinical studies indicate purified corn syrup is hypoallergenic. Corn starch, which contains less than 0.5% protein, has produced reactions. However, clear corn syrup contains no intact protein and minute amounts of nonprotein nitrogen. Advantages of eliminating corn-derived CHO may be questionable

Fat Adjustment. *Lowered Fat Content*	Probana (MJ)	1 Celiac syndrome (As assoc. with CF) 2 Gluten-induced enteropathy 3 Idiopathic celiac disease 4 Diarrhea, acute and recovery stages 5 Poor protein absorption	High protein content to meet increased needs. CHO as simple sugars and banana powder	24% calories derived from protein. Additional water may be indicated
	Similac 13	Uncomplicated infectious diarrhea	Provides higher levels of protein & minerals than would be available from diluted regular formula	Insufficient calories for growth; intended for temporary use
	Advance (Ross)	Anemia assoc. with cow's milk intake (enteric blood loss assoc. with too early introduction of cow's milk)	Protein is heat-denatured	Lower in calories than standard formula or whole milk. Highly polyunsaturated. Not appropriate for infants under 6 mo. Transition from breast to formula should coincide with increasing intake of solid food to maintain recommended caloric distribution from CHO, PRO, and fat (PRO, 7–16% fat, 30–50%, remainder from CHO) Formula should not be discontinued earlier than 5–6 mo
	Skim Infant Formula	Use of skim milk during infancy *is not recommended*		10 kcal/oz insufficient to support growth. Provides poor caloric distribution of CHO, PRO, and fat. Fat essential to myelination of CNS. Lack of satiety value may predispose infant to obesity by initiating an abnormally large compensatory intake of solid food

Incorporation of MCT	Portagen (MJ)	1 Defect in hydrolysis of fat
		  ↓ Pancreatic lipase (CF, pancreatic insuffic.)
		  ↓ Bile salts (chronic liver disease, biliary atresia, or obstruction)
		2 Defect in absorption of fat
		  ↓ Permeability (Sprue, idiopathic steatorrhea)
		  ↓ Gut surface (resection, blind loop syndrome)
		  Defective lipoprotein-lipase system (hyperchylomicronemia)
		  Faulty chylomicron formation (β-lipoproteinemia)
		3 Defects in fat transportation (Intestinal lymphatic obstruction, lymphangiectasia, chylothorax, chyluria, chylous ascites exudative enteropathy)
			MCT more readily hydrolyzed and absorbed. The 8–10-carbon fatty acids comprising MCT require less pancreatic lipase & bile salts for digestion. They can be absorbed and hydrolyzed within mucosal cells, and do not require micellar or chylomicron formation. They are transported unesterified via the portal system	Not recommended with advanced cirrhosis (impaired clearance of fatty acids absorbed via portal system)
				
				Inclusion of sucrose and intact casein in formulation limits use to conditions without disaccharidase deficiency or milk protein sensitivity milk protein sensitivity

(continued)

TABLE 12-4 (continued)

Purpose	Available products	Indications for use	Rationale	Considerations
	Pregestimil (MJ)	1 Neonates & infants with malabsorption (Disaccharidase Defic., intractable diarrhea, idiopathic defects in digestion & absorption) 2 Cystic fibrosis 3 Nutritional management following intestinal resection 4 Food allergies	All nutrients in easily absorbable form. (glucose hydrolyzed casein, and MCT)	Supplemental K necessary with prolonged use of antibiotics. Metabolic acidosis known to occur with use of hydrolyzed casein. Reversed by use of 2–3 meq sodium bicarbonate/ kg per day High osmolarity requires acclimation; initial use of 1/4-, 1/2-, then 3/4-strength recommended *Note:* Terminal sterilization results in marked color change but protein efficiency ratio is not appreciably affected.

Source: Courtesy Nutrition Service, Dietary Department, Children's Hospital Medical Center, Boston, Mass.

Abbreviations used: CHO = carbohydrate, PRO = protein, MCT = medium-chain triglycerides, CF = cystic fibrosis, CNS = central nervous system, GI = gastrointestinal, MJ = Mead Johnson.

TABLE 12-5 ENERGY AND PROTEIN VALUES OF SELECTED BABY FOODS

Type	Amount	Energy kcal	Energy kJ	Protein, g
Baby rice cereal (dry)	1 tbsp	3	12.6	trace
Baby oatmeal cereal (dry)	1 tbsp	9.3	39	0.33
Strained rice cereal with applesauce and bananas	1 tbsp	10	42	0.05
Strained beef*	1 tbsp	13.8	58	1.9
Strained chicken*	1 tbsp	18.8	79	1.9
High-meat dinner* beef with vegetables	1 tbsp	12	50	0.8
Strained beets	1 tbsp	5.2	22	0.1
Strained carrots	1 tbsp	3.8	16	0.1
Strained applesauce	1 tbsp	6	25	
Strained peaches	1 tbsp	11	47	

* Compare the protein in high meat dinner to the protein in strained beef and chicken.

Source: *Nutrient Values of Gerber Baby Foods,* 1977.

and smells will stimulate their interest and promote food learning experiences. Cooked vegetables, meats, cheddar cheese sticks, fruit, and enriched cereals are good choices. Stringy foods, nuts, and raisins can cause choking and should not be offered. Table 12-6 summarizes the transition of infant feeding during the first year of life.

The Transition to Whole Milk

Somewhere between the end of the fourth month and six months of age the child will make the transition to whole milk and the need for sterilization will cease. There is no specific timing. Fomon suggests that the infant should make the transition when consuming two 4.5-oz jars of commercially prepared strained foods or the equivalent in home-prepared table foods.[27]

With the introduction of whole milk, the infant may regurgitate a sour vomitus, because of the presence of butyric acid (a volatile fatty acid) in the butter fat. Also, constipation may occur because of a change in the curd tension of the protein.

Skim milk is not recommended throughout the first year because the lack of the essential fatty acid, linoleic acid, and the low caloric density prompt the infant to compensate by an increased consumption of solid baby food to meet appetite needs, thereby causing a disproportionate distribution of energy from carbohydrate and protein.

The introduction of whole milk into the infant's diet has been identified as a factor in the occurrence of iron-deficiency anemia. The mechanism is associated with microscopic changes in the gastrointestinal tract, leading to impaired iron absorption.[28]

Some pediatricians are recommending the continued use of iron-fortified formulas through the first year to meet the infant's growth needs for iron and to prevent iron-deficiency anemia, especially in high risk infants, namely, those in low socioeconomic strata who are likely to be born with low iron stores and infants born to teenage mothers.

Weaning

By definition, weaning is to detach affections from something long desired. Weaning a child marks that period of transition from breast or bottle feeding to a more solid-food diet and cup drinking. Preparation for weaning begins in the second half of the first year. By the time of 5 to 6 months of age, infants are beginning to be able to approximate their lips to the rim of a cup, and by the time they are 1 year old, they can hold and drink from a cup with assistance. As the infant can take more from the cup, less will be needed from the bottle. Somewhere between 1 and 2 years, the transition from the bottle is usually complete. While there is no specific age for weaning, it is suggested that weaning be a gradual process accomplished over a period of time, not overnight. The early practice of bottle propping, leading to empty feeding experiences, and excessive breast or bottle feeding, promoting dependency, may negatively affect the weaning process. During the weaning process, some children will refuse to drink milk from the cup, causing the con-

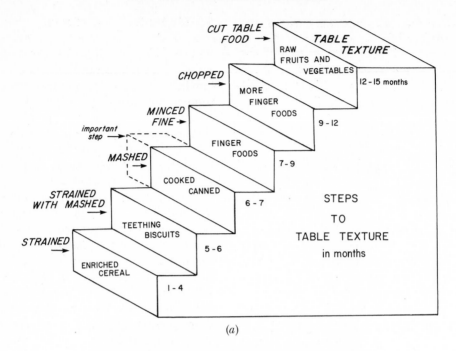

(a)

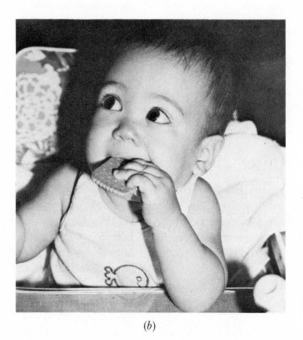

(b)

Figure 12-7

The steps to table-food texture at the 6- to 7-month level.
(Adapted from Nutrition Service, Children's Hospital
Medical Center, *Steps to Table Texture*, Boston, Massa-
chusetts.)

cerned parent to continue with the bottle. Offering alternate milk substitutes (cheese, yogurt, milk puddings, milk-based soups) to replace the calcium source can alleviate the concern without interfering in the weaning process.

Infant Feeding Problems

The feeding process undergoes many changes in the first year as the child progresses from 6 to 8 breast or bottle feedings to the cup, table foods, and three meals. This process of food input and elimination is subject to an enormous range of management issues which are commonly manifested as "classic infant feeding problems" (e.g., colic), which exclude all those problems emanating from any underlying pathological conditions or disease states. Simple inquiries into the amount of formula or food intake, the technique of feeding or formula preparation, and the emotional climate in the home can help to identify the problem area.[29] Table 12–7 suggests some practical approaches to infant feeding problems.

TODDLER (1 TO 3 YEARS)

As the rapid growth of the pre- and postnatal period subsides, the ego identity of the toddler becomes the thrust of this next developmental period. Decreasing energy requirements (90 kcal or 378 kJ/kg of body weight) and appetite reflect this period of slow progressive growth as mealtime negativism with food "jags" become the prevailing theme in the toddler's bid for autonomy.

With the increasing refinement of hand and finger movements and the appearance of most of the primary teeth, the toddler can be allowed more independence at mealtimes and can be presented with most table foods. However, meat and stringy vegetables may still pose a problem, as good tongue lateralization and rotary chewing, skills necessary to facilitate good chewing, do not develop until somewhere between 18 and 21 months of age. Also, the ritualistic toddler may prefer plainer food to mixed dishes and may designate specific places for the various food items on his or her plate.

Figure 12-8
Weaning, a gradual process. As the child takes more from the cup, less will be required from the bottle.

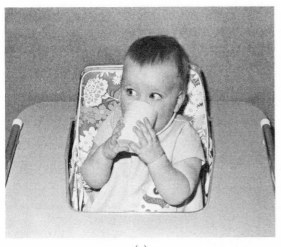

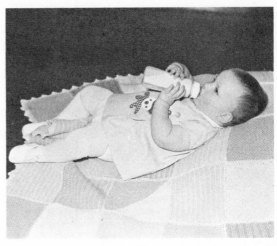

(a)   (b)

TABLE 12-6 FEEDING GUIDELINES

	0–2 weeks	2 weeks–2 months	2 months	3 months*	4–5 months	5–6 months
Formula						
Ounces per feeding	2–3 oz	3–5 oz	4–6 oz	4–6 oz	5–7 oz	5–7 oz
Average total ounces	22 oz	28 oz	29 oz	30 oz	32 oz	30 oz
Number of feedings	6–8	5–6	4–5	4–5	4–5	4–5
Food texture	Liquids	Liquids	Liquids	Baby soft	Baby soft	Baby soft
Food additions						
Orange juice		Give diluted juice 1 oz juice and 1 oz water	2 oz, undiluted	3–4 oz	3–4 oz	3–4 oz
Baby cereal, enriched				1 tsp, B & S	2 tbsp, B & S	2 tbsp, B & S
Strained fruits				1 tsp, B & S	1 tbsp, B & S	1½ tbsp, B & S
Strained vegetables					1–2 tbsp, L	2 tbsp, L
Strained meats						1 tbsp, L
Egg yolk or baby egg yolk						½ med or 1 tbsp
Teething biscuit						½–1
Total calories	440	475	610	659–674	751–772	777–843
Recommended calories 117 kcal/kg	410	410–608	608	667	725–784	784–878
Oral and neuromuscular development related to food intake	Rooting, sucking, swallowing ⟶			Extrusion reflex diminishes; sucking becomes voluntary	Learning to reach hands to mouth: develops grasp	Chewing begins; can approximate lips to the rim of cup

	6–7 months	7–8 months	8–9 months	9–10 months	10–11 months	11–12 months
Whole milk						
Ounces per feeding	7–8 oz	8 oz	8 oz	8 oz	8 oz	8 oz
Average total ounces	28 oz	28 oz	24 oz	24 oz	24 oz	24 oz

Number of feedings	3–4	3–4	3	3	3	3
Food texture	Gradual increase ――――→		Mashed table ――――→			→ Cut fine
Food items						
Orange juice	4 oz	4 oz	4 oz	4 oz	4 oz	4 oz
Fortified cereal	⅓ cup, B	⅓ cup, B, L, & S	½ cup, B	½ cup, B	½ cup, B	½ cup, B
Fruit, canned or fresh	4 tsp, B L, & S	4 tsp, B, L, & S	2 tbsp, L & S	2 tbsp, L & S	3 tbsp, L & S	3 tbsp, L & S
Vegetables	1½ tbsp, L & S	2 tbsp, L & S	2 tbsp, L & S	2 tbsp, L & S	3 tbsp, L & S	3 tbsp, L & S
Meat, fish, poultry	1 tbsp, L & S	2 tbsp, L & S	2 tbsp, L & S	2 tbsp, L & S	2½ tbsp, L & S	2½ tbsp, L & S
Egg yolk or baby egg yolk	1 medium yolk, or 2 tbsp	1 medium yolk, or 2 tbsp	1 medium yolk, or 2 tbsp	1 whole egg	1 whole egg	1 whole egg
Teething biscuit or bread	1 biscuit	1 biscuit	½ slice bread	½ slice bread	½ slice bread	½ slice bread
Starch—potato, rice, macaroni				2 tbsp, S	2 tbsp, S	2 tbsp, S
Dessert—custard, pudding						
Butter			1 tsp	1 tsp	1 tsp	1 tsp
Total calories	859	876	937	974	1037	1069
Recommended calories 108 kcal/kg	810–864	864–918	918–972	972–1015	1015–1048	1048–1083
Oral and neuromuscular development related to food intake	Begins using cup	Sits erect with support Feeds self biscuit		Without support ――――→ Holds bottle	Picks up small food items & releases	Will hold and lick spoon after dipped into food; self feeding

* Current opinion recommends that the introduction of the baby foods be delayed until 5 months of age.

Abbreviations used: B = breakfast, L = lunch, S = supper

Source: Getchell and Howard, "Nutrition in Development", chap. 15 in G. Scipien et al., *Comprehensive Pediatric Nursing*, McGraw-Hill Book Company, New York, 1975.

TABLE 12-7 PRACTICAL APPROACHES TO INFANT FEEDING PROBLEMS

Problem	Signs and symptoms	Management
Intake of formula too large	Regurgitation Vomiting Diarrhea or frequent large stools Normal or excessive weight gain History of excessive intake for age	Reduce formula intake at feedings Explain the problem in detail to the parents and give reassurance
Intake of formula too small	Irritable Underweight Hungry Constipated History of inadequate intake for age	Increase the amount and frequency of formula and possibly the calorie content of the feedings
Improper technique of feeding	Any of the above signs and symptoms Following errors frequently encountered: 1 Hole in rubber nipple too small (providing too long feeding period) or too large (causing excessive swallowing of air, discomfort, and regurgitation)	A puncture with a needle will not increase the size of aperture; discard and use a new one
	2 Formula too hot	Moderately cold or room temperature formulas are well tolerated
	3 Improper placement of nipple in mouth	Place nipple far enough back in mouth
	4 Failure to bubble the infant	After feeding, hold the infant erect against shoulder to expel swallowed air
	5 Improper position of infant during feeding, such as horizontal or with propped pillow	The position should be inclined to at least a 45-degree angle
	6 Nursing from an empty bottle	Formula should fill the nipple throughout feeding, and ½ to 1 oz should be left in the bottle at termination of feeding
	7 Improper sterilization technique	Check sterilization technique Terminal sterilization technique consists of 1 Scrub bottles, nipples, equipment 2 Measure and mix formula 3 Pour mixture into bottles 4 Place bottle on rack in sterilizer and boil gently for 25 minutes 5 Store capped bottles in refrigerator
Improper composition of formula	*Carbohydrate:* Excessive amounts may produce diarrhea	Added carbohydrate in the form of corn syrup to evaporated milk formula need rarely exceed 1 oz or 2 tbsp per 24-hour volume
	Protein: Allergy to protein in cow's milk; allergic infants may have vomiting, irritability, diarrhea, with or without blood in the stool; onset 2–4 weeks after initiating of formula; history in other family members is significant	A few days' trial with a cow's milk substitute such as soybean milk, Nutramigen, or Cho-Free, with subsequent alleviation of symptoms, indicates milk allergy

(continued)

TABLE 12-7   (continued)

Problem	Signs and symptoms	Management
	Fat: Improper fat digestion causes large bulky stools; digestion of cow's milk butterfat may be less complete than that of fat of breast milk	Substitute a formula free of butterfat, such as Similac, Enfamil, etc.
Emotional problems in the family	Irritability Colic Spitting up Vomiting Failure to gain weight	Explanation, education, patience, and understanding are needed along with constant reassurance and considerable tact

Source: Getchel and Howard, "Nutrition in Development," chap. 15 in G. Scipien et al., *Comprehensive Pediatric Nursing,* McGraw-Hill Book Company, New York, 1975, p. 221; adapted from W. T. Hughes and F. Falkner, "Infant Feeding Problems: A Practical Approach," *Clinical Pediatrics,* 3:65, 1964.

Figure 12-9
The toddler: Able to drink from a straw and eat with a spoon but still apt to resort to his hands.

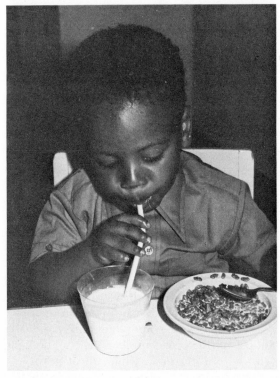 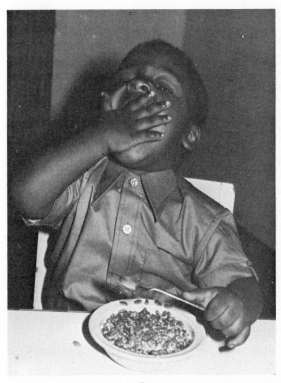

(a)   (b)

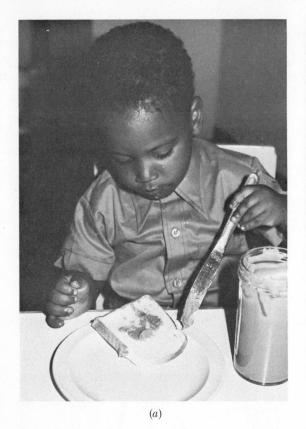

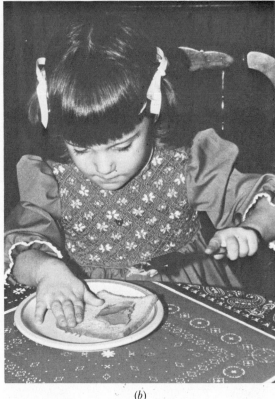

(a)   (b)

Figure 12-10
The difference between being 22 months and 36 months of age.

During this period, parents need to understand that the characteristic small, finicky appetite is part of this stage of development. Overreacting to the situation by forcing, bribing, or punishing to make the child eat only reinforces the child's negative behavior. Parents need help in maintaining reasonable limits on the child's behavior while allowing the child some freedom of control. The toddler's negativism can be met by phrasing questions so as to elicit a positive response; for example, "Do you want milk or juice first?" This approach maintains parental control yet fosters toddler independence. Servings of a reasonable size are also needed to encourage the toddler whose appetite is easily overwhelmed, especially by frequent drinks or between-meal snacks. Still-uncoordinated fine motor control

makes spills a common occurrence and unrealistic social expectations should not be made of the toddler at the family dinner table.

Frequent spills, finicky appetite, and underdeveloped chewing skills leave the toddler open to nutrient deficiencies. Vitamin A, calcium, phosphorus, riboflavin, and iron deficiencies would be the concern with a child who may be refusing to drink milk or who has difficulties in chewing meat. Meat and vegetables are the foods most frequently refused during this period, which further compromises the toddler's zinc and folate nutriture.

Powdered or evaporated milk, added to soups, can help as supplements for the child who is refusing milk, while wheat germ and peanut butter are folate-containing foods that are readily acceptable to the toddler. Meat that is easy to chew (chicken, turkey) and minced, moist meat can help to solve the meat dilemma.

Another concern is the toddler who drinks milk to the exclusion of solid foods, leaving the diet particularly deficient in iron, zinc, vitamin C, and folate. Iron-deficiency anemia (see Chap. 7) and encopresis (see Chap. 18) are common findings in this age group.

Pica

Increasing mobility leads to greater environmental exploration, and a great deal of exploration revolves around oral examination of both edible and nonedible objects. Pica, an aberration of appetite leading to the consumption of inedible objects such as dirt, soap, or paint chips, commonly occurs in young children between the ages of 18 and 24 months. The cause is unknown and seems related to environmental deprivation rather than to a deficiency of any specific nutrient, although diets of these children are often deficient in iron.[30] Pica can be the cause of lead poisoning from the ingestion of plaster or other objects that are saturated or coated with lead-based paint. Treatment includes the use of chelating agents. Many children are iron-deficient and may be receiving iron therapy when the diagnosis of lead poisoning is made. Iron binds the chelating agents, and must be discontinued during chelation therapy.

THE PRESCHOOL CHILD

The preschool child, now mostly independent at the table, continues to make slow steady gains in weight and height of approximately 2 kg (4.5 lb) and 6 to 8 cm (2½ to 3½ in) per year. Although growth is at a slower rate, it imposes demands on the young body that are further enhanced by the constancy of activity. Psychosocially, the child struggles to develop a sense of initiative, taking an eager and inquisitive approach to the surroundings. Size, form, color, shape, time, and space now take on a new meaning.

As conversation skills improve, questions become more relevant and demand more than a simple response. The child mimics adult conversations and behaviors, television personalities and advertisements. A nutrition education program that recognizes these influences and the psychosocial characteristics of the preschool child can help to form the basis of a lifetime of good eating practices. This type of program does not need the structure of a preschool, day-care, or head-start center but can be conducted by the parent in the kitchen during meal preparation or at the table or even in the aisles of the supermarket, a trip of special significance to the preschooler.

A survey of the nutritional status of the preschool child was conducted between 1968 and 1970. Evidence of nutritional risk, lower

Figure 12-11

The preschool child: Interested, inquisitive, and especially receptive to nutrition education when offered as part of meal-time preparation.

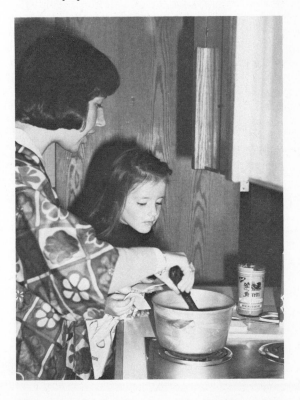

biochemical indices, smaller physical size for age, and lower dietary intake was found clustered among preschool children of lower socioeconomic status because of the insufficiency of food. (See Chap. 15.) Iron-deficiency anemia and dental caries crossed all socioeconomic barriers, however, although they showed a high preponderance in the lower socioeconomic group. Many preschool children continued to take a vitamin-mineral supplement despite an adequate diet—a waste, as large quantities of the water-soluble vitamins are excreted in the urine daily. Convenience foods such as frozen pot pies, canned beef stew, chili con carne, spaghetti, macaroni and cheese, pizza, and foods from fast-food establishments were identified by this survey as staples in the preschool diet to the extent that a broader selection of well-balanced foods may have been precluded.[31]

SCHOOL YEARS (6 TO 12 YEARS)

These years, described as the middle childhood, are the product of early growth and development and the preparatory period for adolescence. The adaptation to the school experience and peer identification are significant developmental tasks as the child begins a life that is increasingly independent from the family.

Permanent teeth begin to appear and growth proceeds at a moderate rate of about 3 to 3.5 kg (7 lb) and 6 cm (2½ in) per year, as bodily resources are laid down in preparation for adolescence. Growth during these years is characterized by spurts and plateaus, with a pronounced spurt toward the end of this period. Energy needs decrease per kilogram of body weight but total energy requirements continue to increase.

Figure 12-12
The school-aged child learns through this nutrition game that the "big mouth" only accepts nutritious foods with no room for junk foods.

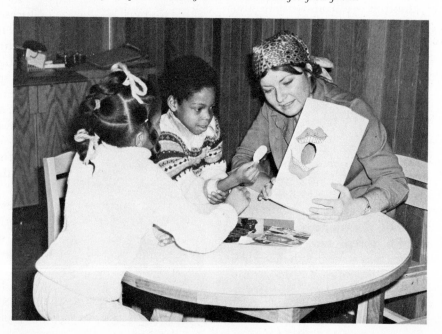

**TABLE 12-8 NOURISHING SNACKS
FOR CHILDREN**

Thirst quenchers	Jucies, milk, protein shake (½ cup milk, ½ cup orange juice, ¼ cup powdered milk)
Finger fruits	Orange, tangerine, banana discs, apple, pear, peach slices, pineapple wedges, dried apricots, dates, raisins, grapes, plums, cherries, berries
Finger vegetables	Cherry tomatoes, carrot and celery sticks, cucumber and zucchini wedges, green pepper strips
Spread-ons	Peanut butter, cream cheese, yogurt dips, butter
Other	Yogurt, cottage cheese, cold meat cubes, whole-grain crackers and cookies, whole-grain bread, fortified cereals

Although the child aspires to the adult world, some of the prerogatives of childhood are maintained and food behavior vacillates accordingly. School activities and pressing schedules impose stress, and hurried or skipped breakfasts and lunches are common complaints of this age group. These meals often go unnoticed and replacement of needed nutrients is forgotten. School breakfast and lunch programs may mean new foods and ways of food preparation, and acceptance is now increasingly governed by peers as food habits take on new social influences and the lure of the vending machines and the corner store is felt for the first time.

The hungriest time of the day for the school-age child is after school. Nutritious snacks (see Table 12-8) should be made available to sustain hunger while maximizing nutrient intake. Forethought in snack preparation is particularly important for the working parent, since many children left to their own devices or in the care of a baby sitter will forage for cookies and candy in attempts to satiate their appetite. Parents must consider themselves as "gatekeepers" who will only allow nutritious foods through the doors of their homes. They will need much support to withstand television, peer, and family pressures to buy certain foods.

It is during this period that childhood obesity becomes apparent. Riding to school and sitting in front of the television after school for an average of 5 hours per day afford little opportunity for physical expenditure. Children living in the inner city have even less opportunity for activity because of limited recreational programs and a high-crime environment that imposes risks on personal safety. Games and toys that require movement, family outings directed to exercise, sports interests which rely more on individual than on team participation and can be maintained throughout life (skating, swimming, tennis, jogging) should all be encouraged. Children must learn to program activity into their daily life style, for herein lies the key to the prevention of adult obesity. (See Chap. 21.)

ADOLESCENCE—THE PREADULT YEARS

The developmental experience of adolescence and the increased velocity of growth are two characteristics shared by boys and girls, and both with nutritional consequences.

During this period the adolescent body undergoes a transition from immature to adult size and shape, changing the configuration of breasts in females and external genitalia in males. With this change in body image comes the new search for identity and the assertion of independence. Moods vacillate from passiveness to rebellion, which can be considered the hallmark of adolescence. Confused, impatient, impulsive are all adjectives that can describe the questioning adolescent.

Although emerging differences in growth and body composition alter the nutrient needs of the two sexes, boys and girls share their overriding concern for body image and peer group identification. New eating patterns may evolve, some of which are extreme, faddish, eccentric, or grossly restricted, and cola, chips, pizza, and doughnuts may become the main-

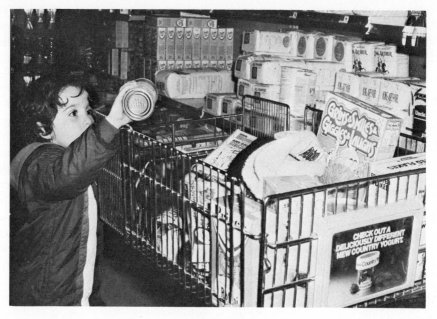

Figure 12-13
In the aisles of the supermarkets. Parents need support to maintain their
stance as "gatekeepers" of their families' nutrition—parents who have no
room in their shopping carts for junk foods. How would you cope with this
situation?

stay of the diet. The adolescent vegetarian, fruitarian, macrobiotic, or "health-food freak" is a somewhat disruptive influence at the family meal table, causing both parental and in some instances professional concern. Nevertheless, the diet is the adolescent's own personal choice and should be treated accordingly. The preadult will be more receptive to information on how to incorporate the appropriate nutrients (e.g., vitamin B_{12} into the vegetarian's diet) into his or her chosen diet than to suggestions of a change in life style in order to incorporate needed nutrients.

Drugs, marijuana, psychedelics, barbituates, amphetamines, cocaine, volatile aerosol sprays, heroin, alcohol, cigarettes are mediums of rebellion, connoting feelings of status, pleasure, and comfort,[32] and also imparting nutritional risks, either directly through the effect on nutrient metabolism or indirectly through effects on appetite. Nutritional therapy be-

comes a vital part of the rehabilitation of the drugs or alcohol-dependent adolescent.

At the time of puberty, there is an increased demand for thyroxine to support growth. Enlargement of the thyroid gland is indicative of iodine deficiency, a finding among the adolescent population. In the Hanes survey of 1971–72, both grade I and grade II goiters, indicators of moderate and high-risk deficiency states, were found in 11 percent of Negro youths between the ages of 12 and 17 years.[33] (See Chap. 20, "Endemic Goiter.")

Acne, a consequence of changing hormones, adds but another stress to the adolescent experience. Treatment with drugs (e.g., tetracycline) and vitamins A or B_6 have a palliative effect and, in the case of vitamin A, can lead to toxicity states. A prudent diet (see Chap. 2), with avoidance of caffeine (coffee, tea, cola, chocolate), and good hygiene may

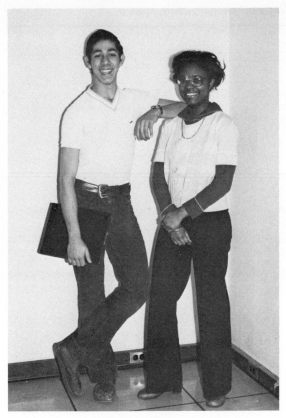

Figure 12-14
The adolescent: Searching for identity, looking for answers: "Why should I eat a well-balanced diet? Prove it!" As a future health professional are you able to?

help to ameliorate symptoms but is without guarantee.

Adolescent Girls

For girls, the adolescent growth spurt occurs somewhere between 10 and 14 years with the onset of menarche when critical body weight, as proposed by Frisch, is achieved.[34] There is great variability in the patterns of growth and hormonal changes, and standards that are related only to age are misleading.

During the active growth period between ages 10 and 14 years, energy requirements reach 55 kcal (231 kJ)/kg of body weight and

thereafter drop to 39 kcal (163 kJ)/kg. Iron to replace menstrual losses and provide for growth, along with protein in the vicinity of 1 g/kg, folate, and B vitamins, should be stressed.

The normal physiological fat deposition around the abdomen and pelvic girdle raises adolescent concerns about weight. Inactivity can accelerate normal deposition and can lead to an overweight condition which leaves the body-conscious girl an easy prey to fad diets. The aesthetic pursuit of thinness can then result in a malnourished state during the very period when her need for nutrients is the greatest and in some extreme cases leads to anorexia nervosa, a neurotic feeding disturbance (see Chap. 22). Weight control programs appear to be more successful among girls either in the preadolescent period or after age 15. The years between 10 and 15 are fraught with change and motivation becomes extremely complex.

The use of oral contraceptives and intrauterine devices among the teenage population is an additional influence to be considered in determining nutritional needs. Despite the widespread use of contraceptives, teenage pregnancies are escalating, and the juvenile gravida is fast becoming the new obstetrical problem, as the developing fetus places yet additional demands on the body of the still-developing adolescent. (See Chap. 13.)

Adolescent Boys

Like their sexual counterparts, boys manifest adolescence with a great range of variability. Some begin early, usually by age 12, and have completed their sexual maturation when others are commencing, at 15. The adolescent male with greatly expanding muscle mass and energy needs has been identified as being at nutritional risk by the Ten State Nutrition Survey of 1968–1970. (See Chap. 15.) Prior to this time the adolescent male was largely overlooked in deference to the teenage girl.

Between the ages of 11 and 14 years, 63

TABLE 12-9 THE BASIC FOUR FOOD GROUPS THROUGHOUT THE GROWING YEARS

Food group	Servings per day	Average-size servings for age			
		Toddler	Preschool	School	Adolescent

Milk or equivalent
½ cup milk equals
  2 tbsp powdered milk
  1 oz of cheese
  ¼ cup evaporated milk
  ½ cup cottage cheese
  1 serving custard (4 servings
  from 1 pt milk)
  ½ cup milk pudding
  ½ cup yogurt
	4	½–¾ cup	¾ cup	¾–1 cup	1 cup

Meat, fish, poultry or equivalent
1 oz meat equals
  1 egg, 1 frankfurter
  1 oz cheese,* 1 cold cut
  2 tbsp peanut butter, cut meat
  ¼ cup tuna fish or cottage
  cheese*
  ½ cup dried peas or beans
	2 or more	3 tbsp	4 tbsp	3–4 oz (6–8 tbsp)	4 oz or more

Vegetables and fruits to include	4 or more				

Citrus fruit or equivalent
    1 citrus fruit serving equals
    ½ cup orange or grapefruit juice
    ½ grapefruit or cantaloupe
    ¾ cup strawberries
    1 medium orange
  ½ citrus fruit serving equals
    ½ cup tomato juice or tomatoes,
    broccoli, chard, collards,
    greens, spinach, raw cabbage,
    brussels sprouts
    1 medium tomato, 1 wedge
    honeydew
	1 or more	4 oz	4 oz	4–6 oz	4–6 oz

Yellow or green vegetable or
equivalent
  1 serving equals
    ½ cup broccoli, greens, spinach,
    carrots, squash, pumpkin
    5 apricot halves
    ½ medium cantalope
	1 or more	4 tbsp	4 tbsp	⅓ cup	½ cup

Other fruits and vegetables	2 or more				
Other vegetables including *potatoes*		2–3 tbsp	4 tbsp	⅓–½ cup	¾ cup
Other fruit including apples, *banana, pears, peaches*		½ med apple	½–1 med apple	1 med apple	1 med apple

(continued)

TABLE 12-9 (continued)

Food group	Servings per day	Average-size servings for age			
		Toddler	Preschool	School	Adolescent
Breads and cereals or whole grain or enriched equivalent	4 or more				
1 slice bread equals		½ slice	1 slice	1–2 slices	2 slices
¾ cup dry cereal		½ cup	¾ cup	1 oz	1 oz
½ cup cooked cereal, rice, spaghetti, or macaroni		2 tbsp	¼–½ cup	½–1 cup	1 cup or more
1 roll, muffin, or biscuit					

* If cottage or cheddar cheese is used as a milk equivalent, it should not also be counted as a meat equivalent.

Source: Getchel and Howard, "Nutrition in Development," chap. 15 in G. Scipien et al., *Comprehensive Pediatric Nursing,* McGraw-Hill Book Company, New York, 1975, p. 223. Adapted from *Infant Feeding Guide,* for use by professional staffs, Washington State Department of Social and Health Services, Health Services Division, Local Health Services, Nutrition Unit, 1972.

kcal (265 kJ)/kg of body weight are needed to support growth, with a decrease to 49 kcal (206 kJ)/kg by age 15 to 18. As with the girl, energy needs must be interpreted according to physiological stage rather than chronological age. Sexual maturity ratings can help to identify the stage of development, a better indicator of energy needs than age. (The scale of sexual maturity ranges from 1 to 5; a rating of 1 represents the prepubertal stage and 5, adulthood.) Growth needs are further met by 1 g/kg of high-biological-value protein. Iron, folate, B vitamins, and iodine also merit attention.

The high school athlete is particularly interested in diet. Programs to both gain and lose weight are undertaken in attempts to achieve a desired ratio of muscle strength to body weight. With weight loss a reduction only in body fat is desired and should be achieved at a rate of no more than 1 kg per week through a moderate decrease in food accompanied by a moderate increase in exercise. Regimens to promote gains in weight should increase not fat but muscle, which is achieved through an increase in muscular exercise supported by an appropriate increment in food intake.[35]

There has been a particular mystique associated with the athlete's diet. In reality, a well-balanced, prudent diet (see Chap. 2) during the training period with sufficient energy to meet the athletic needs, which typically range to as much as 5000 to 6000 kcal (21 to 25.2 mJ) per day, is all that is necessary. The young athlete from an economically disadvantaged family will have difficulty in meeting his requirements and should be given special consideration, such as additional servings of the school breakfast or lunch.

During the 6-day pre-game period, a high-performance diet is utilized by some athletes who require maximal exertion of muscles, such as the long-distance runner, the wrestler, or the middle-distance swimmer. This diet initially limits carbohydrate to approximately 100 g and the specific muscles to be used in the competition are exercised to deplete glycogen stores. After 3 days, the athlete is switched to a high-carbohydrate, low-salt, low-residue diet. The diet is high in carbohydrate to build muscle glycogen stores, low in salt to ensure optimal availability of water to maintain hydration during the event, and low in residue to help contribute to a light feeling in the abdomen, a factor some athletes associate with optimum fitness during the event.[36] Caffeine-containing beverages (coffee, tea, cola, cocoa) act as diuretics and are therefore restricted. Table 12-9 summarizes the needs for foods from the basic four food groups throughout the growing years (see Chap. 2).

Both the adolescent male and female are

particularly prone to nutritional insult. Nutritional education should be part of every student's curriculum. "Rap sessions" on food facts, fads, and foods in space science, and slide talks on food buying, can help to stimulate a lifetime interest in nutrition that is needed to optimize their own and their future family's health. However, a positive food interest is initially formulated as the infant is placed to the breast or given a bottle and provided a nutrient feeding experience with self-expression and good prototypes to follow. The infant, toddler, preschooler, school-aged child, and adolescent perpetuate the cycle in much the same way as their parents and their grandparents before them. Only through a family approach can nutritional education hope to be successful.

STUDY QUESTIONS

1 Describe the processes and mechanisms underlying growth.
2 What are the extrinsic factors influencing growth?
3 During which periods of development would you expect accelerated growth?

4 How would you go about the assessment of a child's growth pattern?
5 Through each stage—infant, toddler, preschooler, school-age child, adolescent—there are certain psychosocial traits which influence food and feeding. Identify and describe these traits and their influence on mealtime behavior.
6 The oral and neuromuscular development of an infant progresses rapidly in the first year of life. How would you associate this development with the progression of food and feeding during this time? What type of food would you offer to a 3-month-old, 6-month-old, and 1-year-old child?
7 What does the phrase "classic infant feeding problem" mean? How would you identify this problem area?
8 Which would you recommend, home-prepared or commercially prepared baby foods?
9 What adolescent characteristics could be utilized as motivational forces for a nutritional education program?

CASE STUDY 12-1

Jennie, a 14-year-old girl, was brought to the adolescent unit of the Children's Hospital Medical Center by her parents, who were concerned about her attempts to control weight by periodic fasting at family meals, and about her complaints of lethargy.

On physical examination, Jennie was found to be a pretty, healthy adolescent with a sexual maturity rating of stage 5, a height of 64 in and a weight of 114 lb. Of significance in the laboratory analysis was a hematocrit of 35.3.

The social worker noted that Jennie was a somewhat shy confused adolescent with overprotective and anxious parents who spent her time after school listening to records in her room. She has no friends. Because of conflicting reports between parents and daughter, no reliable diet history was obtained. Based on Jennie's withdrawal, the diagnosis of adjustment reaction to adolescence was made and the family was referred to a local mental health facility for counseling. Before the family left the unit, the parents and Jennie were seen both alone and together by the nutritionist.

Case Study Questions

1 Judging from the information presented, does Jennie have a nutritional problem?

2 How would you associate Jennie's feeding behavior with the developmental experience of adolescence?

3 What would you recommend to Jennie, and to her parents, to normalize mealtimes?

REFERENCES

1 Donald B. Cheek, *Human Growth: Body Composition, Cell Growth, Energy and Intelligence,* Lea and Febiger, Philadelphia, 1968, p. 3.

2 G. J. Bowles, *New Types of Old Americans at Harvard,* Harvard University Press, Cambridge, Mass., 1932.

3 National Center for Health Statistics, *NCHS Growth Charts, 1976, Monthly Vital Statistics,* **25,** Suppl. 3, U.S. Dept. Health, Education, and Welfare Publ. No. (HRA)76-1120, 1976.

4 C. Yarborough et al., "Length and Weight in Rural Guatemalan Ladino Children: Birth to Seven Years of Age," *American Journal of Physical Anthropology,* **42:**439–448, 1975.

5 A. Prader, J. M. Tanner, and G. A. Von Harnack, "Catch-up Growth Following Illness or Starvation: An Example of Developmental Canalization in Man," *Journal of Pediatrics,* **62:**646, 1963.

6 Donald B. Cheek and Donald Hill, "Changes in Somatic Growth after Placental Insufficiency and Maternal Protein Deprivation," in Donald B. Cheek (ed.), *Fetal and Postnatal Growth: Hormones and Nutrition,* John Wiley & Sons, Inc., New York, 1975, p. 299.

7 S. Babson and G. I. Benda, "Growth Graphs for the Clinical Assessment of Infants of Varying Gestational Age," *Journal of Pediatrics,* **89:**814–820, 1976.

8 L. O. Lubchenko et al., "Intrauterine Growth as Estimated from Live-born Birth Weight Data at 24 to 42 Weeks of Gestation," *Pediatrics,* **32:**793, 1963.

9 Myron Winick, "Malnutrition and Brain Development," *Journal of Pediatrics,* **74:**667–679, 1969.

10 John Dobbing, "Human Brain Development and Its Vulnerability," in *Mead Johnson Symposium on Perinatal and Developmental Medicine,* 6, Evansville, Indiana, 1974.

11 John Dobbing and Jean Sands, "Quantitative Growth and Development of Human Brain," *Archives of Disease in Childhood,* **48:**757, 1973.

12 Donald Cheek, A. B. Holt, and E. D. Mellits, "Malnutrition and the Nervous System," *Nutrition, the Nervous System and Behavior,* Pan American Health Organization Sci. Publ. 251, Washington, D.C., 1972, pp. 3–14.

13 J. Hirsch, J. L. Knittle, and L. B. Salan, "Cell Lipid Content and Cell Number in Obese and Nonobese Human Adipose Tissue," *Journal of Clinical Investigation,* **45:**1023, 1966.

14 J. Knittle and J. Hirsch, "Infantile Nutrition as a Determinant of Adult Adipose Tissue Metabolism and Cellularity," *Clinical Research,* **15:**323, 1967.

15 Virginia Knott, "Stature, Leg Girth and Body Weight of Puerto Rican Private School Children," *Growth,* **27:**157–174, 1963.

16 *Skinfold Thickness of Children 6–11 Years,* U.S. Dept. Health, Education, and Welfare Publ. No. (HSM) 73-1602, Vital and Health Statistics Series 11 No. 120, 1974.

17 *Skinfold Thickness of Youths 12–17 Years,* U.S. Dept. Health, Education, and Welfare Publ. No. (HRA) 74-1614, Vital and Health Statistics Series 11 No. 132, 1974.

18 J. M. Tanner and R. H. Whitehouse, "Standards For Subcutaneous Fat in British Children," *British Medical Journal,* **1:**446, 1962.

19 S. M. Garn and C. G. Rohmann, "Interaction of Nutrition and Genetics in the Timing of Growth," *Pediatric Clinics of North America,* **13:**353, 1966.

20 T. G. H. Drake, "Pap and Panada," *Annals of Medical History,* **3:**289–295, 1931.

21 W. Schmidt, "Health and Welfare of Colonial American Children," *American Journal of Diseases of Children,* **130:**694–701, 1976.

22 R. Kron, M. Stein, and K. Goddard, "Newborn Sucking Behavior Affected by Obstetric Sedation," *Pediatrics,* **37:**1012–1016, 1966.

23 V. Beal, "Termination of Night Feeding in Infancy," *Journal of Pediatrics,* **75:**690–692, 1969.

24 S. Fomon, "What are Infants Fed in the United States?" *Pediatrics,* **56:**350–354, 1975.

25 S. J. Fomon, *Infant Nutrition,* W. B. Saunders Company, Philadelphia, 1974, p. 484.

26 R. Illingsworth and J. Lister, "The Critical or Sensitive Period with Special Reference to Certain Feeding Problems in Infants and Children," *Journal of Pediatrics,* **65:**839–848, 1964.

27 Fomon, *Infant Nutrition,* p. 166.

28 C. Woodruff, "The Role of Fresh Cow's Milk in Iron Deficiency Anemia," *American Journal of Diseases of Children,* **124:**18–23, 1972.

29 W. T. Hughes and F. Faulkner, "Infant Feeding Problems: A Practical Approach," *Clinical Pediatrics,* February 1964, pp. 65–67.

30 M. F. Gutelius et al., "Nutritional Studies of Children with Pica: 1. Controlled Study Evaluating Nutritional Status; 2. Treatment of Pica with Iron Given Intramuscularly," *Pediatrics,* June 1962, pp. 1012–1022.

31 G. Owen et al., "A Study of Nutritional Status of Pre-School Children in the United States, 1968–1970," *Pediatrics,* **53:**597–646, 1974.

32 S. Blades, "Clinical Notes on Adolescent Drug Abuse," in G. Scipien and M. Barnard, *Issues of Comprehensive Pediatric Nursing,* McGraw-Hill Book Company, New York, 1976, pp. 60–64.

33 U.S. Department of Health, Education and Welfare: *Preliminary Findings of the First Health and Nutrition Examination Survey, United States, 1971–2. I. Anthropometric and Clinical Findings,* DHEW Publ. No. (HRA) 75-1229 1973.

34 R. Frisch, "Weight at Menarche: Similarity for Well Nourished Girls at Different Ages and Evidence for Historical Constancy," *Pediatrics,* **50:**445, 1972.

35 N. J. Smith, "Gaining and Losing Weight in Athletics," **236:**149–151, 1976.

36 N. J. Smith, *Food for Sport,* Bull Publishing Co., Palo Alto, Calif., p. 81.

CHAPTER 13

PREGNANCY AND NUTRITION THROUGH THE LATER YEARS

Nancie H. Herbold

KEY WORDS
Primigravida
Amniotic Fluid
Hydramnios
Toxemia
Preeclampsia
Oxytocin
Colostrum
Aging

Introduction

Adequate nutrition during pregnancy has proven to be one of the most important factors influencing its outcome.

A restricted diet during pregnancy may lead to inadequate weight gain, intrauterine malnutrition, or a shorter gestational period, factors which may result in low-birth-weight infants (either small for gestational age or premature) and infants who have lower survival rates. The studies of Burke at the Boston Lying-In Hospital in the 1940s revealed that poor maternal nutrition was associated with a higher incidence of prematurity, stillbirths, neonatal deaths, and congenital malformations.[1] These findings were supported by prospective data from Leningrad and Holland, where fertility rates, birth rates, and perinatal survival were decreased after the starvation that was experienced in these areas during World War II.[2,3] Genetic, biological, social, and psychological factors affect the course and outcome of pregnancy as well as nutrition, which will be the focus of this chapter.

Biochemical and Physiological Changes

During the course of pregnancy many biochemical and physiological changes take place.

1 Plasma volume begins to increase at the end of the third month of pregnancy.
2 Red cell volume begins to increase toward the end of the first trimester and continues to expand through the second trimester. However, the red cell volume does not increase proportionately to the plasma volume, so that an apparent hemodilution occurs, causing a decrease in the hemoglobin concentration. This is a normal physiological anemia of pregnancy, occurring in all women regardless of their previous iron nutriture. However, the effect of hemodilution will be more severe if the pregnant

woman has low iron stores. Normal hemoglobin values for a nonpregnant woman are 12 to 15 g/100 ml; during pregnancy the average values are 11g/100 ml or greater.

3 Protein concentrations fall during pregnancy. One biochemical measure of protein is the serum albumin level. Normal serum albumin values for the nonpregnant female are 4 g/100 ml, and for the pregnant female, 2.5 g/100 ml. The reason for this decline in albumin is not known.

4 Serum cholesterol rises during pregnancy from a norm of 200 mg/100 ml to 250 to 300 mg/100 ml.

5 Cardiac output increases because of an accelerated heart rate and a larger stroke volume.

6 There is a rise in venous pressure. The high venous pressure in the legs may explain the lower leg edema that is commonly seen during pregnancy. While venous pressure is rising arterial blood pressure decreases, returning to normal during the last 2 to 3 months of pregnancy.

During pregnancy the heart enlarges; it is uncertain if this enlargement is a true myocardial hypertrophy or is due to a greater diastolic filling. There is an increased blood flow to the uterus, skin, and kidneys. The GFR (glomerular filtration rate) increases, depressing the urea and creatinine levels in the plasma. Improved renal clearance causes waste products to be excreted more efficiently. Sugar is excreted more rapidly and is often seen in the urine of pregnant women, as a result of the increased GFR. Amino acids and iodine are excreted in the urine as well. This excretion of iodine lowers the circulating iodine, which in turn leads to an increase in the size of the thyroid gland. Folic acid deficiency during pregnancy may be the result of an increased loss of renal folate caused by the more efficient clearance of nutrients during pregnancy.

During the early stages of pregnancy there is an increased urine flow; however, by late pregnancy urine excretion is below normal. This decrease of flow is probably due to the pooling of water in the lower limbs. The water is mobilized when the woman is in the supine position perhaps explaining the nocturia that many women experience. There is an increase in total body fluid of 8.5 l. All the water that is gained up to 30 weeks of pregnancy can be accounted for by the products of conception and the increase in blood volume. Increased appetite and thirst, particularly during the first trimester (and not necessarily inconsistent with nausea), are frequently reported once nausea has subsided.

Nutrient digestion and absorption is generally more efficient during pregnancy. There is no evidence that the old wives' tale of "a tooth for every child" is true. Scientific data do not support an increase in caries or a demineralization of the tooth. However, gum involvement may occur. Gingival edema with consequent gingivitis is not uncommon.

Many women complain of heartburn. This is due to a relaxation of the cardiac sphincter, which permits the stomach contents to reach the esophagus, thus causing heartburn. During pregnancy gastric acid and pepsin production is depressed, slowing the emptying time of the stomach; this accounts in part for the nausea associated with pregnancy. The relaxation of the smooth muscles in the large intestine may produce constipation (discussed under "Complications of Pregnancy," below).

Weight gain The recommended weight gain for a pregnant woman is 10 to 13 kg (22 to 28 lb). This weight gain encompasses the fetus, uterus, placenta, amniotic fluid, expanded blood volume, extracellular fluid, breast tissue, and fat (see Table 13-1). The lowest incidence of preeclampsia, prematurity, and perinatal mortality is seen with an average weight gain of 12.5 kg. The pattern of weight gain is most important. A gain of 1 to 2 kg during the first trimester followed by a gain of approximately 0.4 kg/week throughout the last two trimesters of

TABLE 13-1 WEIGHT GAIN DURING PREGNANCY

Tissue	Weight	
	lb	kg
Fetus	7.5	3.4
Uterus	2.0	.90
Placenta	1.5	.68
Amniotic fluid	2.0	.90
Blood volume	3.0	1.36
Extracellular fluid	2.0	.90
Breast tissue	1.0	.45
Fat	9.0	4.0
Total	28.0	12.59

pregnancy is the recommended pattern (see Figs. 13-1 and 13-2). Equally important is the type of weight gained; i.e., tissue accretion vs. fluid retention. Restricting the diet in order to limit the weight gain to less than 10 to 13 kg is not advisable. Limiting the weight gain increases the risk of a low-birth-weight infant, especially if the regimen is instituted during the third trimester of pregnancy when the fetus is growing most rapidly in size.

Young pregnant women tend to gain more than 12.5 kg, whereas older women tend to gain less. Primigravidas (women in their first pregnancy) gain slightly more than multigravidas, and thin women gain more than obese women.

Nutritional Requirements

The recommended daily dietary allowances (RDAs) for pregnancy are calculated for a semi-sedentary population. It should be remembered that the RDAs are not intended for evaluation of individual diets. They are meant to serve as guides for evaluating diets of large populations.

Energy

Energy requirements vary, depending upon age, activity, height, prepregnancy weight, stage of pregnancy, and ambient temperature.

Energy needs are greatest during the second and third trimesters of pregnancy because of the accelerated growth of the fetus. These needs are in part offset by the decrease in physical activity during late pregnancy. New tissue that is being laid down plus the storage of fat accounts for approximately 80,000 kcal (336 MJ). However, a decrease in energy expenditure by the mother, because of her heavier body weight, amounts to 40,000 kcal (168, MJ), leaving 40,000 kcal (168 MJ) as the total cost of pregnancy. The recommended

Figure 13-1
Normal weight gain pattern during pregnancy. (U.S. Dept. Health, Education, and Welfare, Social and Rehabilitation Service, Children's Bureau. Reprinted from Clifford B. Lull and R. A. Kimbrough (eds.), Clinical Obstetrics, J. B. Lippincott Company, Philadelphia, 1953.)

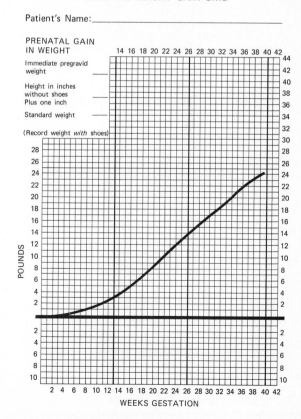

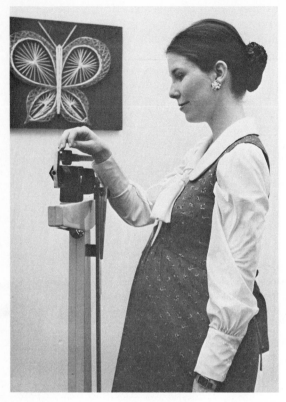

Figure 13-2
A weight gain of 1 to 2 kg during the first trimester and of 0.4 kg per week throughtout the last two trimesters of pregnancy is recommended.

minimum energy intake is 36 kcal/kg (151 kJ/kg) of ideal body weight, with a recommended *average* intake of 40 kcal/kg (168 kJ/kg) of ideal body weight. The pregnant woman does not need to eat for two. She must increase her nutrient intake above the nonpregnant state but she need only increase her caloric consumption by 300 kcal (1260 kJ) per day.

Protein

The recommended protein intake[4] is:

1.3 g/kg of ideal body weight for the mature woman

1.5 g/kg of ideal body weight for 15- to 18-year-olds

1.7 g/kg of ideal body weight for those younger than 15

Approximately two-thirds of the protein requirement should be of high biological value (meat, fish, eggs, cheese). An increased protein intake is needed for fetal growth and maintenance of maternal tissues. Low protein intakes may lead to nutritional edema. An adequate caloric intake is also essential, in order to avoid protein utilization for energy.

Vitamins and Minerals

Studies have been carried out to investigate the effect of vitamin supplements on the outcome of pregnancy. There has been no evidence to suggest that pregnant women in developed countries benefit from vitamin supplementation.[5] In fact, in some cases supplements may be a detriment, in that they provide a false sense of nutritional security. The pregnant woman does not realize that vitamin supplements do not contain all the nutrients obtained in a well-balanced diet. On the other hand, too much of a vitamin, especially the fat-soluble ones, can be harmful (see Chap. 6). Although vitamin supplementation as a routine practice has not been proven to be beneficial, there are some women for whom supplementation is necessary, such as the patient who is at nutritional risk because of her diet or a poor previous nutritional status.

Iron   The amount of elemental iron needed for the full-term fetus is approximately 300 to 370 mg/100 ml. The increase in maternal erythropoiesis requires approximately 300 to 500 mg of iron. The cessation of menstruation provides a saving of approximately 120 to 240 mg of iron. Therefore, the total amount of iron needed during pregnancy is approximately 480 to 630 mg.[6,7]

The amount of iron consumed in the diet is approximately 6 mg/1000 kcal (6 mg/4200 kJ). If a pregnant woman is consuming 2400 kcal/day (10,080 kJ/day), she is ingesting approximately 12 to 15 mg of iron. However, only 10 to 20 percent of dietary iron is absorbed. The RDA for the pregnant woman is 18+ mg of iron. Since most women do not consume this amount, it is necessary to supplement dietary iron with other sources. The recommended daily supplementation is 30 to 60 mg of ferrous iron during the last two trimesters of pregnancy. Iron can cause black stools, constipation (see under "Complications," below), and, less frequently, diarrhea. Increased vitamin C intake has been shown to improve iron absorption. The pregnant woman should therefore be encouraged to include in her diet foods that are high in vitamin C.

Folic acid Folic acid deficiency during pregnancy is not as common as iron deficiency but may develop because of a low prepregnancy folacin status (oral contraceptives can cause decreased serum folic acid), severe vomiting, or excess excretion. Some physicians and nutritionists recommend folic acid supplementation as a prophylactic measure. If a folate supplement is to be administered, the recommended dose is 400 to 800 μg/day. The RDA for folacin is 800 μg/day.

Calcium, phosphorus, and vitamin D Calcium absorption is more efficient during pregnancy. The RDA for calcium is 1200 mg/day. When the pregnant woman is not ingesting sufficient amounts of calcium, the fetal requirements will be met by demineralization of maternal bones. Approximately 128 to 130 g of calcium are present in the infant at birth. If protein and calcium requirements are met, phosphorus requirements (1200 mg/day) will most likely be satisfied. The vitamin D requirement (400 IU/day) can usually be met with the use of vitamin D–fortified milk. However, if the patient is not consuming milk fortified with vitamin D, a supplement will be necessary.

Sodium Sodium intake during pregnancy should be allowed ad libitum. The kidneys are more efficient during pregnancy and maintain the body's sodium balance. *Excessive* sodium intake is not recommended for any individual as a general health measure. (See "Toxemia," below, for further discussion.)

Iodine There is an increased need for iodine during pregnancy because of the increased metabolic demands of the thyroid gland. The RDA (125 μg) can generally be met if the pregnant woman is using iodized salt. Other sources of iodine are seafoods, breads, and milk.

The Patient at Nutritional Risk

Nutritional risk during pregnancy is associated with age, socioeconomic status, and a history of past medical and obstetrical problems.

Not all the women within these groups will have inadequate diets. However, nutritional screening and assessment will identify those who will need more intensified nutritional counseling and follow-up. Nutritional assessment should be carried out for each new prenatal patient seen in the clinic or health center. Assessment should be done as soon as possible, preferably during the patient's initial visit. This will allow the health professional to identify those patients at high nutritional risk and begin appropriate nutritional counseling.

Adolescence The metabolic demands for growth during adolescence plus the additional requirements of pregnancy place teenage mothers at high nutritional risk.

Age alone does not generally reflect obstetrical complications except with the very young (under the age of 14). Race and socioeconomic status are stronger determinants.[8] Adolescent mothers have a higher incidence of premature births and toxemia of pregnancy than older mothers have. When nonwhite race and low socioeconomic status are combined with adolescence, the incidence of prematurity and toxemia is greatly increased.[9] Neonatal mortality rates are higher for both white and nonwhite mothers under the age of 15 than for older women.

Even without the metabolic and physiologic demands of pregnancy, adolescent females are known to be a group vulnerable to poor nutrition. Many teenage girls are concerned about their weight and restrict their dietary intakes inappropriately; others have generally poor eating habits. Studies have revealed that the nutrients which are most poorly supplied by the pregnant teenage diet are calcium, iron, vitamin A, and energy.[10–12]

The adolescent girl is subject to many psychological stresses during her pregnancy. Even though the number of teenage pregnancies is increasing, societal mores are not accepting of the adolescent girl who is pregnant and may need to leave school. All of these concerns may be so overriding that her nutritional well-being may be overlooked.

High parity and frequency of conception   It is necessary for women to have sufficient time to rebuild or replenish nutrient stores after pregnancy. High parity and frequency of conception can result in iron deficiency, premature labor, and low-birth-weight infants.

Low prepregnancy weight and insufficient weight gain   Low prepregnancy weight (10 percent or more below ideal weight for height) and inadequate weight gain during pregnancy (see Table 13-1) are associated with low-birth-weight infants.

Anemia, obesity, and diabetes   These medical problems may also place the patient at nutritional risk; they are discussed under "Complications," below.

Obstetrical record   Particular attention should be paid to the past obstetrical record of the patient. Preeclampsia, miscarriage, anemia, premature labor, and low-birth-weight infants are all conditions which can be associated with nutritional inadequacies.

Smoking and alcoholism   The use of cigarettes may cause a decrease in nutrient intake. Women who smoke deliver infants of lower birth weights than those of nonsmokers. The alcoholic woman must be monitored closely to ensure that alcohol is not replacing necessary nutrients. Particular attention should be paid to the B vitamins, especially thiamine, as it is not uncommon for the alcoholic to be deficient in this particular nutrient.

Inadequate income   Women with inadequate income may not be able to purchase those foods needed to meet their nutritional requirements. If they are from another country, they may not be able to find culturally acceptable foods or may not be able to afford them once found and therefore may eat less nutritious substitutes. These pregnant women should be encouraged to utilize the Food Stamp program and the Special Supplemental Feeding Program for Women, Infants, and Children (the WIC program) to help improve the quality of their diets (see Chap. 14).

Pica   Pica refers to the ingestion of nonfood substances. During pregnancy women may eat clay or dirt (geophagia), or laundry starch (amylophagia). These substances usually replace other nutrients in the diet and can interfere with iron absorption. Anemia can result if the amounts consumed are significant. Reasons for this particular behavior are usually custom, culture, superstition, and a liking for the taste.

Psychological conditions   Psychological problems may also interfere with nutrient intake and place the woman at high nutritional risk. (See Chap. 10.)

Vegetarians   Lacto-ovo vegetarians (those who drink milk and eat eggs and milk products but do not eat meat) will have little difficulty in meeting most of the nutrient requirements of pregnancy. Women who follow a vegan diet (no milk or milk products, and no meat, poultry, or fish) should have their dietary intakes assessed to ensure that all nutrient needs are met. Protein requirements can be met only if a variety of plant foods are eaten. Certain combinations of food are necessary in order to provide complete protein, containing all the essential amino acids in proper proportions (see Chap. 3).

Vegetarians who do not eat any animal protein or drink cow's milk may need a vitamin B_{12} supplement as these foods are the primary source of this nutrient. If the cow's milk that is consumed is not fortified with vitamin D, the diet should be supplemented, since vitamin D is necessary for the utilization of calcium. If no milk or milk products of any kind are consumed, calcium intake is likely to be inadequate. Plant foods contain some calcium but its availability for absorption is limited, making supplementation necessary. Vegetarian diets, like the diets of nonvegetarians, are likely to be inadequate in iron. A ferrous salt should be prescribed. Although riboflavin can be found in such foods as whole grains, enriched breads and cereals, legumes, nuts, and various vegetables, the vegetarian diet must be assessed to ensure an adequate intake of this vitamin as milk and meat are the chief sources. Iodized salt should be encouraged; sea salt does not contain iodine. (See Chap. 14.)

Food Selection During Pregnancy

Daily Food Guide

The food guide (see Table 13-2) has been planned to meet the RDA for pregnancy. The foods are grouped according to the nutrients they provide. The patient should be encouraged to eat the recommended number of servings in each food group daily. It is difficult to consume an adequate intake of iron and folic acid. Therefore, it is recommended that the diet be supplemented with 30 to 60 mg of iron and 400 to 800 μg of folacin.

Complications of Pregnancy with Nutritional Implications

Anemia

Iron-deficiency anemia is common in pregnancy. It should not be confused with the seeming hemodilution that occurs naturally during pregnancy. Those patients who are found to have iron-deficiency anemia (hemoglobin less than 11 g/100 ml or hematocrit less than 33 percent) are treated with 200 mg of iron per day as three 0.2-g tablets of either ferrous sulfate or ferrous fumarate. Women who are at higher risk of developing iron-deficiency anemia are those of high parity and a short interval between pregnancies. If the mother's iron intake is inadequate, the infant may have a low hemoglobin at birth and insufficient iron stores for use during the first several months of life. Those women should be counseled to increase not only the amount of iron-rich foods (see Chap. 7) in their diet, but also the protein sources, which provide amino acids for globin formation. An increase in vitamin C may aid iron absorption.

Folic acid deficiency is sometimes seen during pregnancy. It is not as prevalent as iron-deficiency anemia. Folic acid supplementation may be needed in women with hemolytic anemia or multiple fetuses. Usually 400 to 800 μg is prescribed to decrease the likelihood of megaloblastic anemia of pregnancy.

Nausea and Vomiting

Women will frequently complain of nausea during the first trimester of pregnancy. The nausea usually starts to subside after the twelfth week. A fewer number of patients experience excessive vomiting (pernicious vomiting) which is severe enough to cause a weight loss. These patients must be followed closely to prevent dehydration and ketonuria. (See Table 13-3.)

Obesity

Weight reduction is *not* recommended during pregnancy. Research has shown that when

TABLE 13-2 DAILY FOOD GUIDE

	Amounts	
Food group	*Pregnancy*	*Lactation*
Protein foods		
Animal protein: In addition to protein, supplies iron, riboflavin, niacin, B_6, B_{12}, phosphorus, zinc, and iodine	two 3-oz servings	two 3-oz servings
Vegetable protein: In addition to protein, supplies iron, thiamine, folacin, B_6, E, phosphorus, magnesium, and zinc	Serving size varies. Plan with nutritionist.	
Milk and milk products *		
Supply calcium, phosphorus, vitamin D, riboflavin, A, E, B_6, B_{12}, magnesium, and zinc, protein	4 servings	4 servings
	serving equals 8 oz of milk or its equivalent	
Grain products		
Supply thiamine, niacin, riboflavin, iron, phosphorus, zinc, magnesium (whole grains provide more magnesium and zinc and should be encouraged). and fiber	3 servings	3 servings
	serving equals 1 slice of bread or ½ cup of macaroni, rice, or hot cereal	
Vitamin C–rich fruits and vegetables		
Supply ascorbic acid; when fresh supply fiber	1 serving	1 serving
	serving equals approximately ½ cup fruit or ¾ cup of vegetables	
Leafy green vegetables		
Supply folacin, A, E, B_6, riboflavin, iron, magnesium, and fiber	2 servings	2 servings
	serving equals approximately 1 cup raw or ¾ cup cooked	
Other fruits and vegetables		
Include yellow fruits and vegetables, which supply large amounts of vitamin A as well as B complex, E, magnesium, phosphorus, zinc, and fiber	1 serving	1 serving
	serving equals approximately ½ cup	

* Vitamin D is necessary for the utilization of calcium. Milk is fortified with vitamin D most other sources of calcium are not. A supplement to ensure an adequate vitamin D intake may be necessary if milk is not consumed.

Source: Adapted from Maternal and Child Health Unit, California Department of Health, *Nutrition during Pregnancy and Lactation,* 1975, pp. 34–40.

TABLE 13-3 DIETARY SUGGESTIONS FOR THE ALLEVIATION OF NAUSEA AND VOMITING

Frequent small meals

Crackers or dry cereal at bedside to eat before rising

Drink liquids one-half to one hour before or after meals*

Avoid heavy fried foods*

Avoid strongly flavored vegetables (onions, cabbage, turnips, etc.)*

Avoid highly spiced foods*

Use skim milk in place of whole milk if fat is not tolerated

Eat whatever will stay down until intake can gradually be increased to a complete meal

* May also be suggested for patients suffering from heartburn

maternal weight gain is limited, there is a greater chance of delivering a low-birth-weight infant, especially if the weight gain is restricted during the third trimester. Severe restriction of calories—to 1500 kcal (6300kJ) or less per day—even with adequate protein, can result in the body's use of protein for energy requirements rather than for growth and development of the fetus. If fat stores are catabolized for energy, ketosis and acetonuria may result, leading to neuropsychological damage of the fetus.[13] The increased nutrient needs of pregnancy are difficult to meet when food is restricted.

Excessive weight gain, more than 7 lb per month, must be evaluated and edema ruled out. Excessive weight (fat) gain during pregnancy can lead to subsequent obesity. Weight reduction should only be initiated after delivery. The obese pregnant patient must be encouraged to consume the recommended amounts of food as specified in the food guide, to avoid or decrease such foods as candy, cake, soft drinks, potato chips, and other high-energy snack foods, and to eat snacks of fruit and fruit juice, vegetables, and cheese and crackers instead.

Underweight

The patient who enters pregnancy with a low weight for her height and who gains less than 2 lb per month after the first trimester has an increased risk of delivering a low-birth-weight infant. Frequently, the underweight patient goes unnoticed by health professionals in their concern for the excessive gainer. Frequent meals and high-protein, high-energy snacks should be encouraged.

Constipation

Constipation is a common complaint of the pregnant woman. During the latter part of pregnancy constipation may be due to the pressure on the digestive tract exerted by the fetus. Many women experience constipation after iron therapy has been initiated. The diet should be evaluated for fiber content. Foods high in fiber and foods with a natural laxative effect should be increased if necessary. Fluid intake should be evaluated as well. A fluid intake of at least 6 or 8 glasses daily is recommended. If the patient is consuming 8 glasses of fluid per day, the efficacy of increasing intake beyond this amount for the treatment of constipation is questionable.

Diabetes and Pregnancy

There is a relatively high perinatal mortality among pregnant diabetics. It is important that prenatal care start as early as possible. The physician, nurse, and nutritionist must work together to maintain a "normoglycemic" patient. Early in pregnancy hypoglycemia may occur. This is due to the transfer to glucose to the fetus. The mother may develop hypoglycemic symptoms and a reduction in insulin may be necessary.[14] This hypoglycemia is often intensified by the nausea and vomiting of early pregnancy and by a consequent decrease in food intake. Nausea and vomiting with a decrease in intake may produce "starvation ketosis." This can be differentiated from diabetic ketoacidosis since hyperglycemia exists with diabetic ketoacidosis but is not present with starvation ketosis. Decreased mental development can occur in the offspring of mothers who developed starvation ketosis during pregnancy.[15]

Insulin requirements increase during the second half of pregnancy. There is an increase in placental hormones with effects that are antagonistic to insulin, contributing to the greater insulin demand. Ketoacidosis is more common during the second trimester of pregnancy and can be fatal to the fetus. During the third trimester of pregnancy, ketoacidosis is less life-threatening to the fetus.

Hydramnios (excessive amniotic fluid accumulation) is often seen in the pregnant diabetic. This fluid accumulation represents an excessive urine output by the fetus, resulting from an overstimulation of the fetal kidneys caused by the mother's elevated blood sugar. Hydramnios can endanger the fetus by causing premature rupture of the membranes and consequently early delivery. Hydramnios has also been associated with preeclampsia and eclampsia.

The infant's birth weight tends to be higher than normal when the mother is diabetic. A relationship exists between maternal hyperglycemia and the infant's birth weight. Maternal hyperglycemia results in fetal hyperglycemia, which causes an excess of fetal insulin secretion. This increased insulin secretion in turn causes an increase in fat and glycogen storage, thus increasing fetal weight. A large baby can cause difficulties during labor or may necessitate a cesarean section.

The recommended nutrient requirements for the pregnant diabetic mother are the same as for the nondiabetic pregnant woman.

On the day of delivery nutrition is provided by intravenous glucose; 6 to 8 g of glucose/kg of body weight is administered.[16] After delivery the diabetic mother is gradually progressed to her normal diet. Postpartum there is a brief remission of diabetes for 3 to 5 days.

Toxemia

Toxemia literally means "poison" and can be applied to any build-up of a toxic substance, although the term is generally associated with pregnancy. The cause of toxemia of pregnancy is not known, though many theories have been postulated, such as large weight gain, low weight gain, low protein intake, and lack of vitamin B_6. Toxemia can be divided into two phases: preeclampsia and eclampsia.

Preeclampsia is defined by the American College of Obstetricians and Gynecologists as "hypertension with proteinuria or edema or both, appearing after the twentieth week of pregnancy."[17] *Eclampsia* is defined by the same group as "the occurrence of one or more convulsions in a patient with the criteria for the diagnosis of preeclampsia."[18]

Preeclampsia is associated with a rapid, sharp increase in weight after the twentieth week, caused by fluid retention. However, there is no evidence to suggest that a large sharp weight gain, whether in the form of fat or water, will cause toxemia. Preeclampsia is more frequently seen in:

Primigravidas
Young adolescents
Women over the age of 30
Low-income populations
Women with multiple pregnancies

The important factor in the weight gain is the pattern of weight gain (see Fig. 13-1). Blood pressure rises to over 140/90 mmHg, albumin is present in the urine, and patients may complain of headaches and jitteriness.

The role of nutrition continues to be a controversial subject. The major controversy focuses around the issue of sodium restriction. Sodium has long been one of the elements restricted from the diets of women with preeclampsia. A reappraisal of the use of sodium-restricted diets has recently been conducted. One investigation has shown that during pregnancy there is an increased need for sodium and even though sodium restriction may help to alleviate edema, a reduced sodium intake may actually exacerbate toxemia.[19] An adequate sodium intake is essential during the summer months when greater amounts of sodium are being lost in the perspiration. Also, by restricting sodium in the pregnant woman's diet, one may inadvertently be restricting other nutrients as well.

An increased amount of sodium is needed during pregnancy to accommodate for the expanded blood volume. If sodium is limited in the diet, the kidneys will try to conserve sodium via the renin-angiotensin system and sodium will be reabsorbed by the renal tubules.[20] (See Chap. 8.)

Studies that altered the levels of sodium intake in women with toxemia of pregnancy have not demonstrated an improvement in their condition, and in light of the physiological need for increased amounts of sodium during pregnancy, sodium should be allowed ad libitum.[21] Nutritional treatment should remain as a well-balanced diet, adequate in calories (Joules) and all nutrients.

Fortunately, most cases of preeclampsia do not reach the eclampic stage. Eclampsia requires hospitalization and complete bed rest. Cesarean section is advisable in most cases. Nutritional treatment follows the guidelines outlined in Chap. 24 for surgery if a cesarean section is performed.

Diet during Labor

During the initial phases of labor carbohydrate foods may be allowed as they remain in the stomach for the shortest amount of time. However, when active labor has begun no food is usually allowed. This is to prevent the possibility of vomiting and aspiration.

LACTATION

Introduction

Whether or not to breast-feed should be decided by the parents during the prenatal period. Information, encouragement, and reassurance provided by the nurse, nutritionist, and obstetrician are extremely important factors in determining whether breast feeding will be the feeding method chosen. Breast feeding should be encouraged for any infant who has a strong familial history of allergy. The intestinal wall is more permeable to cow's milk than breast milk, thereby increasing the risk of allergy.

Only one percent of the women who decide to breast-feed are unsuccessful, and since breast feeding has many positive qualities (see Table 13-4) it is unfortunate that we are witnessing a general decline in its usage. However, in certain segments of the population—college-educated women and women in the upper middle class—breast feeding is gaining support; this increase appears to be related to the "back-to-nature" movement.

Many developing countries have had a falling off in the practice of breast feeding. In terms of national development and nutritional planning this decline in breast feeding is a loss of a valuable natural resource that is a major force in the prevention of malnutrition. (See Fig. 13-3.)

The Physiology of Lactation

The female breast is composed of fat, glandular tissue, and connective tissue. The mammary glandular tissue contains many lobules which are composed of alveoli or acinar cells where the breast milk is actually formed.

The "letdown" of milk, or the *ejection reflex,* is a neurohumoral reflex brought about by the sucking of the infant. Proprioceptors in the nipple and areola are stimulated by the sucking. Nerve impulses are transmitted to the hypothalamus which stimulates the anterior pituitary to secrete prolactin, the hormone needed for milk production. The posterior pituitary is stimulated to secrete oxytocin, which travels via the blood to the alveoli or acinar cells, causing them to rupture and contract, forcing the milk into the lactiferous ducts. The lactiferous ducts then transport the milk first to storage spaces (ampullae) located under the areola, and finally out the nipple.

TABLE 13-4 BREAST MILK VS. INFANT FORMULA: A COMPARISON

Breast milk: comparison with cow's milk	Advantages and contraindications	Additional information
Water, solids, and fat content similar to cow's milk. Protein and ash content only about one-third that of cow's milk. Lactose content is approximately 1½ times that of cow's milk. (Colostrum, a yellowish secretion which appears 2–4 days after delivery, is not mature milk.)	1 Human milk is a natural food for infants; however, the psychological advantages are difficult to demonstrate	Milk is more mature at the end of the first month than earlier
	2 Human milk is better tolerated; a small flocculent curd is formed instead of a large casein curd.	Great variability in amount secreted by different women from one day to another, and from one breast to another; however, volume averages out over a period of time
	3 Protein utilization is somewhat higher because of the lactose content and amino acid pattern	When a woman is poorly nourished, the volume of milk secreted will decrease but the percent of carbohydrate, protein, and fat will be little affected. However, vitamin content does reflect intake
	4 Lower renal solute load is due to lower levels of protein and minerals in human milk	Most drugs taken by a nursing mother, including anesthesia used in dental treatment, may inhibit milk production
	5 May prevent tendency to overfeed	Cigarette smoking also reduces the amount of milk produced
	6 No sanitation or preparation problems	
	7 Usually fewer and less serious feeding problems	
	8 Constipation occurs less frequently	
	9 May provide antibody immunization, though this is questionable -since antibodies do not survive ingestion. However, it is felt that maternal antibodies exert some production of local immunity	

in the gastrointestinal tract but cannot be expected to influence the frequency or severity of infections due to organisms that enter the body through other portals

10 A substance present in some women's milk appears to be responsible for persistent elevation of indirect-reacting bilirubin. In such cases breast feeding should be interrupted for 24–48 h, which generally permits the bilirubin concentration to fall below 10 mg/100 ml with no increase in bilirubinemia on resumption of breast feeding

11 Discontinue if mother supplies less than half the infant's needs

12 Discontinue if mother has chronic illness (cardiac disease, tuberculosis, severe anemia, nephritis, chronic fevers)

13 May be necessary to discontinue if mother returns to work

14 Discontinue if infant is weak or unable to nurse because of oral anomalies

15 Discontinue temporarily during acute maternal infections. Milk should be pumped so that supply will not dwindle

Source: Adapted from G. M. Scipien et al., *Comprehensive Pediatric Nursing*, McGraw-Hill Book Company, New York, 1975, p. 214.

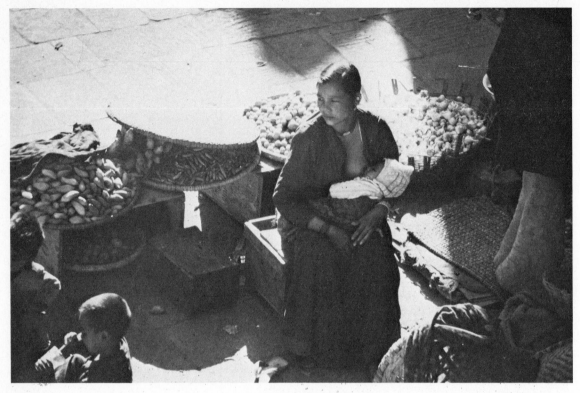

Figure 13-3
Breast feeding, a natural resource, is a diminishing phenomenon in developing countries. (Photo courtesy of Jane McCotter O'Toole.)

The infant's continuous sucking empties these ducts of milk.

Women sometimes experience uterine cramps while first nursing. These cramps are caused by the contraction of the uterus brought about by the hormonal changes of lactation. These contractions are helpful to:

1   Expel the placenta if it has not already occurred
2   Reduce the chances of postpartum hemorrhage
3   Bring about involution of the uterus

Milk may be expelled from the breast at the mother's sight of the infant, and once nursing has begun milk may drip from the breast that is not being suckled. A tingling sensation or nipple pain is experienced by some women but soon dissipates after nursing has begun.

Types of Milk

Breast milk can adequately nourish the infant for the first 4 to 6 months of life, but should be supplemented with 400 IU of vitamin D (a fluoride supplement should also be used in the areas where the water supply is not fluoridated). For a comparison of nutrients in human milk and commercial formulas see Chap. 12.

Colostrum   Colostrum develops after the sixteenth week of pregnancy. It is produced for the first 2 to 4 days postpartum. Colostrum is thicker and more yellow than mature breast milk (milk produced after colostrum has ceased). Colostrum has less energy value (67 kcal/100 ml or 281 kJ/100 ml) than mature milk (75 kcal/100 ml or 315 kJ/100 ml) but has a higher protein, sodium, potassium, and chloride content. Colostrum contains secretory immunoglobins; i.e., antibodies to poliomyelitis and coliform microorganisms.

Mature milk Mature milk is composed of foremilk and hindmilk. Foremilk is a low-fat milk that is secreted immediately at the initiation of feeding.[22] Hindmilk makes up approximately two-thirds of the total volume of milk produced and is secreted shortly after the infant commences sucking.[23]

Nutrient Needs during Lactation

Except in cases of extreme malnutrition, an inadequate maternal diet, will affect the volume of milk produced but apparently will have little effect on the nutritional composition of the breast milk. Maternal nutrient stores are used to maintain the nutritional value of the milk.

Table 13-2 lists the food groups and number of servings necessary to provide a nutritionally adequate diet for a lactating woman.

Energy An additional 500 kcal (2100 kJ) per day is recommended for the lactating woman to produce 850 ml of milk (the average amount produced per day). This is based on the premise that 80 percent of maternal energy is converted to milk energy and that the production of 100 ml of milk requires 90 kcal (378 kJ). In addition, the 4 kg of body fat laid down during pregnancy will provide an additional 200 to 300 kcal (840 to 1260 kJ).[24] If a mother continues to breast-feed beyond 3 months (so that fat stores will be used up) or if she is breast feeding more than one child at once, her energy needs will be further increased.

Protein The recommended daily intake is 20 additional grams of high-biologic-value protein. Protein is necessary for maternal needs as well as to supply the amino acids in the breast milk.

Calcium The requirement during lactation is 1200 mg per day; 800 ml of breast milk contains approximately 300 mg of calcium. Since calcium absorption is not 100 percent efficient, an intake of 1200 mg is necessary to ensure sufficient absorption.

Iron The recommended dietary iron intake for the lactating woman is 18 mg/day. This amount of iron is difficult for most women to consume via the diet, and iron stores may be depleted during pregnancy and after delivery. Therefore, iron supplementation, initiated during pregnancy, should be continued for several months postpartum.

Fluids The lactating woman should drink 2 to 3 qt of liquid per day. This increase in fluid intake is necessary to provide the liquid volume of breast milk.

Other Nutritional Concerns

Most foods, including spicy foods and chocolate, do not need to be restricted from the mother's diet as they are not gastrointestinal irritants to the infant.[25]

Both alcohol and coffee are excreted in the breast milk; therefore, moderation is recommended. (See Table 13-5 for a list of drugs excreted in human milk.)

How to Breast-Feed

Some authorities recommend breast massage and manual expression of milk during the last 2 months of pregnancy. This is thought to increase the protractibility of the nipple, which aids good nursing grasp by the infant. Infants can be breast-fed with the mother in either a sitting or reclining position. If the mother is sitting while nursing, a chair with low arms is helpful. If the mother is reclining she should

TABLE 13-5 DRUGS EXCRETED IN HUMAN MILK

Alcohol	Erythromycin	Ergot	Potassium
Allergens	Flabayl	Estrogens	Sodium
Ambenonium chloride (Mytelase)	Furadantin	Ethinamate (Valmid)	Sulfur
Aminophylline (theophylline with ethylenediamine)	Isoniazid (more than twenty trade names)	Ethyl biscoumacetate (Tromexan)	Nicotine
Amphetamines	Mandelic acid	Cyclophosphamide (Cytoxan)	Papaverine
Amphetamine salts (Benzedrine and numerous other trade names)	Neomycin (Mycifradin, Neobiotic)	DDT (chlorophenothane)	Phenylbutazone (Butazolidin)
Dextroamphetamine salts (Dexedrine and numerous other trade names)	Nitrofurantoins	Dicumarol (bishydroxycoumarin, Melitoxin)	Phenytoin (diphenylhydantoin, Dilantin)
	Novobiocin (Albamycin, Cathomycin)	Ephedrine	Propylthiouracil
Analgesics (nonnarcotic)	Para-aminosalicylic acid and salts (numerous trade names)	Hexachlorobenzene	Pseudoephedrine (Sudafed)
Acetaminophen (numerous trade names, including, Amdil, Anelix, Apamide, Elixodyne, Febrolin, Fendon, Lestemp, Lyteca Syrup, Metalid, Nacetyl, Nebs, Tempra, Tylenol)	Penicillin G	Imipramine hydrochloride (Tofranil)	Pyrimethamine (Daraprim)
	Streptomycin	Iodides including ^{131}I	Quinidine
	Sulfonamides (breast concentration may exceed maternal plasma level; this represents a small oral dose for infant)	Iopanoic acid (Telepaque)	Quinine
		Laxatives and cathartics	Reserpine (many trade names)
Aspirin	Sulfamethoxazole (Ganthanol)	Aloin	Salicylates
Dextropropoxyphene (Darvon)	Sulfadimethoxine (Madribon)	Calomel (mild mercurous chloride)	Scopolamine (hyoscine)
Phenacetin	Tetracycline	Cascara	Sodium chloride
Sodium salicylate	Antihistamines (most pass into milk)	Danthron (Dionone, Dorbane, Istizin)	Thiazides
Analgesics (narcotic)	Brompheniramine (Dimetane)	Rhubarb (said either not to pass or, conversely, to purge infant)	Thiouracil
Mefenamic acid (Ponstel)	Diphenhydramine (Benadryl)	Levopropoxyphene (Novrad)	Thyroid
Methadone (Adanon, Althose syrup, Dolophine)	Methdilazine (Tacaryl)	Mephenoxalone (Trepidone)	Tolbutamide
Morphine (trace)	Atropine	Methimazole (Tapazole)	Tranquilizers
Heroin	Barbiturates	Methocarbamol (Robaxin)	Chlorpromazine (Thorazine)
Anesthetics	Amobarbital (Amytal)	Metals, salts, minerals	Hydroxyzine (Atarax, Vistaril)
Chloroform	Methohexital (Brevital)	Arsenic	Phenaglycodol Ultran)
Cyclopropane	Phenobarbital (Luminal)	Calcium	Trifluoperazine (Stelazine)
Ether	Secobarbital (Seconal)	Chloride	Vitamins
Antibiotics and chemotherapeutics	Thiopental (Pentohal)	Copper	A, B₁, B₁₂, D, C, E, K
Chloramphenicol (Chloromycetin)	Bromides	Iodides	Folic acid
Cycloserine (Seromycin)	Caffeine	Lead	Niacin
	Chloral hydrate	Magnesium	Pantothenic acid
	Cortisone	Mercurous chloride (see Calomel)	Riboflavin
		Mercury	Thiamine
		Phosphate	

Synonyms and combinations may be found in Charles O. Wilson and Tony E. Jones (eds.), *American Drug Index*, J. B. Lippincott Company, Philadelphia, 1975. Concentrations may be found in J. A. Knowles, "Excretion of Drugs in Milk—A Review," *Journal of Pediatrics*, 66: 1068, 1965.

Source: J. M. Arena, "Contamination of the Ideal Food," *Nutrition Today* magazine, 101 Ridgely Avenue, Annapolis, Maryland 21404, Winter 1970, p. 8.

lie on her right side to feed from the right breast. The baby should lie on its side, facing the mother and cradled in her arms.

When nursing is to begin the mother must stroke the cheek of the infant with her nipple to produce the "rooting" reflex, which causes the infant to turn its head in that direction and open its mouth. Contact can then be made with the nipple. By grasping the nipple with her second and third fingers, the mother can increase the nipple's protractibility. This allows the infant to place its lips on the areola and not the nipple; room must be made between the breast and the infant's nose so that breathing is not hindered. (See Fig. 13-4.)

The infant should be allowed to suckle at both breasts for approximately 5 min on the first day, 10 min on the second day, and 15 on the third day. Maximum ejection of milk takes place approximately 2 to 3 min after sucking has begun; therefore a minimum of 5 min at the breast is essential, and feeding should continue for even longer, approximately 15 min. The infant should be nursed at both breasts to prevent engorgement. The subsequent nursing session should start with the breast that was suckled last to ensure emptying. Feedings should not be rushed and a calm pleasant environment is essential.

Nipple care   The sweat glands of the nipple provide sweat which mixes with the oils of the skin to produce an antibacterial agent; therefore nipples need only to be washed with water. A nursing brassiere may provide support and comfort. However, plastic liners should not be used since they hinder air circulation and hold in moisture, which can contribute to sore nipples.

Nipple Engorgement   Engorgement may be caused by a poor "let down" reflex. If the milk is not ejected the breasts are not adequately emptied and engorgement can result. This is generally the result of emotional influences or infrequent nursing. It may also be caused by an infant with poor sucking strength. Women

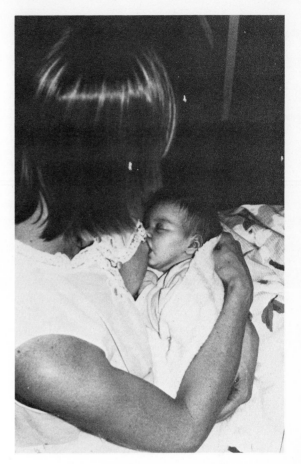

Figure 13-4
Proper technique ensures a positive feeding experience, which includes proper placement of the infant's lips on the areola and not on the nipple. (Photo courtesy of Jane McCotter O'Toole.)

who receive large amounts of anesthesia during childbirth may deliver infants who are not fully alert and therefore initially have a weak suckle-swallow reflex. The discomfort of nipple engorgement can be relieved by applying ice packs to the breast.

Hyperbilirubinemia

Hyperbilirubinemia is a build-up of bilirubin in the blood, causing jaundice. Conjugation of bilirubin is essential for its excretion. In unconjugated hyperbilirubiemia there is a deficiency or inadequacy of glucuronyl transferase, which is needed for bilirubin conjugation and hence its excretion. Maternal milk may contain an inhibitor of bilirubin conjugation. Therefore, if the breast-fed infant develops hyperbilirubinemia it will be necessary to discontinue breast feeding for several days until the infant's plasma bilirubin levels have returned to normal. Breast feeding can then be restarted without the return of elevated serum bilirubin. During the interim, the woman should manually express her milk to prevent breast engorgement.

Weaning

Most American women tend to discontinue breast feeding after the first 2 to 3 months. Weaning should be done gradually in order to prevent nipple engorgement and to allow the baby to become accustomed to the bottle. If breast feeding has continued until the baby is 6 months of age, weaning can proceed directly from the breast to a cup. Older babies may actually wean themselves.

NUTRITION THROUGH THE CONTINUING YEARS OF THE LIFE CYCLE

The Middle Years

The nutritional status of the middle adult is a continuum of the early years of the life cycle. As with the infant, toddler, preschool child, school-age child, and adolescent, the adult is subject to physiological and psychological influences. Little research has been directed toward nutrition during this period nor to the psychological stresses inherent in working and child rearing. Unlike the well-documented turmoil of adolescence, the crisis of middle years is now being discovered, as the middle adult must integrate generativity and prevent stagnation in order to prepare for the later years of the life cycle.[26]

These are productive years when the adult makes a significant contribution to society. The type of employment may influence nutrient intake as hectic schedules leave little time to eat, and cocktails with clients over lunch greatly expand energy intake. Women who may no longer be part of the work force but may be at home caring for children, now have ready access to the refrigerator and extra calories. The financial burden imposed by raising a family, especially with college-age children, may necessitate an additional source of income from a second job. Busy schedules can lead to stress and mealtime disorganization, hardly an environment for a family dinner.

Both men and woman will need to decrease their energy intake at this stage of life; growth is complete, basal metabolic rate is decreasing, and activity is generally reduced. Because of this diminished energy requirement less food should be consumed; however, foods with a high nutrient density must be selected so as to meet other nutrient needs which have not decreased significantly. Many men and women begin to gain excessive amounts of weight during these years. Participation in sports diminishes, life styles become more sedentary without a concomitant reduction in food energy intake, and hence weight gain occurs. Obesity has been associated with atherosclerosis and diabetes, which are already more prevalent during the adult years. Families with a positive history for these diseases should be carefully monitored. An increase in alcohol consumption adds unnecessary energy to the diet and also leads to more serious problems such as liver disease. Modifying diet and life style during the early stages of the life cycle, before these problems develop, may prevent or diminish the severity of these conditions.

A special concern for women during these years is the effect of contraceptives on nutritional status. The woman using oral contraceptives may be at nutritional risk for the following nutrients: folic acid, vitamin C, riboflavin, vitamin B_6, and vitamin B_{12},[27] and she should be monitored accordingly. The use of an intrauterine device (IUD) can cause an increase in blood loss during menstruation, leading to iron-deficiency anemia. Women who are using the IUD as a method of birth control should be monitored for iron status and iron nutriture.

Careful selection of foods with the use of the daily food guide to ensure the prudent diet (see Fig. 2-2) can help meet nutrient requirements and maintain a positive nutritional status for the continuing life cycle. Activity and exercise should be emphasized as an integral part of nutritional well-being. The amount and type of activity should be determined by past physical fitness and present tolerance.

The Older Adult

Many older adults in the United States today are not adequately nourished. Reports from the Ten State Nutrition Survey indicated that persons over the age of 60 had low intakes of calories, protein, iron, and vitamin A.[28]

Four million six hundred thousand older adults are part of the poverty population of the United States, or approximately one-fifth of all people over the age of 65.[29] Income is probably the strongest determinant affecting the nutritional status of the older adult.[30] If an older person does not have an adequate income or does not utilize food programs and resources appropriately, the diet can be inadequate. For many senior citizens, grocery shopping is difficult or inaccessible and buying for one person is expensive. Other factors known to influence nutrition are nutritional knowledge, health, environment, and emotional status. Frequently, older individuals do not like to cook a meal if they must eat alone.

Physiological and Psychological Aspects of Aging

Aging is not a process that begins late in life; it is initiated at conception and continues throughout life. Although the aging process is not thoroughly understood, we do know that reduced cell metabolism and cellular loss seem to play a role. Physiological changes that may

be influenced by these phenomena are a decreased rate of nerve impulse transmission, decreased blood flow to the kidneys, and a decreased resting cardiac output.

Often the older adult will complain that food has no taste. An altered sense of taste and smell due to a decrease in the number of taste buds/or to interference from a dental plate is a common problem. A recent theory has been postulated that this decrease in taste acuity may be the result of deficient zinc nutriture.[31] However, to date there is no evidence to support this hypothesis. Poor teeth or poorly fitting dentures, necessitating the use of soft, bland foods that are easy to chew, further exacerbate this problem.

Dental disease is common in the older population. It may be a result of natural loss of teeth due to the aging process, or may result from poor oral hygiene. (See Chap. 23.) In the population over the age of 65, 50 percent have lost all their teeth and only 75 percent have adequate dentures.[32] This may be one factor in the development of malnutrition.

Gastric esophageal reflux (heartburn) and hiatus hernia are common in the older population as a result of dilatation of the esophagus. (See Chap. 18.) The stomach may have a reduced acid secretion, making digestion more difficult. With age there is a decrease in enzyme production in the small intestine, leading to problems of malabsorption, obstruction, and diverticulitis. Diverticulitis is further aggravated by the lack of fiber in the diet since fibrous foods such as raw fruits and vegetables and whole grains are difficult to chew. The incidence of cholelithiasis (gallstones) increases with age and a reduced secretion of bile results in a lower tolerance for fatty foods. The older adult also suffers from chronic disorders such as obesity, diabetes, atherosclerosis, hypertension, arthritis, and orthopedic problems.

Perhaps even more important than the physiological influences are the psychological factors which affect the nutritional well-being of the older adult. Many older adults experience feelings of inadequacy or loss of self-worth. Spouses and friends have died and family members may no longer live near by. Physical disabilities may prevent the individual from accomplishing activities once taken for granted. Isolation, loneliness, and fear of death are common among the elderly and frequently affect food intake. Many older adults will not prepare a meal for themselves or having prepared one will not eat, if they must eat alone. In a study conducted by Davidson et al. the diets of isolated elderly persons were much poorer than the diets of socially gregarious older adults.[33]

The fear of death and dying is often repressed because of the social stigma attached to it.[34] The older individual may need to discuss death and frequently it is the health professional who is turned to, as the family finds the subject too painful and is unable to lend support.

The nutrition educator must respect the wishes of the older patient and not adopt a condescending attitude. Dietary habits have developed over many years and are a source of security; therefore, it is important to initiate change gradually.

Nutrient Requirements

Energy As individuals grow older their basal metabolic rate decreases as well as their level of activity. (See Fig. 13-5.) Therefore, it is necessary to decrease dietary energy requirements. The RDA for individuals over the age of 51 is 2400 kcal (10,080 kJ) for men and 1800 kcal (7560 kJ) for women. However, this recommended allowance may be too high for the adult over the age of 60. A recent study revealed that 30 percent of the elderly persons surveyed in the study were overweight, even though reported energy intakes were below the recommended dietary allowance.[35]

Carbohydrate Carbohydrates such as breads, cakes, and cereals make up a large portion of the older individual's diet. Mildly flavored carbohydrate foods are generally easy to chew,

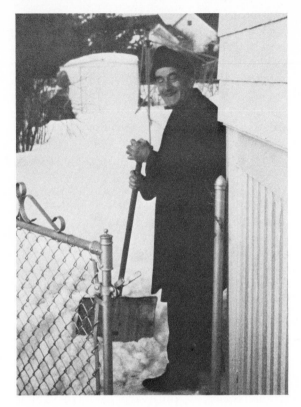

Figure 13-5
While many older adults remain very active, nutritional energy requirements have diminished because of a decreased basal metabolic rate, and food intake must be adjusted with consideration of this fact and of the psychosocial effects of aging. (Photo courtesy of Richard F. Herbold.)

easy to prepare, and packaged in small quantities, and the taste acuity for sweets is still strong among most older individuals. Wholegrain breads and cereals should be encouraged to increase fiber intake.

Protein Protein foods may be scarce in the diets of the elderly. The cost of protein foods may make them prohibitive. Meat may be difficult to chew and appropriate substitutions such as cheese, peanut butter, and eggs are often not made. Protein requirements for the older individual are the same as for the younger adult (0.8 g/kg of ideal body weight) since protein is needed to offset the catabolic processes of aging.[36]

Fat Since many older individuals have coronary artery disease, the amount and type of dietary fat may need to be modified. (See Chap. 17.) Older adults who are overweight should decrease the amount of fat in their diets.

Iron Elderly individuals are at nutritional risk for iron-deficiency anemia. Because their diet tends to be low in protein it is also low in iron. The nutrition educator should recommend as sources of iron, foods that are inexpensive and easy to chew, such as iron-fortified cereals, eggs, legumes, and dark green leafy vegetables.

Calcium Diets low in calcium have been associated with osteoporosis, a disease of aging. Osteoporosis afflicts 25 percent of postmenopausal women.[37] Liberal amounts of high-calcium foods such as milk and milk products, which are easy to chew, are relatively inexpensive, and provide protein as well, should be encouraged. However, lactose intolerance may be a problem for some individuals and other sources of calcium may need to be recommended; e.g., dark green vegetables, beans, and nuts.

Vitamins Older adults make up a large percentage of the health food market. The use of vitamins and other "cure-alls" is a common practice among this age group. In one study, 30 percent of the elderly participants believed that in order to remain healthy, vitamin and mineral supplements were necessary,[38] while 88 percent believed that natural vitamins were better than synthetic ones.[39] Vitamins C and E are frequently used by the older adult striving to remain young.

Vitamin E became known as an anti-aging vitamin because of its property as a natural antioxidant. Antioxidants are protective forces against the effects of free radicals and oxygen, which cause normal cell aging. Vitamin C may act as a synergist to the antiperoxidative activity of vitamin E.[40] However, no evidence to date has shown that *increased* intakes of vitamin C or E will delay the aging process.

Many older individuals use mineral oil as a laxative, which use is not recommended since vitamins A, D, E, and K will not be absorbed. Foods high in roughage and with natural laxative properties should be encouraged to aid in elimination.

Community Services for the Older Adult

Home-delivered meals ("Meals on Wheels") is one type of support service being offered to meet some of the special needs of the older adult and disabled individual. The program is designed for those persons who for physical or mental reasons are unable to prepare their own food. Meals prepared at a central location are delivered to the homes of the clients, thus enabling these individuals to remain in their own homes. Group meals for senior citizens are another service being offered by many communities under Title VII of the Older Americans Act. (See Table 14-4.) These programs are currently being run under the auspices of various agencies: councils on aging, antipoverty organizations, hospitals, and various volunteer groups.

The meals provided are planned to meet part of the nutritional requirements of adults over the age of 60. Since the meal that is furnished only supplies one-third of the RDA, there is a need for nutritional education. The senior citizen should be taught how to augment the home-delivered meal with other foods available in the home. Special educational emphasis should be given to those nutrients that are found to be low in the diets of the older adult. Meal planning, budgeting, and cooking for one are potential areas for nutritional education. The nutritional educator must help the senior citizen to plan and maintain a diet of adequate quality.

STUDY QUESTIONS

1 What is an appropriate weight gain for a pregnant woman? Why?

2 Why is an iron supplement recommended during pregnancy?

3 Why is the adolescent at nutritional risk during pregnancy?

4 What are the various types of milk produced by the lactating woman? How do they differ?

5 Why should the middle and older adult decrease energy intake?

CASE STUDY 13-1

C. P. is a 21-year-old primigravida at 30 weeks gestation. C. P. has had a weight gain of 10 lb in 1 month, bringing her total weight gain to 27 lb. Until this visit to the health center, C. P. had an appropriate weight gain for gestational date. Clinical examination and laboratory data revealed:

> *Blood pressure 140/98*
> *Proteinuria 2+*
> *Edema 2+*
> *Weight 145 lb*
> *Height 5 ft 2 in*

C. P. is experiencing symptoms of preeclampsia and is referred to the nutritionist.

Case Study Questions

1 *Should a weight-reducing program be instituted? What is an appropriate energy level?*

2 *Should sodium be restricted?*

3 *What other general nutritional recommendations would you make?*

REFERENCES

1 B. C. Burke et al., *Journal of Nutrition,* **38**:453, 1949.

2 A. M. Antonov, "Children Born During the Siege of Leningrad in 1942," *Journal of Pediatrics,* **30**:250–259, 1947.

3 D. Baird, "Variations in Fertility Associated with a Change in Health Status," *Journal of Chronic Diseases,* **18**:1109–1124, 1965.

4 American College of Obstetricians and Gynecologists, *Nutrition in Maternal Health Care,* 1974.

5 Committee on Maternal Nutrition, Food and Nutrition Board, *Nutrition and the Course of Pregnancy,* Summary Report, National Academy of Sciences National Research Council, Washington, D.C., 1970, p. 133.

6 Ibid., p. 68.

7 American College of Obstetricians and Gynecologists, op. cit.

8 John Grant and Felix Heald, "Complications of Adolescent Pregnancy. Survey of the Literature on Fetal Outcome in Adolescence," *Clinical Pediatrics,* October 1972, p. 567.

9 Ibid., p. 567.

10 Harold Kamenetzky et al., "The Effects of Nutrition in Teenage Gravidas on Pregnancy and the Status of the Neonate," *American Journal of Obstetrics and Gynecology,* **115**:639–646, 1973.

11 Janet King, S. Cohenour, S. Calloway, and H. Jacobson, "Assessment of Nutritional Status of Teenage Pregnant Girls. I. Nutritional Intake and Pregnancy," *American Journal of Clinical Nutrition,* **25**:916, 1972.

12 W. J. McGanity et al., "Pregnancy in Adolescence. I. Preliminary Summary of Health Status," *American Journal of Obstetrics and Gynecology,* **103**:77, 1969.

13 Committee on Maternal Nutrition, op. cit., p. 123.

14 J. Tyson and P. Felig, "Medical Aspects of Diabetes in Pregnancy and the Diabetogenic Effect of Oral Contraceptives," *Medical Clinics of North America,* **55**(4):952, 1971.

15 Ibid., p. 954.

16 R. Francois, "The Newborn of Diabetic Mothers," *Biology of the Neonate,* **24**:28, 1974.

17 American College of Obstetricians and Gynecologists, op. cit.

18 American College of Obstetricians and Gynecology, op. cit.

19 Ruth Pike and H. Smiciklas, "A Reappraisal of Sodium Restriction during Pregnancy," *International Journal of Obstetrics and Gynecology,* **10**(1):1–8, 1972.

20 Ibid., p. 4.

21 Roy Pitkin et al., "Maternal Nutrition," *Journal of Obstetrics and Gynecology,* **40**:773–785, 1972.

22 R. M. Applebaum, "The Modern Management of Successful Breast Feeding," *Pediatric Clinics of North America,* **17**(1):222, 1970.

23 Ibid.

24 Food and Nutrition Board, National Research Council, *Recommended Dietary Allowances,* 8th ed., National Academy of Sciences, Washington, D.C., 1974, p. 32.

25 Applebaum, op. cit., p. 218.

26 E. H. Erikson, *Identity: Youth & Crisis,* W. W. Norton and Company, Inc., New York, 1968.

27 American College of Obstetricians and Gynecologists, op. cit.

28 U.S. Department of Health, Education, and Welfare, Health Services and Mental Health Administration, *Ten State Nutrition Survey 1968–1970, V. Dietary,* Washington, D.C., DHEW Publ. no (HSM) 72–8133, 1976.

29 Commonwealth of Massachusetts Commission on Elderly Affairs, *A Profile of Massachusetts Elderly,* 1971.

30 N. W. Shock, "Physiologic Aspects of Aging," *Journal of the American Dietetic Association,* **56**:491–496, 1970.

31 J. L. Greger and B. S. Sciscae, "Zinc Nutriture of the Elderly," *Journal of the American Dietetic Association,* **70**(1):37–41, 1977.

32 R. A. Notzold, "Geriatric Nutrition," *Osteopathic Annals,* March 1974, pp. 32–47.

33 S. Davidson et al., "The Nutrition of a Group of Apparently Healthy Aging Persons," *Journal of Clinical Nutrition,* **10**:191–199, 1962.

34 P. Cameron et al., "Consciousness of Death across the Life Span," *Journal of Gerontology,* **28**(1):92–95, 1973.

35 Joseph Carlin, "Nutritional Study of Elderly Women in the Inner City," paper presented at the American Dietetic Association annual meeting, Boston, Mass., October 1976.

36 A. Albanese, "Nutrition and the Health of the Elderly," *Nutrition News,* **39**(2):5,8, 1976.

37 Ibid., p. 8.

38 J. Roundtree and M. Tinklin, "Food Beliefs and Practices of Selected Senior Citizens," *The Gerontologist,* December 1975, p. 548.

39 Ibid., p. 540.

40 Albanese, op. cit., p. 5.

CHAPTER 14

COMMUNITY NUTRITION

Nancie H. Herbold

KEY WORDS
Food Patterns
Yin & Yang
Kashruth
Kosher
Food Stamps
WIC
Organically Grown Food
Zen Macrobiotics

INTRODUCTION

It is important for the nutrition educator to become familiar with the myriad of factors which affect the nutritional behavior of a community—factors such as cultural patterns and ethnic background, food fads, income and spending patterns, and food resources (e.g., the Food Stamp and School Lunch programs). Before nutritional intervention programs are planned a great deal of groundwork must be done. The nutrition educator should identify the diversified ethnic groups located in the community. It is important to understand the eating practices in the mother country and the effect of immigration and Americanization on food habits. For example, foods that were available in the mother country may have provided all necessary nutrients, but in the United States such foods, if imported, may be too expensive or they may simply not be available. Other foods are then often substituted, resulting in a decreased nutritive value of the diet.

The nutrition educator also needs to identify the major health problems in the community and to determine the areas where poor nutrition is adversely affecting health. Priorities for nutrition education can then be set and nutrition intervention programs can be planned accordingly. For active outreach programs to be effective, it is necessary to assess community needs. Identification of community leaders and obtaining input from community groups can be of great help in planning and implementing such programs.

CULTURAL FOOD PATTERNS

Every culture has an accepted standard of food practices. What is eaten, when, with whom, and how much are all factors which establish food patterns or food ways within a society. These food ways, which have developed over centuries (see Chap. 1) and have many meanings (religious, symbolic, emotional), are

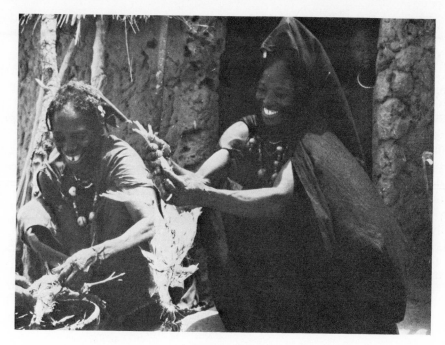

Figure 14-1
Food ways are influenced by physiological and psychological needs as well as a number of other factors—food availability, economics, politics, and food symbolism—psychological needs. (Photo courtesy of Jane McCotter O'Toole.)

not easily changed. Food ways are influenced by a variety of conditions, such as food availability, economics, politics, food symbolism, and physiological and psychological needs. (See Fig. 14-1.) It is more difficult for older individuals to change long-established food habits than it is for younger persons. When food practices are changing it is important to consider the effect this may have on the nutritional quality of the diet.

Within a given culture there are subcultures with unique eating practices which differ from the typical diet. For example, within the United States, individuals who live in the North eat differently than individuals who live in the South. Differences may be due to climate, natural resources, and food availability. Food patterns may even differ within a family unit. An individual's food habits are the

characteristic and repetitive acts that he performs under the impetus of the need to provide himself with nourishment and simultaneously to meet an assortment of social and emotional goals.[1]

Individual food habits are learned and begin early. The child is influenced by the providers of food who already have preconceived ideas, values, beliefs, and attitudes regarding food and convey these to the child.

It is possible to say that the particular way children of any society are fed and weaned has significance for the food behavior of that society.[2]

The nutrition educator must be aware of those culturally accepted norms which affect food ways. Only by working within this established framework can the nutritionist make the appropriate recommendations that will bring about behavioral change. Change is a gradual process and too many recommendations or too drastic a suggestion may overwhelm the individual. The nutrition educator must concentrate on the positive aspects of an individual's diet and encourage the strengthening of these positive habits. The following section will describe some of the common food patterns of several different cultures found within the United States. The student should be reminded, however, that the longer an individual or family has lived in the United States and has become acculturated to the United States the more their food ways will resemble those of the American diet.

Chinese

As with most peoples, the eating habits of the Chinese vary, depending upon the region of the country from which they originate. The northern area (Mandarin style cooking) has many sweet and sour dishes, noodles, and steamed breads. Shanghai is coastal and the eating habits include many fish and seafood dishes. Inland China (Szechwan style cooking) is known for its "hot" foods seasoned with pepper. Southern China (Cantonese) uses pork, chicken, and a dumpling filled with meat, Dim sum.

The Eastern philosophy of yin and yang is probably the major influence on Chinese eating habits. Some foods are thought to be more yin (cold; feminine), and others more yang (hot; masculine). The hotness or coldness has no relationship to the actual temperature of the food, but rather to its hypothesized action within the body. This theory is also used for medicinal purposes. When an individual is sick more yin or more yang foods may be recommended according to the ailment.

Milk and milk products Milk is not used as a beverage but may be used on cereal. Cheese is not

a common item in the Chinese diet, but ice cream is popular.

Protein Bean curd (tofu) is used frequently and is a good source of protein and calcium. All types of meat are used but in smaller amounts than are found in the typical American diet. Meats are usually mixed with vegetables. Chicken, duck, and pigeon eggs are preserved or fermented, as well as used fresh in cooking.

Vegetables and fruits A large variety of vegetables are used: Chinese cabbage, bok choy, broccoli, spinach, bamboo shoots, bean sprouts, snow peas, winter melon, mushrooms, and onions (see Fig. 14-2). Fruits are usually eaten fresh but some are salted or dried. Plums, dates, pineapples, oranges, and litchi (lichee) nuts are eaten.

Bread and cereals Rice is the staple of the Chinese diet. Enriched rice should be encouraged. Noodles, millet, and steamed buns are also consumed.

Miscellaneous Soy sauce, ginger, garlic, scallions, peppers, vinegar, and monosodium glutamate are used for seasoning. Peanut oil, soybean oil, and lard are used in cooking. Green tea is the usual beverage.

Nutritional Concern

The Chinese use the stir-fry method of cooking and are therefore able to retain the maximum amount of nutrients in their food. The Chinese diet may be inadequate in calcium and vitamin D because of the low intake of milk and milk products. (This low intake may be due to the high prevalance of lactose intolerance among the Oriental population.) Tofu, soy beans, mustard greens, collard greens, and kale should be encouraged to improve calcium intake. A vitamin D supplement may be needed. Protein intake should be

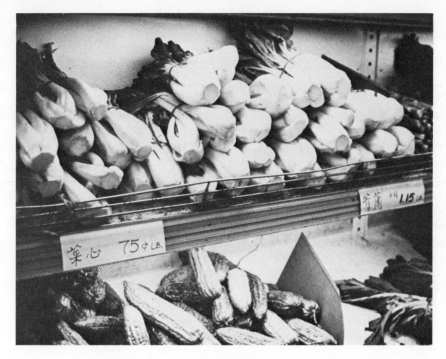

Figure 14-2
Chinese vegetables, bok choy upper right; winter melon, lower left. Recognition of the various cultural foods is important in nutritional planning for various ethnic groups. For example, vegetables such as bok choy and winter melon are significant foods in the Chinese diet. (Photo courtesy of Richard F. Herbold.)

checked for adequacy, since the serving size of meats is small.

Some individuals experience sensations of flushing, tingling, dizziness, and tachycardia after eating Chinese food. This is known as "Chinese restaurant syndrome" and is due to a sensitivity to monosodium glutamate, which tends to dilate blood vessels, thereby causing the cited effects.

Japanese

Many Japanese foods are similar to Chinese foods. Rice is a staple and tea is the common beverage. Foods are marinated, broiled, and stir-fried.

Milk and milk products Little milk or cheese is eaten; however, bean curd (tofu) is eaten.

Protein The Japanese diet contains much seafood, fresh, smoked, and raw (sashimi). Meat is used in combination with vegetables and is spiced with soy sauce. Eggs may be used in soups as well as boiled or scrambled. Miso (soy bean paste) is used in cooking.

Vegetables and fruits Spinach, broccoli, mustard greens, snow peas, taro (Japanese sweet potato), cucumbers, tomatoes, and eggplant are eaten. Vegetables may be steamed with soy sauce, pickled, or dipped in batter and fried in deep fat (tempura). Oranges, tangerines, and melons are eaten raw.

Breads and cereals White rice (short-grained) is preferred. Wheat products, such as wheat noodles cooked in broth, are also used.

Miscellaneous Dried seaweed is eaten as a snack food. Soy sauce, sweet and sour sauce, mustard sauce, and plum sauce are used in cooking.

Nutritional Concern

The Japanese diet, like the Chinese, may be low in milk and milk products, and the same nutritional concerns and suggestions apply.

Puerto Rican

The Puerto Rican people, like the Chinese, have a hot-cold theory related to food and health. Foods are grouped as either hot or cold and are eaten in different proportions depending upon the state of health. The staples of the Puerto Rican diet are salted cod, lard, coffee, sugar, rice, and beans. The main meal for most Puerto Rican people is the midday meal. It is a hot meal and the largest of the day.

Milk and milk products Coffee with a large amount of hot milk added (cafe con leche) is the major source of milk in the Puerto Rican diet. Some cheese (queso blanco), is eaten; it is similar to farmer's cheese.

Protein Chicken is frequently used, along with beef, pork, and salted cod (bacalao). Meat is used for seasoning in stews composed of vegetables rather than as a food by itself. Chickpeas, small black beans, and red kidney beans are mixed with rice and a sauce (sofrito, made from tomatoes, onion, garlic, green peppers, salt pork, and lard) and eaten almost daily.

Vegetables and fruits *Vianda* is the name given to starchy vegetables common to the Puerto Rican diet. Examples of viandas are plantain (green starchy bananas), yucca (cassava), malanga, and blanco name (white sweet potato). Salads consisting of lettuce and tomatoes with olive oil and vinegar as dressing are served frequently. Fresh pineapples, bananas, oranges, and acerola cherries (an excellent source of vitamin C) are eaten, as well as canned fruits.

Breads and cereals Rice is a staple of the Puerto Rican diet. Although breads and cereals are gaining in use, they are not yet generally accepted. Bread is sometimes eaten for breakfast.

Miscellaneous Lard and salt pork are common flavorings. Sugar is used in large amounts to sweeten beverages. Guava and mango paste may be eaten for snacks. Black malt beer (malta) is a nonalcoholic beverage believed to be very nourishing and is given to pregnant women and underweight children.

Nutritional Concern

Many pregnant Puerto Rican women develop megaloblastic anemia.[3] Generally, their diets meet the recommended dietary allowance (RDA) for folacin.[4] Therefore, they may require an intake which is higher than the RDA for folic acid. Foods high in folacin (see Chap. 6) should be encouraged.

Obesity is another problem among the Puerto Rican population. Decreasing the amount of fat used in cooking as well as decreasing the sugar consumption should be stressed.

Mexican-American

The Spanish-American eating habits are a blend of several different cultures—those of the Spanish settlers, the Indians, and the Anglos. The resulting food pattern is common among the Mexican-Americans living in the Southwestern United States.

Milk and milk products Limited amounts of milk are used, usually in the form of custards or rice puddings. Cheese is a common item in the diet.

Protein Meat is eaten only a few times per week, usually as hamburger or chicken mixed with vegetables. Beans (pinto and garbanzo) are eaten at every meal. They may be prepared by boiling and then frying (refried beans; frijoles refritos), or may be boiled and added to hamburger seasoned with chili, peppers, and garlic (chili con carne).

Vegetables and fruits Chili peppers, tomatoes, and corn are the most popular vegetables. Oranges, apples, bananas, and some canned fruits may be used.

Breads and cereals Corn is the basic grain of the Mexican diet. Tortillas, a dietary staple, are flat cakes made from ground corn that is soaked in lime water and then baked on a griddle. Enchiladas and tacos are made by filling the tortillas with a variety of meat mixtures. Cornmeal gruel and oatmeal are sometimes eaten with milk.

Miscellaneous Lard is used freely. Seasonings include chili pepper, onion, garlic, oregano, and coriander. Coffee is the common beverage and may be given to children.

Nutritional Concern

The Ten State Nutrition Survey found a low vitamin A intake among the Mexican-American population,[5] however, this finding is now suspect of being a laboratory error. Nevertheless foods that are high in vitamin A such as chili peppers, carrots, and avocados can be encouraged. The folacin content of the diet may be low and dark green vegetables must be increased. There is a high incidence of obesity in the Mexican-American population. Decreasing the amount of fat used in cooking should be suggested as well as omitting any high-energy foods which are low in nutrients.

Black

"Soul" food, a name now associated with black eating habits, had its origins in the South where both poor blacks and poor whites followed the same eating patterns.

Milk and milk products Limited amounts of milk are used; this may be due to a high preva-lance of lactose intolerance. Buttermilk (sour milk) is used in cooking and as a beverage. Cheese is eaten in dishes such as macaroni and cheese.

Protein All types of meat, fish, and chicken are eaten and are frequently fried. Pig's feet, neck bones, ham hocks, chitterlings (intestines), hog maws (stomach), and spareribs are popular. Bacon and sausage are commonly eaten at breakfast.

Vegetables and fruits Vegetables are cooked for long periods of time, with salt pork, ham hocks, or bacon fat used as seasoning. Water-soluble vitamins will be lost in the cooking water; therefore individuals should be encouraged to decrease the amount of water and the cooking time in order to conserve nutrients. The liquid from these vegetables is known as 'pot liquor' and is eaten with cornbread. Popular vegetables include turnips, mustard greens, collard greens, black-eyed peas, okra, green beans, corn, lima beans, white potatoes, and sweet potatoes. Sweet potatoes may be fried, baked, candied, or used to make pies. Oranges, apples, bananas, peaches, and watermelon are popular fruits.

Breads and cereals Grits, cornbread, biscuits, and muffins are eaten. Rice is more frequently used than potatoes.

Miscellaneous Gravies are used on rice, potatoes, and meat. Cakes and pies are popular desserts. Molasses is used as a sweetener. Large amounts of soft drinks and fruit drinks are consumed.

Nutritional Concern

Obesity is a problem among black women of lower socioeconomic status. Encouragement should be given to reduce snack foods, sweets, soft drinks, and fats. The Ten State Nutrition Survey found a high incidence of low hematocrits and hemoglobins in the black population.[6] Foods high in iron should be encouraged. Hypertension is another health problem for this group. Foods high in sodium such as salt pork, ham hocks, bacon, and sausage should be limited as a preventive measure against hypertension.

Jewish

The Jewish dietary laws, Kashruth, are observed by many members of the Jewish faith. The extent to which these laws are followed or interpreted will depend upon which religious group the individual may belong to:

Orthodox Jews observe the laws strictly.

Reform Jews do not place great emphasis on the dietary rules.

Conservative Jews are somewhere in the middle.[7]

Kosher, which means clean or fit, includes foods such as grains, fruits, vegetables, tea, and coffee which are considered naturally kosher foods. Those foods which are not naturally kosher (meats, poultry) must undergo a "koshering" process before they can be eaten by those individuals observing Kashruth. In this process the animals must be slaughtered in accordance with a particular ritual; the meat is then soaked in salted water to remove all blood. Only certain types of animals can be koshered. Animals that are cloven-hoofed quadrupeds and chew a cud can be used (beef, lamb). Pork and pork products and fish without scales and fins (i.e., shellfish) are prohibited.

Milk and meat may not be eaten together. Milk should be consumed immediately before or 6 hours after eating meat. Seperate plates must be used for dairy and meat meals.

Many foods will have the emblem Ⓤ on the package, which signifies endorsement by the Union of Orthodox Jewish Congregations of America, indicating that the food was packaged under rabbinical supervision. The letter **K** appearing on foods also indicates rabbinical supervision.

The Jewish sabbath starts at sundown Friday and continues until Saturday evening. No cooking is allowed on the sabbath; therefore food is prepared ahead to be used on Saturday.

Passover is a religious week when no leavened bread products are used. A special set of dishes is used during this week, again with different plates for meat and for dairy foods. Therefore, the Jew observing Kashruth has four sets of dishes, everyday dishes for meat and for dairy, and a separate set for use during Passover.

Yom Kippur (Day of Atonement) is a religious holy day when fasting is observed for 24 h.

Milk and milk products All types of milk and milk products are used.

Protein Orthodox Jews will eat only the forequarters from allowed animals. All types of beef, lamb, chicken, and fish are used. A few specialties include chopped liver, lox (smoked salmon), gefilte fish (fish filet chopped and seasoned and stuffed), and herring.

Vegetables and fruits All types of fruits and vegetables are eaten. Borscht (beet, cabbage, or spinach soup) is served hot or cold with sour cream. Potato pancakes (latkes), carrot pudding (tzimmes), and cooked dried fruits (prunes, raisins, and apricots) are other favorites.

Breads and cereals Bagels, egg bread (challah), dark breads (which contain no milk and can be eaten with meat) and matzo (an unleavened bread product allowed during Passover) are bread products commonly consumed.

Nutritional Concern
The Jewish diet contains many foods high in saturated fat and cholesterol. Individuals should be counseled to modify their intake of these foods.

NONTRADITIONAL FOOD PRACTICES

It is important for the student to remember that food fulfills a number of needs beyond physiological nourishment—psychological, emotional, religious, and symbolic (see Chap. 10). In this section nontraditional food practices will be reviewed to sensitize the student of nutrition to the varied motivational factors that influence these eating practices. An understanding of these factors will enable the nutritional educator to better counsel these clients.

Food Fads

The public is exposed to many types of food misinformation via the media. Food fads usually meet one or more of the following criteria:[8]

1 Rapid rise and fall in popularity
2 Stretching facts or using them out of context
3 Special appeal to certain segments of the population
4 Simplistic
5 Promotion of special virtues of a food
6 Restriction of certain foods in the belief that they are harmful

In addition to characterizing the types of food fads the individuals drawn to them can be described as well. Beal has grouped these individuals into eight categories that specify the type of need which the food practice fulfills.[9] They are as follows:

1 Miracle seeker—food fad fulfills the need of self-worth and stability regarding health
2 Antiestablishmentarian—food provides a vehicle to express values
3 Super-health seeker—food is used as an ego defense to delay the aging process
4 Distruster of medical profession—food is used to control one's own body and eliminate dependence upon others

5 Fashion follower—food is used as a means for acceptance
6 Authority seeker—food is used as an area of expertise
7 Truth seeker—must experience first hand claims regarding food
8 One concerned about the uncertainties of living—needs stability regarding the world

It is important for the nutrition counselor to be aware of the various needs that food fads fulfill. In this way, food substitutions of a more nutritious nature can be suggested while supporting the social and psychological needs of the individual.[10] Table 14-1 outlines some of the more common food fads.

Natural, Organically Grown, and Health Foods

Natural foods Natural foods are generally regarded as those foods which remain in their original state. Natural foods have a minimum of processing and contain no artificial ingredients.

Organically grown foods The term *organic food* is a misnomer—all foods are organic. *Organically grown food* is more accurate. It refers to food grown without the use of pesticides, fumigants, or synthetic fertilizers, and containing no preservatives or synthetic coloring agents. Individuals who favor organically grown food may eat meats only from animals that receive no antibiotics or hormones and that are fed only organically grown grains.

There is no evidence that organically grown food offers any extra nutritional benefit. Growing food organically cannot produce a large crop yield and consequently the consumer must pay anywhere from 30 to 100 percent more for organically grown food.[11] Presently, there are no federal regulations governing the labeling of organic food. Therefore, it is important for the consumer to become acquainted with the stores in their neigh-

TABLE 14-1 COMMON FOOD FADS

Name	Description	Comment
Mayo Clinic diet (*not related to the Mayo Clinic in Rochester, Minn.*)	Promotes quick weight loss. High-protein diet consisting of grapefruit, meats and vegetables	Promotes grapefruit as having fat-burning properties. No scientific evidence to back up this claim
Stillman diet	Promotes quick weight loss. High-protein, high-fat diet consisting of unlimited amounts of meat, fish, eggs, low-fat cheese, 8 glasses of water, plus a vitamin supplement	Unbalanced. May be harmful for anyone with gout, diabetes, or kidney problems. High in cholesterol and saturated fat. No metabolic advantage over a well-balanced low-calorie diet
Atkins diet	Promotes quick weight loss. No carbohydrate for first week, to produce ketosis; carbohydrate gradually added to reach a maximum of 50 g. Amount of protein and fat unlimited	Unbalanced. High in saturated fat and cholesterol. May be harmful for anyone with gout, diabetes, or kidney problems. No metabolic advantage over a wall-balanced low-calorie diet
Simeon diet	Injections of the hormone human chorionic gonaditropin (HCG) plus a 500-kcal diet	No scientific evidence to suggest HCG is useful for the treatment of obesity
Mucusless diet	Allows only raw and cooked fruits, "starchless" vegetables, and cooked or raw leafy green vegetables. All are considered "mucus" free. Diet, fasting, or both can cure all disease by preventing mucus formation	Unbalanced. Claims are not substantiated scientifically
Adele Davis	Recommends massive doses of vitamins for all. Recommends a variety of foods to cure ills—brewer's yeast, dessicated liver, etc.	Scare tactics are used. Scientific information, often out of context, is mixed with author's own theories
Hypoglycemia Foundation	Claims that millions of people have hypoglycemia and are undiagnosed. Advocates many expensive lab tests and use of injections of whole adrenocortical extracts to treat hypoglycemia	According to the American Medical Association "these claims are not supported by medical evidence"*
Jerome Rodale	Owner of Rodale Press (which prints *Prevention Magazine* and *Organic Gardening and Farming*); makes such fallacious statements as that pumpkin seeds will cure prostatic disease;† opposed to organized medicine and the food industry	Many erroneous statements with no scientific backup
Orthomolecular Therapy	Advocates use of megavitamins (large quantities, usually of the water-soluble type) for the treatment of a variety of mental disorders	To date there is no evidence that this is an effective mode of treatment

* American Medical Association, "Statement on Hypoglycemia," 223:682, 1973.

† J. I. Rodale *Prostate*, Rodale Press, Emmaus Pa., 1969.

borhood in order to know which stores are reputable and to be sure that the food is indeed organically grown. The positive aspects of organic gardening include a reduction of pollution and a concern for our environment as well as a reminder of how many additives we are using in our food.[12]

Health Foods Health foods may or may not include natural or organically grown foods.

They are foods usually thought to impart good health and are generally purchased in health food stores. Health foods may be advertised as preventing or curing illness. Examples of some commonly used health foods include tiger's milk, brewer's yeast, blackstrap molasses, desiccated liver, kelp, and sea salt.

Natural and Synthetic Vitamins

There is no scientific or legal definition for the term "natural" vitamin. Two common fallacies associated with natural vitamins are:

1 Natural vitamins are better than synthetic vitamins.
2 Natural vitamins contain no synthetic ingredients.[13]

The chemical properties of synthetic and natural vitamins are the same.[14] One manufacturer of a "natural" vitamin C compound uses rose hips with added chemical ascorbic acid; "natural" B vitamins have been made with brewer's yeast and synthetic B vitamins. Consumers may pay considerably more for natural or organic vitamins since they are more difficult to produce than synthetic ones, but they offer no extra nutritional benefit.

Zen Macrobiotics

Zen macrobiotics was introduced to the United States by George Ohsawa. Followers of the macrobiotic philosophy believe that the individual should live off his or her "natural" environment and achieve harmony by a healthful existence from the balance of yin and yang. Foods are grouped as having more yin or more yang:

Yang = meats—eggs—fish—grains—
    vegetables—fruits—dairy products—
    sugar—alcohol—drugs—chemicals = Yin

Yin and yang are used to determine appropriate food combinations. Climate and gender as well as the emotional, physical, and spiritual state of an individual influence the dietary proportions of yin and yang.

There are ten dietary stages incorporated into the macrobiotic philosophy which become progressively more restrictive (see Table 14-2). The lower level diets contain cereals, vegetables, fruits, seafoods, and desserts; the higher level diets consist of 100 percent cereal, usually brown rice. Fluids are limited at all levels. The higher level diets are not nutritionally adequate. Scurvy, anemia, hypoproteinemia, hypercalcemia, emaciation due to starvation, and death can result.[15] Fortunately most macrobiotic enthusiasts follow the lower level diets, which can be planned to meet nutrient needs. Brown and Bergan, studying the nutrient intakes of macrobiotic individuals, found their diets to be adequate in most nutrients.[16] Those nutrients that were found to be limited were energy, calcium, riboflavin, and iron (in women only). They also studied a small group of children eating macrobiotic diets and found their energy and calcium intakes to be low.[17]

Followers of the macrobiotic philosophy believe that illness can be cured through proper eating. This is a dangerous assumption which can prove fatal if more traditional medical care is not sought for an illness.

Vegetarianism

Although vegetarianism has been practiced for many years by Seventh-Day Adventists and Trappist monks it is only within the past 10 years that it has gained in popularity among young Americans.[18]

Individuals choose to become vegetarians for a number of reasons, the most common being:

Religious preference
Health concerns
Environmental considerations
Humanitarian issues
Economics
Political reasons

TABLE 14-2 MACROBIOTIC DIET

| Diet level | Content, % | | | | | | | Drinking liquid |
	Cereals	Vegetables	Soup	Animal products	Fruits, salads	Desserts	
7	100	—	—	—	—	—	Sparingly
6	90	10*	—	—	—	—	Sparingly
5	80	20	—	—	—	—	Sparingly
4	70	20	10	—	—	—	Sparingly
3	60	30	10	—	—	—	Sparingly
2	50	30	10	10	—	—	Sparingly
1	40	30	10	20	—	—	Sparingly
−1	30	30	10	20	10	—	Sparingly
−2	20	30	10	25	10	5	Sparingly
−3	10	30	10	30	15	5	Sparingly

* Refined vegetables. In other regimens vegetables are not refined.

Source: R. Frankle and F. K. Heussenstamm, "Food Zealotry and Youth, New Dilemmas for Professionals," *American Journal of Public Health,* January 1974, p. 15.

The term *vegetarian* is applied to those individuals who do not eat meat. However, within this group there are several different types:

1 Vegans: strict vegetarians who eat or drink no animal or dairy products

2 Lacto-ovo vegetarians: those who drink milk and eat eggs but consume no other animal product

3 Lacto vegetarians: those whose only source of an animal product is milk

4 Ovo-vegetarians: those who eat eggs but no other animal product

5 Pesco-vegetarians: those who eat fish but no other animal product

6 Vegetarians who eat fish and chicken but no red meat

7 Fruitarians: those whose diet is composed chiefly of fruits and nuts

Vegetarian diets will be nutritionally sound if they include a wide variety of nuts, legumes, grains, fruits, vegetables, milk, and milk products. The diets of vegans and fruitarians are the only diets which offer no source of complete protein. It is important for the nutrition educator to teach these individuals the use of complementary proteins—beans and rice, tacos and beans, etc. (see Table 14–3).

Most young vegetarians do not use textured vegetable protein as it resembles meat in some products and the cost is prohibitive. Seventh-Day Adventists, however, may use these products.

Meat and meat products are the chief sources of vitamin B_{12} in our diet. Vegetarians therefore may need a B_{12} supplement. Calcium intake should be evaluated for adequacy and dark green vegetables, especially kale, collards, mustard, turnip, and dandelion greens, and soybeans should be encouraged.

Milk is fortified with vitamin D and is the major dietary source of this nutrient. Vitamin D is also supplied by the action of the sun on the skin. If milk is not used and the individual is only outdoors occasionally a vitamin D supplement may be needed.

Following a vegetarian diet offers several advantages. It is lower in cholesterol and saturated fat than the ordinary diet, and high in fiber. Most vegetarians are not overweight, perhaps because of the high fiber and water content of vegetables as well as the avoidance of high-fat snack foods.

TABLE 14-3 COMPLEMENTARY PROTEINS

Food group	Complementary proteins
Legumes	Legumes and rice
	Soybeans, rice, and wheat
	Beans and wheat
	Soybeans, corn, and milk
	Beans and corn
	Soybeans, wheat, and sesame seeds
	Soybeans, peanuts, and sesame seeds
	Soybeans, sesame seeds, and wheat
Grains	Rice and legumes
	Corn and legumes
	Wheat and legumes
	Rice and milk
	Wheat and cheese
	Wheat and milk
	Wheat, peanuts, and milk
	Wheat, sesame seeds, and soybeans
	Brewer's yeast and rice
Vegetables	Lima beans ⎫
	Peas ⎪ and Sesame seeds
	Brussels sprouts ⎬ Brazil nuts
	Cauliflower ⎪ Mushrooms
	Broccoli ⎭
Nuts and seeds	Peanuts, sesame seeds, and soybeans
	Sesame seeds and beans
	Sesame seeds, soybeans, and wheat
	Peanuts and milk
	Peanut and sunflower seeds
	Peanuts, wheat, and milk
	Sesame seeds, wheat, and soybeans

Source: Adapted from F. M. Lappe, *Diet for a Small Planet*, Friends of the Earth/Ballantine Books, Inc., New York, 1971.

COMMUNITY RESOURCES

Knowledge of food resources is essential, particularly in low-income communities. Helping clients to enroll in the Food Stamp Program, the Special Supplemental Feeding Program for Women, Infants, and Children (WIC), or Elderly Feeding programs will help them to stretch limited incomes. Government programs and community agencies attempt to provide people with a minimum quality of life and it is up to the health professional to help people, especially those with limited incomes, to utilize available resources to the utmost.

Addressed in this section are two examples of community resources, their purpose, their target population, and a general description of their function. Others are summarized in Tables 14–4 and 14–5.

Food Stamp Program

The Food Stamp program (see Table 14–4) began in 1964 and has grown to become a food program servicing a large segment of the population—18.5 million Americans[19] (although approximately 30 million individuals are eligible[20]).

It is important that the nutrition educator become familiar with the eligibility requirements and how the Food Stamp program operates.

Food stamps are coupons that can be used in place of money to buy food. The individual is free to select any type of food (alcohol, tobacco, and pet food are excluded). Food stamps cannot be used to purchase cleaning items, soap, detergent, or paper goods. Food stamps can be used in any store, supermarket, or food cooperative that has registered to accept food stamps. Almost all large grocery stores and many small stores are registered.

Individuals or families who are eligible for food stamps include anyone who receives public assistance and households where incomes and financial resources are limited. All households of the same size receive the same amount of food stamps. However, the cost of the food stamps will vary, depending upon income (i.e., the smaller the income, the less paid for the food stamps). Therefore, a family of four can receive approximately $155 worth of food stamps, but depending upon income one family might pay $100 while another family may only pay $50 for the same $155 worth of food stamps.

Individuals can apply for food stamps at a variety of locations which vary from state to state. As previously mentioned, those individuals or households receiving public assistance are automatically eligible, and fill out a sim-

TABLE 14-4 FOOD PROGRAMS

Program	Legislation	Funding	Eligibility	Services provided	Other
School Lunch program	National School Lunch Act of 1946 and Section II amendment to the National School Lunch Act and the Child Nutrition Act of 1966	USDA reimbursement for partial cost of food. Federal funds aid schools in poverty areas to purchase equipment	All public and private nonprofit schools	Type A school lunch: 8 oz milk, 2 oz protein, 1 starch serving, ¾ cup vegetable, ¾ cup fruit. Operates on a nonprofit basis. Provides free or reduced-price lunch for those unable to pay	USDA authorized to buy food through the Surplus Removal and Price Support program to distribute to schools. Schools must agree to participate in school lunch or breakfast program
School Breakfast program	The Child Nutrition Act of 1966 funded the program for 2 years. An amendment in 1971 extended the program further	USDA reimbursement for food cost. In areas of severe need 80% of operating costs, food expense, and labor are covered. 1971 amendment extended this benefit to 100% reimbursement	Schools in poverty areas where children travel long distances to school; all children in these areas are eligible	Breakfast: 8 oz milk, 1 slice of bread or equivalent grain product, ½ cup fresh fruit or full-strength fruit or vegetable juice. Schools are asked to provide a protein food as often as possible	USDA authorized to buy food via the Surplus Removal and Price support program
Food Stamp programs	Food Stamp Act of 1964 (there had been pilot programs prior to this law)	USDA and state funding. Food Stamp program at the state level is usually run by the Dept. of Public Welfare	All individuals who meet financial criteria	Food stamps or coupons that can be used like money to buy food. Increases purchasing power by reducing the cost of food	

Program	Legislation	Funding	Eligibility	Benefits	Requirements
The Special Supplemental Food Program for Women, Infants, and Children (WIC)	1972 amendment to the Child Nutrition Act of 1966	Federal funds provide cash grants to states	Health centers in areas of high risk because of inadequate nutrition & income Individuals eligible—Pregnant women; mothers up to 6 months postpartum; nursing mothers up to 1 year; children to age 5; if at nutritional risk and income as determined by a professional	Mothers and children receive monthly: 3 l q milk 2½ doz eggs 4 (8-oz) pkgs iron-fortified cereal 6 (46-oz) cans fruit or vegetable juice Equal amounts of Swiss, American and cheddar cheese may be substituted for milk at the rate of 1 lb cheese for 3 qt milk Infants receive: 31 (13-oz) cans of iron fortified formula 3 (8-oz) pkgs or iron fortified cereal 15 (4-oz) or 2 (46-oz) cans of fruit juice Nutritional education also provided	Health center must collect the following data: weight height head circumference hematocrit hemoglobin
Elderly Feeding program	Title VII of the Older Americans Act	USDA and state funds reimburse for partial cost of food	All nonprofit organizations; all individuals over the age of 60	Hot Meal: 8 oz milk 2 oz meat 1 starch serving 2 (¾-cup) servings fruit & vegetable	May provide 10% of the meals served to home-bound elderly

TABLE 14-5 COMMUNITY RESOURCES

Resource	Comment
Headstart program	Educational enrichment and nutritional services for children aged 3–5 years from low-income areas
Visiting Nurse Association	Provides nutritional information to clients— many have a nutritionist as a consultant
American Heart Association American Diabetes Association American Cancer Society	Local chapters run screening clinics, pro- vide educational material for the public and professionals
American Dietetic Association	Many state chapters sponsor Dial-a-Dietitian whereby public may call and ask questions regarding nutrition
National Dairy Council	State branches provide educational material, run workshops in schools, employ nutritionists and home economists
Departments of Public Health (state & local)	Conduct clinics, health screening programs; provide educational materials. Nutritionists work to set up needed nutritional programs in the community
Agricultural Extension Service	Provides nutrition educa- tion to the community. Runs workshops and trains individuals from the community to work as nutrition aides
Consumer councils (state, voluntary)	Provide nutrition informa- tion and help individuals take legal action against misrepresentation
Schools, churches, agencies	May provide meals to special age groups

ple application form. Non–public assistance households are required to complete a much more lengthy application and must be interviewed. This is necessary to verify income and financial resources, in order to determine how much must be paid for the food stamps. To facilitate the food stamp application procedure, the individual should bring proof of income (pay stubs) and proof of expenses (rent receipts, medical bills, utility bills, etc.) when applying. Once eligibility has been established, an identification card, which is needed for purchase and use of the food stamps, will be issued. Then an Authorization-to-Purchase card (ATP) will be received in the mail 1 or 2 times per month, notifying the individual of the amount of food stamps that can be purchased and how much they will cost.

Food stamps are sold in a variety of locations that differ from state to state. Some of the more common sites include banks, post offices, food stamp offices, and community action agencies. These groups are paid by the government for each food stamp transaction. The individual goes to one of these locations, presents the identification card and the ATP card, pays the appropriate amount of money, and then receives the stamps. One of the problems encountered at the inception of the Food Stamp program was that recipients found it difficult to gather the full amount of money needed to purchase a month's food stamps. To help alleviate this problem food stamp recipients can now buy all, three-fourths, one-half, or one-fourth of the monthly supply of stamps. Once the food stamps are purchased they can then be used to buy food.

A common misconception about the Food Stamp program is that many middle-income families are receiving food stamps. According to the U.S. Department of Agriculture, 50 percent of food stamp households have a take-home pay of less than $3,000 per year and 92 percent of all food stamp recipients are in households which earn less than $7,000 per year.[21]

The Special Supplemental Feeding Program for Women, Infants, and Children

The Special Supplemental Feeding Program for Women, Infants, and Children (WIC) was established in 1972 as an amendment to the Child Nutrition Act of 1966. The purpose of the program is to prevent as well as correct nutritional deficiencies, thereby abating the physical and mental damage to infants that can be caused by malnutrition. To achieve this goal, approved health centers provide food to pregnant and lactating women (up to 1 year), postpartum women (up to 6 months), and infants and children (until age 5). Eligibility for the program is determined by the following criteria:

1 Individuals must reside in a low-income area serviced by an approved health care center which administers the WIC program.
2 Individuals must be eligible for free or reduced-rate health care at this facility.
3 Individuals must be considered by a health professional to be at nutritional risk because of inadequate nutrition and income.

Nutritional risk has never been clearly defined; however, those criteria for pregnant women, postpartum women, (up to 6 months), and lactating women (up to 1 year) usually include:

Nutritional anemia
Inadequate dietary intake
Inappropriate growth patterns (overweight, underweight, stunting)
High-risk pregnancy (premature or low-birth-weight infants, miscarriage, high parity, short interconceptual time)

The criteria for nutritional risk in an infant or child usually include:

Nutritional anemia
Inadequate dietary intake
Poor growth pattern (obesity, failure to thrive)

The foods that are provided by the program (see Table 14–4) were selected for their specific nutrient content: high-biological-value protein, iron, calcium, and vitamins A and C. These are nutrients known to be lacking in the diets of populations at nutritional risk.[23]

Each WIC program center decides on the method it will use to provide these foods to the participants. The most commonly used method is the voucher system, whereby participants are given coupons that are redeemable for food at particular stores. Other methods include home delivery, and warehousing by the health center (which then distributes the food items).

The participants in the program usually return monthly to receive their vouchers for food and return periodically for medical check-ups. The minimal medical data that must be collected by the health center include height, weight, head circumference, hematocrit, and hemoglobin. It is hoped that having the participants return regularly will encourage and familiarize them with the use of the health care system.

If the community has a WIC program it is important for the nutrition educator to initiate outreach. Federal funds are not provided for this activity; therefore the nutrition educator will need to publicize the program via word of mouth, media, community leaders, church groups, the Visiting Nurse Association, day care centers, headstart programs, and community action agencies. It should also be emphasized that the WIC program does not take the place of the Food Stamp program. Women who are participating in the WIC program may also be eligible for food stamps. The WIC program is designed to supplement the diet with food.

Evaluation is an important component of any program if effectiveness is to be ascertained. There has been an evaluation of the WIC program; however, few conclusions can be reached. This is due to:[24]

1 A lack of uniformity in health and nutritional data collected by each WIC program
2 No universally accepted nutritional and health standards
3 Lack of exact determination of nutrient requirements which will improve or maintain nutritional status
4 Inadequate indicators to determine an infant's mental development
5 Difficulty in finding and using a control group

The preliminary findings did reveal (though their accuracy is questionable due to the aforementioned problems) the following: an increase in height, weight, and head circumference among infants enrolled in the program; a decrease in anemia among both infants and mothers; an increase in the consumption of protein, calcium, phosphorus, iron, vitamin A, thiamine, riboflavin, niacin, ascorbic acid, and folacin; increased weight gain by pregnant women; and increased birth weight among minority-group infants.[25]

STUDY QUESTIONS

1 Why is it important for the nutritional educator to understand cultural food patterns?
2 The Mexican-American diet may be inadequate in what nutrients?
3 Explain the Jewish dietary laws.
4 Describe the process that an individual must follow in order to obtain food stamps.
5 What are the various types of vegetarian diets? What nutrients may be inadequate in these diets?

CASE STUDY 14-1

S. C. is a 3-months-postpartum mother who immigrated to the United States from China 1 year ago. She is currently unemployed, as is her husband. This is her first visit to the health center and she is referred to the nutritionist for dietary evaluation.

Her typical meal plan includes:

Breakfast
Roll
Tea

Lunch
Dim sum
Rice

Orange
Tea

Supper
Chicken with bok choy, bamboo shoots, broccoli, and rice
Pineapple
Tea

Case Study Questions

1 *What nutrients appear to be inadequate in S. C's diet?*
2 *What recommendation would you make?*
3 *What food programs would you suggest?*

REFERENCES

1 H. Gift et al., *Nutrition Behavior and Change,* Prentice-Hall Inc., Englewood Cliffs, N.J., 1972, pp. 29–30.

2 M. Mead, "Food and the Family," in *Food and People,* UNESCO, New York, 1953, p. 7.

3 V. Herbert, "Symposium: Folic Acid Deficiency," *American Journal of Clinical Nutrition,* vol. 23, 1970, p. 841.

4 S. Parker and J. Bowery, "Folacin in Diets of Puerto Rican and Black Women in Relation to Food Practices," *Journal of Nutrition Education,* vol. 8, no. 2, 1976, pp. 73–76.

5 U.S. Department of Health, Education, and Welfare, Health Services and Mental Health Administration, *Ten State Nutrition Survey, 1968–1970,* DHEW Publ. no. (HSM) 72-8133, 1970.

6 Ibid.

7 A. Natow et al., "Integrating the Jewish Dietary Laws into a Dietetic Program," *Journal of the American Dietetic Association,* vol. 67, 1975, p. 14.

8 R. Schaffer and R. Yetley, "Social Psychology of Food Faddism," *Journal of the American Dietetic Association,* vol. 69, 1975, p. 129.

9 V. Beal, "Food Faddism and Organic and Nautral Foods," paper presented at the National Dairy Council Food Writers Conference, Newport, R.I., May 1972.

10 R. Schaffer and E. Yetley, op. cit., p. 133.

11 Review, *Nutrition Reviews,* vol. 32, Suppl., July 1974, p. 53.

12 F. Clydesdale and F. J. Francis, *Food, Nutrition, and You,* Prentice-Hall, Inc., Englewood Cliffs, N.J., 1977. p. 89.

13 Consumer's Union, *The Medicine Show,* Consumer's Union, Mt. Vernon, N.Y., 1974.

14 A. Kamil, "How Natural Are Those Natural Vitamins," *Nutrition Reviews,* vol. 32 Suppl., July 1974.

15 Presentation of the Passaic, N.J., Grand Jury, "Zen Macrobiotic Diet Hazardous," *Public Health News,* New Jersey Department of Health, June 1966, pp. 132–135.

16 P. T. Brown and J. G. Bergan, "The Dietary Status of 'New' Vegetarians," *Journal of the American Dietetic Association,* Vol. 67, 1975, pp. 455–459.

17 Ibid.

18 J. T. Dwyer et al., *"New Vegetarians," Journal of the American Dietetic Association,* vol. 64, 1974, p. 376.

19 Food Stamp Committee, "The Facts About Food Stamps," Washington, D.C., November–December 1975, p. 1.

20 Ibid. p. 6.

21 U.S. Department of Agriculture, "Food Stamp Program: A Report in Accordance with the Senate Resolution 58," presented to the Senate Agriculture Committee, June 30, 1975.

22 Massachusetts Community Action Program Directors Association, "WIC, a Guide to the Women, Infants and Children Feeding Program, January 1976, p. 3.

23 Comptroller General of The United States, *Report to Congress: Observation on Evaluation of the Special Supplemental Food Program,* Food and Nutrition Service, USDA RED-75-310, December 1974, p. 2–3.

24 Ibid., pp. 23–24.

25 J. C. Edozien et al., *Medical Evaluation of the Special Supplemental Food Program for Women, Infants and Children,* Vol. II, *Results,* Department of Nutrition, School of Public Health, University of North Carolina, Chapel Hill, N.C., July 15, 1976.

PART THREE

THE CONSEQUENCES
OF DISEASE ON
NUTRITIONAL STATUS

Advances in technology have tempered the effect of disease in many cases, but unfortunately the routine and policies of hospitals and clinics have allowed little change in the total care of the patient. Upon hospitalization, patients lose their individual control as they face the ever-present threat of death and dying and the awareness of finality. Mood swings, from withdrawal to denial, to anger, to bargaining, to depression, and, in children, acceptance with regression, are all characteristic of this process. It is in the midst of such conflict and in the maze of hospital or clinic routines—laboratory tests, x-rays, physical examinations, medications—that you will interact with your patient. The patient in a debilitated state that is conditioned by age, emotions, culture, and past general health must marshal physiological and psychological resources to offset the disease and adapt to being sick, treated, and possibly hospitalized (see "The Psychology of Diet," in Chap. 10).

The individual's response to food, both physiological and psychological, is altered by the disease state. The disease itself or the drugs used in treatment may interfere with nutrient effectiveness or alter taste sensations. (see Table III-1), and the food presented to the patient or the special therapeutic diet may now be rejected as the patient maintains his or her last vestige of control. Nutrition is essential in the treatment and rehabilitation of the patient and the cause of indifferent appetite and food complaints (legitimate in some instances) must

TABLE III-1 COMMONLY USED DRUGS WITH NUTRITIONAL IMPLICATIONS

Drug	Potential nutrient interference	Side effects with nutritional implications
Adrenal corticosteroids	Vitamins C, A, D; folic acid, pyridoxine, calcium, potassium, zinc	Gastric inflammation; may produce ulcers
Antibiotics		
Chloramphenicol	Folic acid, pyridoxine, riboflavin, vitamins B$_{12}$, A; iron	Aplastic and hypoplastic anemia, nausea, vomiting, diarrhea may occur; glossitis and stomatitis
Erythromycin		Inhibits protein synthesis; gastrointestinal discomfort, cramping. Nausea, vomiting, and diarrhea occur occasionally. May form salts with acids—avoid orange, lemon, cranberry juices and other acid drinks
Neomycin	Vitamins B$_{12}$, A; iron, calcium, potassium	Glossitis, stomatitis, nausea, vomiting, diarrhea. May produce malabsorption with increased fecal fat
Penicillin	Potassium	Nausea, vomiting, occasionally hemolytic anemia
Tetracycline	Vitamins C, K; folic acid, riboflavin, calcium, zinc, magnesium	If used during tooth development may cause permanent staining. May cause increased blood urea nitrogen, anorexia, nausea, vomiting, diarrhea, glossitis, dysphagia, hemolytic anemia. Should not be taken with milk, since calcium impairs absorption
Anticoagulants		
Coumarin derivatives	Vitamin K, alcohol	Gastrointestinal bleeding, nausea, vomiting, diarrhea
Anticonvulsants		
Phenobarbital	Folic acid, pyridoxine, vitamins B$_{12}$, D, K; calcium	Nausea, megaloblastic anemia
Antidepressants (Monoamine oxidase inhibitors) Phenelzine Tranylcypromine		Foods high in tyramine should be avoided as they may precipitate a hypertensive crisis. Foods to avoid: aged cheddar cheese, alcohol, yogurt, sour cream, yeast, bananas, broad beans, canned figs, raisins, chicken liver, chocolate, cola, coffee, tea, pickled herring, licorice
Antihypertensives Diuretics		
Chlorothiazide	Pyridoxine, riboflavin, zinc, potassium, sodium	Fluid and electrolyte imbalance
Furosemide		Fluid and electrolyte imbalance
Hydralazine		Anorexia, nausea, vomiting, diarrhea, constipation, reduction in hemoglobin
Antilipemic agents		
Cholestyramine	Vitamins A, B$_{12}$, D, K; calcium, iron	Binds bile acids, may interfere with normal fat absorption. Constipation, flatulence, nausea, diarrhea
Clofibrate	Vitamins A, B$_{12}$; iron	Nausea, diarrhea, vomiting, anemia
Cardiac glycosides		
Digitalis	Calcium, magnesium	Nausea, vomiting
Levodopa	Vitamin C, pyridoxine, potassium	Drug effectiveness decreased by increased intakes of protein. Anorexia, nausea, vomiting, burning sensation of the tongue, bitter taste
Uricosuric Agents		
Allopurinol	Riboflavin, calcium, magnesium, potassium	Increased fluid intake is desirable. Nausea, vomiting, diarrhea
Probenecid		Anorexia, nausea, vomiting, anemia

Sources: D. C. March, *Handbook: Interactions of Selected Drugs with Nutritional Status in Man*, American Dietetic Association, October 1976; Physicians' Desk Reference, 31st ed., Medical Economics Company, Oradell, N.J., 1977.

be discerned. A number of factors should be explored to ensure the success of a nutritional care plan:*

Physical factors   General physical condition (too weak or too ill to eat)

Position in which the patient is fed

Comfort (need to void, comfortably dressed, cleanliness of hands and teeth, treatments given before or after meals, environment with unpleasant objects in sight, odors or inappropriate room temperature)

Presentation of food (unattractive tray, inappropriately sized utensils, rushed meals with too little time to chew and swallow between mouthfuls)

Medications (some cause drowsiness, nausea, alterations of taste and appetite—e.g., amphetamines cause decreased appetite, steroids increase appetite)

Forced feedings

Emotional factors

Anxiety

Depression

Stress

Loneliness

This last part of the book is directed to the effect of disease on the human condition. Diseases, like nutrients, do not operate in a vacuum, and the total patient, along with his or her family, must be considered in planning the special diet, for there are no special diets, only special people.

---

*E. Getchel and R. Howard, "Nutrition in Development," in G. Scipien et al., *Comprehensive Pediatric Nursing,* McGraw-Hill Book Company, New York, 1975, p. 239.

CHAPTER 15

THE EVALUATION
OF NUTRITIONAL
STATUS

Nancy S. Wellman

KEY WORDS
Nutritional Status
24-Hour Recall
Nutrition History
Problem-Oriented Medical Record (POMR)

INTRODUCTION

The general term *nutritional status* describes the overall state of the nutrition of a person. Nutritional status is defined by Christakis (1973) as the "health condition of an individual as influenced by his intake and utilization of nutrients, determined from the correlation of information obtained from physical, biochemical, clinical, and dietary studies."

There is no single rapid reliable test which measures nutritional status. It is currently accepted that a true assessment of nutritional status requires collection and correlation of four types of data, *anthropometric, biochemical, clinical,* and *dietary.* An unacceptable or deficient finding in any single area, such as short stature or a low serum ascorbic acid level, is not indicative of malnutrition per se. Detection of subclinical malnutrition remains difficult because of complexities in the definition of "optimal nutrition." Also, the progressive nature of deficiency diseases (from desaturation of blood stores, to a lesion at the molecular level, to the overt clinical lesion), the wide range of individual nutrient requirements, the general inability of biochemical tests to assess body stores, and the lack of comparative standards further compound the problem. Therefore determination of nutritional status is dependent upon assessments of the total individual.

ANTHROPOMETRIC METHODS

Taking body measurements constitues a relatively simple assessment procedure that is useful in nutritional screening. Since physical measurements are partially dependent upon nutrient intake, they are of help in assessing nutritional status. In children, a fall-off or an acceleration in the rate of gain in both height and weight is a sensitive indicator of malnutrition, which may be due to either inadequate or excessive food intake and of underlying disease conditions. In adults, weight is a useful indicator of change.

In addition to food intake, genetic and environmental factors influence growth and development. However, nutrition is one of the critical factors, as evidenced by a significant dissimilarity in the growth of children in developed versus developing countries where there are differences in the availability of food.

Longitudinal measurements provide a system for monitoring nutrient effectiveness in infants, children, and adolescents, particularly when plotted on percentile curves. With care, measurements of body size, height, weight, and skinfold thickness can be taken efficiently and accurately. Standardized equipment and procedures should be used (see Chap. 12).

BIOCHEMICAL METHODS

Laboratory techniques have been developed to determine levels of various nutrients in the blood and urine and to examine some metabolic functions that depend on an adequate intake of certain nutrients. Such tests provide an objective means of monitoring aspects of nutritional status. The purpose of laboratory assessments is to detect subclinical deficiencies prior to the onset of overt clinical signs, in order to allow early intervention for those at risk.

Blood constituents include nutritional, excretory, and intrinsic (functional) substances. *Nutritional substances* are either nutrients absorbed from the intestinal tract or intermediate products being transported for cellular utilization elsewhere. Examples include amino acids, glucose, minerals, vitamins, lipids, lactic acid, pyruvic acid, creatinine, and circulating hormones. Homeostasis controls their concentrations, which are therefore fairly stable under basal conditions. *Excretory substances* are en route for elimination by the kidneys, lungs, or liver. Examples include carbon dioxide, creatinine, urea, bilirubin, and some enzymes such as amylase and phosphatase. Normal concentrations may be influenced by food intake (urea), breakdown rate (bilirubin), or bodily content (creatinine). *Intrinsic or functional sub-*

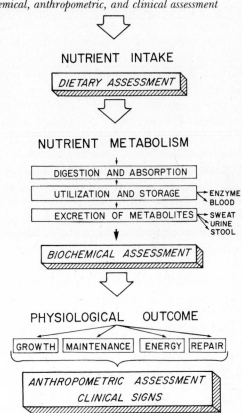

Figure 15-1

The evaluation of nutritional status includes dietary, biochemical, anthropometric, and clinical assessment

stances are inherent fundamental blood components such as hemoglobin, glutathione, adenosine triphosphate (ATP), plasma proteins, fibrinogen, some minerals, hydrogen ions, and cations. They exhibit a narrow range of normal concentration, as in the case of electrolytes.

Three stages of gradual depletion take place in the body when nutrient intake is deficient over a prolonged period:

First, the nutrient or its metabolites is homeostatically conserved by a slight decrease in the urinary excretion level or the plasma concentration.

Second, tissue concentration and storage forms are reduced.

Third, as the internal nutrient supply is exhausted, clinical symptoms appear.

When considering the *normalcy* of circulating nutrient levels, it should be recognized that, in general, urinary excretion levels fluctuate more than plasma levels and reflect immediate rather than usual intake. Most circulating nutrient levels are not indicators of storage quantities. For example, a urinary ascorbic acid level is directly related to recent dietary intake and is, therefore, an unreliable indicator of nutritional status. On the other hand, some tests, such as serum protein, may reflect long-term dietary influences.

Tests which measure a step in the metabolism or use of a nutrient are commonly referred to as *functional tests*. They usually provide more sensitive indications of nutritional status. Measuring the erythrocyte activity of transketolase to determine thiamine status and the level of glutathione reductase in red blood cells as a test of riboflavin are two examples of these newer indirect, more specific functional laboratory tests. For other nutrients (e.g., iron), the actual storage form level (ferritin) can now be determined. As standards are developed, early identification of decreasing levels of storage forms will aid in identifying inadequate dietary intakes, absorption, or utilization of specific nutrients. Depletion of some nutrients, such as water-soluble vitamins, is accurately reflected in diminished plasma levels because the total body content is normally low in relation to utilization.

Attempts to find a single specific biochemical test to measure nutritional status have been unsuccessful. Some laboratory tests, such as the hydroxyproline index (urinary hydroxyproline creatinine ratio), have no clear advantage over height and weight as an indicator of nutritional status. The biochemical tests that are chosen depend upon the situation. For a hospitalized patient, several routine laboratory procedures are readily available which can provide valuable information when integrated with data concerning the patient's condition and medicinal intake. Such tests include serum protein and albumin, creatinine and creatinine-height index, serum iron, transferrin saturation, plasma ascorbate, serum electrolytes, etc. In large-scale screening surveys, the laboratory analyses that are chosen should measure those nutrients which are suspected or known to be marginally available. For example, the high prevalence of iron-deficiency anemia among preschool children mandates measurement of iron, preferably in its storage form, for that population group.

Interpretation of biochemical data is not without problems. Assuming adequate laboratory quality control, neither dietary nor clinical findings may correlate with the laboratory findings. As previously indicated, reproducibility and reliability of results may be difficult to achieve even with one individual because of the relationship of findings to current dietary intake rather than to actual nutritional status. Coexisting illnesses, malabsorption, medications, and diurnal variation may also obscure results. Moreover, the classification of *normal* biochemical levels is not universally agreed upon. Standards for the lower limits of hemoglobin in children which indicate anemia vary between 10 and 12 g/100 ml. Because hemoglobin levels may decrease because of protein insufficiency, the test is nonspecific for iron intake. Thus, immunoassays of serum ferritin are more valuable in detecting dietary deficiencies of iron. For some nutrients, normal limits are arbitrary decisions awaiting more sophisticated specific laboratory procedures. Current guidelines for the interpretation of laboratory data for various nutrients are provided in Table 15-1.

Individuals can also be at nutritional risk for certain nutrients which can accumulate to toxic levels in the body. Blood levels of vitamin A greater than 100 mg/100 ml are indicative of hypervitaminosis A. Vitamin D toxicity is evidenced by hypercalcemia (more than 12 mg/100 ml).

TABLE 15-1 CURRENT GUIDELINES FOR CRITERIA OF NUTRITIONAL STATUS FOR LABORATORY EVALUATION

Nutrient and units	Age of subject, years	Criteria of status		
		Deficient	Marginal	Acceptable
Hemoglobin* (g/100ml)	6–23 mos.	Up to 9.0	9.0– 9.9	10.0+
	2–5	Up to 10.0	10.0–10.9	11.0+
	6–12	Up to 10.0	10.0–11.4	11.5+
	13–16M	Up to 12.0	12.0–12.9	13.0+
	13–16F	Up to 10.0	10.0–11.4	11.5+
	16+M	Up to 12.0	12.0–13.9	14.0+
	16+F	Up to 10.0	10.0–11.9	12.0+
	Pregnant (after 6+ mos.)	Up to 9.5	9.5–10.9	11.0+
Hematocrit* (packed cell volume in percent)	Up to 2	Up to 28	28–30	31+
	2–5	Up to 30	30–33	34+
	6–12	Up to 30	30–35	36+
	13–16M	Up to 37	37–39	40+
	13–16F	Up to 31	31–35	36+
	16+M	Up to 37	37–43	44+
	16+F	Up to 31	31–37	33+
	Pregnant	Up to 30	30–32	33+
Serum albumin* (g/100ml)	Up to 1	—	Up to 2.5	2.5+
	1–5	—	Up to 3.0	3.0+
	6–16	—	Up to 3.5	3.5+
	16+	Up to 2.8	2.8–3.4	3.5+
	Pregnant	Up to 3.0	3.0–3.4	3.5+
Serum protein* (g/100ml)	Up to 1	—	Up to 5.0	5.0+
	1–5	—	Up to 5.5	5.5+
	6–16	—	Up to 6.0	6.0+
	16+	Up to 6.0	6.0–6.4	6.5+
	Pregnant	Up to 5.5	5.5–5.9	6.0+
Serum ascorbic acid* (mg/100ml)	All ages	Up to 0.1	0.1–0.19	0.2+
Plasma vitamin A* (mcg/100 ml)	All ages	Up to 10	10–19	20+
Plasma carotene* (mcg/100 ml)	All ages	Up to 20	20–39	40+
	Pregnant	—	40–79	80+
Serum iron* (mcg/100ml)	Up to 2	Up to 30	—	30+
	2–5	Up to 40	—	40+
	6–12	Up to 50	—	50+
	12+M	Up to 60	—	60+
	12+F	Up to 40	—	40+
Transferrin saturation* (percent)	Up to 2	Up to 15.0	—	15.0+
	2–12	Up to 20.0	—	20.0+
	12+M	Up to 20.0	—	20.0+
	12+F	Up to 15.0	—	15.0+
Serum ferritin† (ng/ml)	16+M			77+
	16+F			36+
Serum folacin† (ng/ml)	All ages	Up to 2.0	2.1–5.9	6.0+
Serum vitamin B_{12}† (ng/ml)	All ages	Up to 100	—	100+
Thiamine in urine* (mcg/g creatinine)	1–3	Up to 120	120–175	175+
	4–5	Up to 85	85–120	120+
	6–9	Up to 70	70–180	180+

(continued)

TABLE 15-1 (continued)

Nutrient and units	Age of subject, years	Criteria of status		
		Deficient	Marginal	Acceptable
	10–15	Up to 55	55–150	150+
	16+	Up to 27	27–65	65+
	Pregnant	Up to 21	21–49	50+
Riboflavin in urine* (mcg/g creatinine)	1–3	Up to 150	150–499	500+
	4–5	Up to 100	100–299	300+
	6–9	Up to 85	85–269	270+
	10–16	Up to 70	70–199	200+
	16+	Up to 27	27–79	80+
	Pregnant	Up to 30	30–89	90+
RBC transketolase-TPP-effect† (ratio)	All ages	25+	15–25	Up to 15
RBC glutathione reductase-FAD-effect† (ratio)	All ages	1.2+	—	Up to 1.2
Tryptophan load† (mg xanthurenic acid excreted)	Adults (Dose: 100 mg/kg body weight)	25+(6 hrs.) 75+(24 hrs.)	— —	Up to 25 Up to 75
Urinary pydridoxine† (mcg/g creatinine)	1–3	Up to 90	—	90+
	4–6	Up to 80	—	80+
	7–9	Up to 60	—	60+
	10–12	Up to 40	—	40+
	13–15	Up to 30	—	30+
	16+	Up to 20	—	20+
Urinary N′methyl nicotinamide* (mg/g creatinine)	All ages	Up to 0.2	0.2–5.59	0.6+
	Pregnant	Up to 0.8	0.8–2.49	2.5+
Urinary pantothenic acid† (mcg)	All ages	Up to 200	—	200+
Plasma vitamin E† (mg/100ml)	All ages	Up to 0.2	0.2–0.6	0.6+
Transaminase index† (ratio)				
SGOT‡	Adult	2.0+	—	Up to 2.0
SGPT§	Adult	1.25+	—	Up to 1.25

* Adapted from the Ten State Nutrition Survey. ‡ Serum Glutamic Oxalacetic Transaminase.
† Criteria may vary with different methodology. § Serum Glutamic Pyruvic Transaminase.

Source: G. Christakis, "Nutritional Assessment in Health Programs," American Journal of Public Health, vol. 63, pt. 2, November 1973.

CLINICAL METHODS

Classic physical signs of deficiency disorders occur late in the continuum of events associated with malnutrition. Such signs of malnutrition may be nonspecific because they are often caused by multiple nutrient deficiencies or by nonnutritional factors such as poor hygiene or excessive sun exposure. Generally a malnourished person has multiple nutrient deficiencies. A clinical diagnosis alone is inadequate and other nutritional status assessments (biochemical, anthropometric, dietary) must be given consideration. However, direct correla-

TABLE 15-2 PHYSICAL SIGNS AND CAUSES OF MALNUTRITION

Body area	Signs associated with malnutrition	Nutrition-related causes
Hair	Lack of natural shine; dull, dry, sparse, straight, color changes (flag sign); easily plucked	Protein-calorie deficiency; often multiple co-existent nutrient deficiencies
Face	Dark skin over cheeks and under eyes (malar and supraorbital pigmentation), scaling of skin around nostrils (nasolabial seborrhea)	Inadequate caloric intake; lack of B complex vitamins, particularly niacin, riboflavin, pyridoxine
	Edematous (moon face)	Protein deficiency
	Color loss (pallor)	Iron deficiency, general undernutrition
Eyes	Pale conjunctivae	Iron deficiency
	Bitot's spots*, conjunctival and corneal xerosis*, soft cornea (keratomalacia)	Vitamin A deficiency
	Redness and fissuring of eyelid corners (angular palpebritis)	Niacin, riboflavin, pyridoxine deficiency
Lips	Redness and swelling of mouth or lips (cheilosis)*, angular fissure and scars	Niacin or riboflavin deficiency
Tongue	Red, raw and fissured, swollen (glossitis)*	Folic acid, niacin, B_{12}, pyridoxine deficiency
	Magenta color	Riboflavin deficiency
	Pale, atrophic	Iron deficiency
	Filiform papillary atrophy	Niacin, folic acid, B_{12}, iron deficiency
	Fungiform papillary hypertrophy	General undernutrition
Teeth	Carious or missing	Excess sugar (and poor dental hygiene)
	Mottled enamel (fluorosis)	Excess fluoride
Gums	Spongy, bleeding*, may be receding	Ascorbic acid deficiency
Glands	Thydroid enlargement (goiter)	Iodine deficiency
	Parotid enlargement	General undernutrition, particularly insufficient protein
Skin	Follicular hyperkeratosis*, dryness (xerosis) with flaking	Vitamin A deficiency; insufficient unsaturated and essential fatty acids
	Hyperpigmentation*	B_{12}, folic acid, niacin deficiency
	Petechiae*	Ascorbic acid deficiency
	Pellagrous dermatitis*	Niacin or tryptophan deficiency
	Scrotal and vulval dermatosis*	Riboflavin deficiency
Nails	Spoon nails (koilonychia), brittle or ridged	Iron deficiency
Muscular and skeletal systems	Muscle wasting	Protein-calorie deficiency
	Frontal and parietal bossing; epiphyseal swelling; soft, thin infant skull bones (craniotabes), persistently open anterior fontanelle; knock-knees or bow-legs	Vitamin D deficiency
	Beading of ribs (rachitic rosary)	Vitamin D and calcium deficiency

(continued)

TABLE 15-2 (continued)

Body area	Signs associated with malnutrition	Nutrition-related causes
Internal systems		
Gastrointestinal	Hepatomegaly	Chronic malnutrition
Nervous	Mental confusion and irritability	Thiamine, niacin deficiency
	Sensory loss, motor weakness, loss of position sense, loss of vibration, loss of ankle and knee jerks, calf tenderness	Thiamine deficiency
Cardiac	Cardiac enlargement, tachycardia	Thiamine deficiency

* See color plates located inside back cover.

tions may not be evident. For the diagnosis of mild deficiency, the clinical examination is ineffective. The low general prevalence of clinical signs of malnutrition in developed countries often results in an overlooking or misinterpreting of such signs.

Certain characteristic physical signs which are associated with malnutrition, and which are valuable in nutritional assessment, are given in Table 15-2. (See also color plates located inside back cover.) Health care professionals should be able to recognize these dramatic signs, although there is some variation among population groups and according to age. Any suggestive physical finding should be pursued further through laboratory tests, dietary assessments, or other tests, such as x-rays for confirmatory evidence of rickets. The clinical examination should note other acute illnesses, chronic diseases, and disorders which could interfere with nutrient ingestion, absorption, or utilization. The oral cavity and teeth should be evaluated for signs of malnutrition and to note factors which may restrict the variety or amount of food intake, such as decayed or missing teeth, gum hypertrophy, ill-fitting dentures, or glossitis.

DIETARY METHODS

Information describing what an individual or a population group is in the habit of eating can help to determine dietary patterns that affect nutritional status and can enhance the understanding of socioeconomic and cultural influences involved in food selection. A variety of methods are used in the collection of dietary information: *24-h recall, 3- or 7-day food records, a nutritional history,* and *a household survey.* The methods vary in reliability, validity, and depth. The method of choice depends upon whether information is being gathered for an individual diet assessment or a population survey, the extent of dietary information required, the time and money available, and the cooperation of the subjects.

Interviewing Techniques

Skillful interviewing is the foundation necessary for acquiring accurate information. Care must be taken to avoid distorting what is heard because of one's own perceptions, prejudices, and assumptions. Questions should be asked which elicit meaningful responses. The questions and the tone of voice should not give clues to the expected answers. "Does your son drink a quart of milk every day?" and "How many eggs do you eat a week?" both imply positive answers. Even asking "What did you have for breakfast this morning?" includes an assumption. A better question is "What is the first thing you ate or drank today?" After a food item, such as bread, has been mentioned, follow-up questions should delineate the type, amount, preparation method (such as "buttered"—which itself must be further defined). Assumptions should not be made about serving size. "A hamburger" and "a glass of milk" may each vary threefold in size. All glasses do not contain 8 oz or 1 cup. Food models of known sizes should be available to aid the interviewee in estimating portion sizes. The amount eaten may differ from the amount served.

The interviewer should be aware that distortion of amounts consumed may occur because those eating small amounts may think they should eat more and those eating large amounts may be well aware that they should eat less. Details may be missed when the interviewer neglects to ask about food practices that are different from his own. Not everyone butters a hot dog roll, uses mayonnaise in sandwiches, or "cream" in coffee. Probing for details, such as snack habits and fluid intake, will often significantly change the day's reported total intake. Constant awareness of variables and biases which interviewers can introduce into data collection will help to control the problem.

The 24-Hour Recall

The most frequently used dietary survey procedure to measure current food intake is the 24-h recall. Collecting data via a 24-h recall requires a trained person to obtain accurate estimates of the quantity of all foods eaten during the previous 24 h or for the entire day preceeding the interview. This simple, rapid method can be completed in 15 to 20 min. However, quantities consumed may be over- or underestimated and food intake on a single day may not be representative of the usual intake. For these reasons, the information obtained from an individual will not necessarily correlate with physical or laboratory findings. When the 24-h recall is used as a screening tool in dietary surveys of population groups, the trends detected provide information about specific nutrient intake that is useful when measuring and comparing differences between large groups.

The interviewer should use glasses, spoons,

bowls, and food models of various sizes to help the respondent estimate the quantities consumed as accurately as possible. Some foods, such as beverages, margarine, gravy, sauces, and salad dressing, are often accidentally omitted and the day's nutrient and caloric (kilojoule) totals may be underestimated.

The 3- or 7-Day Food Record

Another commonly used dietary tool is a written record of all food eaten which is kept by an individual for a specified period of time. Instructions are given regarding weighing and measuring food and the need to indicate cooking methods and brand names. A standard set of measuring cups and spoons along with simple record forms should be provided to the recorder. Home visits by a trained person during the recording period will help to clarify serving portion size, recipes used, etc. As a minimum, the food record should be reviewed with the respondent to refine the information provided. The accuracy of the record is dependent upon the cooperation and ability of the respondent, along with the adequacy and clarity of the prior instructions that were given about how to complete the record.

The Nutritional History

The nutritional history is a record of the amount and frequency of food consumption during a longer period of time, usually 1 to 6 months. It is a valuable tool for correlation with physical and biochemical data. Biweekly and semiannual histories are the most satisfactory method of obtaining continuous dietary data for longitudinal studies. Periodic histories from the same individual increase the accuracy. The initial nutritional history should be seen as a trial effort rather than as a valid record. The food history compensates for the wide daily variations that are possible in eating habits and for fluctuations in food intake that occur over a period of time, as in the changing eating patterns during the first year of life.

The nutritionist must be trained in effective techniques and the subject must also be trained to become a careful observer of food intake. Ideally, the nutritional history is completed in the subject's home to permit measurement of glasses, cups, and serving size and to check recipes and brand names. A sample form for recording the nutritional history for children is given in the Appendix.

The Household Survey

Household surveys measure all the food consumed by a family over a period of time, usually a week. The procedure includes initial weighing of all food in the home, recording all food purchases made during the time period, and deducting any food remaining in the home at the end of the survey. Food wastage is also deducted. The age, sex, and occupation of household members are recorded, as is the number of meals eaten away from home. Nutrient intake can be calculated for the household as a group. Data are not available for any one individual because food distribution among family members is not distinguishable. The household survey is useful for differentiating food consumption patterns for varying economic and cultural groups. Marked seasonal variations may occur in some population groups, particularly in developing countries.

EVALUATION OF DIETARY DATA

The records of foods that have been eaten are usually converted into nutrient quantities as a first step in the evaluation of dietary records. Food composition tables, such as *Nutritive Value of American Foods* (Agriculture Handbook No. 456, United States Department of Agriculture, 1975) and *Food Values of Portions Commonly Used* (J. B. Lippincott Company, Philadelphia, 1975), provide actual or estimated nutrient data for foods. Although these are frequently updated, current values for nutrient content can be found in nutrition journals.

Problems are frequently encountered in the calculation of dietary data and may result in questionable validity. For this reason, there is often a poor correlation between dietary histories and other parameters studied in nutritional surveys. Common sources of error leading to miscalculation of dietary data include:

1 Mistakes in converting a household portion size to a weighed amount (e.g., 1 cup to 100 g)
2 Arithmetic mistakes converting food intake into nutrient values
3 Use of food table values which are estimated rather than actual laboratory analysis amounts for nutrient content
4 Use of food table average values which may not reflect nutrient variations due to seasonal differences and methods of processing, cooking, and storage
5 Frequent ingredient changes in processed food products
6 Wide variability and combination-dish recipes for items such as baked goods, casseroles, etc.

In metabolic balance studies, laboratory analyses of an aliquot of all foods consumed can accurately measure the actual nutrient intake. This is useful in providing a basic knowledge of nutrient metabolism in order to establish minimum requirements or to study metabolic disorders.

Calculating the nutrient content of dietary records by hand may be a lengthy, tedious process. Therefore, manual calculations usually include only a small number of nutrients. Deciding which nutrients to calculate is based upon other indices of nutritional problems of a population group or individual. For example, it would be appropriate to calculate the energy and protein intake for a failure-to-thrive infant, while estimating the usual energy intake would be adequate when counseling an obese adolescent.

Computer analysis of dietary records provides a rapid means of calculating a large number of nutrients. However, considerable time must be spent in preparing the dietary record information for computer processing. Programs have been devised for use with a data bank of the known nutrient content in foods. Updating the nutrient data bank is necessary at frequent intervals. The limitations and sources of error with computer analysis are similar to those for manual calculations.

To assess the adequacy of dietary intake, it is necessary to compare dietary data with established standards. Comparing the record of foods consumed with the recommended number of daily servings from each of the basic four food groups (see Chap. 2) helps to provide a general impression regarding the nutritional adequacy of the diet. Consistent omission of one or more food groups focuses attention on a group of nutrients whose intake may be suboptimal.

The international standards that are used to judge dietary adequacy vary widely in their levels of recommended intake. The standard most frequently used in the United States is the Recommended Dietary Allowances (RDA) of the National Academy of Sciences—National Research Council. The inherent limitations of the RDA must be recognized when comparing it to an individual's intake. (See Chap. 2). A person's nutrient intake may be expressed as the percent of that nutrient's RDA, qualified for the age and sex of the individual. Certain nutrient intakes are evaluated on the basis of body size, such as calories and protein per kilogram of body weight in infants, or on the basis of quantity per 1000 kcal (4200 kJ) for niacin and thiamine. Such measurement standards indicate metabolic relationships which may vary considerably.

Since the RDA includes a margin of safety, a person not consuming 100 percent of all the RDA nutrients may not necessarily be deficient in a nutrient and should not be considered malnourished without the support of biochemical, clinical, and anthropometric data.

NUTRITIONAL STATUS OF THE UNITED STATES POPULATION

Since 1967, three major nutrition surveys have attempted to define the nutritional problems that beset our population. The first of these, the Ten State Nutrition Survey (1968–1970) was mandated by the U.S. Congress in response to testimony on the existence of hunger in America. The demographic, dietary, clinical, anthropometric, and biochemical data collected in this survey revealed that undernutrition was causing growth failure in children and that it tended to be more prevalent in low-income populations. Iron-deficiency anemia, obesity, dental caries, and hyperlipidemia were additional findings. Groups at risk of developing malnutrition were noted to include elderly and adolescent males, in addition to infants, children, and pregnant women. The relatively high prevalence of vitamin A deficiency found among low-income Spanish-Americans is now suspected of having been a laboratory error.

Other studies including the Pre-School Nutrition Survey (1968–1970) and the Health and Nutrition Examination Survey (Hanes) (1971–72) have essentially identified the same problems. It is interesting to note that the classic clinical signs of malnutrition are practically nonexistent. As a result of survey findings, the National Center for Disease Control has recently inaugurated a Nutrition Surveillance program. The center utilizes already existing data (e.g., height, weight, hemoglobin, hematocrit) from agencies such as the Early Periodic Screening, Diagnosis, and Treatment (EPSDT) programs, Headstart, Special Supplemental Feeding Program for Women, Infants, and Children (WIC), well-baby clinics, and family planning clinics. The participating states and counties submit the data for computer analysis and comparison with standards. These enable the states and counties to identify and follow-up individuals and target populations and then to allocate services to high-prevalence areas at nutritional risk.

Preliminary nutritional surveillance has shown that iron-deficiency anemia, as measured by hemoglobin and hematocrit, continues to be a major problem as are obesity and poor growth in a number of children. In the United States, the surveillance program has yet to identify third-degree malnutrition.

PROBLEM-ORIENTED MEDICAL RECORD

The *problem-oriented medical record system* (PMOR) developed by Weed is a modern professional tool. It provides a logically organized method for recognition of all of a patient's problems. The POMR coordinates members of the entire health team and therefore improves patient care. The *data base* includes the patient's chief complaints, present illness, past medical history, patient profile, physical examination findings, and basic laboratory studies. Following completion of the data base, a numbered *master problem list* is drawn up, composed of items demanding attention of a diagnostic, therapeutic, or educational nature. A problem may be a symptom, a physiologic abnormality, an abnormal laboratory test, a diagnosis, or a social, nutritional, psychiatric, or demographic factor. A plan is developed as part of each problem's analysis. The acronym *SOAP,* derived from the first letters of the words *subjective, objective, assessment,* and *plans,* provides the format for the problem formulation, as follows:

Date, Problem Number, Title

Subjective Brief summary of pertinent history for this problem

Objective Pertinent hard facts such as physical findings, laboratory data

Assessment Precise interpretation of the problem and related factors

Plans Diagnostic, therapeutic, and patient education plans

Progress notes, which follow the same SOAP format, document further developments within the problem situation.

An example follows showing the original problem formulations by the physician and the dietitian of a child seen in an ambulatory pediatric clinic.

7-9-77 #2 Nutritional Anemia

S 17-month-old girl appears pale to mother recently—drinks 1 ½ qt milk daily—no history of pica—child still eats mainly pureed foods; doesn't like to chew

O Questionably pale, no hepatomogaly or splenomegaly. Hemoglobin 9.1 g/100 ml, white blood cells and platelets normal, reticulocytes 1.4 percent. Height, 80 cm, weight, 10.5 kg

A History and findings compatible with iron-deficiency anemia

P Rx Fer-In-Sol 1.2 ml bid for 1 month (approximately 5 mg elemental iron/kg body weight per day)

Patient education

1 Mother instructed to decrease daily milk intake and to increase iron-containing foods.

2 Appointment made for counseling by dietitian regarding poor iron intake

Repeat hemoglobin at return visit in 1 month

_____M.D.

7-9-77 #2 Nutritional Anemia

S Large intake of milk daily, questionable iron intake from food sources, diagnosis of iron-deficiency anemia confirmed; mother considers the child underweight

Daily food intake consists of 48 oz milk, one 4 ½-oz jar strained cereal with fruit, and one 7-oz jar junior vegetables and meat. Over 90 percent of total calories come from milk

O Child observed eating: drinks liquids from a bottle, is spoon-fed, does not chew well. No other developmental delays. Dentition is normal for age. Height, weight, and weight-for-stature are at the 25th percentile

A 1 Iron deficiency appears to be caused by low iron intake, which is less than one-third the RDA

2 Delayed feeding skills seem caused by mother's overprotectiveness

3 Intake of other nutrients such as ascorbic acid is suboptimal because of limited dietary variety. Appetite for other foods is diminished by excessive milk intake

P Parent education—Nutritional counseling included

1 explanation of average milk requirements for young children.

2 discussion of normal feeding skills for age

3 demonstration of techniques to encourage development of self-feeding skills,

4 discussion of iron-rich sources of culturally acceptable foods and suggestions to increase food variety

5 reassurance regarding the child's adequate physical development utilizing anthropometric graph for visual enhancement

6 reinforcement of the need to give the prescribed medicinal iron as directed Follow-up appointment with dietitian at time of return clinic visit 1 month hence

_____R.D.

The POMR has interesting implications for health care professionals. The team approach is encouraged by the use of the medical record as a communication vehicle which focuses on the patient's problems. All health professionals involved in the patient's diagnosis, therapy, or education document their input in the patient's record. The "total patient" is more likely to receive care in a facility utilizing the POMR since the anthropometric, biochemical, clinical, and dietary data are clearly observable and readily available to determine nutritional status. The hospitalized patient is at special risk

TABLE 15-3 CONDITIONS RESULTING IN NUTRITIONAL FAILURE

1. _Inadequate intake—quantity_
   Mechanical feeding problems or undeveloped feeding skills
   Anorexia (due to emotional problems, disease process, drugs)
2. _Inadequate intake—quality_
   Education of parents or caretaker
   Institutionalized setting
   Poor food habits
   Allergies
3. _Increased metabolism_
   Fever
   Infections
   Malignancy
   Hyperthyroidism
   Athetosis
   Surgery, stress, burns
4. _Increased loss_
   Vomiting
   Diarrhea
   Decreased food transit time through the gut
5. _Defective utilization_
   Metabolic diseases (aminoacidopathies, galactosemia, lipidoses)
   Disturbed metabolic states (hepatic insufficiency, renal tubular acidosis, nephrogenic diabetes insipidus, adrenal cortical hyperplasia with salt loss)
   Drug interference with nutrients
6. _Defective absorption_
   Intrinsic disease states (regional enteritis, Hirschsprung's disease)
   Exogenous states (intestinal parasitosis, celiac disease, surgical removal of the small bowel)
   Drugs
7. _Defects in the function of major organ systems_
   Severe congenital heart disease
   Severe chest disease
   Severe liver disease
   Kidney disease
   Brain damage
8. _Excessive food or vitamin intake_
   Obesity
   Vitamin intoxication—fat-soluble vitamins

for nutritional failure; the predisposing conditions are presented in Table 15-3. Such a patient warrants close nutritional surveillance, which is expedited by the use of the POMR.

STUDY QUESTIONS

1 Define the term *nutritional status*.
2 Identify the type of information obtained in each of the four assessment areas which is helpful when evaluating the nutritional status of a person or a population group.
3 Despite the difficulty in diagnosing subclinical malnutrition, explain why it is important to identify persons at nutritional risk prior to the onset of clinical signs.
4 Discuss the factors involved in the calculation and interpretation of dietary data which affect the reliability and validity of the data.
5 List the most common nutritional problems of the American population.
6 In the problem-oriented medical record system, explain the type of information contained in each area of the *SOAP* format.

CASE STUDY 15-1

The nutritional problems of a hospitalized cancer patient are written in a SOAP format below. The **Subjective** *and* **Objective** *sections provide anthropometric, biochemical, clinical, and dietary data related to the patient's nutritional status. Complete the* **Assessment** *and* **Planning** *portions for the patient's nutrition-related problems as you would enter them in the chart.*

#1 **Poor nutritional status due to resectable cancer of the pancreas**

Subjective **Elderly female patient, very fearful about eating because of constant diarrhea following surgery. Patient reports decreased appetite and has noticed that "even ice cream makes her run"**

Objective **Hospital diet prescription is 1800 kcal (7560 kJ) with 100 g fat. Pa-tients height is 160 cm.; Weight on hospital admission was 82 kg; weight prior to surgery was 68.5 kg.; weight at present is 59 kg. Serum potassium is 3.0 meq/l; sodium, 120 meq/l. Fasting blood glucose was 175 mg/100 ml; patient currently receiving NPH insulin. Appears lethargic and exhibits overall weakness**

Assessment

Plan

Case Study Question

1 Based on subjective and objective data presented, develop both the assessment and plans section of the problem-oriented record.

BIBLIOGRAPHY

Beal, V. A.: "The Nutritional History in Longitudinal Research," *Journal of the American Dietetic Association*, **51**:426–532, 1967.

Butterworth, C. E. and G. L. Blackburn: "Hospital Mal-nutrition," *Nutrition Today*, **10**:8–18, March-April 1975.

Christakis, G.: "Nutritional Assessment in Health Programs," *American Journal of public Health*, **63**: 80–82, November 1973.

Hoffman, W. S.: *The Biochemistry of Clinical Medicine,* 4th ed., Year Book Medical Publishers, Inc., Chicago, 1970, chaps. 1 and 7.

Madden, J. P., S. J. Goodman, and H. A. Guthrie: "Validity of the 24-hour Recall," *Journal of the American Dietetic Association,* **68:**143–147, 1976.

Nichaman, M. Z.: "Developing a Nutritional Surveillance System," *Journal of the American Dietetic Association,* **65:**15–17, 1974.

Owen, G. M., K. M. Kram, P. J. Garry, J. E. Lowe, and A. H. Lubin: "A Study of Nutritional Status of Preschool Children in the United States, 1968–1970," *Pediatrics,* **53:**597–646, April 1974.

U.S. Dept. Health, Education, and Welfare: *Highlights, Ten State Nutrition Survey, 1968–1970,* DHEW Publ. no. (HSM) 72–8134.

U.S. Dept. Health, Education, and Welfare: *Preliminary Findings of the First Health and Nutrition Examination Survey, United States, 1971–72, I. Anthropometric and Clinical Findings,* DHEW Publ. no. (HRA) 75–1229; *II. Dietary Intake and Biochemical Findings,* DHEW Publ. no. (HRA) 76–1219-1.

U.S. Dept. Health, Education, and Welfare: *Screening Children for Nutritional Status: Suggestions for Child Health Programs,* DHEW Publ. no. (PHS)2158, 1971.

Voytovich, A. E., F. M. Walters, and M. DeMarco: "The Dietitian/Nutritionist and the Problem-oriented Medical Record," *Journal of the American Dietetic Association,* **63:**639–643, 1973.

Weed, L. L.: *Medical Records, Medical Education and Patient Care,* The Press of Case Western Reserve University, Cleveland, 1970.

CHAPTER 16

THE MALNOURISHED CHILD AND THE IMMUNE RESPONSE

Robert M. Suskind

KEY WORDS
Marasmus
Kwashiorkor
Antigen
Cell-mediated Immune Response
Humoral Immunity
Polymorphonuclear Leukocytes
Complement System

INTRODUCTION

A recent study of childhood mortality in Latin American countries cited malnutrition as either the direct or the indirect cause of death of over one-third of the children under 5 years of age.[1] Up to 80 percent of over 190,000 children surveyed in 46 Asian, African, and South American communities between 1963 and 1972 suffered moderate or severe forms of protein-calorie malnutrition (PCM).[2] Judging from these figures, roughly 100 million children under 5 years of age are now severely or moderately malnourished.

Malnutrition strikes children in well-fed developed nations as well as in the developing world (see Case Study 16-1). Primary protein-calorie malnutrition is not commonly seen in American hospitals, but physicians are becoming increasingly aware that malnutrition may develop from other disease states such as renal, liver, or cardiopulmonary illness. Children with these secondary nutritional deficits must be considered in studies of the nutritional status of children throughout the world.

ETIOLOGY OF MALNUTRITION

The development of malnutrition depends on a complex of interactions among nutrient, host, and environment.[3]

In deficiency states, nutrients act as if they were present in insufficient quantities at a cellular level to satisfy metabolic needs.[4] When considering protein intake, it is important to determine whether the composition of the protein, in terms of essential amino acids, is adequate for body requirements. If the dietary protein lacks one essential amino acid, the body reacts as if all essential amino acids were deficient in the food. The biological value of a protein food depends not only on its amino acid composition, but on the degree to which the amino acids are liberated during digestion, since complete protein utilization will not occur until all the essential amino acids are available at approximately the same time.[5] In addition, the caloric value of the diet affects the biological value of the protein. If the diet lacks calories, protein will be used for energy, with the eventual result being similar to the effects of a protein-deficient diet. Conversely, excess calories will spare the utilization of protein for energy. In many parts of the world, the foods children consume for calories, such as casava or sweet potato, are grossly deficient in essential nutrients and contribute to protein deficiency.[6,7]

Host factors affecting nutritional status include age, sex, activity, growth, pregnancy, lactation, and various pathological states. The nutrient requirements of a growing child are much different from those of an adult. Pregnancy and lactation increase the nutrient requirements. Activity and genetic variability must also be considered. Environmental factors which affect the availability of nutrients include food production, cost, processing, distribution, and population density.[8] Temperature, humidity, and sunlight affect nutrient requirements.

Cultural influences are among the most important environmental determinants of what an individual eats.[9] For example, Northern Thai children from birth are started on supplemental rice and bananas, which are often given prior to breast feeding. This practice leads to a decreased consumption of breast milk. As a result, these children often develop permanent protein deficits from early infancy. Prejudices such as withholding cow's milk from young infants for fear that it causes diarrhea lead to decreased utilization of important protein sources in certain parts of the world. Religious taboos, such as the Hindu prohibition of beef in India, have greatly affected efforts to improve nutritional status. When a child has acute diarrhea or an infection and parents withdraw food, kwashiorkor (protein malnutrition) often develops from the metabolic loss of nitrogen. The nutritional status of the child further deteriorates when he receives strong purgatives to eliminate parasites which the mother believes are causing the diarrhea.

CLASSIFICATION OF PROTEIN-CALORIE MALNUTRITION

In 1955, Gomez et al.[10] defined childhood malnutrition in terms of deficits in the weight that would be appropriate for the child's age (weight for age). Using local standards, they categorized first-, second-, and third-degree malnutrition in terms of 75 to 90 percent of weight for age, 60 to 75 percent of weight for age, and less than 60 percent of weight for age, respectively. Today Gomez's classification has been modified to use internationally accepted standards derived from the mean weights and heights of healthy children from North America or Europe.[11] Since genetic differences apparently do not affect growth potential during the early years of life,[12] norms from developed countries also apply to communities with widespread malnutrition.

Height for age and weight for height are often more useful tools for defining an individual's nutritional status than weight for age, which fails to consider the height deficit caused by chronic malnutrition. The child with a decreased weight for height is wasted or acutely malnourished, while the child with a decreased height for age is stunted or chronically malnourished. Often the malnourished child is both wasted and stunted.

Waterlow's table classifies children according to their degree of malnutrition and retardation (Table 16-1).[13] Studies from several developing countries commonly show both wasting and stunting in children between the ages of 1 and 2 years. By age 3 or 4, underweight-for-age children are chiefly stunted rather than wasted.[14] In other words, they have stopped growing linearly but have a normal weight for height. Table 16-2 summarizes the effects of malnutrition on height and weight. The above classification of wasting and

TABLE 16-1 CLASSIFICATION ACCORDING TO DEGREE OF MALNUTRITION AND RETARDATION

		Retardation grade			
		0	*1*	*2*	*3*
*% Expected height for age:**		over 95%	95–90%	90–85%	under 85%
Malnutrition grade	*% Expected weight for height**				
0	over 90%	*52†	32	3	1
1	90–89%	2	7	1	0
2	80–70%	1	2	0	0
3	under 70%	0	0	0	0

* Expected values = Boston 50th percentile; 95% expected height for age = approximately Boston 3d percentile.

† % of sample population studied.

Source: Adapted from J. C. Waterlow, "Some Aspects of Childhood Malnutrition as a Public Health Problem," *British Medical Journal,* 4:88, 1974.

stunting provides a guide for use in the development of public health or community intervention programs. Wasted children require nutritional rehabilitation, either as inpatients or outpatients, while stunted children need a total community program with public health intervention and child feeding programs.

SEVERE MALNUTRITION: MARASMUS AND KWASHIORKOR

Children develop *marasmus* following severe deprivation of both protein and calories, resulting in growth retardation, weight loss, muscular atrophy, and severe decrease of sub-cutaneous tissue (Fig. 16-1). Children with *kwashiorkor,* caused by acute protein loss or deprivation, are characterized by edema, skin lesions, hair changes, apathy, anorexia, an enlarged fatty liver, and decreased serum total protein and serum albumin (Fig. 16-2). These children have abundant subcutaneous fat and recover rapidly on a high-protein diet.[15]

Marasmus and kwashiorkor may be superimposed on one another at any stage. Patients with combined marasmus-kwashiorkor are undersized and underweight, with markedly diminished subcutaneous fat, mild to moderate fatty infiltration of the liver, and a much greater degree of muscular wasting than is seen with kwashiorkor alone. They may have

TABLE 16-2 THE EFFECT OF MALNUTRITION ON HEIGHT AND WEIGHT

Type of malnutrition	Weight compared to age	Height compared to age	Weight compared to height
Chronic (past, long-term)	Low	Low	Normal
Current acute	Low	Normal	Low
Chronic and acute	Low	Low	Low

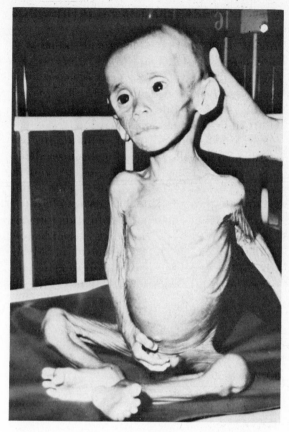

Figure 16-1

Marasmic child with evidence of growth retardation, weight loss, muscular atrophy, and severe decrease of subcutaneous tissue. (Courtesy of Medical Staff, Anemia and Malnutrition Research Center, Chiang Mai, Thailand. From R. M. Suskind, O. Thanangkul, D. Damrongsak, C. Leitzmann, L. Suskind, and R. E. Olson. "The Malnourished Child: Clinical, Biochemical, and Hematological Changes," in R. M. Suskind, (ed.), *Malnutrition and the Immune Response*, Raven Press, New York, 1977.)

mild to moderate edema which disappears within a few days of nutritional therapy, leaving only signs of marasmus. Children with marasmic-kwashiorkor have considerably lower total serum protein and serum albumin values than marasmic children, whose values are usually only slightly below normal.

Because of variations in feeding practices and body requirements, the various states of malnutrition have characteristic age distributions. Marasmus usually occurs in children under 1 year of age when the mother's breast milk provides insufficient protein and calories for the growing child and when the supplementary feeding is inadequate.[16] Kwashiorkor, on the other hand, most commonly occurs after age 1 when a borderline diet becomes deficient in protein relative to calories, as a result of superimposed infection.[17] Gopalan has outlined the differences between children with marasmus and kwashiorkor[18] (Table 16-3). His observations are similar to those of others who have described these syndromes from various parts of the world.

INFECTION AND MALNUTRITION

Scrimshaw et al.[19] noted that infection worsens the individual's nutritional status by reducing appetite, creating a tendency for solid foods to be withdrawn (especially those of animal origin), increasing metabolic losses of nitrogen, and (when infection involves the gastrointestinal tract) decreasing nitrogen absorption. Purgatives and various home remedies may also adversely affect absorption.[20] The prevalence rates for infectious disease range from 50 to 60 percent during the 6- to 24-month age period.

The child who gains weight more or less normally during the first 4 to 6 months, but thereafter develops recurrent infectious diseases, will show a leveling off in both weight and height gain. During the period of no significant weight gain there is usually no increase in height, leaving the child's weight for height unchanged. However, if an intercurrent infection develops, a resultant decrease in weight for height occurs simultaneously as the child's nutritional status deteriorates.

Reyna-Barrios et al.[21] evaluated the frequency of infectious diseases in an Indian village in the Guatemalan highlands. Upper respiratory infections and acute diarrheal diseases were major problems for some children up to 7

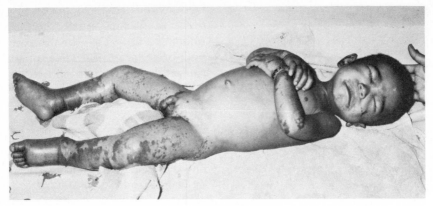

Figure 16-2

Child with kwashiorkor, with evidence of edema, skin lesions, hair changes, and apathy. Anorexia, an enlarged fatty liver, and decreased serum total protein and albumin are also present. (Courtesy of Medical Staff, Anemia and Malnutrition Research Center, Chiang Mai, Thailand. From R. M. Suskind, O. Thanangkul, D. Damrongsak, C. Leitzmann, L. Suskind, and R. E. Olson. "The Malnourished Child: Clinical, Biochemical, and Hematological Changes," in R. M. Suskind, (ed.) *Malnutrition and the Immune Response,* Raven Press, New York, 1977.)

TABLE 16-3   CLINICAL AND BIOCHEMICAL DETERMINANTS OF MARASMUS AND KWASHIORKOR

	Marasmus	*Kwashiorkor*
Age of maximal incidence	6–18 months	12–48 months
Emaciation	3+	1–2+
Edema	None	1–3+
Fatty infiltration of liver	None to 1+	3+
Skin changes	Infrequent	Frequent
Serum albumin	Almost normal	Markedly decreased
Serum enzymes		
Lipase	Normal	Markedly decreased
Amylase	Normal	Decreased
Esterase	Slightly decreased	Decreased
Serum Lipids		
Triglycerides	Normal	Normal
Cholesterol	Normal	Lowered
Nonesterified fatty acids	Increased	Increased

Source: Adapted from C. Gopalan, "Kwashiorkor and Marasmus: Evolution and Distinguishing Features," in R. A. McCance and E. M. Widdowson (eds.), *Calorie Deficiencies and Protein Deficiencies,* Little, Brown and Company, Boston, 1968.

years old, with both diseases peaking between 6 and 24 months of age. Other researchers report similar observations on the frequency of infectious diseases in developing countries. Scrimshaw et al.[22] outlined very clearly the consequences of infection on human nutritional status. Even the mildest infectious diseases increase urinary nitrogen excretion,[23] because of an increased mobilization of amino acids from peripheral muscle for gluconeogenesis in the liver, with deamination and the excretion of nitrogen in the form of urea. Unless an augmented dietary intake compensates for the lost nitrogen, the depletion will precipitate a kwashiorkorlike syndrome.

Besides nitrogen, metabolic losses also include potassium, magnesium, zinc, phosphorus, sulphur, and vitamins A, C, and B_2.[24] There is increased utilization, sequestration, or diversion from normal metabolic pathways of several nutrients. In spite of the mobilization of amino acids from the peripheral muscle, whole-blood amino acids decrease after exposure to an infectious agent.[25] Increased gluconeogenesis is accompanied by an increased diversion of amino acids for the synthesis of acute-phase proteins such as haptoglobin C-reactive protein, alpha$_1$-antitrypsin and alpha$_2$-macroglobulin in response to the infection.[26]

MALNUTRITION AND THE IMMUNE RESPONSE

The malnourished child is susceptible to infections because the child's immune defense system is depressed. The child's already poor nutritional status further deteriorates after the infection, making the child more susceptible to a secondary infection.

The term *immune* is derived from the Latin word *immunis,* meaning "safety." Several host defenses of the body's immune response system have been shown to be affected by malnutrition; these include the cell-mediated immune response antibody production, phagocyte and killing function of the leukocytes, and the complement system.

Cell-Mediated Immunity

The cell-mediated immune response is controlled through the *thymus-dependent lymphocytes* (T-cells). It plays a major role in the body's defense against viruses, mycobacteria, and fungi.[27] Thymus-dependent lymphocytes are present in the peripheral blood, thymus, spleen, and peripheral lymph nodes.

Jackson was the first to call attention to lymphoid atrophy associated with severe protein-calorie malnutrition (PCM) when he noted at autopsy that the thymus glands of children with kwashiorkor were reduced to only a few strands of tissue.[28] In addition to atrophy of the thymus, lymph nodes, and tonsils, the spleen appeared smaller in malnourished children.[29-31] Malnourished children have fewer circulating T-cells,[32,33] but this thymus-dependent lymphopenia improves with nutritional recovery.[34] Lymphocytes account for 30 percent of the normal differential white count (6.300/mm^3 average value for a 2-year-old

child),[35] and a lymphocyte count below this value in a child of two may be indicative of an impaired cellular defense mechanism.

The cell-mediated immune response is evaluated in individuals by intradermal skin testing and in culture mediums by the enumeration of T-lymphocytes and by the antigen and mitogen stimulation of isolated lymphocytes. [Antigen—any protein not normally present in the body which, when introduced into the bloodstream, stimulates production of a protein (antibody) that reacts specifically with it. Mitogen—a substance causing or inducing mitosis.] When an individual is exposed to a new antigen such as mycobacteria or BCG, the uncommitted lymphocytes become sensitized to the new antigen. With reexposure to the antigen, the lymphocytes proliferate, releasing lymphokines which produce the inflammatory response and a positive skin test.

Several investigators have noted decreased numbers of positive tuberculin skin tests in children with PCM, although the defective skin test response improves after nutritional rehabilitation.[36] The depressed reactivity to skin test antigens in the malnourished child correlates well with depression of lymphocyte function in culture mediums. This in vitro evaluation of lymphocytes reveals a decreased rate of DNA synthesis. After nutritional recovery, in vitro lymphocyte transformation also becomes normal.[37]

The depressed cell-mediated immune response may be secondary to deficiencies of protein, calories, vitamins, or minerals, or may be due to the suppressive effect of the superimposed infection. These nutritional factors interact with and depress the cell-mediated immune system, leading to increased susceptibility to those infections which the system normally handles.

Polymorphonuclear Leukocytes and Macrophages

The polymorphonuclear leukocytes (PMNs) and macrophages are phagocytic cells with functions related to three major areas:[38]

1 Chemotaxis (the ability of the cell to be attracted to a foreign subject)
2 Phagocytosis (engulfment of particles)
3 Postphagocytotic events, including:
   a phagocytic vacuole formation and degranulation
   b microbial killing
   c concomitant metabolic changes

Under normal conditions, PMNs constitute 65 percent of the differential leukocyte count, of which 59 percent are segmented polymorphs and 5 percent are nonsegmented. With certain infections a polymorpholeukocytosis occurs and the number of nonsegmented polymorphs increases.

Phagocytosis of various particles by the PMNs is not affected by the child's nutritional state.[39,40] In addition the opsonic activity of the plasma in protein-calorie malnutrition does not appear depressed.[41] (Opsonic activity refers to the presence of opsonin in the serum, a substance which attacks bacteria, rendering them more susceptible to the action of phagocytes.)

Humoral Immunity-Immunoglobin and Antibody Response

A second population of circulating lymphocytes, the B-cells (bursa cells) or thymus-independent lymphocytes, is responsible for immunoglobulin production. In humans there are five major structural types or classes of immunoglobins called IgG, IgM, IgA, IgD, and IgE.

Although the majority of malnourished children have elevated circulating immonuglobulins secondary to an intercurrent infection, many children cannot respond to various antigenic stimuli when they enter the hospital.[42] In addition to the depressed antibody response to foreign antigens, the malnourished child has depressed secretory IgA in nasopharyngeal and salivary secretions.[43] Chandra et al. have demonstrated that malnourished children have a reduced secretory IgA antibody response to poliomyelitis vaccine. Other changes accompanying the decreased secretory immunoglobulins include reduced digestive enzymes, atrophy of the gut wall, and an impaired hepatic reticuloendothelial system, all of which affect the body's susceptibility to gram-negative organisms, especially those from the gastrointestinal tract.[44]

It has not been determined which of the specific nutrient deficiencies in malnourished children is responsible for the depressed antibody response.

Complement System

This system comprises several protein fractions, known as *complement* components, which are involved in several host defenses:[45]

Viral neutralization

Chemotaxis of polymorphs, leukocytes, monocytes, eosinophils

Opsonization of fungi (a process related to opsonin activity)

Endotoxin inactivation

Lysis of virus-infected cells

Bacteriolysis

Sirisinha et al. found that most of the complement components and hemolytic activity were depressed in children with PCM. In addition, malnourished children had anticomplementary activity in their serum.[46] It is well known that several substances, including endotoxin and immune complexes, activate complement or have anticomplementary activity. There is evidence that a circulating endotoxin exists which may be one source of the anticomplementary activity found in 50 percent of the children with PCM on hospital admission.[47] (Table 16-4 summarizes the changes in the immune system in PCM.)

INTRAUTERINE MALNUTRITION

Severe nutritional deficits during pregnancy affect intrauterine growth. Intrauterine growth is indicative of maternal well-being as

TABLE 16-4 CHANGES IN THE IMMUNE SYSTEM IN PROTEIN-CALORIE MALNUTRITION

Cell-mediated immunity (T-cell-mediated)	Depressed
Humoral immunity (B-cell-mediated)	
1 Serum immunoglobulins	Normal or elevated
2 Antibody response	Depressed or negative
3 Secretory immunoglobulins	Depressed
Polymorphonuclear leukocyte response	
1 In vivo	Normal
2 In vitro	Depressed or normal
Complement system	
1 Complement proteins	Depressed
2 Hemolytic complement activity	Depressed

well as socioeconomic status.[48] The effects of malnutrition on fetal growth depend on the timing, severity, and duration of the nutritional insult. Subacute fetal distress occurs when the fetus is overdue and is deprived of appropriate supplementation for days prior to birth; this leads to a wasted infant of normal length. In chronic fetal distress, deprivation extends over weeks and arrests growth at an earlier period. Inasmuch as the fetus has not acquired any excess body fat, deficits occur in weight proportional to length. The post-term sequelae of chronic fetal intrauterine malnutrition include height and weight retardation, in which the neonate tends to remain small for his age, in addition to defects in immunocompetency similar to those seen in postnatally malnourished children.

Several etiologic factors contribute to the development of intrauterine malnutrition. The influence of maternal nutrition on ultimate fetal weight has been pointed out by Lechtig et al.,[49] who found that when short women from the lower socioeconomic group were given caloric supplementation during pregnancy, neonatal birth weight was significantly increased.

THE TREATMENT OF THE MALNOURISHED CHILD

Severely malnourished children usually have either diarrhea, pneumonia, otitis media,

urinary tract infection, or septicemia. It is important to determine the site of infection and the etiologic agent. The malnourished child should have a complete blood count; serum electrolyte determination; and cultures of stool, urine (by suprapubic tap), blood, ear exudate, throat and nasopharnygeal specimens, and cerebrospinal fluid where clinically indicated. Therapy should be rigorous in the treatment of infection.

Initial intravenous rehydration is with Ringer's lactate with 50 percent dextrose added to make a 10 percent solution. A child with severe potassium depletion should receive up to 6 to 7 mq of supplemental potassium/kg of body weight per day. Intravenous fluids may contain up to 40 mq/l of potassium. The remainder of the potassium supplementation is given orally. A severely dehydrated child may receive up to 20 ml of fluids/kg during the first hour of therapy in order to increase the intravascular volume and renal blood flow. Following initial rehydration, the patient's fluid balance can be maintained through the use of $1/4$ normal saline in 10 percent dextrose solution.

After initial rehydration, the patient continues to receive supplemental potassium at a maintenance dose of 5 mq/kg per day. Magnesium is given at a dose of 0.4 mq/kg intramuscularly daily for 7 days, followed by daily oral magnesium doses of 1.4 mq/kg. Once a patient has reached a daily oral intake of 175 kcal (735 kJ)/kg and 4 g of protein/kg, magnesium and potassium are usually met by diet alone.

Patients with severe diarrhea are kept NPO (nothing per os—by mouth) for up to 24 to 48 h. Following the first 24 to 48 h, the patient is placed on gradually increasing protein and calorie intakes. By the end of the first week, the patient usually tolerates 100 kcal (420 kJ)/kg and 4 g of protein/kg of body weight. Initially, the needed calories and protein may be supplied by a diluted milk-based formula supplemented with Dextri-Maltose and corn oil, which can be readily given by tube feeding. A formula which provides 175 kcal (735 kJ)/kg and 4 g of protein/kg would have 9.5 g of fat and 18.3 g of carbohydrate. When cow's milk is used as a formula base it is important to consider the addition of essential vitamins and minerals.[50] Iron supplementation should be given when indicated.[51]

After the patient's course has stabilized, solid food may be gradually introduced into the diet. When children with protein-calorie malnutrition are offered solid food ad lib., they soon take up to 160 to 180 kcal (672 to 756 kJ)/kg by the second or third week of hospitalization. This intake is maintained for the first month and then gradually is decreased to 140 to 150 kcal (588 to 630 kJ)/kg. After the child has reached the optimal weight for height, intake usually decreases to 110 to 120 kcal (462 to 504 kJ)/kg of body weight per day.

THE PREVENTION OF MALNUTRITION

Before initiating preventive measures, one must define the objectives of such a program, such as:[52]

1 Detection of early signs of malnutrition in order to take remedial action
2 Reduction of the frequency and severity of infectious disease
3 Improvement of the nutritional status of women of childbearing age, particularly through adolescence, pregnancy, and lactation
4 Reduction in the number of low-birth-weight infants and in perinatal mortality and morbidity
5 Spacing pregnancies at reasonable intervals

Ignorance of nutritional requirements and of the nutritive value of foods often plays an important role in the etiology of malnutrition.[53] Nutritional information should be included in all educational activities. However, if educational measures ignore the population's existing food habits and prejudices, proposed nutritional changes are likely to be unrealistic and unacceptable.[54] Improvements through relatively small alterations in established food habits are easier to institute than radical changes. Nutrition education programs should recommend locally available foods.

To prevent malnutrition, the basic principles of nutrition must be taught to teachers, nurses, social workers, agricultural extension workers, home economists, and other professionals who use their knowledge in community activities.[55] In addition, political authorities and professionals at the university level in medicine, public health, biological sciences, agriculture, economics, and other subjects directly or indirectly related to health and nutrition should be included in educational programs.

Education and intervention programs should be aimed at improving the children's nutritional status. Early weaning risks in developing countries[56] arise largely from infection associated with poor hygiene, especially in formula preparation, and from the lack of knowledge and money to prepare a nutritious substitute for breast milk. Mothers should be encouraged to breast-feed for as long as possible.

Supplementary feeding programs have been widely used for improving nutrition. Pregnant and lactating women are frequently the recipients of such food distribution. School lunch programs and nutritional rehabilitation centers help to carry out supplementary feeding programs.[57] These low-cost day-care center programs are particularly intended to rehabilitate malnourished children without the expense of full hospitalization. Day-care centers have also been set up in different parts of the world for children over 2 years of age; they receive supplementation at these centers as well as in home visits. In terms of maternal- and family-child interaction, the supplemented child often receives more stimulation, rewards, and deferences than the unsupplemented child, and becomes an active, independent, playful youngster who frequently verbalizes and demands. This behavior appears to stimulate the parent, resulting in more frequent and varied two-way interaction between child and parent, and between child and environment.

Adding a relatively small quantity of animal products to the diet of predominantly vegetarian populations can be beneficial. Animal protein supplementation corrects the lysine deficiency of wheat and the tryptophan and lysine deficiency in corn. INCAP studies demonstrated that adequate combinations of vegetable products result in protein values that are comparable to the protein content of animal foods.[58]

Control of infectious disease should be given the highest priority because infection adversely affects the nutritional status of the child. Two essential programs for preventing the consequences of infection are immunization programs and the rehydration of children with diarrhea to minimize the detrimental metabolic response.

Family planning is of paramount importance in most developing countries,[59] since a strong relationship exists between malnutrition and close spacing of pregnancies.[60] The cumulative effect of multiple pregnancies starting very early in life often leads to maternal nutritional depletion. Therefore, family planning should be given its proper role in the prevention of protein-calorie malnutrition.[61]

Successful implementation of the above programs should decrease the prevalence of protein-calorie malnutrition.

The synergism between poor nutritional status, the body's depressed immune response, and infection has been established. There remains now to establish a program which combines food, medicine, nutritional education, and sanitation to interrupt this continuous synergetic interaction and ensure total health and well-being. This particularly applies to the developing nations where hundreds of millions of subsistence farmers and many millions of the absolute poor living in exploding cities are constantly menaced by hunger and malnutrition.

STUDY QUESTIONS

1 Distinguish between the clinical states of kwashiorkor and marasmus.
2 How does infection affect the individual's nutritional status?
3 Explain the cell-mediated immune response. What effect does protein-calorie malnutrition have on this response?
4 Explain humoral immunity. How is it affected by protein-calorie malnutrition?
5 Describe the functions of the complement system.

CASE STUDY 16-1

The following case history is that of a severly malnourished infant whose clinical picture, course, and treatment, may be used as a model to better understand the significance of malnutrition in pediatrics today.

The patient was a 26-day-old malnourished

white male admitted to the Boston Children's Hospital Medical Center with severe isotonic dehydration, shock, and apnea. He was born to a gravida 2, para 1, 25-year-old woman after a normal pregnancy, labor, and delivery. The baby was breast-fed 10 or 12 times daily at home and was given no supplemental foods or vitamins. The mother denied any feeding problems, but noted that the baby was often fussy. Eventually the parents did realize that the baby was thin, but he still seemed to be feeding well. On the day before hospitalization, the infant began sleeping longer than usual, and by the time of admission he was limp and unresponsive. He had no history of fever or vomiting, but several loose stools were noted during the week prior to admission.

Admission data showed the following:

Anthropometric measurements

Birth weight	3270 g
Admission weight	2280 g (79% of birth weight)
Length	45 cm
Head circumference	34 cm (after rehydration)

Laboratory values

Hematology

Hematocrit	46%
White blood cells	10,000

(included 13 PMNs, 15 band cells, 56 lymphocytes, 11 monocytes, 3 myelocytes, and 2 metamyelocytes)

Platelets	increased on peripheral smear

Urinalysis

Specific gravity	1.013
Protein	1+
Glucose	negative
Red blood cells	0
White blood cells	5–10
Hyaline casts	1–2

Chemistries

Sodium	142 meq/l
Potassium	6.0 meq/l
Chloride	115 meq/l
Bicarbonate	17 meq/l
Blood urea nitrogen	136 mg/100 ml
Creatinine	1.7 mg/100 ml
Creatinine	1.7 mg/100 ml
Calcium	6.8 mg/100 ml
Phosphorus	12.0 mg/100 ml
Total protein	4.8 g/100 ml

After initial resuscitation in the emergency clinic, the pale, emaciated, moribund infant was transferred to the intensive care nursery, and an indwelling central venous cannula was inserted. Following initial emergency hydration, his blood pressure was measured at 98/66 mm Hg and central venous pressure at 5 cm H_2O. He had loose, wrinkled skin and decreased subcutaneous tissue. His anterior fontanelle was depressed and his sutures were overriding. Additional physical findings on admission included decreased breath sounds over the left lung field, decreased cardiac sounds, lethargy, and limp reflexes.

Blood, urine, cerebrospinal fluid, and nasopharyngeal, throat, and stool cultures were all negative for pathogens. A chest x-ray revealed a partial left pneumothorax secondary to the attempted placement of the central venous pressure catheter. Long bone x-rays and an upper gastrointestinal x-ray series were normal.

Case Study Questions

1 What criteria would you use to classify this infant nutritionally?

2 How may infection have compromised his nutritional status?

3 Explain the way in which the patient's nutritional status may have affected his immune response and ability to combat infection.

REFERENCES

1 Pan American Health Organization, *Inter-American Investigation of Mortality in Childhood, First Year of Investigation, Provisional Report,* Pan American Health Organization, Washington, D.C., 1971.

2 J. M. Bengoa, "The Problem of Malnutrition," *WHO Chronicle,* **28**:3, 1974.

3 N. S. Scrimshaw, "Causes and Prevention of Malnutrition," in G. H. Beaton (ed.), *Nutrition, a Comprehensive Treatise,* Academic Press, New York, 1964.

4 Ibid.

5 Ibid.

6 D. B. Jelliffe, "Infant Nutrition in the Subtropics and Tropics," World Health Organization Monograph Series, no. 25, 1955.

7 M. Behar, "Principles of Treatment and Prevention of Severe Protein Malnutrition in Children (Kwashiorkor)," *Annals of the New York Academy of Science,* **69:** 954, 1958.

8 Scrimshaw, op. cit.

9 Scrimshaw, op. cit.

10 F. Gomez, "Malnutrition in Infancy and Childhood with Special Reference To Kwashiorkor," *Advances in Pediatrics,* **7**:131, 1955.

11 J. C. Waterlow, "Some Aspects of Childhood Malnutrition as a Public Health Problem," *British Medical Journal,* **4**:88, 1974.

12 J. P. Habicht, "Height and Weight Standards for Preschool Children—How Relevant are Ethnic Differences in Growth Potential?" *Lancet,* **1**:611, 1974.

13 Waterlow, op. cit., p. 88.

14 Habicht, op. cit., p. 611.

15 Behar, op. cit., p. 954.

16 J. C. Waterlow, *Advances in Protein Chemistry,* **15**:138, 1960.

17 Scrimshaw, op. cit.

18 C. Gopalan, "Kwashiorkor and Marasmus: Evolution and Distinguishing Features," in R. A. McCance and E. M. Widdowson (eds.), *Calorie Deficiencies and Protein Deficiencies,* Little, Brown and Company, Boston, 1968.

19 N. S. Scrimshaw, C. E. Taylor, and J. E. Gordon, "Interactions of Malnutrition and Infection: Advances in Understanding," World Health Organization Monograph Series, no. 57, 1968.

20 Ibid.

21 J. M. Reyna-Barrios, "Methods to Increase Coverage and Improve the Quality of Ambulatory Patient Care in Rural Areas of Guatemala, Using Medical Auxiliaries," *Revista del Colegio Medico de Guatemala,* **22**:134, 1971.

22 N. S. Scrimshaw, C. E. Taylor, and J. E. Gordon, "Interactions of Malnutrition and Infection."

23 W. R. Beisel, "Malnutrition as a Consequence of Stress" in R. M. Suskind (ed.), *Malnutrition and the Immune Response,* Raven Press, New York, 1977.

24 W. R. Beisel, "Non-Specific Host Defense Factors," in R. M. Suskind (ed.), op. cit.

25 R. D. Feigin, "Whole Blood Amino Acids in Experimentally Induced Typhoid Fever in Man," *New England Journal of Medicine,* **278**:293, 1968.

26 W. R. Beisel, "Nutritional Effects on the Responsiveness of Plasma Acute Phase Reactant Glycoproteins," in R. M. Suskind (ed.), op. cit.

27 R. Edelman, "Cell Mediated Immune Function," in R. M. Suskind (ed.), op. cit.

28 C. M. Jackson, *The Effects of Inanition and Malnutrition upon Growth and Structure,* P. Blakiston's Son and Co., Philadelphia, 1925, p. 285.

29 J. W. Mugerwa, "Lymphoreticular System in Kwashiorkor," *Journal of Pathology,* **105**:105, 1971.

30 T. H. Work, "Tropical Problems in Nutrition," *Annals of Internal Medicine,* **79**:701, 1973.

31 P. M. Smythe, "Thymic Lymphatic Deficiency and Depression of Cell Mediated Immunity in Protein Calorie Malnutrition," *Lancet,* **2**:939, 1971.

32 R. K. Chandra, "Rosette-Forming T Lymphocytes and Cell-Mediated Immunity in Malnutrition," *British Medical Journal* **3**:608, 1974.

33 P. Kulapongs, "In Vitro Cellular Immune Response in Thai Children with Protein Calorie Malnutrition," in R. M. Suskind (ed.), op. cit.

34 Ibid.

35 J. Wallach, *Interpretation of Diagnostic Tests,* Little, Brown, and Company, Boston, 1974, p. 5.

36 R. Edelman, "Cell-Mediated Immune Function," in R. M. Suskind (ed.), op. cit.

37 Ibid.

38 S. D. Douglas, "Disorders of Phagocyte Formation; Analytical Review," *Blood,* **35**:851–866, 1970.

39 E. U. Rosen, "Leukocyte Function in Children with Kwashiorkor," *Archives of Diseases of Children* **50**:220, 1975.

40 A. Seth, "Opsonic Activity of Phagocytosis and Bactericidal Capacity of Polymorphs in Undernutrition," *Archives of Diseases of Children,* **47**:282, 1972.

41 Ibid.

42 R. K. Chandra, "Immunoglobulins and Antibody Response in Malnutrition," in R. M. Suskind (ed.), op. cit.

43 S. Sirisinha, "Secretory and Serum IgA in Children with Protein Calorie Malnutrition," *Pediatrics,* **55**:166, 1975.

44 R. K. Chandra et al., "Reduced Secretory Antibody Response to Live Attenuated Measles and Polio Virus Vaccines in Malnourished Children," *British Medical Journal,* **2**:583, 1975.

45 R. B. Johnston, "The Biology of the Complement System," in R. M. Suskind (ed.), op. cit.

46 S. Sirisinha et al., "The Complement System in Protein Calorie Malnutrition," in R. M. Suskind (ed.), op. cit.

47 R. M. Suskind, "Endotoxemia, A Possible Cause of Decreased Complement Activity in Thai Children with Protein Calorie Malnutrition," in R. M. Suskind (ed.), op. cit.

48 P. Gruenwald, "Fetal Growth as an Indicator of Socioeconomic Change," *Public Health Reports,* 83:867, 1968.

49 A. Lechtig et al., "Influence of Maternal Nutrition on Birth Weight," *American Journal of Clinical Nutrition,* **28:**1223, 1975.

50 R. Suskind, "The In-Patient and Out-Patient Treatment of the Child with Severe Protein-Calorie Malnutrition," in R. E. Olson (ed.), *Protein Calorie Malnutrition,* Academic Press, New York, 1975.

51 Ibid.

52 J. M. Bengoa, op. cit.

53 N. S. Scrimshaw, "Causes and Prevention of Malnutrition."

54 Ibid.

55 J. C. Waterlow, *Advances in Protein Chemistry.*

56 J. M. Bengoa, "Prevention of Protein Calorie Malnutrition," in R. E. Olson. (ed.), op. cit.

57 Ibid.

58 N. S. Scrimshaw, "All Vegetable Protein Mixture for Human Feeding. V. Clinical Trials with INCAP Mixtures 8 & 9 and with Corn and Beans," *American Journal of Clinical Nutrition,* **9:**196, 1961.

59 J. M. Bengoa, "Prevention of Protein Calorie Malnutrition,"

60 R. Bisewara, "Nutrition and Family Size," *Journal of Nutrition and Diet,* 1969, p. 258.

61 J. M. Bengoa, "The Problem of Malnutrition."

CHAPTER 17

THE CARDIOVASCULAR SYSTEM

Margaret L. Mikkola

KEY WORDS
Ischemic Heart Disease
Atherosclerosis
Cholesterol
Hyperlipoproteinemia
Hypertension
Congestive Heart Failure
Diuretic

INTRODUCTION

The heart and blood vessels comprise the cardiovascular system, and together establish and maintain the circulation. The heart is a muscular organ which functions as a pump. The blood vessels are a successively dividing series of progressively smaller tubes beginning with the aorta, progressing to arteries, then to arterioles, and finally reaching the capillaries. At this point they gather successively into venules, veins, and the vena cava to return to the heart. The aorta is primarily an elastic structure; the arteries and arterioles, muscular; and the capillaries, thin-walled (one-celled) structures. The venules, veins, and vena cava lack, in large part, the elastic and muscular tissue of the arteries. The heart and blood vessels are so arranged as to link the systemic circulation (peripheral blood vessels) and the pulmonary circulation (blood vessels of the lungs) in series, thus providing a continuous system for blood flow (Fig. 17-1).

The primary functions of the cardiovascular system are to deliver oxygen, required for aerobic metabolism, from the lungs to the other organs (brain, kidneys, liver, skeletal muscle), and, on return, to transport carbon dioxide, as metabolic waste, back to the lungs. These functions are autoregulated by a complex feedback mechanism between the heart and blood vessels on the one hand and the metabolic demands of the organism for oxygen on the other hand.

Diseases of the cardiovascular system affect the heart and its components (heart valves, conduction system, and myocardium) and the blood vessels, primarily the arteries.

In 1973, diseases of the cardiovascular system accounted for approximately 53 percent of all deaths in the United States.[1] Fig. 17-2 shows the death rates from ischemic heart disease and degenerative heart disease from all causes in selected countries. (*Ischemic heart disease* and *coronary artery disease* are inclusive terms for conditions that imply deprivation of the blood supply to the heart and include ath-

Blood flow	Area
Blood returns from the general systemic circulation through the inferior and superior venae cava to the right atrium	Inferior and superior venae cava Right atrium
It then flows to the right ventricle through the tricuspid valve and then is ejected by the right ventricle through the pulmonary valve into the pulmonary artery and to the lungs.	Right ventricle Pulmonary artery ↓ Lungs
Oxygenated blood returns to the left atrium via the pulmonary veins. It then passes through the bicuspid valve to the left ventricle and is pumped through the aortic valve into systemic circulation through the systemic capillary beds where the oxygen and nutrients are distributed.	Pulmonary veins Left atrium Left ventricle Aorta ↓ Systemic capillary beds

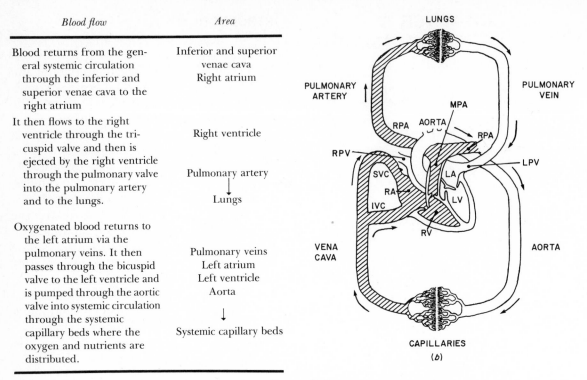

Figure 17-1

Diagram of the cardiovascular system. The heart and blood vessels are so arranged as to link the systemic circulation and the pulmonary circulation in a series, thus providing a continuous system for blood flow.

erosclerosis, angina pectoris, and myocardial infarction.) These figures represent death rates; there are many people alive who are affected by one or more of these diseases. Many of these people are asymptomatic and undiagnosed, while others are handicapped. Because of the high incidence of cardiovascular diseases, many investigations have been initiated to develop effective and feasible means of prevention and treatment.

Cardiovascular disorders that affect human morbidity and mortality in the United States are ischemic heart disease, hypertensive heart disease, congestive heart failure, rheumatic heart disease, and congenital heart disease. In this chapter, ischemic heart disease will be emphasized both because of its high in-

cidence and because of the direct implications for dietary management in prevention and treatment.

ISCHEMIC HEART DISEASE

Atherosclerosis is a degenerative disease of the large and medium arteries. It results from a loss of elasticity (*sclerosis*) that occurs when the inner layer of the arterial wall becomes thickened by atheromatous plaques, consisting first of lipid (mainly cholesterol) followed by fibrous tissue. As these plaques increase in size they may inhibit blood flow through the affected arteries, leading to the clinical manifestations of the disease, primarily ischemic (de-

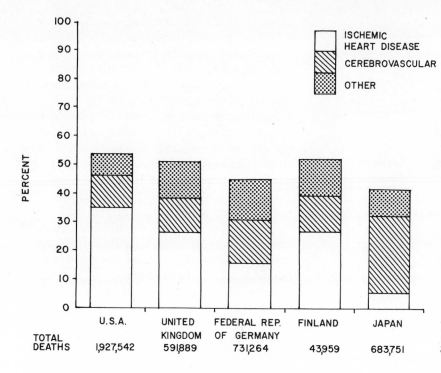

Figure 17-2
Death rates for ischemic heart disease and degenerative heart disease in selected countries. (Adapted from World Health Statistics Annual, vol. 1, World Health Organization, Geneva, Switzerland, 1972.)

prived of blood supply) heart disease. The mechanisms by which these plaques progress is not completely understood. The suspected mechanisms are:[2]

1. Thrombus formation (clot formation on the surface of the plaque followed by fibrous organization of the thrombus)
2. continued lipid accumulation
3. hemorrhage into the plaque

A question frequently posed in regard to plaque formation and atherosclerosis is whether atherosclerosis is a pediatric problem. Fatty streaks in the major arteries have been identified in the first years of life.[3-5] (A fatty streak is a superficial yellowish-gray lesion, similar in composition to the lipids in blood and the earliest accumulation of lipid found in the intima of medium-sized and large arteries.) However, because these streaks have been shown to have about the same severity and prevalence in the first decades of life among many races and countries no matter what the

incidence of ischemic heart disease in these countries, their causative role in the later formation of adult lesions is not clear. Adult lesions evolve from fatty streaks, but the streaks found in the early decades of life do not necessarily predict liability to the disease. Presently, this question must await further research before it can be answered. Figure 17-3 is a diagrammatic illustration of the natural history of atherosclerosis.

Anticoagulants are often used in the treatment of atherosclerosis in addition to diet therapy. The purpose of anticoagulants is to prevent clot formation. The most commonly used anticoagulants are heparin, warfarin, and Dicumarol. When a patient is receiving anticoagulant therapy, specifically Dicumarol, the dietary intake of vitamin K and supplements providing this vitamin should be monitored. This monitoring is necessary since vitamin K promotes clotting of the blood by increasing hepatic synthesis of prothrombin. (Vitamin K sources include spinach, alfalfa, cabbage, and egg yolk.)

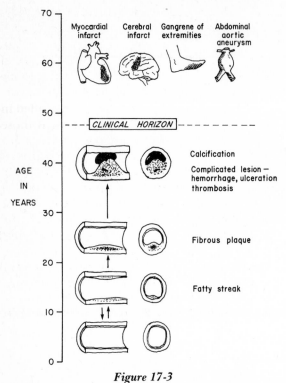

Figure 17-3

Diagram of the natural history of atherosclerosis. Adapted from H. C. McGill, J. C. Geer and J. P. Strong, "Natural History of Human Atherosclerotic Lesions," in M. Sandler and G. H. Bourne (eds.), Atherosclerosis and Its Origins, Academic Press, New York, 1963, p. 42.

The most serious form of atherosclerosis is ischemic heart disease. Its major clinical manifestations are angina pectoris, acute myocardial infarction, sudden death, disturbance in heart rhythm, and congestive heart failure.

Angina pectoris may be defined as a symptom complex consisting of acute substernal chest pain, usually with a characteristic radiation to the left arm, resulting from transient ischemic deprivation of blood flow to the subendocardial layers of the ventricular myocardium. This may occur when the blood supply to the heart is diminished by stenotic obstructive atheromatous lesions in the walls of the coronary arteries. The symptoms of angina frequently may be precipitated by exertion or exercise, when the coronary blood flow, be-

cause of the atheromatous plaques, is unable to meet the oxygen requirements of the exercising heart. Angina pectoris is a common warning signal of coronary artery disease. It can exist for many years in a stable form or may be altered and thus signal the onset of a myocardial infarction.

Myocardial infarction (heart attack) is the extension of diminished coronary blood flow from a transient phenomenon to a state of total permanent deprivation of blood supply to various areas of the heart by complete obstruction of the coronary artery. The severity of the heart attack is related to the site and extent of the interruption of coronary flow, the state of unaffected coronary arteries (the collateral circulation), and the condition of the heart muscle (e.g., from previous heart attacks).

Treatment for angina pectoris includes avoidance of activities which produce its occurrence (often excessive exertion), the use of nitroglycerin and other drugs, maintenance of ideal body weight, and appropriate prescribed exercise. During the past 5 years, intractable angina pectoris (unresponsive to nitroglycerin or propranolol), with operative stenotic lesions demonstrated by coronary angiography, has been surgically treated by inserting an autogenous saphenous vein graft from the aorta to the involved coronary artery, bypassing the obstructive lesions. Symptomatic results are encouraging although a certain percentage of the grafts have become obstructed after surgery.

Treatment for myocardial infarction requires hospitalization for proper management. This will include diet therapy when the patient's condition is stable. The emphasis of dietary therapy immediately after hospitalization is of course to aid in attaining a stable condition by utilizing a nutritionally adequate diet which is usually soft, bland, and easily tolerated. If this can be done with the type of diet (i.e., fat-controlled, low-cholesterol) that the patient will be following after discharge, dietary teaching will be more effective.

Complications that may develop after a myocardial infarction are cardiovascular shock, arrhythmias, and congestive heart failure. These complications are treated with medical therapy, which includes digitalis, anticoagulants, diuretics, and dietary salt restriction as well as mechanical methods to aid the pumping function of the heart.

Sudden death may occur during an acute myocardial infarction but also may occur in a patient with no symptoms or with stable angina, or when there has been a previous myocardial infarction. The immediate mechanism is probably ventricular fibrillation (total disorganization of heart contractions). Recently mortality from myocardial infarction has been decreasing in areas where there are mobile and hospital coronary care units.

It is important that patients be educated about the warning signs of myocardial infarction (for example, chest pain) and about the risk factors, which are discussed below.

Cerebrovascular disease is another major form of atherosclerosis. It includes the complex clinical symptoms of *transient cerebral ischemic attacks* and *strokes*. The symptoms that occur depend on the artery involved, the area of the brain supplied, the nature of the collateral circulation, and the pathologic process in the artery. Strokes may be associated with atherosclerosis, resulting in cerebral infarction (the brain is deprived of blood), or may be associated with hypertensive disease, resulting in brain hemorrhage.

Other types of atherosclerosis include aortic, renovascular, peripheral vascular, and pulmonic. Each type has symptoms manifested in the organ or area supplied by the affected arteries. Treatment depends on the extent and location of the plaque and may consist of medical therapy, including medication, diet (e.g., weight reduction, sodium restriction), and exercise, or surgical intervention.

Risk Factors

Several risk factors, identified through extensive epidemiologic studies, have been associated with an increased rate of atherosclerosis and ischemic heart disease. Of the factors iden-

tified none is believed to be solely responsible; they are thought to be multiply causal, each playing an interrelated role. The risk factors cited by the American Heart Association can be separated into (1) overt problems and personal attributes, and (2) environmental factors (see Table 17-1). From the factors identified in the table one can separate into groups those which cannot be modified, those which are difficult to adjust, and those which can be altered or are subject to intervention (see Table 17-2). In the future, epidemiologic studies of populations in whom these risk factors have been changed may define the extent to which the progression of atherosclerosis and ischemic heart disease can be altered.

Dietary intervention is especially important in the adjustment of three risk factors, namely, *obesity, hypertension,* and *hyperlipidemia.* Since hyperlipidemia has been identified as one of the major risk factors and is particularly responsive to diet therapy, its role in ischemic heart disease will now be considered.

TABLE 17-1   RISK FACTORS AND CORONARY DISEASE

Overt problems and personal attributes	Environmental factors
Familial occurrence of coronary disease at an early age	Cigarette smoking
Hypertension	Lack of physical activity
Electrocardiographic abnormalities	Emotionally stressful situations
Diabetes mellitus	
Lipid abnormalities involving serum cholesterol and triglycerides and their lipoprotein vehicles	
Obesity	
Gout (hyperuricemia)	
Certain personality and behavior patterns	

Source: Risk Factors and Coronary Heart Disease: A Statement for Physicians, American Heart Association Publ. No. EM451, 1968. Reprinted with permission.

TABLE 17-2 ALTERABILITY OF RISK FACTORS IN ATHEROSCLEROSIS AND ISCHEMIC HEART DISEASE

Possible	Difficult	Impossible
Hyperlipidemia*	Underlying disease	Heredity
Hypertension*	Stress	Advancing age
Obesity*	Personality	Sex
Smoking		
Exercise		

*Dietary implications.

Hyperlipidemia

Hyperlipidemia is an elevation of serum cholesterol, triglycerides, or both. Cholesterol, triglycerides, and phospholipids are carried in the plasma bound to specific proteins, the alpha-globulin and beta-globulin fractions of plasma protein. These lipoproteins vary as to the amount of protein and fat they contain and can be identified according to their density and electrophoretic mobility. The four major classes of lipoproteins are:

Chylomicrons

Pre-beta (very-low-density) lipoprotein (VLDL)

Beta (low-density) lipoprotein (LDL)

Alpha (high-density) lipoprotein (HDL)

Figure 17-4 shows the composition of the various lipoproteins. Low-density lipoproteins (LDL) and very-low-density lipoproteins (VLDL) are those lipoproteins which contain the most lipid and the least protein; high-density lipoproteins (HDL) are those containing the most protein and the least lipid. Table 17-3 gives the normal limits of the plasma lipids and lipoproteins. Generally, the HDL level is higher in women than in men,[6] and the level is thought to remain relatively constant in all individuals. Factors that might affect an individual's HDL level (e.g., diet, exercise, and medication) and the role of HDL in coronary heart disease are being investigated. The plasma LDL, VLDL, and chylomicrons, on the other hand, reflect dietary changes.

The occurrence of another lipoprotein has been proposed, that of a transient intermediate-low-density lipoprotein (ILDL) appearing during conversion of VLDL to LDL.[7] This lipoprotein has not been shown to have any dietary significance.

Each of the lipoproteins has a different

Figure 17-4

Composition of lipoproteins.

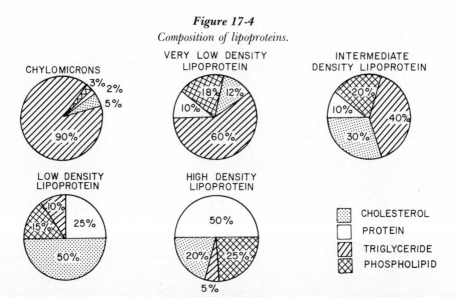

TABLE 17-3   PLASMA LIPID AND LIPOPROTEIN CONCENTRATIONS
Suggested normal limits*

Age	Total cholesterol mg/100 ml	Triglyceride, mg/100 ml	Pre-beta cholesterol, mg/100 ml	Beta cholesterol, mg/100 ml	Alpha cholesterol, mg/100 ml Males	Females
0–19	120–230	10–140	5–25	50–170	30–65	30–70
20–29	120–240	10–140	5–25	60–170	35–70	35–75
30–39	140–270	10–150	5–35	70–190	30–65	35–80
40–49	150–310	10–160	5–35	80–190	30–65	40–85
50–59	160–330	10–190	10–40	80–210	30–65	35–85

* Based on 95 percent fiducial limits calculated for small samples—all values rounded to nearest 5 mg. (It will be noted that, for practical purposes, differences between the sexes have been ignored except for alpha-lipoprotein concentrations.)

Source: D. S. Fredrickson, "Fat Transport in Lipoproteins—An Integrated Approach to Mechanisms and Disorders," *New England Journal of Medicine* **276:**151 1967.

charge which enables it to be separated by electrophoresis, on paper or agarose gel, into a nonmigrating lipoprotein band (Fig. 17-5). The lipoproteins can also be identified by ultracentrifugation, which separates them according to their density. These two methods have been used to determine the lipoprotein

Figure 17-5

Normal lipoprotein band on electrophoresis.

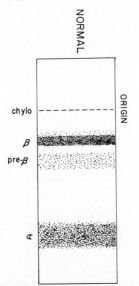

values in plasma and to identify five major types of hyperlipoproteinemias, which are discussed in detail below.

Since diet is essential in the treatment of the hyperlipoproteinemias, those dietary factors influencing the lipoproteins will now be discussed.

Dietary treatment involves alteration in the following dietary components: cholesterol, fat, saturated fat, polyunsaturated fat, carbohydrate, and alcohol.

Cholesterol

Changes in the diet can cause predictable changes in the plasma cholesterol level. The cholesterol level in the red blood cells remains very constant, approximately 138 mg/100 ml of cells, and the effects of diet exert their influence on the serum.[8] Most of the cholesterol in the plasma is carried in the LDL. Keys has reported that the usual American diet averages approximately 250 mg cholesterol/1000 kcal (or 250 mg cholesterol/4200 kJ) and that at this level of intake substantial changes in the serum cholesterol level are difficult to detect.[9] Table 17-4, below, gives the average amount of cholestrol in some common foods.

Fat

The normal metabolic pathways of fat are described in Chap. 5. The ingested long-chain free fatty acids (chain length of C_{12} or greater) are reesterified with glycerol to form triglycerides in the intestinal mucosa. These triglycerides combine with cholesterol esters, phospholipids, and protein to form the chylomicrons of plasma. These macroparticles serve as a vehicle for transport of fatty acids within the plasma. In the human body chylomicron levels rise after meals; the amount of chylomicron formation is determined by the amount of fat ingested. Chylomicrons eventually move from the plasma into the body's fat depot, a process facilitated by the enzyme lipoprotein lipase. There are certain individuals who do not adequately clear the chylomicrons and even after a 12 to 16 hour fast their plasma levels remain elevated. This is known as *exogenous hyperlipidemia* and indicates a deficient clearing mechanism, possibly resulting from decreased lipoprotein lipase activity.

Dietary fat has a less understood effect on the VLDL. Both the liver and intestine synthesize VLDL from glucose and free fatty acids. An elevation of VLDL from this source is known as *endogenous hyperlipidemia*. The free fatty acid availability is determined by several factors, one of which and of primary importance is obesity.

Saturated Fats

Saturated fatty acids, primarily those with 12 through 17 carbon atoms and especially lauric acid, elevate the plasma cholesterol. Saturated fats are primarily of animal origin, although several nonanimal sources are highly saturated, for example, coconut oil. Table 17-4 lists some of the common sources of saturated fats.

Polyunsaturated Fats

Polyunsaturated fatty acids, primarily linoleic acid, in contrast to saturated fatty acids, have a lowering effect on the plasma cholesterol, but approximately 2 g of polyunsaturates are needed to counteract the effect of 1 g of saturates; thus, a dietary ratio of 2 to 1 (polyunsaturates to saturates) is recommended. Polyunsaturates are primarily of vegetable origin, the greatest source being vegetable oil. Table 17-4, below, lists the linoleic fatty acid content of some selected foods. Food processing may induce partial hydrogenation of polyunsaturated fat, decreasing the total amount available. Another change that may occur following food processing is isomerization of some of the naturally occurring *cis* fatty acids into *trans* fatty acids. The effect of larger amounts of *trans* fatty acids in the diet is controversial; there are conflicting reports of their effect on plasma lipids, on essential fatty acid requirements, and on cell membranes.[10] Other questions have been raised regarding possible adverse effects of diets with high levels of polyunsaturated fats on the incidence of cancer,[11] but the evidence is inconclusive.

Vitamin E requirements are thought to be increased with higher intakes of polyunsaturated fats.[12] Some sources high in polyunsaturated fats also have higher levels of the vitamin but many do not. Of special concern is the infant receiving formulas high in polyunsaturated fats. The recommended dietary allowance of 4 to 5 IU of vitamin E[13] can be met by these formulas but the adequacy of this amount with some formulas is still questionable. Studies in adults living at home and eating diets high in polyunsaturated fat have not demonstrated a decrease in serum vitamin E levels or conclusive evidence of any harmful effect. The effects on populations who have consumed large amounts of polyunsaturated fats for extended time periods are unknown.

One needs to exert clinical judgment in the amount of polyunsaturated fat to be recommended. Too often patients have taken excessive quantities of polyunsaturated fat to counter their intake of saturated fat, resulting in an excessive caloric intake and therefore in weight gain.

Monounsaturated Fats

Monounsaturated fatty acids, primarily oleic and erucic acids, have no known effect on plasma cholesterol levels. Table 17-4 lists some of the most common oleic acid food sources.

Carbohydrate

The liver and intestine make VLDL from glucose and free fatty acids. It is believed that the primary effect of excess carbohydrate on plasma lipids is the elevation of VLDL. Normal individuals, when on a high-carbohydrate diet, will exhibit a degree of elevated plasma VLDL but this will usually disappear gradually. However, some persons have persistently elevated VLDL levels. Low-carbohydrate diets cause a significant reduction in the mean levels of triglyceride and VLDL in men who previously exhibited elevated levels. There remains controversy as to the effect of simple carbohydrates (sugars) versus more complex carbohydrates (starches) on the plasma lipids. It is generally accepted that simple sugars seem more lipemic (increasing the VLDL) in patients who have hyperlipoproteinemia. This is most likely because of the increased quantity that is frequently ingested.

Alcohol

In many types of hyperlipoproteinemia alcohol produces or exacerbates hyperglyceridemia.[14,15] The exact mechanisms by which this is produced are unclear.

The Hyperlipoproteinemias

Having presented the dietary factors which affect the lipoproteins, the five major types of hyperlipoproteinemia (Table 17-5) will now be discussed, with emphasis on their dietary treatment as recommended in Table 17-6.

Type I Hyperlipoproteinemia

Type I hyperlipoproteinemia is manifested by the inability to clear chylomicrons from the plasma. It is believed to be due to a deficiency of the enzyme lipoprotein lipase. It is usually diagnosed in childhood.

Clinical and laboratory signs Chylomicrons are present in the serum (expressed in a triglyceride value often in the thousands) and give a creamy appearance to the blood. Eruptive xanthomas may be seen. Patients may complain of abdominal pain and suffer from pancreatitis.

Dietary treatment Type I is treated with a diet very low in fat (25 to 35 g in adults, 10 to 15 g in infants),[16,17] to aid in keeping the plasma chylomicron level low. Medium-chain triglycerides (MCT), i.e., fatty acids of 8 to 10 carbon atoms in length, are available commercially and are often used to make the diet more palatable. MCT are absorbed directly via the portal circulation and do not increase chylomicron formation. Calories, carbohydrate, protein, and cholesterol are not restricted, but alcohol should be avoided as it may produce hypertriglyceridemia (the exact mechanism by which this is produced is unclear).

Type II Hyperlipoproteinemia

Type II hyperlipoproteinemia, also known as familial hyperbetalipoproteinemia or familial hypercholesterolemia, is characterized by an elevated cholesterol of LDL origin. Type II is one of the severest types in regard to its arterial involvement and is believed to account for a large degree of premature morbidity and mortality from ischemic (coronary) heart disease. Type II is further differentiated into type IIa and type IIb. In type IIa triglycerides are normal while in type IIb they are elevated, as shown by increased VLDL. The fundamental defect, which appears to be inherited, is unknown.

Clinical and laboratory signs In *type IIa* serum cholesterol is elevated, frequently to 300 to 600 mg/100 ml, and on electrophoresis the beta-lipoprotein band is enlarged. The homozygous

TABLE 17-4 CHOLESTEROL AND FAT CONTENT OF SELECTED FOODS

Food	Measure	Weight, g	Fat, g	SFA, g	Linoleic acid, g	Oleic acid, g	Cholesterol, mg
Egg yolk	1 large	50*	5.7	1.7	0.6	2.1	252
Liver (beef, calf, lamb, pork)		100					438
Kidney		100					804
Brains, raw		100					>2000
Veal		100	5.4	2.3	0.1	2.4	99
Beef, round	lean	100	6.4	2.7	0.25	2.3	91
Lamb, leg	only	100	7.1	4.0	0.2	2.6	100
Pork:							
Loin		100	13.9	4.7	1.15	5.8	88
Cured ham		100	8.8	3.0	0.7	3.7	
Poultry: (chicken, turkey)							
light		100	3.7	1.1	0.7	1.4	78 average
dark		100	7.3	2.2	1.5	3.0	96 average
Fish:							
Flounder	raw	100					50
Haddock		100	1.0	0.6	tr	0.3	60
Halibut		100					60
Tuna, canned water pack		100	0.8	0.2	0.01	0.1	63
Salmon, canned pink		100	5.2	0.85	0.1	0.8	35
Shellfish		100					45–150 varies widely
Milk:							
3.5% Fat	1 cup	244	8.5	5.4	0.2	2.1	34
1% Fat	1 cup	246	2.5	1.5	0.05	0.6	14
Skim	1 cup	245	<1				5
Butter	1 tbsp	14	11.2	7.0	0.3	2.8	35
Cream:							
Light	1 tbsp	15	3.1	1.9	0.1	0.8	10
Half & half		15	1.8	1.1	tr	0.4	6
Heavy		15	5.7	3.5	0.1	1.4	20
Sour		12	2.2	1.4	0.1	0.6	8
Cottage cheese:		100					
4% Fat			4.0	2.6	0.09	0.9	19
1% Fat			1.0				9
Cheddar and American cheese	1 oz	28	8.6	5.4	0.2	2.2	27
Cream cheese	1 tbsp	14	4.7	3.0	0.1	1.1	16
Yogurt:							
Whole milk		100	3.4	2.2	0.07	0.8	
Partially skim		100	1.5	1.0	0.03	0.3	8
Ice cream, 16% fat	1 cup	148	23.8	13.1	0.7	7.9	85
Oils:							
Safflower		100	100	9.4	73.3	11.9	—
Sunflower		100	100	10.6	56.5	27.4	—
Corn		100	100	12.7	57.4	24.6	—
Soybean		100	100	15.0	50.8	22.8	—
Cottonseed		100	100	26.1	50.3	18.1	—
Olive		100	100	14.2	8.2	71.5	—
Peanut		100	100	19.1	28.9	46.0	—
Coconut		100	100	86.3	1.8	5.7	—

(continued)

TABLE 17-4 *(continued)*

Food	Measure	Weight, g	Fat, g	SFA, g	Lino-leic acid, g	Oleic acid, g	Cholesterol, mg
Nuts:							
Walnuts	1 cup	100	63.4	6.9	34.9	9.7	—
Peanuts	⅔ cup	100	49.7	9.4	14.4	22.9	—
Cashews	⅔ cup	100	45.6	9.2	7.3	26.2	—
Margarines	1 tbsp						
Corn oil:		14	11.2	2.0	5.3	3.6	—
Tub		14	11.2	2.1	4.1	4.6	—
Partially hydrogenated		14	11.2	2.4	2.0	6.2	—
Shortening, vegetable	1 tbsp	12.5	12.5	3.1	2.7	6.3	—
Mayonnaise	1 tbsp	14	11.2	2.0	5.6	2.4	10
Avocado	⅔ cup	100	16.4	3.3	2.1	7.4	—
Chocolate	1 oz	28	15.0	8.4	0.3	5.6	—
Lard		100	100	38	10.0	46	95

SFA = saturated fatty acids; tr = trace; > = more than; < = less than.

* Whole egg.

Sources:

1 R. M. Feeley, "Cholesterol Content of Foods," *Journal of the American Dietetic Association,* **61:**134–149, 1972.

2 L. P. Posati, "Comprehensive Evaluation of Fatty acids in Foods. I. Dairy Products," *Journal of the American Dietetic Association,* **66,** 482–488, 1975.

3 B. A. Anderson, "Comprehensive Evaluation of Fatty Acids in Foods. II. Beef Products," *Journal of the American Dietetic Association,* **67:**35–41, 1975.

4 L. P. Posati, "Comprehensive Evaluation of Fatty Acids in Foods. III. Eggs and Egg Products," *Journal of the American Dietetic Association,* **67:**111–115, 1975.

5 G. A. Fristrom, "Comprehensive Evaluation of Fatty Acids in Foods. IV. Nuts, Peanuts and Soups," *Journal of the American Dietetic Association,* **67:**351–355, 1975.

6 C. A. Brignoli, "Comprehensive Evaluation of Fatty Acids in Foods. V. Unhydrogenated Fats and Oils," *Journal of the American Dietetic Association,* **68:**224–228, 1976.

7 B. A. Anderson, "Comprehensive Evaluation of Fatty Acids in Foods. VII. Pork Products," *Journal of the American Dietetic Association,* **69:**44–49, 1976.

8 J. Exler, "Comprehensive Evaluation of Fatty acids in Foods. VIII. Finfish," *Journal of the American Dietetic Association,* **69:**243–248, 1976.

9 C. F. Adams, *Nutritive Value of American Foods,* U.S. Dept. of Agriculture Handbook No. 456, November 1975.

10 B. K. Watt, *Composition of Foods,* U.S. Dept. of Agriculture Handbook No. 8, December 1963.

11 R. M. Leverton, *Fats in Food and Diet,* U.S. Dept. of Agriculture Information Bulletin No. 361, January 1974.

child may exhibit clinical signs at birth or within the first few years of life, but the heterozygous child often is not diagnosed until environmental factors such as diet have exacerbated the clinical symptoms in later years or adulthood. The clinical signs include corneal arcus (cholesterol deposits surrounding the cornea), xanthelasma (cholesterol deposits around the eye such as on the eyelid) tendinous and tuberous xanthomas (cholesterol deposits on tendons, heel, and elbow) and premature vascular disease involving the coronary, lower limb, and cerebral arteries.

In *type IIb* triglycerides of VLDL origin as well as cholesterol of LDL origin are found to be elevated. Severe forms of type IIb may exhibit the same clinical features as type IIa; however, IIb is often of a milder form. Patients with mild IIb tend to be obese and glucose-intolerant.

TABLE 17-5 THE TYPES OF PRIMARY HYPERLIPOPROTEINEMIA

Type	Lipoprotein abnormalities	Usual age of expression	Familial forms	Some clinical features
I	Severe chylo-micronemia	Infancy and childhood	Rare and usually familial (recessive)	Bouts of abdominal pain, pancreatitis, eruptive xanthomas, hepatosplenomegaly
IIa	LDL increased	At birth, if genetic	Most obvious genetic form is expressed in heteroxygote, but is more severe in homo-zygote; many mild examples are not obviously familial	Premature vascular disease; in familial forms, tendon and tuberous xanthomas
IIb	LDL and VLDL increased	At birth, if genetic	Pattern alternates with IIa in families affected with "monogenic" type II; milder defects are sporadic or due to other genetic defects	Severe forms are like IIa; milder IIb patterns tend to be accompanied by glucose intolerance, obesity
III	VLDL and LDL of abnormal composition	Third decade; often after menopause in women	Frequently familial, genetic mode uncertain	Glucose intolerance, tuberoeruptive or planar xanthomas, pre-mature vascular dis-ease (especially peri-pheral vascular disease); worsened by alcohol excess
IV	VLDL increased	Usually third decade or later, can occur in children	Often half of adult close relatives will also have type IV; number of mutants or frequency of familial involvement unknown	Glucose intolerance in about 50%, excess caloric intake common; occasionally eruptive xanthomas, hyperuri-cemia; worsened by alcohol excess
V	VLDL increased, chylomicrons present	Adulthood, very rare in children	When familial, more than half of close relatives have either type IV or type V	Bouts of abdominal pain and pancreatitis, erup-tive xanthomas, hepato-splenomegaly, excess caloric intake common, hyperuricemia; most patients have glucose intolerance; worsened by alcohol excess

LDL = low-density lipoproteins; VLDL = very-low-density lipoproteins.

Source: R. I. Levy, "Dietary and Drug Treatment of Primary Hyperlipoproteinemia," *Annals of Internal Medicine,* **77**:273, 1972.

TABLE 17-6   SUMMARY OF DIETS FOR TYPES I–V HYPERLIPOPROTEINEMIA

	Type I	Type IIa	Type IIb & Type III	Type IV	Type V
Diet prescription	Low-fat (25–35 g)	Low-cholesterol; polyunsaturated fat increased	Low-cholesterol calories approx. 20% from protein 40% from fat 40% from carbohydrate	Controlled carbohydrate—approx. 45% of calories. Moderately restricted cholesterol	Restricted fat—30% of calories. Controlled carbohydrate—50% of calories. Moderately restricted cholesterol
Calories	Not restricted	Not restricted	Achieve and maintain "ideal" weight; i.e., reduction diet if necessary	Achieve and maintain "ideal" weight; i.e., reduction diet if necessary	Achieve and maintain "ideal" weight; i.e., reduction diet if necessary
Protein	Total protein intake is not limited	Total protein intake is not limited	High protein intake*	Not limited other than control of patient's weight	High protein intake*
Fat	Restricted to 25–35 g; type of fat not important	Saturated fat intake limited; polyunsaturated fat intake increased	Controlled to 40% of calories (polyunsaturated fats recommended in preference to saturated fats)	Not limited other than control of patient's weight (polyunsaturated fats recommended in preference to saturated fats)	Restricted to 30% of calories (polyunsaturated fats recommended in preference to saturated fats)
Cholesterol	Not restricted	As low as possible; only source of cholesterol is the meat in the diet	Less than 300 mg; only source of cholesterol is the meat in the diet	Moderately restricted to 300–500 mg	Moderately restricted to 300–500 mg
Carbohydrate	Not limited	Not limited	Controlled; concentrated sweets restricted	Controlled; concentrated sweets restricted	Controlled; concentrated sweets restricted
Alcohol	Not recommended	May be used with discretion	Not more than 2 servings (substituted for carbohydrate)	Not more than 2 servings (substituted for carbohydrates)	Not recommended

* High protein: 18–21% of calories in type IIb and III, 21–24% type V. This is well above the recommended allowances for protein and is aimed at keeping the total fat and carbohydrate in the diet restricted.

Source: D. S. Fredrickson, Dietary Management of Hyperlipoproteinemia, A Handbook for Physicians and Dietitians, Dept. Health, Education, and Welfare Publ. No. (NIH) 76–110.

Dietary treatment   Cholesterol intake is restricted to less than 300 mg per day, ideally to 100 to 150 mg per day in children and 200 mg per day in adults when possible.[18,19] Saturated fats should be restricted to 6 to 10 percent of total calories (joules) and the polyunsaturated fats should be adjusted to attain a polyunsaturates/saturates ratio of 2 to 1 (see the further discussion of this ratio on page 324). Maintenance of ideal body weight, which may require weight reduction, is recommended. Protein, carbohydrate, and total fat from the allowed sources are not limited in type IIa if ideal body weight is maintained, and alcohol may be used with discretion. In type IIb, concentrated sweets should be restricted as well as alcohol since both have an effect on the triglyceride level.

Type III Hyperlipoproteinemia

Type III hyperlipoproteinemia is characterized by an abnormal lipoprotein with the electrophoretic mobility of a beta-lipoprotein but with a very low density. The defect is thought to be in the conversion of VLDL to LDL.

Clinical and laboratory signs   Both the cholesterol and triglycerides are elevated and both are close to the same value. The plasma often appears lipemic. A "broad beta" band is found on electrophoresis. Clinical signs include planar xanthomas, tuberoeruptive lesions, xanthelasma, premature corneal arcus, and tendon xanthomas. Abnormal glucose tolerance and hyperuricemia may be found. Ischemic coronary artery disease and peripheral vascular disease are common.

Dietary treatment   Maintenance of ideal body weight is very important, so that weight reduction is frequently necessary. Dietary cholesterol should be restricted to approximately 300 mg per day or less with a concurrent substitution of polyunsaturated for saturated fats.[20] Concentrated sweets and alcohol intake should be restricted and total carbohydrate intake should make up approximately 40 percent of calories (joules).

Type IV Hyperlipoproteinemia

Type IV or hypertriglyceridemia is characterized by an elevation of endogenous pre-beta-lipoprotein (VLDL).

Clinical and laboratory signs   Triglycerides are elevated and a slight elevation of cholesterol may be found. Plasma may appear clear, cloudy, or milky depending on the degree of triglyceride elevation. A pre-beta-lipoprotein band appears on electrophoresis. Patients with type IV hyperlipoproteinemia often have eruptive xanthomas. Obesity, hyperuricemia, and glucose intolerance are frequently present.

Dietary Treatment   Type IV responds well to attainment of ideal body weight, controlled carbohydrate intake (specifically restriction of concentrated sweets), alcohol limitation, moderate cholesterol restriction (usually 300 to 500 mg per day), and substitution of polyunsaturated for saturated fats.[21]

Type V Hyperlipoproteinemia

Type V hyperlipoproteinemia is characterized by an increased concentration of pre-beta-lipoprotein (VLDL) and an increase in chylomicrons in the fasting patient, which results in a lipemic plasma.

Clinical and laboratory signs   Triglycerides are elevated, frequently into the thousands, and concurrent elevated cholesterol is often found. Patients with type V may have eruptive xanthomas, lipemia retinalis, recurrent abdominal pain, acute and chronic pancreatitis, and hepatosplenomegaly. Type V is frequently associated with obesity and hyperuricemia, and glucose intolerance is common.

Dietary treatment   Restriction of total fat is recommended because of the appearance of some chylomicrons and the high VLDL levels. Type V requires a moderate restriction of carbohydrate since both fat and the glycerol from carbohydrate metabolism influence VLDL formation. Cholesterol is usually moderately restricted and maintenance of ideal weight is stressed.[22] Alcohol is not recommended. The use of MCT is not recommended for type V because it also increases the VLDL levels.

Dietary Principles for Reducing Blood Lipids

Since there are some conflicting views regarding the age at which diet therapy should be started, questions arise regarding the role of cholesterol in the developing infant and whether a low-cholesterol diet could be harmful. It is not yet known whether a low-cholesterol diet in the infant has any beneficial effects. Maternal milk is much higher in cholesterol than many infant formulas, and so the advisability of a low-cholesterol diet is even more complicated since mother's milk is the prototype in infant feeding.

Glueck has been able to demonstrate that infants with familial type II hyperlipoproteinemia can have their cholesterol normalized in the first year of life with dietary intervention;[23] however, it is not yet known what effect this early normalization of cholesterol means in terms of general health or of preventing the development of atherosclerosis.

Typing of the hyperlipoproteinemias has helped to determine the best treatment. There are rare occasions when typing may not be feasible. In these situations, general recommendations common to all types of hyperlipoproteinemia may be justified.

TABLE 17-7 COMPOSITION OF FAT-CONTROLLED DIETS RECOMMENDED BY THE AMERICAN HEART ASSOCIATION

	Preventive diet (3)*	1200 kcal (5.04 mJ)	1800 kcal (7.56 mJ)	Therapeutic diets 2000–2200 kcal (8.4–9.24 mJ)	2400–2600 kcal (10.08–10.92 mJ)
Nutrients:					
Carbohydrate (g)	273	120	200	270	335
Protein (g)	114	75	85	95	110
Fat (g)	83	42	68	70	84
Saturated fatty acids (g)	18	7	10	11	12
Linoleic (g)	26	14	26	26	33
Cholesterol (mg)	356	258	258	279	286
Iron (mg)	21.6	14	14	17	19
Dietary patterns:					
% Calories (joules) from carbohydrate	47	41	45	51	52
% Calories (joules) from protein	20	26	20	18	17
% Calories (joules) from fat	33	32	35	30	30
% Calories (joules) from saturated fatty acids	7	5	5	4	4
% Calories (joules) from linoleic acid	10	10	13	11	11
P/S ratio†	1.4:1	2:1	2.6:1	2.4:1	2.8:1

* 2300 kcal (9.66 mJ).

† Ratio of linoleic acid to saturated fatty acids.

Source: J. F. Mueller, "A Dietary Approach to Coronary Artery Disease," *Journal of the American Dietetic Association,* **62:**614, 1973.

The American Heart Association has made dietary recommendations for the prevention of coronary heart disease (ischemic heart disease) in the general population. These recommendations are available to health professionals and the public in their publication, *The Ways to a Man's Heart.*[24] Their purpose is to prevent the disease process before it becomes apparent at a more severe stage. The nutrient composition and energy patterns of the American Heart Association's preventive diet and therapeutic diets are shown in Table 17-7. These diets are not geared to any particular type of hyperlipoproteinemia but are available in different energy levels since obesity is common and is a risk factor in itself. The exact foods that would fit into these patterns are covered in the American Heart Association's booklets.

The American Heart Association's recommendations to physicians and health professionals are:[25]

1 Adjustment of the caloric content of the diet to achieve and maintain optimal weight
2 Reduction of the total fat content of the diet to no more than 35 percent of total calories, with restriction of saturated fat to less than 10 percent of total calories and inclusion of polyunsaturated fat to comprise up to 10 percent of total calories.
3 Restriction of dietary cholesterol to approximately 300 mg per day
4 Limitation of concentrated "empty" calories, simple sugars, etc., which provide only calories without vitamins and other essential nutrients
5 "Prudent" use of salt until its role in hypertension is defined

In addition to these general recommendations, the therapeutic diets of the American Heart Association (Planning Fat-Controlled Meals) (Table 17-7) make some adaptations: the inclusion of polyunsaturated fats to achieve a polyunsaturates/saturates ratio of 2 to 1 or better and a further reduction in dietary cholesterol to less than 300 mg per day.

Table 17-8 lists recommendations for one week's intake that is low in cholesterol and saturated fat. Egg yolks are the highest common source of cholesterol; persons on cholesterol-restricted diets should either limit or avoid them and use various egg substitutes if necessary. If egg yolks are avoided the diet can offer much more variety by including other cholesterol-containing foods.

Meat (lamb, pork, beef) and dairy products (whole milk, butter, cream, cheese, etc.)

TABLE 17-8 RECOMMENDATIONS FOR ONE WEEK'S DIETARY INTAKE LOW-CHOLESTEROL, LOW-SATURATED-FAT

2 eggs per week (egg whites freely)

56 oz meat, fish, and poultry to include:	20 oz meat
	20 oz poultry
	16 oz fish

3 oz cheddar cheese or equivalent
2 cups low-fat (1%) cottage cheese
14 cups skim milk
Approximate cholesterol content: 2000 mg per week

Approximate fatty acid content:	Saturated fatty acid	Linoleic acid
	41.6 g	9.3 g

Polyunsaturated fats (safflower, corn oil, and margarines made from these oils, etc.): add to give the desired Polyunsaturates/saturates (P/S) ratio; amount will also depend on the energy level desired.

	Saturated fatty acid	Linoleic acid
14 teaspoons corn oil	8.9 g	40.2 g
7 teaspoons corn-oil margarine	5.0 g	13.3 g
Total	13.9 g	53.5 g
fat from above items	41.6 g	9.3 g
Total	55.5 g	62.8 g

Approximate P/S ratio = 1.1 to 1

The P/S ratio can be increased by the use of safflower oil rather than corn oil if desired. If the energy allowance for the individual is high, more polyunsaturated fat can be added to achieve a higher P/S ratio.

are the primary sources of saturated fats and need to be controlled. In addition, there are some highly saturated vegetable fats, such as coconut oil and shortenings, that are found in many prepared products which need to be avoided. Animal meats, because of their saturated fat content, should be limited and greater emphasis should be placed on the inclusion of fish, poultry, low-fat dairy products, and vegetables as protein sources. Table 17-9 lists those foods which should be avoided on a low-cholesterol, low-saturated-fat diet.

The method of preparing allowed meats, by trimming of fat and by baking or broiling, is essential to fat control. Several cheeses made partially or totally from skim milk as well as skim, nonfat, and fat-free milks in powdered, liquid, and evaporated forms are encouraged in the diet. The patient should be aware of the difference between the many fat-free and low-fat products available. When making these changes in the diet, such as avoiding egg yolks and limiting red meats, the diet should be checked for nutrient adequacy since in this case the excluded foods may cause the diet to be low in vitamin A and iron content.

The most common sources of polyunsaturated fats are safflower, sunflower, corn, soybean, and cottonseed oils and the marga-rines made from these oils (see Table 17-4). There are many textured vegetable-protein products being marketed today which are good sources of polyunsaturated fat. The use of oils in cooking and the use of margarines only when spreads are desired ensures a higher polyunsaturates/saturates ratio without the consumption of large amounts of fats and calories (joules).

Many investigators are in disagreement regarding the 2 to 1 polyunsaturates/saturates ratio previously recommended. Often it is not considered necessary when the total saturated fat intake can be kept very low; moreover, with weight reduction diets that necessitate the control of total fat intake, the use of large amounts of polyunsaturates is impossible. In the future, changing the fat composition of beef by means of variations in the feed of cattle, leading to a product that is higher in polyunsaturated fat and lower in saturated fat, may be the answer to providing variety on a fat-controlled diet.

The patient should be aware of the product label as a source of information (see "Labeling," in Chap. 2). Local and regional heart associations can be contacted for dietary booklets dealing with commercial products for fat-controlled diets.

There are several other dietary factors which have received and still are receiving attention in the search for causes of ischemic heart disease and hyperlipidemia. These include coffee, vitamin C, and hard water. However, there has been no conclusive evidence of any harmful effects of these factors.

Lack of dietary fiber has been proposed as a factor in atherosclerosis. It has been postulated that dietary fiber may exert a cholesterol-lowering effect. Various investigations have demonstrated a hypocholesterolemic effect with a high-fiber diet but it is not known whether this effect is due to an increase in the fiber or to the complex carbohydrate content of the diet. Trowell has presented data to support the hypothesis that dietary fiber decreases reabsorption of bile salts, increases fecal excretion, and reduced hyperlipidemia.[26]

TABLE 17-9 FOODS TO AVOID ON LOW-CHOLESTEROL, LOW-SATURATED-FAT DIETS

Eggs yolks—except as allowed on diet

Organ meats

Fatty meats, luncheon meats, frankfurter, bacon, sausage, poultry skin, duck, caviar

Whole milk, evaporated and condensed whole milk, filled milks with coconut oil, cream, ice cream, sour cream, whole milk cheeses and yogurt

Butter, lard, gravies made with animal fat, hydrogenated vegetable shortenings

Coconut, chocolate, palm oil

Mixed nuts, cashews, potato chips

Commercially prepared baked goods which may contain the above foods

Medical Treatment of Hyperlipidemia

Diet is the cornerstone of therapy for any of the primary or familial disorders. Diet therapy should always be tried before any drug is used. If the addition of drugs proves necessary, diet should be continued, for in essentially all cases, the effects of diet and drugs are additive and more effective than either alone.[27]

Unfortunately there are those patients in whom diet alone cannot normalize the lipid abnormalities and those who fail to comply with the dietary recommendations advised. The effects of adequate diet and medication are additive, so the patient who adheres to a diet is more successfully treated with medication. If the patient chooses not to follow a diet, medical management is usually more difficult and the patient may also fail to comply with prescribed medical therapy.

As in dietary treatment, each type of hyperlipoproteinemia responds most effectively to specific medications. However, different patients with the same type of hyperlipidemia often respond differently to medications, so each patient needs to be considered individually to achieve optimal benefit. There are several medications available which have been shown to treat certain lipid abnormalities effectively. These are usually grouped into two types: those that decrease lipoprotein synthesis (nicotinic acid, clofibrate), and those that increase lipoprotein catabolism (cholestyramine, sitosterol and D-thyroxine).[28]

HYPERTENSION AND HYPERTENSIVE HEART DISEASE

Hypertension is defined as a sustained increase in the arterial blood pressure, either diastolic, systolic, or both. The prevalence of hypertension in adults is estimated to be somewhere between 15 and 20 percent of the population. Disparities in this estimate occur because of observer bias, because of inappropriate equipment, and because many people remain undiagnosed. Furthermore, there is not a natural cutoff point between normal and elevated blood pressures. Table 17-10 gives the generally accepted upper limits of "normal" blood pressure for different age groups. A hypertensive individual is one who has had at least three consecutive blood pressure values which are elevated by two or more standard deviations above the normal for the appropriate age group. Blood pressure readings should be done while the person is at rest and the values should be taken several days apart. Even the normotensive person may have elevated blood pressure at times of excitement or when involved in physical activity. Labile hypertension is diagnosed if the blood pressure is intermittently elevated. (*Labile:* subject to free and rapid change.)

There are several factors which influence the prognosis of the hypertensive patient. The factors of primary importance are age, sex, and race. The prevalence of hypertension among blacks in the United States is almost twice as high as it is in whites. Blacks also have more severe hypertension and under the age of 50 have a death rate approximately 6 to 7 times higher than whites. This rate decreases to about 2½ times higher after the age of 50.[29] At any age level the hypertensive individual has a worse prognosis than the normotensive person

TABLE 17-10   UPPER LIMITS OF NORMAL BLOOD PRESSURE BY AGE GROUP

Age group	Blood pressure
Infants	90/60 mmHg
3–6 years	110/70 mmHg
7–10 years	120/80 mmHg
11–17 years	130/80 mmHg
18–44 years	140/90 mmHg
45–64 years	150/95 mmHg
65 and older	160/95 mmHg

Source: B. Batterman, "Hypertension. Part 1: Detection and Evaluation," *Cardiovascular Nursing,* **11**:38, July–August 1975.

of the same age. More adult men have hypertension than adult women until age 50. After menopause the incidence of elevated blood pressure in women rises and remains higher. Women have a better prognosis than men at any level of blood pressure.[30] Any elevation of blood pressure, systolic or diastolic, is associated with an increased risk of morbidity and mortality from cardiovascular disease.[31,32]

Hypertension may either be *essential* (of unknown cause) or *secondary* (of known cause). Essential hypertension, i.e., without any known cause, accounts for about 90 percent of hypertensive patients. Causes of secondary hypertension include renal parenchymal disorders, peripheral vascular disease, endocrine abnormalities, and coarctation of the aorta. The family history of hypertensives suggests genetic factors; however, the bulk of evidence indicates that in the origin of hypertension genetic tendencies are modified by environmental factors. Obesity, cigarette smoking, stress, and sedentary life styles have all been associated with the occurrence of hypertension,[33] although none of these factors alone has been shown to cause hypertension. Morbidity from cardiovascular diseases also increases when hypertension occurs in conjunction with these conditions.

Diet, specifically sodium intake, is receiving more attention in the search for the cause of essential hypertension.[34–36] Many studies, both in human populations and in animal experiments, have implicated a high sodium intake as a causative factor.[37] The Committee on Nutrition of the American Academy of Pediatrics has estimated that approximately 20 percent of the children in the United States are at risk of developing hypertension when they reach adulthood.[38] Because of this high number, much attention has focused on the dietary sodium intake of infants and children. With the early introduction of solid foods into the infant's diet, sodium intake has increased substantially and exceeds by severalfold the minimum requirements of the amount provided by human milk. In the last few years manufacturers have reduced the total salt content of baby foods. However, the diets of older children and adolescents continue to exceed the minimum daily requirement for sodium,[39] since we consume a large amount of commercially prepared foods that are high in sodium content. Also, certain cultural food patterns, such as kosher and Chinese, provide large amounts of sodium.

Hypertension may occur in mild forms and often remains undiagnosed for years. When undiagnosed or left untreated, hypertension, if severe, may result in damage to the heart, eyes, kidneys, or brain. If the hypertension is diagnosed before complications occur, treatment may delay end-organ manifestations. As in the hyperlipidemia syndrome, the problem of early treatment in the child with a predisposition for essential hypertension remains a quandary. Treatment of children with elevated blood pressure is based on the hypothesis that therapy will reduce morbidity and mortality rates later in life. Studies have recently been established that will follow up early hypertensive children into adulthood to determine if this is correct. Factors such as obesity, diet, and life style of the adolescent probably play a role.

Treatment

Treatment of the hypertensive individual includes both medications and diet. Diet may include sodium restriction and weight reduction, depending on the condition of the patient.

Sodium Restriction

Sodium restriction lowers arterial blood pressure by producing a negative salt and water balance, which prevents the development of sodium and water retention. Currently there is much discussion in the literature with respect to the appropriate level of sodium restriction. While various levels of sodium restriction are often advised, most advocates of sodium deprivation agree that to be effective in long-term treatment of essential hypertension, dietary sodium intake must be limited to 200 to 250 mg (approximately 9 to 10 meq) per day.[40,41] There are individuals with hypertension who respond well to milder sodium restriction, so that its value should not be discounted. An intake of 250 mg is very restricted and often impractical when renal function is adequate enough to allow diuretic drugs to be effective. Strict sodium restriction is advised at the beginning of diuretic treatment in patients with cardiac failure or decreased kidney function, in order to hasten the establishment of negative sodium and water balance. Any treatment of hypertension should include the avoidance of obviously salted foods and other forms of excessive sodium intake. This is advised to avoid overriding the ability of the diuretic to prevent sodium retention.

TABLE 17-11 SODIUM CONTENT OF SELECTED FOODS* AND SODIUM-RESTRICTED DIET PLANS

Food	Amount	Sodium, (approximate values)	Levels of sodium restriction (amounts per day)			
			500 mg	1000 mg	2000 mg	4000 mg
Milk						
Regular	8 oz (240 g)	125	—	2 cups	2 cups	2 cups
Low-sodium		less than 5	2 cups			
Egg	1 average	60	1	1	1	1
Butter, Margarine	1 tsp (5 g)					
Salted		50	4	2	4	4
Unsalted		0–1	freely	freely	freely	freely
Cheese	1 oz	200–300	—	—	—	1
Meat, Fish, Poultry						
Salted	1 oz	300	—	—	—	5
Unsalted		20	6	8	8	—
Vegetables						
Salted	½ cup	250	—	—	—	1
Unsalted		10	3	4	4	3
Fruit	½ cup	0–5	4	4	4	4
Bread						
Salted	1 slice (approx. 25 g)	125–150	—	2	6	6
Unsalted		5–10	4	2		
Cereals						
Salted	1 cup	200–300	—	—	1	1
Unsalted		5	1	1		
Beverages (beer, wine distilled spirits, carbonated beverages, coffee, tea)	8 oz	0–20				
Desserts						
Jello	½ cup	125	—	—	—	1 dessert
Ice cream	1/6 qt		—	—	—	
Baked goods	Amount varies widely. Any containing regular baking power or baking soda should be omitted on strict sodium-restricted diets.					

**Source:* C. F. Adams, *Nutritive Value of American Foods*, U.S. Dept. of Agriculture Handbook No. 456, November 1975.

For help in planning a sodium-restricted diet, Table 17-11 lists the sodium content of selected foods and suggested amounts for use in sodium-restricted diet plans. In planning diets, it should be remembered that cultural food habits with predilections for salt may prevail (e.g., kosher, Chinese), along with acquired taste from years of usage, so that expectations for sodium restrictions must be realistic. Salt substitutes may help to make diets more appetizing and various herbs and spices (see Table 19-6, in Chap. 19) can be used in food preparation; however, this is a difficult transition for any patient. Salt is one of the primary tastes—taste buds specific for salt are located on each side of the tongue, and patients accustomed to receiving a lot of taste stimulation from these centers need to be highly motivated and given much support to help them refrain from this basic instinct.

Generally, animal foods and dairy products have a sodium content which varies with the protein content: the higher the protein content, the higher the sodium. Thus, skim milk products and leaner meats have a higher sodium content than whole milk products and fatty meats. Most cheeses and dairy products contain high levels of sodium.

Kosher meats are generally quite high in sodium (approximately 600 to 1000 mg sodium/3 oz). This can be altered to an extent by the type of koshering. Low-sodium meats may be koshered by broiling rather than salting. This permits the blood to drip away from the meat. The sodium content of other fresh meats and fish can be reduced by boiling them in water and discarding the liquid.

The amount of sodium in the drinking water varies considerably. Water treated in most water-softening equipment is often much higher in sodium because the conditioners add sodium to replace the calcium and magnesium in harder water.

There are many medications which contain considerable amounts of sodium and should be avoided on sodium-restricted diets. These include many antacids, laxatives, and

TABLE 17-12 FOODS TO AVOID ON SODIUM-RESTRICTED DIETS

Salt

Obviously salty foods such as salted crackers, potato chips, pretzels, salted nuts, pickles, olives, sauerkraut

Smoked, cured, or pickled meats and fish such as ham, bacon, frankfurters, bologna, salami, other cold cuts, salted fish and pork, corned beef

Seasonings such as catsup, prepared mustard, Worcestershire sauce, celery salt, onion salt, garlic salt, soy sauce, barbecue sauce, monosodium glutamate

Bouillon cubes, concentrated, canned, or frozen soups, dried soup mixes

Baking soda, seltzers, or antacids

Most commercial salad dressings

bromides, such as Alka-Seltzer and Brioschi (see Table 19-7, in Chap. 19).

Many high-sodium compounds are used in food manufacturing and in food preservation. These commonly include baking powder, sodium bicarbonate, sodium propionate, sodium alginate (found in chocolate milk drinks and ice cream), sodium nitrate, and monosodium glutamate.

Table 17-12 lists the most common foods that should be avoided on sodium-restricted diets.

Weight Reduction

Weight reduction is advised in the treatment of the hypertensive patient. The intent is to decrease the extra cardiac load imposed by obesity. It is not clear whether there is a direct relationship between body weight or obesity and blood pressure. However, obese individuals have an increased tendency to develop diabetes or hyperlipidemia, which may influence the morbidity and mortality of the hypertensive patient.

Medications

The medications used in the treatment of hypertension are numerous. The first ones usually employed are the oral diuretics, including the thiazides, ethacrynic acid, and furosemide. Both sodium restriction and these medications produce saluresis (salt loss) and diuresis (water loss), resulting in a reduction in extracellular fluid volume, plasma volume, and total exchangeable sodium, with the desired fall in blood pressure. An associated decrease in cardiac output then occurs. After several weeks of this therapy these factors rise to their previous normal levels but blood pressure usually remains lower. The exact mechanisms which maintain the lowered blood pressure are not known.

Side effects of these diuretics include hypokalemia (low serum potassium), hyperuricemia (high serum uric acid), and hyperglycemia (high blood sugar). Hypokalemia is especially common and can be treated with diet or potassium supplements. When possible, dietary sources of potassium are preferred because of the unpleasant taste of most potassium supplements. Table 17-13 lists some common sources of potassium. If potassium depletion becomes a problem, there are several potassium-sparing diuretics available. Both potassium tablets and some of the potassium-sparing diuretics may irritate the gastric mucosa, so that caution must be exerted with their usage. There are also various salt substitutes on the market which substitute potassium for sodium. These may be contraindicated if there are any kidney problems. The patient should be told to check labels thoroughly as many available substitutes are not completely sodium-free. Chloride depletion may also be a problem for patients taking diuretics. Both the salt substitutes and potassium elixir (one of the common supplements) provide a source of chloride in addition to potassium.

Other antihypertensive medications used include hydralazine, methyldopa, and guanethidine. These drugs and the diuretics are often used in combination to achieve a maximum reduction of blood pressure with a minimum of side effects. These agents, in contrast to the diuretics, produce a decrease in blood pressure by reducing peripheral vascular resistance through blocking of the sympathetic receptor sites in the arterioles and the sympathetic nervous system. Medications should be chosen on an individual basis with respect to dosage, frequency, and side effects, just as diet should be tailored to the individual need by the health professional, with respect to the patient's cultural, physical, and emotional background.

RHEUMATIC HEART DISEASE

Rheumatic fever is an inflammatory disease affecting the heart, connective tissues, and brain that occurs in 3 percent of patients after untreated pharyngitis caused by the group A beta-hemolytic streptococcus. It may be prevented by adequate treatment of "strep throat" (streptococcal pharyngitis) with penicillin. Major complications result from inflammation of the heart valves and heart muscle, leading to chronic rheumatic heart disease. Malnutrition may result in increased rates of infection and therefore may correlate with a higher incidence of rheumatic fever among those that are malnourished. The main nutritional concern in treatment is the provision of a diet with adequate nutrients to replete a prior state of malnutrition and to compensate for losses due to the stress of illness and increased temperature.

TABLE 17-13 POTASSIUM-CONTAINING FOOD

Food	Amount	Potassium, mg
Banana	1 small	350
Broccoli	1 cup	415
Canteloupe	¼ of 5-in melon	340
Grapefruit juice	1 cup	400
Orange	1 medium	270
Orange juice	1 cup	495
Potato	1 medium	555

Source: C. F. Adams, *Nutritive Value of American Foods,* U.S. Dept. of Agriculture Handbook No. 456, November 1975.

CONGENITAL HEART DISEASE*

Congenital heart defects may take many forms—ventricular septal defect, coarctation of the aorta, transposition of the great arteries, tetralogy of Fallot, and aortic stenosis, to name a few (see Table 17-14)—and often may not be diagnosed or detectable at birth. The only known causative factor is maternal rubella, which results in a specific syndrome in approximately 20 percent of affected infants. The many other malformations are probably multifactorial in origin, involving both unidentified genetic and unidentified prenatal environmental factors. Cyanosis (decreased oxygen in the blood), congestive heart failure, pulmonary hypertension, bacterial endocarditis, repeated respiratory infections, and poor physi-

*Contributed by Rosanne B. Howard.

cal growth frequently complicate the lives of children with these malformations.

Surgery is frequently performed, with relief of many of the symptoms. Recent trends in cardiac surgery have been aimed at correction of the defects during infancy, particularly in those with cyanotic ("blue baby") lesions. Survival and relief of symptoms are the immediate goals of treatment. Long-term goals are the provision of optimal physical, intellectual, and emotional growth.[42]

Growth retardation is common in children with congenital heart disease (Fig. 17-6). The mechanism of growth retardation is poorly understood, but a number of hypotheses have been proposed to explain this altered pattern. These include congestive heart failure, chronic hypoxia with acidosis, pulmonary hypertension, repeated infections, or some combination of these. Traditionally, these factors have been grouped into three general categories: (1) Ab-

TABLE 17-14 COMMON CONGENITAL HEART DEFECTS

Type	Description
Ventricular spetal defect (VSD)	A malformation resulting in a hole in the septum between the right and left ventricles.
Coarctation of the aorta	Constriction of the lumen of the aorta at any point—usually at the junction of the aortic arch and descending aorta.
Transposition of the great arteries	A defect in the anatomic relationship of the pulmonary artery and the aorta such that the aorta arises above the right ventricle and the pulmonary artery above the left ventricle.
Tetralogy of Fallot	A combination of four defects: (1) interventricular septal defect (2) stenosis of the pulmonary artery (3) hypertrophy of the right ventricle (4) dextroposition of the aorta so that it overrides the VSD.
Aortic stenosis	A congenital narrowing of the aortic valve, usually with a unicuspid or bicuspid configuration rather than the normal tricuspid morphology.

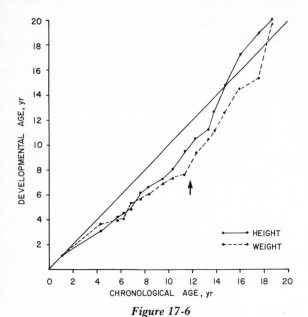

Figure 17-6

Growth curve in congenital heart disease. Growth curve shows catch-up growth after surgery with subsequent normal growth. A. Rosenthal and A. Castaneda, "Growth and Development after Cardiovascular Surgery in Infants and Children," Progress in Cardiovascular Diseases, **18:**27–37, 1975.)

normal metabolism of ingested food substances, (2) an excessive loss of nutrients via the urine and feces, or by removal of body fluids, and (3) quantitatively poor intake.[43]

Hypermetabolism has been proposed as a cause for failure to thrive in these infants on the theory that the following conditions may possibly prevent a basal state: increased metabolic demands of specific tissues, an elevated body temperature, and a level of thyroid activity incompatible with a reduction in cardiac reserve and energy intake.[44]

However, there is research to show that hypermetabolism may be the effect rather than the cause of growth failure.[45] Some investigators have found that infants with congenital heart disease were not hypermetabolic when oxygen consumption was related to lean body mass rather than determined per kilogram of body weight. Huse suggests that the growth failure seen in these infants appears more directly related to chronically inadequate

intake rather than to any other factor studied.[46]

Although the question of a hypermetabolic state is unresolved, it is a well-established fact that many affected infants do not accept a normal volume of food. Voluntary reduction of food is so common that some researchers ascribe this to a compensatory role whereby infants reduce their food intake in order to prevent the additional strain on the failing myocardium that a large meal with its resulting increase in splanchnic (visceral) blood flow would impose.[47] This limited intake, with a questionable state of hypermetabolism, malabsorption, or both, causes these children to be at risk nutritionally.[48]

It has been estimated that these children need somewhere in the vicinity of 29 to 59 extra calories (122 to 248 kJ) per kilogram of body weight over the recommended dietary allowances (RDA) for their age to achieve increments in weight.[33] For example, an infant requiring 117 kcal (491 kJ)/kg of body weight daily according to the RDA would then require 148 to 178 kcal (622 to 748 kJ)/kg of body weight or a midpoint of approximately 160 kcal (672 kJ)/kg.

The normal infant formula, after dilution, provides 20 kcal (84 kJ)/oz. To achieve a diet of high energy density without increasing the renal solute load, infant formulas with low electrolyte and protein values (10 to 11 percent protein) can be supplemented with Karo syrup, Polycose, or medium-chain triglycerides to provide 25 to 30 kcal (105 to 126 kJ)/oz (see Table 17-15). Dietary management for these children needs careful supervision to determine their ability to tolerate increasing levels of carbohydrate without developing diarrhea. Formulas should not be concentrated in energy density by decreasing the amount of water, as this precipitously increases the renal solute load.

Nutritional management of infants with severe congenital heart disease involves providing essential nutrients in a form of food or formula that is easily digestible, without pre-

TABLE 17-15 ENERGY SUPPLEMENTS FOR DIETS OR CHILDREN WITH CONGENITAL HEART DISEASE

Product	Calories/tablespoon (kJ/tablespoon)	Description
Karo syrup (Carbohydrate)	57 (239)	Corn sugar (mainly glucose) in syrup form Taste—sweet
Lipomul Oral Upjohn (Fat)	90 (378)	Corn-oil emulsion White liquid Taste—perfumelike
Polycose Ross (Carbohydrate)	30 (126)	Glucose polymer in powdered and liquid forms with low osmolarity; rapidly absorbed as glucose Taste—less sweet than most sugars
MCT Oil Mead Johnson (Medium-chain triglycerides)	115 (483)	MCT Oil made from fractionated coconut oil containing triglycerides of medium-chain fatty acids. These are rapidly hydrolyzed and absorbed into the intestinal mucosa, not depending on bile salts, chylomicron formation, or lymphatic transport. They travel directly to the liver via the portal circulation. Taste—Bland

Amount to be added to formulas to make 25 kcal (105 kJ)/oz:

To 1 qt of SMA* or Similac PM 60/40* add:

3 tbsp Karo syrup or
6 tbsp Polycose or
1½ tbsp MCT Oil

* See Table 17-16.

senting an excessive renal load. The possibility of excessive fecal loss of fat should be considered and the use of formulas providing fat in the form of easily absorbed vegetable oils is recommended. Formulas that provide a low renal solute load and a form of easily digestible fat are SMA (Wyeth) and Similac PM 60/40 (Ross) (see Table 17-16). It is recommended that the formulas used have an energy distribution of approximately 8 to 10 percent protein, 35 to 65 percent carbohydrate, and 35 to 50 percent fat in order to attain an adequate intake without incurring a high renal solute load.[49] When foods other than formulas are fed, they should be given with attention to their energy density (calories (joules) per teaspoon or tablespoon), sodium content, renal solute load, and digestibility.

The renal solute load is based on the dietary intake of nitrogen and three major minerals—sodium, potassium, and chloride. Fomon has developed a simplified method for calculating the renal solute load whereby each gram of dietary protein is considered to yield 4

TABLE 17-16 FORMULAS PROVIDING A LOW RENAL SOLUTE LOAD AND EASILY DIGESTED FAT

Type	Fat sources	Protein, g/100 ml	Carbohydrate, g/100 ml	Fat, g/100 ml	Na, meq/l	K, meq/l	Cl, g/100 ml	Estimated renal solute load,* mosmol/l
SMA	Oleo (de-stearinated beef fat), coconut, safflower, soybean oils	1.6	7.6	3.5	7	15	10	96
Similac PM 60/40	Corn and coconut oil	1.5	7.2	3.6	6	14	10	90

Na = sodium; K = potassium; Cl = chloride.

*Using Foman's simplified method[36] to calculate renal solute load, 1 g protein equals 4 mosmol; each meq, Na, K, Cl equals 1 mosmol.

TABLE 17-17 SODIUM CONTENT OF COMMONLY USED BABY FOODS

Product	Measure	Sodium, mg
Baby ready-to-serve dry cereal	3 tbsp	1.73–1.87
Baby dry cereal with fruit	3 tbsp	11.0–11.8
Strained cereal with fruit (jar)	3 tbsp	42.6–62.4
Strained fruit (pure fruit)	3 tbsp	0.42–1.26
Strained fruit with tapicoa	3 tbsp	4.26–13.2
Strained dessert	3 tbsp	7.2–58.5
Strained vegetables	3 tbsp	43–79.2
Strained meat	3 tbsp	64.5–94.2
Strained egg yolk	3 tbsp	75.3
Strained dinners (vegetable and meat)	3 tbsp	43.2–99.6
Strained high meat dinners	3 tbsp	54–75
Baby fruit juice (strained orange)	1 oz	0.6
Orange juice (fresh)	1 oz	0.3
Whole milk	1 oz	15.8
Teething biscuit	1	58.5

Source: Gerber Products Company, 1977.

mosmol of renal solute load, and each milliequivalent of sodium, potassium, and chloride is assumed to contribute 1 mosmol.[50]

Small amounts of energy supplements can be added to foods without appreciably changing the renal solute load since those which are recommended are pure fat or carbohydrate and have only trace electrolyte values. These energy supplements (Table 17-15) have a high satiety value and should only be given in small amounts. Large amounts of supplements can decrease the appetite for meals and produce diarrhea.

The sodium content of the diet should not exceed that of normal infants (7 to 8 meq per day).[51] Since commercially prepared strained foods contribute substantial amounts of sodium (see Table 17-17), supervision of both the type and amount used is necessary. With home-prepared baby food the amount of added salt can be controlled; however, foods low in sodium must be selected for preparation.

Water balance must be maintained to compensate for losses through the lungs due to tachypnea and for losses from the skin and lungs during illness or high environmental temperatures. (Normal estimated water requirements for infants are 100 to 120 ml/kg of body weight, and for children, 60 to 80 ml/kg of body weight.)[52] Determinations of urine osmolarity can be used to monitor the renal solute load, and dietary adjustments can be made accordingly. Fomon suggests that urine osmolarity be maintained below 400 mosmol/l.[53]

In children with congenital heart disease, fatigue due to inadequate oxygen transport may appear and may interfere with the child's ability to suck from the bottle or to eat solid foods. In addition, anorexia may interfere with food intake. It may be the result of cardiac decompensation or may be due to psychological factors in both the parent and the child. In the presence of chronic and life-threatening disease, the child may be forced to eat by anxious parents who equate food intake with their child's survival, with the child in turn reacting negatively to food. Feeding a child with congenital heart disease brings into play many uncertainties, leading some parents to respond to their unpredictable child by being unpredictable themselves. Parents may find it difficult to set consistent limits with a child who "turns blue" with prolonged crying. Inconsistent parental management and the child's loss of pleasure in the function of eating may pave the way for neurotic feeding disturbances. Anticipatory guidance centered around feeding and mealtime management should be provided to all parents of children with congenital heart disease. They need to have an understanding of normal feeding behavior (see Chap. 11) so that they can develop a consistent approach that fosters independence at the level appropriate to the child's physical and mental capabilities (e.g., increasing texture in the diet; encouraging self-feeding, weaning, drinking from a cup, etc.). They must avoid infantilizing and overprotection, thwarting the child's psychosocial development, and causing him to react negatively and manipulatively toward food.

An explanation of the child's tolerance levels by the physician and nurse along with a few simple directives for mealtime management can help to alleviate feeding problems.

For example, the parents can learn to reinforce positive food behaviors, using the same words of praise while giving a lot of attention. Usually, it is the crying that receives the attention; this can best be met by withholding attention through calmly and quietly ignoring it without comment. The parents' approach needs to be consistent and in some instances behavior reinforcements other than praise must be found. Also, the parents need the support of all professionals in setting the appropriate limits and in distinguishing real food problems (vomiting, gagging, regurgitation) associated with their child's condition from those related to behavior. The following questions can help to determine difficulties in infant feeding:

Does the infant tire easily with feeding?

Does the infant need to rest while feeding?

Does the infant vomit frequently?

Does the infant consume approximately 3 to 4 oz of formula over a 20- to 30-minute period?

Does the infant's color become increasingly gray with feeding?

The child should be observed in the feeding situation so that these questions can be answered objectively.

Positioning for feeding is an important consideration. The child should be upright and well supported. Also, oral-pharyngeal stimulation of the lips, tongue, and gums can help to stimulate sucking ability.

CONGESTIVE HEART FAILURE

When the various cardiovascular disease states (ischemic, hypertensive, rheumatic, congenital) are sufficiently severe, the patient may manifest a constellation of symptoms and physical signs called *congestive heart failure*. This syndrome may be either acute, occurring over a short period when the insult is sudden and severe (as in massive myocardial infarction), or chronic, developing over a long period of time (this can occur in all forms of heart disease). The primary characteristic of congestive heart failure is the decreased efficiency of the heart as a pump, or decreased contractility of the myocardium. In order to maintain an adequate cardiac output, the heart compensates by increasing both its size (cardiomegaly) and its rate (tachycardia). Despite this effort at compensation, the cardiac output may fall, decreasing in turn the renal blood flow and glomerular filtration rate. Normal excretion of sodium and water is thus impaired, leading to retention of excess salt (sodium) and water; peripheral edema, pulmonary edema, and ascites are the physical signs of the retained solute and fluid. Acute pulmonary edema, related primarily to left ventricular failure, is a medical emergency requiring prompt treatment to prevent the patient from drowning in his own fluids. Other signs and symptoms of cardiac failure are fatigue, shortness of breath (dyspnea), paroxysmal nocturnal dyspnea, rales (abnormal respiratory sounds), hepatic enlargement (hepatomegaly), and weakness.

Treatment of congestive heart failure involves proper use of digitalis, diuretics, and oxygen; sodium restriction; and bed rest. Reduction in body weight decreases the metabolic demands of the patient and thus reduces the work imposed on the failing heart. The objectives of diet therapy in the patient with congestive heart failure are:

1 *Prevention or elimination of edema.* This involves diuretic therapy along with sodium and fluid restriction where indicated.
   a *Sodium restriction:* The range of sodium intake for the acute stage of congestive heart failure is 250 to 1000 mg. In the acute stage, a dietary restriction of 500 mg can be effective, although a lower level of 250 mg of sodium or a higher level of 1000 mg may be indicated. As edema is eliminated, the diet may be liberalized to permit a sodium intake ranging from 1000 to 1500 mg.

   b *Fluid restriction* is usually necessary. If the kidneys have not been injured, fluid restriction does not have to be severe, since the mechanisms regulating sodium concentration in the extracellular fluid do not allow for retention of fluid without sodium. The aim is to avoid causing extra work for the kidneys by the administration of excessive fluids or by restricting sodium so severely that the kidneys cannot adequately excrete waste products. (See Chap. 8.) All food in liquid form and those foods that are liquid at room temperature (e.g., Jello, ice cream, gruel) should be considered as part of the fluid intake, in addition to some fruits with a high water content (e.g., orange, grapefruit, baby-food fruits). These may have to be limited, depending on the severity of the restriction on fluid intake

2 *Provision of easily digestible foods to avoid excessive strain on the heart during digestion.* Foods should be soft in texture (to minimize chewing), bland, and easily digested, although some foods containing fiber (fruits, vegetables, whole-grain breads and cereals) and foods with laxative effect (prunes, prune juice, raisins, apricots) should be included to prevent constipation. Foods that produce flatulence (cauliflower, onions, cabbage, etc.) should be avoided in order to prevent confusion resulting from symptoms of heartburn. Meals should be divided into small, frequent feedings to prevent exertion. The patient should be positioned to prevent aspiration.

3 *Maintenance of nutritional well-being.* During periods of stress such as that imposed by congestive heart failure, the provision of adequate calories, protein, vitamins, and minerals is essential but often difficult to achieve because of loss of appetite and restricted diets. Supplements of vitamins and minerals and the use of high-energy foods (e.g., concentrated carbohydrates such as jams, jellies, and syrups; and polyunsaturated fats) may be indicated. When

foods to increase energy are included, those foods known to be lipogenic, such as fried foods, butter, and rich pastries, should be avoided.

EDUCATION OF PATIENTS

There are many cookbooks available for fat-controlled, low-cholesterol, or sodium-restricted diets; however, most are fairly expensive and often not necessary if the patient already has basic cookbooks. Suggestions for altering recipes and information about commercially available products for use in cooking should be given to the patient. Public libraries often carry a varied selection of cookbooks that can be recommended (*The American Heart Association Cookbook, The Fat and Sodium Controlled Cookbook, The Low-Fat–Low-Cholesterol Diet*). Another point that should be presented to patients is that their diet can be successfully used for the entire family and that they need not prepare separate meals for themselves. When possible, the husband, wife, and other family members should be taught the diet together so that both those who cook and those being served understand the reason for the dietary limitations. If the diet is very restrictive, "extras" can then be added for the rest of the family.

STUDY QUESTIONS

1 What are the three major risk factors of coronary heart disease that have dietary implications and what three major dietary components do they involve?

2 For patients who are at their ideal weight, what difference would the amount and type of fat make if they had type I hyperlipoproteinemia? Type II?

3 Why might it be difficult for an individual on a low-sodium diet to get an adequate calcium intake?

4 Why are many patients with hypertension told to have a large glass of orange juice or a banana every day?

5 What energy requirement might a 10-kg infant with congenital heart disease require? How would this differ from the energy requirement of a normal infant?

CASE STUDY 17-1

Past History

Mr. Smith, a professor of electrical engineering, was 30 years old when he first developed chest pressure. This pressure was without pain and was brought on by physical exercise and anxiety, and occasionally occurred after eating. After these initial episodes of chest pressure he started a fairly active physical exercise program. Over the next few years the chest pressure gradually became less frequent. At age 47, while still remaining very active, he developed a reccurrence of these chest symptoms. Approximately 1 year later Mr. Smith suffered an acute myocardial infarction with ventricular fibrillation and cardiac arrest requiring resuscitation. After discharge from the hospital, his course was stable for the next 6 years. He continued to be physically active by taking nitroglycerin prophylactically before extensive physical exertion and during periods of stress. Mr. Smith's family history was positive for coronary heart disease.

Mr. Smith smoked two packs of cigarettes per day for 16 or 17 years, stopping at approximately age 36. He drank five to six cups of coffee per day and occasional alcoholic beverages.

Diet

He had been limiting the amount of eggs and shellfish he was eating, and used oil and margarine as his primary fat sources. His diet was normal, without excessive fat, protein, or carbo-hydrate.

Initial Physical Examination
Three months after the myocardial infarction a physical examination was unremarkable except for a mild left facial weakness.

Laboratory Findings
All values were within normal limits except for the serum cholesterol and triglycerides, which were 316 mg/100 ml and 139 mg/100 ml respectively.

Case Study Questions

1 *What risk factors for coronary disease did Mr. Smith have?*

2 *Is it possible to classify the type of hyperlipoproteinemia Mr. Smith had? If so, what type was it? If not, what further information is needed?*

3 *What type of diet would be likely to be advised, considering that Mr. Smith was at his ideal body weight? Is it critical that the type of hyperlipoproteinemia be identified in order to advise him regarding his diet?*

REFERENCES

1 U.S. Public Health Service, *Monthly Vital Statistics Report,* vol. 23, no. 11, suppl. 2, p. 16.

2 National Heart and Lung Institute Task Force on Arteriosclerosis, *Arteriosclerosis,* vol. 1, U.S. Dept. Health, Education, and Welfare Publ. No (NIH) 72–137, June 1971, p. 3.

3 W. B. Kannel, "Atherosclerosis as a Pediatric Problem," *Journal of Pediatrics,* **80:**544–554, 1972.

4 G. C. McMillan, "Development of Arteriosclerosis," *American Journal of Cardiology,* **31:**542–546, 1973.

5 J. P. Strong, "The Pediatric Aspects of Atherosclerosis," *Journal of Atherosclerosis Research,* **9:**251–265, 1969.

6 A. Keys, "Blood Lipids in Man—A Brief Review," *Journal of The American Dietetic Association,* **51:**508–516, 1967.

7 R. I. Levy, "Drug Therapy— Treatment of Hyperlipidemia," *New England Journal of Medicine* **290:**1295–1301, 1974.

8 Ibid.

9 Ibid.

10 National Dairy Council, "The Biological Effects of Polyunsaturated Fatty Acids," *Dairy Council Digest,* **46** (6):31–35, 1975.

11 F. Ederer, "Cancer Among Men on Cholesterol-Lowering Diets," *Lancet,* **2:**203, 1971.

12 M. M. Christiansen, "Dietary Polyunsaturates and Serum Alpha-Tocopherol in Adults," *Journal of The American Dietetic Association,* **63:**138, 1973.

13 Food and Nutrition Board, National Research Council, *Recommended Dietary Allowances,* 1974, pp. 56–61.

14 R. I. Levy, "Dietary Management of Hyperlipoproteinemia," *Journal of The American Dietetic Association* **58:**406–416, 1971.

15 D. S. Fredrickson, "Fat Transport in Lipoproteins—An Integrated Approach to Mechanisms and Disorders," *New England Journal of Medicine,* **276:**32–33, 93–103, 148–156, 215–226, 273–281; 1967.

16 D. S. Fredrickson, *Dietary Management of Hyperlipoproteinemia—A Handbook for Physicians and Dietitians,* U.S. Dept. Health, Education, and Welfare Publ. no. (NIH) 76–110.

17 R. I. Levy, "Diagnosis and Management of Hyperlipoproteinemia in Infants and Children," *American Journal of Cardiology,* **31:**547–556, 1973.

18 R. I. Levy, "Diagnosis and Management of Hyperlipidemia in Infants and Children," *American Journal of Cardiology,* **31:**547–556, 1973.

19 R. I. Levy, "Dietary and Drug Treatment of Primary Hyperlipoproteinemia," *Annals of Internal Medicine,* **77:**267–294, 1972.

20 D. S. Fredrickson, *Dietary Management of Hyperlipoproteinemia—A Handbook for Physicians and Dietitians,* op. cit.

21 Ibid.

22 Ibid.

23 C. J. Glueck, "Pediatric Familial Type II Hyperlipoproteinemia: Effects of Diet on Plasma Cholesterol in the First Year of Life," *American Journal of Clinical Nutrition,* **25:**224–230, 1972.

24 American Heart Association, *The Way to A Man's Heart.* Publ. No. EM455, 1972.

25 American Heart Association Committee on Nutrition, *Diet and Coronary Heart Disease, A Statement*

for Physicians and Other Health Professionals, 1973.

26 H. Trowell, "Ischemic Heart Disease and Dietary Fiber," American Journal of Clinical Nutrition, **25:**926–932, 1972.

27 R. I. Levy, "Dietary Management of Hyperlipoproteinemia," op. cit., pp. 406–416.

28 R. I. Levy, "Drug Therapy—Treatment of Hyperlipoproteinemia," op. cit., pp. 1295–1301.

29 E. D. Freis, "Age, Race, Sex and Other Indices of Risk in Hypertension," American Journal of Medicine, **55:**275–280, 1973.

30 Ibid.

31 L. B. Page, "Medical Management of Primary Hypertension," New England Journal of Medicine, **287:**960–965, 1018–1023, 1074–1081, 1972.

32 W. B. Kannel, "Systolic Versus Diastolic Blood Pressure and Risk of Coronary Heart Disease," American Journal of Cardiology, **27:**335–346, 1971.

33 B. Batterman, "Hypertension. Part I: Detection and Evaluation," Cardiovascular Nursing, **11:**38, July-August 1975.

34 American Academy of Pediatrics Committee on Nutrition, "Salt Intake and Eating Patterns of Infants and Children in Relation to Blood Pressure," Pediatrics, **53:**115, 1974.

35 H. A. Guthrie, "Infant Feeding Practices— A Predisposing Factor in Hypertension?" American Journal of Clinical Nutrition, **21:**863–867, 1968.

36 E. D. Freis, "Salt, Volume and the Prevention of Hypertension," Circulation, **53:**589–595, 1976.

37 L. K. Dahl, "Salt and Hypertension," American Journal of Clinical Nutrition, **25:**231–244, 1972.

38 American Academy of Pediatrics Committee on Nutrition, op. cit., p. 115.

39 Ibid.

40 H. R. Dustan, "Diuretic and Diet Treatment of Hypertension," Archives of Internal Medicine, **133:**1007–1013, 1974.

41 A. N. Brest, "Therapeutic Aspects of Hypertension," Angiology, September 1975, pp. 584–591.

42 Rosenthal, A., "The Patient with Congenital Heart Disease After Surgical Repair: An Overview," Progress in Cardiovascular Diseases, **17:**401–402, 1975.

43 Pittman, J. G., "The Pathogenesis of Cardiac Cachexia," New England Journal of Medicine. **271:**403, 1964.

44 L. Martin, J. Bristow, H. Griswold, R. Olmstead, "Relative Hypermetabolism in Infants with Cogenital Heart Disease and Undernutrition," Pediatrics **26:**183, 1965.

45 I. Krieger, "Growth Failure and Congenital Heart Disease," American Journal of Diseases of Children, **120:**497–502, 1970.

46 D. Huse, "Infants with Congenital Heart Disease," American Journal of Diseases of Children, **129:**65–69, 1975.

47 J. G. Pittman, J. G. op. cit., p. 403.

48 J. Hakkilia, "Absorption of 1 Triolein in Congestive Heart Failure," American Journal of Cardiology, **5:**295, 1960.

49 S. Fomon, "Nutritional Management of Infants with Congenital Heart Disease," American Heart Journal, **83:**581–588, 1972.

50 S. Fomon, op. cit., pp. 581–588.

51 Ibid.

52 W. E. Nelson, Textbook of Pediatrics, W. B. Saunders Company, Philadelphia, 1969, p. 129.

53 S. Fomon op. cit., p. 581–588.

CHAPTER 18

THE GASTROINTESTINAL SYSTEM

Christine Adamow Murray
Nancie H. Herbold
Rosanne B. Howard

KEY WORDS
Bland Diet
Cystic Fibrosis
Diarrhea
Disaccharidase Deficiency
Diverticulosis
Gastritis
Hiatus Hernia
Lactase Deficiency
Pancreatitis
Regional Enteritis (Crohn's Disease)
Tropical Sprue
Ulcerative Colitis
Ulcer

INTRODUCTION

The gastrointestinal tract is subject to disorders and diseases states, many of which are first manifested by symptoms of digestive complaints. Often, the individual's complaints first appear during periods of stress or emotional conflict, and arise from changes in gastrointestinal motility. Symptoms such as dysphagia (difficulty with swallowing), nausea, vomiting, abdominal pain, diarrhea, or constipation appear. These alterations in intestinal function which occur under stress are far from understood, although we are now able to associate the relationship of these symptoms with psychogenic changes in the gut. The question of why the gut is sensitive to symptom formation in some individuals during stress remains unanswered. In the past, much speculation has been offered, based upon psychiatric theories. For example, the psychoanalytic school of thought associates the etiology of peptic ulcers to reaction patterns persisting from the first stage of personality development or the "oral phase." Disorders of the colon are similarly related to the persistence of the "anal phase." Diarrhea is seen as an attempt to appease parents and constipation is attributed to the desire to withhold affection.[1] Although anecdotal evidence occasionally supports this theory in individual patients, the lack of solid evidence has tended to discourage attention to this field by the trained clinician.[2]

Traditionally, the failure to find a reason for these complaints on clinical examination has led to an artificial classification of disorders into those that are "functional" and those that are "organic" diseases. This classification does not account for the fact that often symptoms caused by an "organic lesion," such as a neoplasm of the bowel or disaccharidase deficiency, and those caused by emotional reaction to the disease, such as diarrhea or colitis, are additive and intertwined. In some disease states emotional factors appear to be significant elements in the etiology of the disease, and the choice of therapy includes treatment of the psychosomatic components of the illness.

The differential diagnosis between so-called functional and organic conditions, then is less often a matter of "either-or" than "how much of each."[3]

It is important to consider together the psychophysiological aspect of the illness with all pathogenetic mechanisms.

The confusion that exists over classification of diseases of the gastrointestinal tract carries over to the role of diet treatment of gastrointestinal disturbances. For the most part, excluding those conditions where there is a clear physiological basis for dietary modification, dietary regulation is based on tradition and on unsubstantiated information. It is the purpose of this chapter to examine the current use of diet and the clinical expression of the diseases of the gastrointestinal system.

Since there is evidence that many common gastrointestinal symptoms are often produced by biologically ingrained patterns of defense and adaptations to stress,[4] there are strong implications for psychotherapeutic management for many patients. When psychogenic factors predominate in the etiology of the disease, the therapeutic treatment plan should include psychiatric intervention as a priority. Therapeutic diets should be used as a tool within this framework of understanding and the diet should be individually tailored to the patient's tolerance as well as the severity of the disease state. The diet should not act as a target for the patient's manipulation by placing unwarranted restrictions on the patient but rather the dietary regimen should help toward the reestablishment of coping power, as the patient learns to identify his or her own level of food tolerance.

The gastrointestinal system begins with the lips, which serve as a gateway of the system. The finely coordinated movement of the lips, mouth, and tongue prepare and propel food in the waves of muscular contraction that constitute swallowing. An understanding of swallowing is essential to the health professional who is studying the gastrointestinal system, since many patients with gastrointestinal diseases, especially those with esophageal disorders, present with complaints of dysphagia (difficult swallowing) in addition to heartburn, regurgitation, and vomiting. Certain neurological disorders with damage to those cranial nerves that control swallowing will also present with the same complaint (see Chap. 22).

THE PSYSIOLOGY OF SWALLOWING

Swallowing can be considered in three separate stages: the *oral stage,* which is initially under voluntary control, and the *pharyngeal* and the *esophageal* stages, which are reflexive and involuntary.[5]

Oral stage A masticated bolus of food is gathered on the upper surface of the tongue, which rises at the tip. A contraction of the tongue flows backward, pushing the bolus toward the pharynx. At this point the swallowing becomes involuntary and nerve impulses emanating from the fifth, ninth, and tenth cranial nerves produce a series of reflexes that propel the food backward and downward.

Pharyngeal stage In this phase the pharyngeal muscles contract, squeezing the contents downward into the esophagus. Simultaneous reflexes close the mouth, nasopharynx, and respiratory passages. The posterior part of the tongue is pressed upward against the roof of the mouth; the soft palate is elevated, and the posterior wall of the nasopharynx bulges forward. Respiration is halted and the air passages are isolated by elevation of the larynx. Swallowing and voluntary inhalation are virtually impossible when the mouth is open. Therefore, patients who cannot properly seal their lips or close the mouth cannot be expected to swallow.

Esophageal stage During this phase the food is passed along the length of the esophagus and into the stomach. Esophageal contractions commence at the upper end of the esophagus with each conscious swallow and travel uninterruptedly to the lower esophageal sphincter at a rate of approximately 4 to 5 cm per second.[6,7] A second wave of peristaltic contractions then takes over if the primary effort fails to empty the esophagus. A third wave, considered to be segmental and nonpropulsive, plays little part in the normal swallowing reflex. For the most part, esophageal peristalsis is not required for swallowing fluids, as the initial phase of swallowing, along with the action of gravity, is sufficient to deliver food to the stomach.

The reverse of this process, vomiting, begins with the opening of the gastroesophageal sphincter. This is caused by contraction of the pyloric sphincter, which induces the stomach and the esophagus to relax. Respiration is then halted, with a fixation of the diaphragm in the inspiratory position. The air passages are isolated, with closure of the glossitis and elevation of the pharynx. Violent contractions of the abdominal muscles expel the contents of the stomach.[8]

Normally, once food is delivered to the stomach, it becomes the primary function of the lower esophageal sphincter to prevent the reflux of the acid gastric contents. Failure of this mechanism produces symptoms associated with two disorders of the esophagus, namely, achalasia and hiatus hernia.

Diagnosis of disorders of the esophagus can be made by plain x-ray, barium swallow x-ray studies, endoscopy, and pressure recordings of the sphincters and muscle walls of the esophagus.

DISEASES INVOLVING THE ESOPHAGUS

Achalasia

Achalasia is a motor disorder involving the smooth muscle of the esophagus. It causes a double defect in esophageal function. Passage of food and fluids from the esophagus to the stomach is impeded by the lower esophageal sphincter, and there is a failure of the normal progressive peristalsis in the upper two-thirds of the esophagus. The individual experiences dysphagia without pain and a feeling of fullness in the chest after meals. The onset is insiduous, developing over a period of time, and the age of onset is nonspecific. However, there is a tendency for the disorder to occur in young individuals.[9]

Regurgitation is another symptom, and is exacerbated by changes in position or by physical exercise. It is interesting to note that true heartburn is an uncommon manifestation of achalasia, yet this frequent regurgitation of material from the esophagus leads to a marked pulmonary change.

Presently, the etiology of the disease is unknown. The original hypothesis of a psychosomatic origin of the disease has been discarded and the disorder is considered to be primarily neural in origin and to represent a muscular adaptation to a primary nerve disorder. Microscopic examination shows fewer ganglion cells in the body of the esophagus and those present may be engulfed by chronic inflammatory cells. The disturbance dilates the esophagus above the stricture. As the disease progresses, the esophagus assumes a sigmoid configuration. This, coupled with the absence of peristalsis and the failure of the lower sphincter to open, is the combination of events that causes the individual to experience difficulties in swallowing.

Treatment   The treatment of achalasia is aimed at weakening the lower esophageal sphincter so that gravity can facilitate emptying. This is usually accomplished by hydrostatic or pneumatic dilation. In some cases surgery is necessary, involving the incising of the circular muscle fibers down to the mucosa.

Prior to treatment, liquids may present as much of a problem in swallowing as solids because of the closed esophageal stricture. However, since fluids do not require esophageal peristalsis small, frequent feedings of semisolid food at moderate temperature will be tolerated better.

In some patients, alcohol is reported to help food pass into the stomach.[10] Whether this effect is due to the demonstrated ability of alcohol to decrease esophageal pressure[11] or is due to the psychic effect is unknown. Since the competence of the sphincter is now felt to be controlled by gastrointestinal hormones and in particular by gastrin,[12,13] and since patients with achalasia are known to be hypersensitive to gastrin, a diet that would reduce gastrin production might be helpful for patients awaiting medical treatment.

Foods containing protein and carbohydrate liberate gastrin and therefore may be responsible for increasing sphincter pressure. In view of this association, a moderate reduction in such foods may be helpful. Fat stimulates the production of cholecystokinin, a duodenal hormone responsible for lowering sphincter pressure either directly or through competition with gastrin.[14] Therefore, foods with a high fat content (e.g., whole milk rather than skim milk) may be encouraged. Babka and Costell also report[14] that chocolate and coffee are known to decrease sphincter pressure and may therefore be included. Spicy foods and citrus and tomato juice should be avoided to prevent direct insult to the esophageal mucosa.

Weight loss may be noted, especially in patients with advanced esophageal stasis associated with bronchopulmonary aspiration and bouts of bronchopneumonia. In these individuals diet considerations should allow for the repletion of nutrient stores.

Hiatus Hernia

A diaphragmatic or hiatus hernia is the condition resulting from a defect in the diaphragm muscle, around the opening in the diaphragm where the esophagus continues into the abdomen. This allows the stomach to protrude upward or herniate into the thoracic cavity (see Fig. 18-1). Symptoms are related to the esophagitis produced by the reflux of gastric juice into the lower esophagus,[15] and include heartburn, acid regurgitation, vomiting, dysphagia

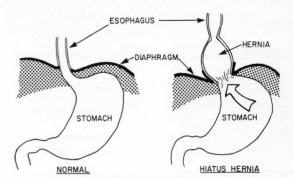

Figure 18-1

The normal esophagus and the mechanism of a hiatus hernia. The diaphragm muscle stretches across the midpoint of the abdomen and the chest cavity. The hernia occurs at the juncture of the stomach and the esophagus as a result of weakness or relaxation of the opening in the diaphragm. (Adapted from J. Pullock, Gaseous Digestive Conditions. Charles C. Thomas, Publishers, Springfield, Ill., 1967.)

(difficulty in swallowing), and odynophagia (painful swallowing).

The etiologic factors are confusing. Congenital weakness of the diaphragmatic muscle, trauma, and the aging process have been considered to contribute to the cause. In addition structural or postural change, as observed in kyphoscoliosis, and conditions that increase abdominal pressure such as obesity, pregnancy, ascites, and tight-fitting clothes have been associated with the etiology.[16]

There are several different types of hiatus hernia (sliding hernia, rolling or parietal hernia, short-esophagus hernia), all of which can be small or large; however, these distinctions are not significant from a clinical nutrition standpoint. Diagnosis depends on radiologic examination.

Treatment Medical treatment is successful in 80 percent of the patients with hiatal hernias. Treatment is aimed at reducing factors which promote reflux of acid juice into the esophagus and at neutralization of the acid.[17] To reduce factors promoting reflux the following measures are recommended:

Removal of tight-fitting garments

Weight reduction (if the patient is obese)

Separation of meals from sleeping time (patient should not eat before retiring—2½ to 3 h should elapse to allow the meal to be digested)

Elevating the head of the patient's bed by placing the bed legs on blocks (the head of the bed should not be elevated in a jacknife position such as occurs in hospital beds)

Giving small meals rather than large meals (6 small feedings are recommended instead of 3 meals)

Small amounts of fluids should be sipped at meals rather than large amounts gulped

Gum chewing should be discouraged to prevent swallowing large amounts of air

To neutralize acid, treatment akin to peptic ulcer management is recommended (see "Gastric and Duodenal Ulcers," below). The following nutritional management is recommended:

Bland diet, which strictly avoids those foods that reduce lower esophageal sphincter pressure, such as coffee and chocolate, and foods that irritate the esophageal mucosa, such as orange, grapefruit, and tomato juice. In addition, since fat lowers pressure of the sphincter, a diet which controls fat may be better tolerated

Small feedings, as described above

Antacids (Maalox, Amphogel)

Anticholinergic drugs (drugs which slow gastric emptying time)

Surgical treatment is indicated when medical treatment fails and complications arise.

Special Feeding Considerations

There are other conditions which may impede the function of the esophagus or certain congenital problems such as esophageal atresia (congenital abnormality of the esophagus with or without tracheoesophageal fistula) which do not necessarily require a special diet per se, but do require special feeding techniques. Special tube feeding (see Chap. 24) are required to maintain or improve nutritional status in conditions that restrict feeding by the oral route. An infant with esophageal atresia requires surgery during the newborn period, and gastrostomy feedings are employed until the function of the esophagus is restored. Children born with congenital abnormalities that affect normal feeding may be maintained until they are as much as 2 years of age on gastrostomy feedings along with amounts of oral food, which are added as tolerated. These children may present further feeding problems after surgical repair because of their lack of food-related experiences. During the period of food introduction, parents need anticipatory guidance on the types, the amount, and the texture of the food to be presented to the infant. They need to understand that the infant's acceptance of food will take time and patience. Some of the techniques of behavior modification may be useful in establishing a positive, well-accepted feeding routine (see Chap. 10).

The same type of feeding problem may also be encountered in the child who has swallowed a corrosive substance such as lye. The recuperative period following ingestion of a caustic agent requires a child to go for long periods without food by mouth. After surgical repair to the damaged esophagus, the child often continues to experience discomfort on swallowing after food ingestion, further slowing the return to oral feeding and increasing reliance on special tube preparations.

DISEASES OF THE STOMACH

The functions of the stomach are threefold: (1) The stomach is a major storage organ in the body, holding large quantities of food until the partially digested mass can be accommodated by the lower portion of the gastrointestinal tract. (2) The organ mixes gastric solutions of hydrochloric acid and food to form a semifluid substance called *chyme*. (3) The stomach regulates the flow of chyme into the intestine to allow for optimal digestion and absorption of ingested nutrients.

Pathologic disorders that affect stomach function will interfere with the breakdown of food entering the organ, with the formation of chyme, or with the passage of the chyme to the intestines for further action by intestinal secretions and bacteria.

Gastritis

Gastritis is an acute or chronic inflammation of the stomach mucosa. The patient may experience anorexia, nausea, vomiting, epigastric pain, and a feeling of fullness. Acute gastritis may be caused by the ingestion of certain drugs (salicylates, antibiotics), excessive intake of alcohol, allergic reaction to foods, food poisoning, and bacterial and viral infections. The etiology of chronic gastritis is unknown.

Treatment   For the first day or two during the acute state of the disease no food is given by mouth (NPO) and parenteral nutrition should be used for nutritional support (see Chap. 24). Liquids are gradually added to the diet as tolerated by the individual patient. When symptom-free the patient can then progress to a bland diet (see page 354 for a discussion of bland diets).

Gastric and Duodenal Ulcers

An ulcer is a circumscribed erosion of mucosal tissue that can occur at various sites in the gastrointestinal tract which are exposed to gastric juice. An ulcer may occur at any of the following sites: esophagus, stomach (gastric ulcer), duodenum (duodenal ulcer), and the jejunum when a gastrojejunostomy has been performed. All ulcers will be considered together, as nutritional intervention and medical treatment are basically similar whatever the location of the lesion.

The exact etiology of peptic ulcers is unclear but hypersecretion of gastric acid (hydrochloric acid, pepsin, and water) by the parietal cells of the stomach has been implicated. Hypersecretion of gastric acid is seen in patients with duodenal ulcers; however, patients with gastric ulcers tend to secrete less acid than normal individuals. The tissue insult in gastric ulcer disease may be due to weakened resistance of the mucosa rather than to the increased amount of gastric acid.

Gastrin, a hormone that is stimulated by the presence of food in the stomach, promotes acid secretion. Investigators have found that fasting levels of gastrin are similar in both normal and ulcer patients. However, ulcer patients had elevated levels of gastrin postprandially, perhaps indicating that hormonal response may be an influencing factor in the development of ulcer disease. Many drugs are known to be "ulcerogenic," for example, salicylates and steroids. These drugs increase gastric acid secretion as well as decreasing mucosal resistance.

Ulcers are more frequently seen in males than females, usually in nervous, tense, aggressive individuals, supporting the theory that the etiology of the disease may be related to emotional factors.

Pain is the major symptom of ulcer disease and is often accompanied by a feeling of hunger. A barium swallow x-ray study is a common procedure used in the diagnosis of ulcer disease. Barium is an opaque dye that will appear on x-rays and reveal a "crater" if an ulcer is present.

Treatment   The major medical treatment for the ulcer patient is rest, both physical and mental, and the use of antacid therapy.

Healing of the ulcer is aided when hydrochloric acid is neutralized or suppressed. Ideally gastric secretions should be between a pH of 4.0 and 5.0.[18] Initially, antacids may be prescribed as frequently as every hour, with subsequent administration reduced to between meals and at bedtime. There are a variety of antacids that may be used. Calcium carbonate, magnesium hydroxide, and aluminum hydroxide are the preferred drugs as they are more palatable and their side effects (constipation and diarrhea) are easier to regulate[19] than those of the other antacids. In addition, the milk-alkali syndrome is a complication that may arise from the excessive intake of milk while on antacid therapy. Besides antacid, antispasmodics or anticholinergic drugs may be used to relieve pain and decrease secretion of acid.

The *bland diet* is the common terminology used in describing the dietary treatment of ulcer disease. For many years the dietary treatment for ulcer disease was based on the premise that all foods which are chemically, mechanically, and thermally irritating to the stomach were to be avoided. However, the foods that were restricted had never been scientifically tested to establish their effect on the stomach. Therefore, each hospital, physician, and nutritionist had their own idea of what should or should not be allowed on a "bland" diet. In the acute phase of ulcer disease it was common practice to provide the patient with small frequent feedings of milk, cream, and antacids. This was known as the *Sippy diet*, named after the physician who introduced it in 1915.[20] The patient slowly progressed to other easily tolerated foods, such as creamed soups, Jello, and poached eggs, and finally to a "bland" diet. (See Table 18-1 below.) This regimen still prevails, although the atherogenic nature of the diet may be altered by substituting skim milk and polyunsaturated fats for the whole milk and cream.

Milk is used in the treatment of the ulcer patient because milk protein, as well as other proteins, neutralizes gastric acid and acts as a buffer. The buffering action of protein is only temporarily effective and necessitates frequent feedings. However, other research indicates that proteins are also gastric stimulants and therefore should be limited. For example, histidine, an amino acid, is decarboxylated to histamine, a gastric stimulant. Fats, on the other hand, are gastric inhibitors and decrease gastric motility, allowing more neutralization of gastric acid and are therefore encouraged.

Large volumes of food can also cause an increase in gastric secretion; hence the need for small meals. Foods and condiments that are presumed to increase secretion, such as black pepper, chili powder, cocoa, alcohol, and caffeine are avoided, and smoking is discouraged since nicotine has this same effect. Traditionally, gas-forming foods (cabbage, onions, brussels sprouts, turnips) and fiber have been eliminated from the daily diet of the ulcer patient.

However, studies[21-23] suggest that the ulcer patient tolerates a wide range of foods and that healing is not aided by the avoidance of foods traditionally listed as irritating, such as foods high in fiber or caffeine. The American Dietetic Association has published a position paper discussing some of the theories of the nutritional management of the ulcer patient.[24]

The use of decaffeinated coffee in place of regular coffee may be unwarranted. Studies have demonstrated that decaffeinated coffee stimulates 75 percent as much hydrochloric acid production as regular coffee.[25,26] This evidence suggests that there are no increased benefits derived from the use of decaffeinated coffee in lieu of caffeinated coffee.

It is difficult to generalize treatment for any patient and all diet therapy must be individualized. Those factors which will influence the nutritional management of the ulcer patient are:

Stage of ulcer disease
Other medical complications
Nutritional status
Food tolerances

The following is a summary of the general principles of dietary treatment which should be considered when individualizing nutritional care.

Diet Progression The various diet progressions that are used for the treatment of ulcer disease are given in Table 18-1. Their purpose is as follows:

Gastric I This diet is used for the patient who is acutely ill and may have internal bleeding.

Gastric II The patient progresses to this diet after bleeding has stopped and convalescence has begun.

Strict bland This regimen is initiated as soon as the patient shows signs of improvement and tolerates all foods allowed in the Gastric II diet.

Liberal bland This diet is used for ambulatory patients, to prevent exacerbation of the ulcer condition resulting from foods that are not well tolerated. The patient is instructed to avoid any foods that are not well tolerated; thus, a diet as tolerated is prescribed. Foods which may cause stress to the patient recuperating from ulcer disease include the gas-forming vegetables, fried foods, and very spicy foods.

This series of diets, especially the Gastric II, strict bland, and liberal bland diets, are used in the treatment of other gastrointestinal disorders, such as gastritis, hiatus hernia, and postoperatively after gastric surgery.

DISEASES OF THE LOWER GASTROINTESTINAL TRACT

The small bowel is the primary site of nutrient absorption. Partially digested food in the form of chyme is emptied from the stomach into the duodenum for further enzymatic action by brush border enzymes and ultimate absorption by the intestinal mucosa.

However, many conditions can alter mucosal function and result in nutrient malabsorption and consequent nutrient imbalance. A review of Chap. 9 is recommended to enhance understanding of normal nutrient digestion and absorption as related to the malabsorption that is characteristic of gastrointestinal diseases of the small bowel.

Diarrhea

Diarrhea is a condition resulting in the passage of loose, frequent stools. Diarrhea stools consist of water, sodium, potassium, and frequently undigested food.

Diarrhea may occur as a functional or organic condition. Frequently, the intestines may be exposed to mucosal irritants such as spices, foodstuffs, or drugs. Overeating, nervous irritability, fermentation of carbohydrates in the gut, and bacterial overgrowth in the gut may result in functional diarrhea. Bacterial food spoilage is also a common cause.

Organic diarrhea is the result of pathogenic bacterial action on the gut and is often associated with such diseases as celiac disease, typhoid fever, dysentery, chronic ulcerative colitis, viral diseases, or tuberculosis. Enzyme-deficient states or disease conditions that cause intestinal lesions can also result in organic diarrhea.

Treatment Because of the rapid passage of the feces through the colon and the resulting water and electrolyte losses, replacement of lost nutrients is crucial to prevent dehydration and fluid and electrolyte imbalances. Fluid replacement is essential to compensate for the osmotic shift of water into the intestinal lumen and rapid excretion in the liquid stools.

The most common dietary treatment is to eliminate the particular food known to be irritating to the intestine. Institution of a diet low in residue will decrease intestinal irritation. The use of hydrophilic vegetable protein compounds to absorb water in the gut may prove beneficial in returning the stool to a soft consistency without the loss of free water.

In the first 24 to 48 h of severe diarrhea it is beneficial to rest the gastrointestinal tract. Giving intravenous therapy to replace fluids and electrolyte losses while allowing nothing by mouth will permit the bowel to rest. When the diarrhea subsides, a clear liquid regimen should be started, with progression to a full liquid diet and then to a diet as tolerated. If the diarrhea is still apparent after the initial 48-h

TABLE 18-1 PROGRESSIVE BLAND DIET FOR TREATMENT OF ULCER DISEASE

Type of food	Food allowed		Foods to be avoided
	Gastric I	*Gastric II*	
Beverage	Milk (skim) at room temperature, 1½ oz each waking hour or at intervals prescribed by the doctor	Gastric I with only these additions: buttermilk, eggnog, milk, milk drinks at room temperature; hot water; and hot milk (fat content may be altered by use of polyunsaturated cream substitute)	Carbonated beverages; coffee; coffee substitute; ice and iced beverages; cocoa; tea
Bread	None	White and toasted; rusk; crackers made with refined flours	Bread and crackers containing whole-grain flour or bran; saltines
Cereal	None	Cooked refined corn, rice, and wheat cereals; strained oatmeal	Dry cereals; whole-grain cereals
Desserts	None	Angel, plain, or sponge cake; plain cookies; custard, gelatin, and rennet desserts; rice, tapioca, and vanilla puddings; melting vanilla ice cream. All desserts must be made without fruits, nuts, or spices	
Fat	None	Butter, sweet and sour cream, cream cheese	All other
Fruits	None	Cooked and strained: apples, apricots, prunes, plums, pears, peaches fruit cocktail, ripe bananas; apple, apricot, prune, and orange juices with or after lunch and dinner only	
Meats, fish poultry, eggs, cheese	None	Eggs baked, boiled, poached, or scrambled in double boiler; cottage or cream cheese; tender chicken and turkey; fresh or frozen fish; canned tuna or salmon, water packed, with bones removed	Fried eggs; any meat or cheese not included on allowed list
Potato or potato substitute	None	Baked or boiled potatoes (**without skin**) macaroni, noodles, refined rice, spaghetti	Fried potato, potato chips, hominy, whole-grain rice
Soup	None	Cream soup made with pureed vegetables: asparagus, green or wax beans beets, carrots, peas (not dried), potato, spinach, squash	All soups prepared from meat, fish, or poultry

Sweets	None	Sugar and jelly in moderation	All other
Vegetables	None	Canned, cooked, and strained: beets, green or wax beans, carrots, peas, pumpkin, squash, whole asparagus tips	All other
Miscellaneous	None	Moderate amount of salt; white sauce	Alcohol, condiments; gravy, herbs, ice, nuts, olives, pickles, popcorn, relishes, spices, vinegar, chocolate

Type of food	Foods allowed *Strict bland*	Foods to be avoided
Beverage	Buttermilk; milk; milk drinks (all at room temperature); Sanka	Carbonated beverages, coffee, strong tea, cocoa
Bread	White, well toasted; rusk; crackers made with refined flours	Whole-grain breads
Cereals	Cooked refined corn, rice, and wheat cereals; strained oatmeal	Whole-grain cereals
Dessert	Angel, plain, or sponge cake; plain cookies; custard, gelatin, and rennet desserts; ice cream and sherbets; rice, tapioca, and vanilla pudding (all without fruits, seeds, nuts, spices, or coconut)	All other pastries
Fat	Margarine, butter; sweet and sour cream; cream cheese	All other
Fruits	Cooked and strained: apples, prunes, plums, fruit cocktail; ripe bananas; whole cooked or canned peaches, pears, and peeled apricots; all fruit juices, including orange juice (strained and diluted) and other citrus juices, taken with lunch and supper meals only	All other
Meat, fish, poultry, eggs, cheese	Eggs creamed, baked, boiled, poached, or scrambled in a double boiler; cottage, cream, mild American cheese; ground or tender beef, lamb, liver, veal; tender or ground chicken and turkey; fresh or frozen fish; canned tuna or salmon, water packed (baked, boiled, or broiled)	Fried eggs, meat, fish, fowl; any not included on allowed list; clams
Potato or potato substitute	Potato; macaroni; noodle; refined rice; spaghetti	Fried potato; potato chips; hominy; whole-grain rice
Soup	Cream soup made with pureed vegetables: asparagus, green or wax beans, beets, carrots, peas (not dried), potato, spinach, squash	
Sweets	Jelly; sugar in moderation; syrup	Jam; marmalade; hard candy; coconut, candy with nuts
Vegetables	Canned or cooked: asparagus tips; strained: beets, green or wax beans, carrots, peas, pumpkin, squash; limit to 1 serving daily	Gas-forming vegetables: onions, turnips, brussels sprouts, cabbage, broccoli, garlic
Miscellaneous	Moderate amount of salt; white sauce	Alcohol, condiments, gravy, herbs, ice, nuts, olives, pickles, popcorn, relishes, spices, vinegar

Source: Adapted from Beth Israel Hospital, *Diet Manual*, Boston, Mass.

period, continuing nothing by mouth and initiating parenteral administration of an amino acid infusion in conjunction with intravenous glucose therapy will achieve bowel rest while supplying the patient with nutrition parenterally.

When oral feeding is allowed, the inclusion of food items containing pectin, a hydrophilic polysaccharide, can prove beneficial. Applesauce and peeled raw apple contain large amounts of pectin and are often given every 2 to 4 h to improve the uptake of free water and the consistency of the stools.

Steatorrhea

Steatorrhea is a diarrhea characterized by excessive fat in the stools and the presence of loose, foul-smelling, infrequent stools that float. Steatorrhea is indicative of the presence of an organic disease and is commonly found as a secondary problem in (1) intestinal mucosal lesions (e.g., celiac disease); (2) structural lesions of the intestine such as short gut, Crohn's disease, or lymphoma; (3) infections such as enteritis; (4) maldigestion, such as occurs with bile acid deficiency, cystic fibrosis, or pancreatitis; or (5) after gastrointestinal surgery such as intestinal resection or gastric surgery.

Steatorrhea results in decreased absorption of most nutrients, and weight loss. Increased loss of fecal nitrogen is common and can contribute to hypoalbuminemia. Fecal fat losses result in concomitant losses of fat-soluble vitamins. Excess loss of vitamin D can interfere with calcium metabolism. This mechanism, coupled with the loss of the calcium that is bound as soaps in the greasy stool, makes calcium depletion a real problem in the patient with severe steatorrhea.

Treatment   Since steatorrhea is a symptom of many organic diseases, treatment of the primary disease will bring secondary relief from fatty stools. It is important to remember that severe losses of fluid, electrolytes, vitamins, minerals, and other nutrients can occur if the underlying disease is not properly treated to ensure a decrease in fecal fat losses.

The use of medium-chain triglycerides (MCT) as a nutrient supplement provides an available source of calories in the form of short-chain fatty acids. MCT can be directly absorbed and utilized and seems to be well tolerated in patients experiencing severe loss of fat through steatorrhea (see Chap. 5).

Malabsorption Syndromes

Malabsorption syndromes are classified according to the age of onset of the disease, and the characteristics of the patient's stools. There is some evidence that malabsorption can occur in the newborn, in relation to congenital abnormalities affecting gastrointestinal structure and function.[27] However, it is more commonly manifested in early infancy and is considered to result from damage to the absorptive areas of the small bowel by enteropathogenic bacteria, viruses, parasites, congenital abnormalities of the gut, or genetic enzymatic malfunctions. Diseases of the small intestine, liver, pancreas, and gallbladder result in primary or secondary malabsorptive states and require specific medical and nutritional therapy.

Malabsorption syndromes clinically present with weight loss, anorexia, abdominal distention, borborygmi (loud bowel sounds), muscle wasting, and passage of abnormal stools. The stools have been described as light yellow to grey, greasy, soft, bulky, bubbling, and glistening, with a tendency to float. Long-standing malabsorption can result in edema, ascites, skeletal disorders, paresthesia, tetany, bleeding, glossitis, cheilosis, and generalized protein-calorie malnutrition. The etiology of these symptoms will be examined here in relation to specific diseases resulting in malabsorptive states.

Gluten-Sensitive Enteropathy (Celiac Sprue)

Dicke[28] first recognized the relationship between dietary wheat products and the course of celiac disease in 1950. Further investigations have demonstrated the efficacy of the gluten-free diet on the anatomy and physiology of the diseased small bowel of patients with this disorder. Therefore, the term *gluten-sensitive enteropathy* best describes the etiological and functional abnormalities found in afflicted patients. Synonymous terms such as *celiac disease, nontropical sprue,* and *idiopathic steatorrhea* have been coined; however, they can be considered to be as accurately descriptive of the disease as the term gluten-sensitive enteropathy.

Gluten-sensitive enteropathy (GSE) is a disease of the intestinal mucosa affecting the proximal portion of the small bowel. Vitamin B_{12} malabsorption may occur because of the severity of steatorrhea and also the severity of the ileal mucosal lesion.

The mechanism whereby gluten causes damage to the intestinal mucosa, resulting in lesions, is not known. However, there are two possible mechanisms which have been proposed. One is that GSE is due to an inborn error of metabolism with a peptidase deficiency, resulting in an accumulation of undigested gluten peptides and consequent mucosal damage.[29] The other suggestion is that an abnormal immune reaction to gluten might be responsible for the damage to the intestinal mucosa.[30] However, neither of these two theories is completely without criticisms.

Celiac disease affects both children and adults and seems to have two peaks in the onset of symptoms. The first is in the very young child, primarily the 1- to 5-year-old, and the other is in the third to fourth decade of life.[31]

The major clinical finding associated with gluten-sensitive enteropathy is diarrhea, characterized by bulky, offensive, greasy, loose, watery stools and caused by the lack of mucosal surface area housing the intestinal enzymes. Green and Wollanger[32] report that 90 percent of patients experience diarrhea at some time during the course of the disease. Edema, nonspecific gastrointestinal symptoms, prolonged pain in the bones due to calcium losses in the stools, osteomalacia, malnutrition, tetany, and hemorrhage from vitamin K malabsorption have been reported. Classic symptoms in afflicted children are failure to gain weight, resulting in failure to thrive; diarrhea; muscle wasting; irritability; and increased appetite due to nutrient depletion. Following treatment there is generally good catch-up growth. Symptoms result from impaired absorption of fat, protein, carbohydrate, fat-soluble vitamins, minerals, electrolytes, and even water. The symptoms may be exacerbated by pregnancy, infection, gastric surgery, and emotional stress.

Common diagnostic tests for gluten-sensitive enteropathy are stool fat determinations, oral tolerance tests, and jejunal biopsy.

Stool fat A 72-h stool collection while the patient is taking a measured fat intake is useful in determining the amount of fat lost in the stool and consequently is assaying the extent of fat malabsorption. Fecal fat excretion is higher in patients with various degrees of malabsorption than in normal subjects. (See Chap. 5.)

Oral Tolerance Tests A glucose tolerance test is a useful indicator of mucosal functioning if no metabolic abnormalities such as diabetes exist. A xylose tolerance test is performed in some centers and is felt to be a valuable diagnostic tool when jejunal biopsy is not available. Glucose and xylose uptake in the cells can be correlated to mucosal integrity and the presence or absence of mucosal lesions.

Intestinal Biopsy Jejunal biopsy is the only definite method for making a diagnosis of mucosal abnormality and is the preferred diagnostic tool. Jejunal biopsy reveals an abnormal jejunal mucosa with a loss of the intestinal villi. The intestinal surface resembles tanned pigskin.

A diagnosis of celiac disease is made on the basis of (1) demonstration of impaired intestinal absorption, (2) finding of histological changes in the duodenal-jejunal mucosa, and (3) definite clinical response to withdrawal of dietary gluten.

TABLE 18-2 GLUTEN-FREE DIET FOR TREATMENT OF CELIAC DISEASE

Type of food	Foods allowed	Foods to avoid
Beverage	Milk (skim may be better tolerated at first) Fruit juice, cocoa (read label to see that no wheat flour has been added) Slowly add: carbonated beverages, coffee, tea, distilled alcoholic beverage	Postum, malted milk, Ovaltine, instant coffee, beer, ale, whiskey, chocolate dairy drink, root beer.
Bread	Only those made from rice, corn, soybean, wheat-starch (gluten-free), potato, lima bean flours, rice wafers	All bread, rolls, crackers made from wheat, oats, rye, barley, wheat graham flours. Rye Krisps, muffins, biscuits, waffles, pancakes, dumplings, rusk, zwieback, baked goods from forbidden grains
Cereals	Cornmeal, hominy, rice, puffed rice, pre-cooked rice) puffed rice, pre-cooked rice)	All wheat, rye, oats, barley, wheat cereal, Grapenuts, bran, kasha, corn flakes, Rice Krispies, malt
Desserts	Gelatins, fruit gelatin, ice, or sherbet; homemade ice cream, custard, Junket, rice or cornstarch pudding, tapioca, cakes, or cookies made from allowed flours	Commercial pies, cookies, pastries, ice cream, ice cream cones, prepared mixes, puddings
Fat	Oil, corn margarine, olive oil (unsaturated fats may be better tolerated initially). Later additions: butter, cream, vegetable shortening, bacon, lard	Commercial salad dressings except pure mayonnaise (read labels)
Fruits	All cooked and canned juices and fruit; include citrus fruit at least once/day. Initially avoid: skins, seeds, frozen fruits, prunes, plums, and their juices	Canned fruit pie filling
Meats, fish, poultry	All lean cuts; better tolerated if baked, broiled, boiled, or roasted	Breaded creamed meat, fish, poultry (e.g., croquette); processed meats (unless pure)
Eggs	As desired; initially avoid frying	
Cheese	All types; add slowly to diet	
Potato or potato substitute	Potato, rice	Noodles, spaghetti, macaroni, some packaged rice mixes
Soups	All clear and vegetable soups, cream soups if thickened with cornstarch or allowed flours	Commercially prepared soups; soups thickened with wheat, rye, oat, barley flours
Vegetables	All cooked and canned. Slowly add: raw vegetables	Creamed if thickened with wheat, oat, rye, barley products
Miscellaneous	Gravies and sauces thickened with cornstarch or allowed flours; vegetable gum	Gravies and sauces thickened with wheat, rye, oat, barley flours

Treatment   The treatment of gluten-sensitive enteropathy is complete withdrawal of gluten from the diet. Gluten is the glutamine-bound fraction (glutenin and gliadin) of protein. In this diet, wheat, rye, barley, oats, and all products containing any of these grains are eliminated. These grains contain a large amount of gluten, which is responsible for the malabsorption associated with the disease. Corn and rice are the only grains permitted on the gluten-free regimen. Table 18-2 gives a diet plan omitting wheat, rye, and oats from the daily intake. It may take several weeks to restore normal jejunal integrity and for symptoms to disappear completely. However, subjective improvement usually occurs within the first few days after gluten withdrawal.

Because the diet is a restrictive one, it is important to provide the patient with a variety of recipes to prevent boredom and lack of compliance. Adequate energy intake may be a problem since the restricted grains are found most often in high-caloric, baked products. Skill is required in meal planning and the importance of label reading needs to be stressed to ensure that commercial products do not contain restricted grains. Close cooperation between the physician, nutritionist, and patient is necessary to increase the probability of strict compliance with the diet. Vitamin and mineral supplements may be prescribed to augment the diet and correct deficient states.

Tropical Sprue

Another of the malabsorption syndromes, most common to tropical and subtropical areas, is tropical sprue. Although the etiology of the disease is unknown it has been postulated that bacteria[33] or a diet deficient in folic acid may be responsible for the damage to intestinal absorption of vitamin B_{12}, for megaloblastic anemia, and for bacterial overgrowth in the proximal small intestine. Because of the extensive microbial overgrowth abdominal distention and loud borborygmia are present; anorexia and vomiting occur frequently. Characteristically, the stools are semiformed or watery and may contain blood and mucus.

Tropical sprue and celiac disease are somewhat related in that both diseases present with villous atrophy of the intestinal mucosa.

Treatment   There is rapid clinical improvement with folic acid and broad-spectrum antibiotic therapy. Vitamin B_{12} therapy is often started because of the megaloblastic anemia. There is prompt response to this treatment.

A gluten-restricted diet does not relieve the symptoms. Rather, a high-energy, high-protein diet in conjunction with vitamin and mineral supplements will counteract the malnutrition and depleted nutrient stores associated with the disease. With treatment patients become asymptomatic and the intestinal mucosa returns to normal.

Disaccharidase Deficiencies

In the Western world a large portion of the daily energy consumed comes from carbohydrates. Kirschmann[34] reports that in the second year of life infants consume an average of 165 g of carbohydrate per day, and by the age of 12 years, the average consumption reaches approximately 350 g of carbohydrate daily. Theoretically, this predisposes the infant to disaccharide intolerance. Approximately 60 percent of the carbohydrate ingested is starch while sucrose accounts for 30 percent and lactose 10 percent of the total amount ingested.[35]

The oligosaccharides and disaccharides (sucrose, lactose, maltose) are hydrolyzed by specific enzymes called disaccharidases which are located in the brush border of the intestinal mucosa. Hydrolysis results in the release of the monosaccharides (glucose, galactose, and fructose) which are absorbed by the mucosa.

When disaccharidases are absent from the brush border, ingested carbohydrates cannot be absorbed and utilized by the body. "Fermentative diarrhea" results—the stools become frequent and are liquid and acidic in character. Abdominal pain and flatulence occur concomitantly with the abnormal stool pattern. The severity of the malabsorption varies with the amount and type of sugar ingested. Symptoms are relieved when a diet free of the problem sugar (e.g., a lactose-free diet) is prescribed.

Disaccharidase deficiencies may be either primary or secondary. Primary deficiencies, which are usually congenital, result in the absence of enzymes although the small intestinal mucosa is normal. Primary lactose and sucrose deficiencies have been described.[36]

Secondary disaccharidase deficiency may occur in any disease involving damage to the small bowel mucosa, such as celiac disease, ulcerative colitis, and cystic fibrosis. Most commonly, secondary disaccharidase deficiency involves lactase.

Lactase Deficiency

Lactose intolerance may be the result of a congenital inborn error of metabolism, resulting in the absence of the enzyme lactase from the intestinal mucosa. Secondary lactase deficiency may result from damage to the small bowel mucosa, as in protein-calorie malnutrition, celiac disease, and infections, or from the administration of colchicine or the antibiotics, neomycin and kanamycin.[37]

Lactase deficiency seems most common to the Negroid, Oriental, and Jewish populations, suggesting that the enzyme-deficient state may be inherited as a recessive trait. Lactose malabsorption may appear as early as the first few days of life or as late as 20 years of age. Clinically, children fail to thrive and appear weak, frail, and irritable, with muscle wasting, chronic diarrhea, vomiting, and dehydration. Stools are characterized as loose, watery, and acid. Adults with the enzyme deficiency experience diarrhea, abdominal discomfort, borborygmi, flatulence, nausea, and general discomfort.

When dietary lactose is not absorbed it remains in the lumen and increases the osmotic load of the contents in the small bowel. As a result, intestinal bacteria act on the sugar, which causes the accumulation of lactic acid in the bowel, giving the stool its characteristic acidity and aiding the production of gas in the gut. In response to the increased osmotic load, fluid is attracted into the bowel in order to decrease the concentration of sugar in the gut, resulting in increased intestinal motility and diarrhea.

The increased fluid load is responsible for the watery, acid stools characterized as having an offensive odor and a pH of less than 6. As a result of the increased peristalsis, malabsorption of protein, fats, carbohydrates, and drugs occurs.

A preliminary screening test can be accomplished by testing the stools for reducing substances with a Clinitest tablet. The presence of 0.5 percent or more of reducing substance in the stool is considered abnormal.

Diagnosis of lactose intolerance is most often made by giving a lactose load of 2 g/kg of body weight (up to a total of 50 g) and then drawing periodic blood samples. A finding of

Figure 18-2

The development of lactose intolerance. Unabsorbed lactose remains in the intestinal lumen and increases the osmotic load. Bacterial fermentation results in the production of lactic acid and gas in the gut. Increased peristalsis and malabsorption occur in consequence.

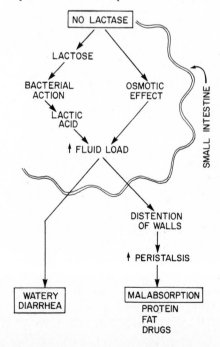

20 mg or less of lactose indicates decreased enzyme activity. Often an exaggeration of symptoms resulting from the lactose load will also indicate a lactase-deficient state. Oral tolerance tests are less satisfactory than a biopsy assay. A small intestinal biopsy taken from the area of the ligament of Trietz can be analyzed for mucosal disaccharidases.[38] This technique is the most accurate and definitive test for disaccharidase deficiency states.

Treatment   Elimination of lactose from the diet brings relief from the symptoms of lactase deficiency. Lactose is primarily found in dairy products. In severe cases of lactose intolerance a totally lactose-free diet is warranted. The elimination of all dairy products increases the susceptibility to calcium deficiency, since dairy products are the best sources of calcium in the daily diet. Birge et al.[39] suggest that the restriction of calcium-rich dairy foods as treatment for lactose intolerance may possibly explain the etiology of at least one type of osteoporosis. The increase in fecal calcium excretion as a result of the chronic diarrhea also suggests that an alternative source of calcium is necessary.

The value of total exclusion of dairy products for the lactose-intolerant individual is under debate. Through the process of fermentation, lactose is removed from aged cheese. The lactose content of cottage cheese is also low because the lactose in the whey is lost during processing (see Table 18-3). Gallagher et al.[40] report that when fermented dairy products are added to the diet a decrease in fecal calcium excretion follows. This suggests that these dairy products may be used as food sources of calcium in the lactose-free diet. However, calcium supplements are recommended in the absence of adequate dietary sources of the mineral.

Infants who are lactose intolerant are given lactose-free formula (e.g., Isomil, Cho-Free) until they are able to tolerate a formula containing the sugar. Certain medications also contain lactose and need to be avoided.

Cystic Fibrosis

Cystic fibrosis (CF) is a chronic disease inherited as an autosomal recessive disorder. The disease afflicts 1 out of every 15,000 live births and is evident early in infancy.

The disease affects the mucosa and sweat glands of the body. The mucosal glands secrete thick mucus and the sweat glands secrete abnormally high concentrations of sodium chloride. Chronic pulmonary disease results from the extensive mucus secretions in airways of the lungs. Fat malabsorption occurs as a result of mucus plugs blocking the pancreatic duct, preventing secretion of pancreatic enzymes. Hypoproteinemia may be seen in childhood because of the expanded plasma volume, which decreases the concentration of protein circulating in the blood. If the pancreatic insufficiency is not treated chronic malnutrition will ensue because of the malabsorption associated with the disease.

The majority of patients diagnosed as having cystic fibrosis have some degree of pancreatic involvement. However, the extent of pancreatic insufficiency depends on the nature and severity of the disease. Shwachman[41] reports that over 10 percent of neonates with CF have meconium ileus, pancreatic insufficiency, steatorrhea, rectal prolapse, growth retardation, and glucose intolerance. Less common but indicative of the cystic condition is liver cirrhosis, esophageal varices, diabetes, fat-soluble vitamin deficiencies and lactase deficiency.

TABLE 18-3   LACTOSE AND PROTEIN CONTENT OF SELECTED DAIRY PRODUCTS

	Amount	Lactose, g	Protein, g
Whole milk	1 cup	11.8	8
Buttermilk	1 cup	12.0	8
Yogurt	1 cup	9.0	8
Cheese			
Cottage	½ cup	1.5	7.5
Aged cheddar	1 oz	0.6	7.0

Children with CF are also described as having voracious appetites, probably as a result of the extensive malabsorption.

Meconium ileus, an obstruction of the small intestine by sticky meconium, occurs in 15 percent of all babies with cystic fibrosis and can be considered diagnostic of the disease. However, the most reliable diagnostic test for cystic fibrosis is a quantitative analysis of the sweat for sodium and chloride. Elevation of sodium and chloride routinely occurs in cystic fibrosis because of abnormal function of the sweat glands. Finger- and toenail analysis for increased levels of sodium and potassium provides an accuracy of 90 percent and is also useful in diagnosing cystic fibrosis. Hair analysis may prove to be of even greater accuracy for sodium and chloride analysis.

Treatment   Involvement of the respiratory and digestive systems and the sweat glands is the basis for medical management of the disease. (See Table 18-4.) Immediately after diagnosis, the patient will frequently require an intense period of hospitalization to stabilize the pulmonary condition and to allow the development of a comprehensive medical care plan to treat the primary systems involved. Antibiotic therapy aids in the treatment of pulmonary lesions

TABLE 18-4   SUMMARY OF MEDICAL PROBLEMS CONFRONTING THE CHILD WITH CYCTIC FIBROSIS AND THE ACCEPTED TREATMENT FOR EACH

Problem	Treatment
Bronchial obstruction	Inhalation therapy Physical therapy
Pulmonary infection	Long-term antibiotic therapy
Exocrine gland dysfunction	Sodium replacement during periods of stress or high environmental temperature
Pancreatic deficiency	Enzyme replacement
Nutritional deficiency	High-caloric, high-protein, low-fat diet; vitamin and mineral supplements

and has significantly increased the life expectancy of CF patients. The pulmonary care program includes the use of inhalation therapy and physical therapy for additional treatment and prevention of the pulmonary lesions.

Dietary regulation and pancreatic replacement therapy are aimed at minimizing the extent of the malabsorption that is likely to occur as a result of the lack of pancreatic enzymes (lipase, amylase, peptidase, cholesterolase). Fat malabsorption seems to present a greater problem than the difficulty in digestion and absorption of carbohydrates and protein caused by the pancreatic insufficiency. In infancy, a formula containing predigested proteins and medium-chain triglycerides (MCT) rather than long-chain fats (e.g., Pregestimil and Portagen) is more readily tolerated.

For the infant, strained or pureed meats are a better source of protein than vegetable and meat combinations. Infant cereals should be given in small amounts and should be of a high-protein formulation because cereals tend to fill the infant and are a lower biological source of protein.

The diet should be adjusted to the age and tolerance level of the individual. Nutrient guides as recommended by the Cystic Fibrosis Foundation are listed in Table 18-5. Calories should be increased 50 to 100 percent above the normal requirements for age because of the increased energy needs related to malabsorption and pulmonary stress. Protein requirements are 2 to 2½ times the normal recommended amounts, while fat intake varies with age, caloric intake, and degree of fat intolerance. Restriction of excess fatty foods is usually desirable in view of the extensive fat malabsorption associated with the disease. A low-fat diet (Table 18-6) is best tolerated, but should be individually tailored. For example, one child may not be able to tolerate the fat in chocolate or peanut butter, while another child may. Due to the decreased pancreatic enzyme secretion, simple carbohydrate sources and protein may be better tolerated.

Vitamin supplementation is necessary.

TABLE 18-5 NUTRIENT GUIDELINES FOR CHILDREN WITH CYSTIC FIBROSIS

Age	Calories (kilojoules)
Infants (to 1 year old)	150–200 kcal/kg/day (630–840 kJ/kg/day)
Children (1–9 years)	130–180 kcal/kg/day (545–755 kJ/kg/day)
Males (9–18 years)	100–130 kcal/kg/day (420–545 kJ/kg/day)
Females (9–18 years)	80–110 kcal/kg/day (335–460 kJ/kg/day)

Age	Protein
Infants	4 g/kg/day
Older children	3 g/kg/day
Young adults	2½–3 g/kg/day

Age	Fat
Infants	
Normal	30–60 g/day
Moderate	30–50 g/day
Low-fat	30–40 g/day
Older children	
Normal	50–120 g/day
Moderate	50–70 g/day
Low-fat	30–50 g/day

Source: Adapted from *Guide To Diagnosis and Management of Cystic Fibrosis,* Cystic Fibrosis Foundation, 1974.

The fat-soluble vitamins, especially vitamins A and D, are prescribed in twice the usually recommended doses. Water-soluble forms of Vitamins E and K are routinely prescribed in view of findings of biliary cirrhosis and Vitamin E deficiency. Vitamin B complex is recommended, especially for patients with cheilosis and those taking broad-spectrum antibiotics. In areas where the local water supply is unfluoridated, fluoride supplementation is also recommended.

Dietary supplements have recently been introduced as a means of increasing the caloric intake of the child with cystic fibrosis. Allan et al.[42] report on the use of a nutritional supplement consisting of beef serum protein hydrolysate, a glucose polymer, and medium-chain triglycerides in a group of 17 patients with cystic fibrosis. Increased rates of weight gain and linear growth were seen in 11 of the children as a result of the increased caloric intake from these supplements.

MCT (medium-chain triglycerides, Drew Chemical Company) provides 9 kcal/ml (38 kJ/ml) and has been used to facilitate the direct absorption of fatty acids in the cystic fibrosis population at Children's Hospital Medical Center in Boston. More recently Polycose (Ross Laboratories), a glucose polymer, has also been employed, as a carbohydrate supplement, in the diet of these children. It provides 0.67 kcal/ml (2.8 kJ/ml) and is tasteless, and colorless when dissolved in solution.

Parenteral hyperalimentation with an amino acid infusion has been used in acute periods of illness when appetitie is poor or the function of the gastrointestinal tract is questionable. Elliot[43] used Intralipid hyperalimentation in 7 children with cystic fibrosis. A weight gain was experienced by all 7 children during the period of infusion and a feeling of well-being was reported concomitantly with the intravenous therapy. The levels of essential fatty acids (linoleic and arachidonic) rose during this time period, suggesting fatty acid deficiency, a concern in the cystic fibrosis population because of fat malabsorption.

Pancreatic enzyme replacement is needed with meals to improve the digestion and absorption of fat and protein. The dosage and the enzyme preparation selected are determined by the individual's fat tolerance and response to the enzyme therapy. Pancreatic enzymes should be taken with all meals and snacks. The quantity is determined by age and body size. In infants, the powdered enzyme is mixed in a small amount of baby fruit and is fed immediately; otherwise enzyme breakdown of the fruit occurs.

The two most common preparations in use in the United States are Viokase and Cotazym. However, several other preparations are also

TABLE 18-6 LOW-FAT DIET PROVIDING APPROXIMATELY 45 TO 50 g OF FAT PER DAY*

Type of food	Food permitted	Foods to avoid
Beverages	Coffee, tea, decaffeinated coffee, cereal beverage, skim milk, skim buttermilk, carbonated beverages	Any others
Breads and cereals	Enriched or whole-grain bread, crackers, plain hard rolls, plain dinner rolls	Very rich breads made with large amounts of eggs or fat, such as quick breads, pancakes, waffles
Desserts	Angel food cake, fruit whips made with foods permitted, gelatin desserts, sherbet, fruit ices, puddings made with skim milk	Pastries and very rich desserts, ice cream, desserts made with egg yolk, chocolate, cream, fat, or whole milk
Eggs, meats, and cheeses	Lean beef, lamb, liver, veal, poultry, fish, canned tuna or salmon (wash off oil carefully); limit eggs to 1 per day (egg whites as desired); uncreamed cottage cheese, pot cheese	Pork; skin of poultry; fried meat, fish, or poultry; fish preserved in oil; bacon; fried eggs; other cheese
Fats	Limit to 1 tsp per meal: butter, fortified margarine, salad oil, cream	Peanut butter, lard, salad dressing, shortening

(continued)

in use (see Table 18-7). The enzymes are available in powder, tablet, and capsule forms and are made from beef or pork sources. Some patients show a better response with the addition of bile salts in conjunction with the enzymes. Clinical signs and symptoms of inadequate pancreatic replacement or excessive fat intake may include the following: abdominal cramps; abdominal distention; light-colored, frequent, mushy stools; foul-smelling flatus; rectal prolapse; and failure to thrive.

DISEASES OF THE LARGE BOWEL

The large intestine functions in the absorption of water and crystalloids from the gut and aids in the passage of the feces to the rectum for excretion.

The large bowel is located in the lower abdomen and starts with the caecum. The appendix projects from this segment. From the lower right quadrant of the abdomen, the large intestine extends upward (ascending colon), crosses underneath the liver and stomach to the spleen (tranverse colon), and turns downward (descending colon) on the left side. The sigmoid segment connects the large bowel to the rectum (Fig. 18-3).

Ulcerative Colitis
Ulcerative colitis is an organic inflammatory disease of the mucosal and submucosal linings of the large bowel. Characteristic lesions or

TABLE 18-6 (continued)

Fruit and juices	All fruits except those listed under *Foods to avoid*, all juices	Watermelon, cantaloupe, honeydew melon, avocado, raw apple
Potatoes and substitutes	White or sweet potatoes, hominy, macaroni, noodles, rice, spaghetti, pretzels	Potato chips; fried rice, noodles, or potatoes; highly seasoned sauces with fat
Soups	Fat-free broth or bouillon, vegetable soup made with allowed vegetables, tomato bouillon, cream soups made with skim milk and allowed vegetables and meat	Cream soups made with whole milk, cream, or butter
Sweets	Sugar, honey, jelly, jam, plain hard candy, syrups	Candy made with cream fat, nuts, or chocolate
Vegetables	All vegetables except those listed under *Foods to avoid*	Vegetables causing gastric distress† such as onion, radishes, sauerkraut, green or red peppers, kohlrabi, cabbage, corn, cucumbers, broccoli, brussels sprouts, turnips, lima beans, dried peas and beans, rutabagas
Miscellaneous	Salt, vinegar, lemon, juice, fat-free gravy	Chocolate, condiments, spices† nuts, olives, pepper†

* This diet should be adapted to individual needs and may not need to be this restrictive.

† May be tolerated unless there is presence of severe abdominal cramping and steatorrhea.

ulcerations are apparent in the left colon and rectum, and often in the entire organ.

Colonic motility is greatly increased, resulting in rapid movements of the small bowel and increased secretions by the colon. The patient has frequent diarrhea, and the stools often contain blood and mucus. Nausea, abdominal pain, anorexia, tachycardia, and anemia are common symptoms.

The etiology of the disease is not known. However, several theories have been proposed. The disease may be due to a nutritional deficiency state, particularly of vitamin B_{12} or protein; or it may be of infectious origin. Many researchers claim that psychogenic disturbances resulting in increased stress will result in the disease. Fried et al.[44] suggest that the disease may be inherited as an autosomal recessive trait.

Ulcerative colitis results in serious local and systemic complications. The disease is characterized by remissions and exacerbations and most frequently appears in youth and early middle age. The disease occurs more frequently among females than males and appears to be predominantly a disease of the Caucasian race with a high incidence in the Jewish population.

The diagnosis of ulcerative colitis is most often based on clinical symptoms. Sigmoidoscopy reveals an abnormal, inflamed colonic mucosa and seems to be the best tool available for diagnosis of the disease. The diagnosis can be supported by rectal biopsy and x-ray examination.

Treatment Medical treatment of the disease includes fluid and electrolyte replacement for

TABLE 18-7 PREPARATIONS AVAILABLE FOR PANCREATIC ENZYME REPLACEMENT IN CYSTIC FIBROSIS

Enzyme preparation (manufacturer)	Source	Dosage*
Cotazym (Organon)	Whole hog pancreas	1–5 capsules/meal ¼–2 pks. powder/meal
Viokase (Viobin)	Whole hog pancreas	2–10 tablets/meal ½–2 tsp/meal
Panteric granules & enteric tablets (Parke-Davis)	Whole hog pancreas	¼–1 tsp granules or 3–5 tablets/meal
Papase tablets (Warner-Chilcott)	Whole hog pancreas	½–3 tablets/meal
Piget-Aide† (Johnson & Johnson)	Whole hog pancreas	1–3 capsules/meal
Ilozyme (Warren-Teed)	Whole hog pancreas	1–5 tablets/meal

* Related to meal or snack size, and age.
† Not available in United States.

the dehydration and water losses from the diarrhea. Blood transfusion, for replacement of losses through rectal bleeding, has decreased the morbidity and mortality associated with the disease. Because ulcerative colitis is an inflammatory bowel disease, administration of

Figure 18-3

The large bowel: Transverse colon, ascending colon, descending colon, sigmoid, ileum, and cecum.

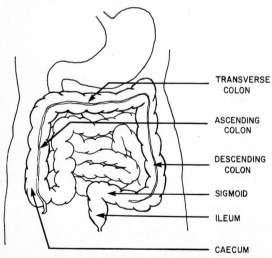

TRANSVERSE COLON

ASCENDING COLON

DESCENDING COLON

SIGMOID

ILEUM

CAECUM

the anti-inflammatory drugs ACTH and cortisone has been used to effect a remission during an acute attack.

Dietary treatment should aim to (1) decrease stool frequency through elimination of irritants to the bowel; (2) provide adequate protein for tissue regeneration and enteric protein losses; (3) provide adequate energy in response to increased catabolic rates; and (4) exclude food substances which careful history reveals may worsen the diarrhea.

Cady et al.[45] have demonstrated a lactase-deficient state in 46 percent of their study population. Therefore a low-lactose, dairy-free diet may improve weight gain in the patient with secondary lactose intolerance.

In general, the diet for patients with ulcerative colitis should be appealing, in order to overcome the anorexia associated with the disease. A diet low in residue (Table 18-8) will eliminate mechanical irritants to the inflamed bowel, while an increased protein and calorie intake will improve clinical response to the chronic diarrhea and tissue breakdown associated with the disease. Elimination of particular food items, especially lactose-containing

TABLE 18-8   LOW-RESIDUE DIET

Type of food	Foods permitted	Foods to avoid
Beverages, milk	Coffee, tea, decaffeinated coffee, cereal beverages, carbonated beverages; 2 cups milk per day (to drink or in cooking)	Milk in excess of 2 cups
Bread and cereals	Enriched white or light rye bread without seeds; cooked refined corn, rice or wheat cereals	Whole-grain or bran flour and cereals
Desserts	Cakes with plain icing, plain cookies, gelatin desserts (all without nuts, coconut, or fruits not listed under *Foods permitted;* smooth and milk-flavored sherbet and ice cream	Pastries, any other not listed
Fats	Butter, margarine, mayonnaise, salad oil, cream (limit to ½ cup per day)	None
Fruits and juices	Strained fruit juice; ripe banana; strained, cooked, and peeled fruits without seeds	Any others
Meats, fish, poultry, eggs, cheese	Crisp bacon; roasted, baked, broiled, or boiled tender beef, ham, lamb, liver, veal, fish, chicken, or turkey; cottage, cream, and mild American cheese; eggs any way except fried	Tough meats, pork, fried meats, highly seasoned meats, strong-flavored fish, sheel & fish, cheese other than those permitted
Potatoes or substitutes	White and sweet potatoes, pasta	Skins of potatoes, fried potatoes, potato chips, highly seasoned sauce
Soups	Bouillon, broth, strained cream soups made with foods permitted and within daily milk allowance	Any others
Sweets	Candy without nuts or chocolate; honey, clear jelly, sugar, molasses, syrup, smooth chocolate in moderation	Candy containing fruits or nuts; jam, marmalade
Vegetables	Tomato juice, canned or cooked pureed vegetables	Any others
Miscellaneous	Gravy, herbs (except garlic), spices in moderation, vinegar, white sauce, smooth peanut butter	Garlic, nuts, olives, pickles, popcorn, pepper, relishes, fried foods, highly seasoned sauces

foods, will improve nutrient absorption and decrease malabsorption due to the inflammatory condition.

Regional Enteritis (Crohn's Disease

Enteritis is an inflammation of the bowel of varying degrees. The condition may be the result of a mechanical or chemical irritation at some point in the bowel. Overeating, poisoning, or bacterial invasion can cause the inflammation. The exact etiology is not known.

When the colon is involved, the resulting disease state is called *regional enteritis* or *Crohn's disease.* However, Crohn's disease has been reported to occur in any portion of the gastrointestinal tract.[46]

Inflammation of the bowel results in a shift of water into the intestine to act as a cleansing and diluting solution. Cramping results from increased intestinal motility. Diarrhea, weight loss, fatigue, and irritability are characteristics of the disease. Frequently steatorrhea will occur, resulting in a loss of large quantities of ingested fat in the stools. Characteristic stools often contain mucus, blood, and pus as a result of the bacterial inflammation.

Treatment Dietary principles for the treatment of regional enteritis include a low-residue diet that is high in protein and rich in vitamins and minerals to promote tissue regeneration. Elimination of residue in the diet reduces mechanical irritation to the gut and provides rest.

Restriction of fat in the diet will aid in controlling the fecal fat losses that occur in steatorrhea. Fat absorption may be improved through the use of medium-chain triglycerides as a source of increased calories.

Diverticulosis

Diverticula are acquired herniations or pocketings of the mucosa through the layers of the bowel wall. *Diverticulosis* is the presence of diverticula which are not inflamed. Infection often occurs as a result of the accumulation of fecal matter within the diverticula, which can become ulcerated or perforated. Inflammation of the diverticula is called *diverticulitis.*

Diverticular disease is the most common colonic disease of the Western nations. The increased incidence of diverticulosis has been attributed to a diet low in fiber. The deficiency of dietary fiber alters the consistency of the feces, causing the sigmoid colon to segment more rapidly. The increased segmentation propels the feces, which generates increased intraluminal pressure, causing herniation of the colonic mucosa. The development of diverticula follows.

Treatment For many years a low-residue diet had been prescribed to help eliminate irritation of the bowel. In view of the recent findings that hypersegmentation of the colonic mucosa is a result of increased intraluminal pressure,[47] a diet high in fiber is the current trend of dietary treatment for the disease, since fiber lowers the intraluminal pressure and shortens the intestinal transit time by providing bulk to the stool.

Kirwan et al.[48] found that unprocessed bran was successful in shortening gastrointestinal transit time. Bran resists digestion by absorbing water, resulting in a soft, bulky stool which is easily passed.

The increased intraluminal pressure associated with diverticular disease develops as a result of increased force exerted by the muscle, increased diameter of the intestinal lumen, and decreased viscosity of the intestinal contents. Burkitt et al.[49] suggest the use of bran in relieving the symptoms associated with diverticular disease that result from increased intraluminal pressure. Findlay et al.[50] report the positive effects of ingesting 20 g of unprocessed bran per day in their population suffering from diverticular disease. Their findings clearly point to the use of coarse bran as therapeutic for (1) shortening intestinal transit time in diverticular disease, (2) increasing stool weight in normal people and to a lesser extent in patients with diverticular disease, (3) modifying fecal flow patterns, and (4) providing a vehicle for interstitial water. They demonstrated a decrease in the intraluminal pressure in response to the bran's stimulus to the distal colon, thus relieving the symptoms associated with increased intraluminal pressure in patients with diverticular disease.

Increased fiber intake has recently been acclaimed as the most appropriate dietary treatment for diverticular disease. However, as many treatments for gastrointestinal disease change, so it is with dietary management of diverticular disease and the dispute over the effectiveness of a low-fiber versus a high-fiber diet.

Bowel Resection

Surgical removal of a section of the ileum (ileectomy) or the colon (colectomy) may be indicated in chronic conditions such as carcinoma, intestinal obstruction, lesions, or ulcerative colitis. Following removal of the bowel segment a permanent opening is made in the abdominal wall to provide for elimination of digestive wastes.

An *ileostomy* results from attaching the proximal end of the ileum to the opening in the abdominal wall. Because the absorptive capacity of the ileum is reduced as a result of the decreased surface area, the ileostomy continuously drains fluid which is often irritating to the surrounding tissue. Proper hygiene and use of a well-fitted appliance is necessary to prevent tissue erosion around the stoma.

Initially, large sodium and water losses occur following an ileostomy procedure because the absorptive capacity of the ileum has been disturbed by the surgery. However within 7 to 10 days postoperatively the losses are adjusted to within normal limits. Extensive resection of the ileum results in fat malabsorption requiring a dietary restriction in fat. Vitamin B_{12} absorption is permanently decreased and is often totally lost. Therefore intravenous fluid and electrolyte replacement is necessary during the convalescent period, while vitamin B_{12} injections are necessary for life to compensate for the isolated defect in vitamin B_{12} absorption. The diet is augmented progressively as tolerated. After complete recovery postoperatively, the ileostomy patient is able to resume a regular diet. However, ingestion of excessive dietary roughage may obstruct the stoma and result in discomfort to the patient.

A *colostomy* results from attaching the proximal end of the colon to the opening in the abdominal wall. The colon retains some capacity to absorb water; therefore, the stools are semiformed. The patient is able to learn to control bowel movements through the colostomy, thus enabling reestablishment of bowel regularity.

Diet is increased progressively as tolerated. The colostomy patient should observe the stools to determine individual tolerances to particular food items and should regulate the diet accordingly. The dietary management of colostomy patients aims to provide adequate energy and nutrition and to allow for good control of bowel movements.

Therapeutic dietary management of ostomy patients must be individualized. The greater the extent of intestinal resection, the greater the degree of secondary malabsorption. In all cases, diet is aimed at providing optimal nutrition through vitamin and mineral replacement and nutrient supplementation in response to the degree of malabsorption.

Constipation

Constipation is a disorder of the colon characterized by infrequent or difficult evacuation of feces. Stools are hard and have a dry consistency. Symptons include dull headache, lazy feeling, lassitude, anorexia, low-back pain, and weakness. Diagnosis is most often made by physical examination of the colon through an anoscope or by a digital rectal examination and proctoscopy.

There are three classifications of constipation: imagined, rectal, and colonic.

Imagined constipation can occur in response to a skipped regular bowel movement. An individual assumes that without a daily bowel movement, constipation exists and treatment must follow. However, skipping a daily defecation may not be a result of constipation but might suggest a reaction to a change in diet or to stress.

Rectal constipation results from delayed elimination and is the most common form of constipation. Most often a routine elimination pattern is formed to coincide with the daily work and life schedule. However, routine elimination schedules may become disturbed and the change may affect the conditioned bowel reflexes. Thus constipation develops.

Colonic constipation is the result of a delay in the passage of residue through the colon. The stool is hard, dry, and difficult to eliminate. Inadequate water intake or a diet rich in food items that are not well tolerated by the individual can result in constipation.

Mechanical obstruction of the colon by a tumor of anal stricture can also influence fecal elimination. Extracolonic pressures during pregnancy, a fibroid uterus, and the aging process can result in poor muscle tone and constipation.

Treatment Drug therapy with a variety of laxatives can improve fecal consistency or increase transit time, thus relieving symptoms associated with constipation. Table 18-9 outlines common types of medications currently in use for the treatment of constipation and their mode of action. Enemas give immediate relief from constipation by softening feces and increasing peristalsis. Increased exercise and the development of regular bowel habits can aid in relieving symptoms of constipation.

Dietary treatment includes the use of a high-fiber diet with increased liquids to promote soft, passable stools. Benson[51] suggests an intake of approximately 1500 ml of water per day to help improve stool consistency. Inclusion of food items known to have a laxative effect such as prunes, figs, raisins, whole grains, and bran can increase stool bulk and bring relief from constipation.

Highly sugared foods will increase fermentation in the gut and aid in the formation of small-chain acids. The resulting acids act as os-

TABLE 18-9 MEDICATIONS COMMONLY PRESCRIBED FOR TREATMENT OF CONSTIPATION AND THEIR MODE OF ACTION

Type of medication	Action
Stimulants Cascara, senna Phenolphthalein (Ex-Lax)	Affects intestinal muscle, increasing motility
Castor oil	Interferes with water absorption thus affecting intestinal motility
Saline cathartics Milk of magnesia Magnesium citrate	Acts as osmotic force in lumen; stimulates peristalsis
Emollient laxatives Mineral oil	Coats stool, prevents absorption of fecal water (Note: interferes with absorption of fat-soluble vitamins)
Dioctyl sodium sulfosuccinate (Colace, Disonate)	Lowers surface tension, allowing water to penetrate feces, thus softening the stool
Bulk-forming laxatives Methycellulose	Absorbs water; softens, thus increases peristalsis
Psyllium hydrophilic mucilloid (Metamucil)	
Osmotic loads Sugar syrup Brown sugar Malt soup (Maltsupex)	Increases fermentation; draws fluid into the gut, distending rectum and leading to defecation

Source: Adapted from L. Olney, *American Family Physician*, March 1976, p. 89.

motic forces and draw fluid into the gut lumen, thus distending the rectum and leading to defecation.

Encopresis

Encopresis is the voluntary withholding of stools, resulting in chronic constipation and rectal leakage of watery fecal matter. The condition occurs in the young child and often arises around issues of bowel training.

Treatment includes education of the

parent and child, training of muscles, and the development of a routine toilet regimen. The use of a high-fiber diet in conjunction with mineral oil is begun and continued until bowel movements are regulated.

Hemorrhoids

Hemorrhoids are ruptured blood vessels located around the anal sphincter. They may be internal or external and may or may not cause pain. Most often hemorrhoids are a result of straining at defecation, of constipation, of prolonged use of cathartics or enemas, or of strain during childbearing.

Treatment Surgical removal is recommended if the condition does not improve.

Dietary modifications are aimed at providing relief from the symptoms rather than at treatment. A low-fiber diet with increased fluid intake and the inclusion of stewed fruits and vegetables most often will prevent constipation and reduce the irritation that may occur from a high-fiber diet. Foods known to cause individual discomfort such as spices should be avoided.

GASTROINTESTINAL CONDITIONS IN INFANCY

A host of conditions occur in infancy that require immediate surgical repair. These congenital conditions affecting the gastrointestinal tract can ultimately alter the nutritional status of the infant and cause failure to thrive as a result of gastric dumping syndromes or intestinal malabsorption.

Many clinical features are common among these conditions, especially the demand for increased nutrients and energy as a result of malabsorption and the metabolic trauma of surgery.

These conditions often cause gastric, intestinal, or colonic obstruction, which requires immediate surgical intervention. Suggested nutritional therapy includes the introduction

TABLE 18-10 GASTROINTESTINAL CONDITIONS IN INFANTS CAUSING SECONDARY NUTRITIONAL PROBLEMS

Condition	Secondary nutritional problem
Gastric	
Gastroschisis	Dumping syndrome
Omphalocele	Diarrhea
Intestinal	
Small bowel obstruction	Malabsorption
Intestinal atresia	Diarrhea
Meconium ileus	Steatorrhea
Colonic	
Necrotizing enterocolitis	Water malabsorption
Hirschsprung's disease	Difficulty with fecal passage
Imperforate anus	Difficulty with fecal passage

of a central venous catheter for delivery of total parenteral nutrition (see Chap. 24). The goal of the nutritional plan is to have the infant progress to an oral formula as soon as the bowel has recuperated and the infant can tolerate the oral feeding.

Table 18-10 is a summary of the special nutritional problems associated with gastrointestinal conditions in the newborn. A full discussion of these conditions and their treatment is beyond the scope of this chapter.

DISEASES OF THE LIVER AND BILIARY TRACT

The liver is the largest organ in the body, with an approximate weight of 1300 g. The normal liver is not palpable; however, when it becomes diseased the liver increases in size and can be palpated. The liver plays an important role in determining an individual's nutritional status as many of its functions relate to nutrient metabolism. The functions of the liver can be summarized as follows:

1 *Formation of bile* Bile is synthesized by the liver and stored in the gallbladder. The major function of bile is to aid in the digestion and absorption of fat and fat-like sub-

TABLE 18-11 LABORATORY TESTS AND INDICES FOR DIAGNOSIS OF LIVER AND BILIARY DISEASE

Diagnostic test	Findings in liver and biliary disease
Bilirubin (serum, urinary)	Elevated
Alkaline phosphatase	Elevated
Cholesterol	Elevated (cholesterol cannot be properly metabolized to bile acids)
Prothrombin time	Decreased (prothrombin and fibrinogen production reduced)
Serum glutamic oxalacetic transaminase (SGOT)	Elevated (as a result of dying liver cells)
Sulfobromophthale in Bromsulphalein, BSP)	Elevated (diseased liver is unable to filter at normal rate)
Albumin (serum)	Decreased (protein synthesis is depressed)

stances. The primary constituent of bile is water. Other components are bile salts (sodium and potassium), bile pigments (biliverdin, bilirubin), cholesterol, fatty acids, lecithin, fat, and alkaline phosphatase.

2 *Detoxification* Of metabolic by-products, poisons ingested in foods, and drugs.

3 *Carbohydrate metabolism* Synthesis of glucose, storage of glycogen, and blood glucose homeostasis.

4 *Protein metabolism* Formation of plasma protein and urea.

5 *Fat metabolism* Synthesis of lipoprotein and ketones.

6 *Vitamin and mineral storage* Of fat-soluble vitamins, B complex, vitamin C, iron, and copper.

A brief description of the more common liver function tests and laboratory indices is summarized in Table 18-11. Familiarization with the diagnostic criteria for liver disease will aid the student in understanding the clinical manifestations of the disease condition.

Diseases of the Liver

Hepatitis

Hepatitis is an inflammation of the liver caused by toxins (chloroform, carbon tetrachloride) and infectious microbes (viruses and bacteria). The term viral hepatitis refers to two conditions: (1) Infectious hepatitis can be transmitted via the oral-fecal route. Other sources of contamination include drinking water, food (many times seafood), and sewage. (2) Serum hepatitis, on the other hand, is transmitted parenterally, from syringes, tubing, and blood. The clinical manifestations are similar for both types; therefore, they can be considered as a clinical entity.

Common clinical symptoms of hepatitis include anorexia, malaise, headache, nausea, vomiting, and the loss of the desire to smoke or drink alcohol. Several days later, jaundice (yellow-appearing skin and eyes) may develop and the urine becomes dark because of the increase in the circulating bilirubin. The liver becomes enlarged (hepatomegaly) and, in some cases, the spleen enlarges (splenomegaly) as well. Laboratory analysis reveals that bilirubin, alkaline phosphatase, and serum glutamic oxalacetic transaminase (SGOT) are elevated.

Treatment Bed rest and diet therapy are the two major components of treatment. In the acute stages of hepatitis when vomiting is severe an intravenous solution of 5 to 10 percent dextrose and water must be administered. If this stage is prolonged protein hydrolysates must be added to the intravenous solution. Parenteral nutrition must be supplied until the patient is able to consume sufficient energy by mouth. (See Chap. 24 for a more detailed explanation of parenteral nutrition.) Since the patient is anorexic and becomes easily nauseated, frequent small meals must be encouraged.

The caloric intake should be 3000 to 4000 kcal (12.6 to 16.8 mJ), of which carbohydrate comprises 300 to 400 g in order to promote glycogen synthesis and spare protein. Protein should be planned to provide 1.4 to 2.0 g/kg of body weight to maintain positive nitrogen balance. This is often difficult to accomplish since the patient has a lack of appetite and may complain of nausea. Fat restriction, once a common practice for hepatitis patients, is no longer indicated. Use of high-caloric drinks and the addition of dry powdered skim milk to regular milk, hot cereals, mashed potatoes and creamed soups not only help to increase energy but protein as well. The use of margarine wherever possible—on vegetables, potatoes, hot cereals, in soups—will also help to increase the energy content of the diet. Vitamin and mineral supplements may or may not be warranted, depending upon the nutrient intake of the patient. Alcohol is to be avoided by all hepatitis patients to prevent any further liver cell necrosis. Disposal precaution trays and dishes should be used during the infectious stages of the disease.

Cirrhosis

Cirrhosis is the end stage of liver injury and is characterized by fibrosis of the connective tissue and degeneration of liver cells with a resultant loss of liver function. The pathophysiologic etiology of cirrhosis is unknown but it is commonly seen in chronic alcoholism and malnutrition as well as in biliary obstruction and infection. The accumulation of fat in the liver (steatosis) may be the first stage of cirrhosis, though some authorities feel that this is not necessarily a sequel of the disease. Fatty liver, which is commonly seen in alcoholics, was originally thought to be due to the accompanying malnutrition rather than to alcoholic consumption. However, Lieber has demonstrated that subjects fed alcohol plus a nutritionally adequate diet still developed fatty liver.[52] Therefore, fatty liver in alcoholics seems to be due to the direct effect of alcohol on the liver and only by the withdrawal of alcohol can the condition be corrected.

The most common form of cirrhosis is Laennec's cirrhosis. It is generally associated with alcoholism, although not all alcoholics will develop Laennec's cirrhosis and it may be seen in nonalcoholics. A variety of metabolic activities are impaired in Laennec's cirrhosis. Scar tissue forms in the liver and the conversion of fat to lipoproteins is impaired; hence the accumulation of fat in the liver. Portal hypertension may develop and blood flow becomes obstructed, with esophageal varices (varicose veins in the esophagus) the end result. Esophageal varices are a serious complication since the danger of rupture with ensuing hemorrhage is an imminent possibility.

The cirrhosis patient has an enlarged liver as a result of fat accumulation and necrosis of the liver cells. Ascites (accumulation of fluid in the abdomen) and edema of the extremities may be present since hepatic filtering is impaired and serum protein levels are low. SGOT is elevated and BSP (sulfobromophthalein) clearing time is reduced resulting in elevated levels. Vitamin deficiencies and depressed hematocrit and hemoglobin values are commonly seen and may be due to malnutrition, gastrointestinal bleeding, or both. Patients may appear jaundiced, lack appetite, and have delirium tremens (DTs).

Treatment Providing a diet which will improve the malnutrition associated with liver disease is the goal of nutritional therapy. A high-energy diet is recommended—approximately 45 to 50 kcal/kg (189 to 210 kJ/kg) of body weight per day.

Protein of high biological value must be provided to enable repair of damaged liver cells. An intake of 1 g of protein/kg of body weight is the ultimate goal. However, optimal protein intake must be attained gradually in response to the patient's tolerance as measured by neurological status. Increased protein intake is contraindicated if hepatic coma is present or imminent (see below).

A diet high in carbohydrate must be provided in order to achieve the desired energy levels and to spare the body protein. A moderately high fat intake is necessary to provide palatable meals and aid in increasing energy. Fat may need to be reduced if there is biliary obstruction or a decrease in bile salt production, or if evidence of fatty liver is present. Medium-chain triglycerides are useful to incorporate into the diet if there is a problem with obstruction and bile salt production; however, in advanced cirrhosis their use is contraindicated. A therapeutic vitamin and mineral preparation is often needed. Vitamin B deficiencies, particularly of thiamine, are commonly seen in alcoholic patients. Other nutrients that are inadequately supplied are iron and folic acid. Vitamin K supplementation may be necessary if the prothrombin time is prolonged. Supplementation of other fat-soluble vitamins may also be necessary if there is a problem with fat absorption.

If ascites is present sodium should be restricted to 10 meq (230 mg) per day. Some physicians may be reluctant to initiate a low-sodium dietary regimen, especially if the patient's serum sodium is low. However, a low sodium intake will promote water excretion, thereby increasing the serum sodium.[53] A diet restricted to this degree will need careful planning in order to incorporate all needed nutrients within the constraints of the sodium limitation. Low-sodium milk such as Lonalac will be a useful adjunct, as are commercially produced supplements which are low in sodium and high in protein and energy. Sodium intake can be gradually liberalized as diuresis occurs. Fluids may need to be restricted (1200 to 1500 ml per day) if the patient's weight does not decrease or if a weight gain is seen.

If esophageal varices are present it is important that small frequent feedings in conjunction with antacids be instituted in order to prevent or minimize bleeding.[54] Nicotine and foods which are known to be gastrointestinal irritants (caffeine, pepper, chili) should be avoided. Foods of a soft or semisolid nature are easier for the patient to swallow and should be incorporated into the diet. Many cirrhotic patients have altered carbohydrate metabolism and a high incidence of diabetes is seen,[55,56] necessitating carbohydrate control.

Hepatic Coma

Hepatic coma can develop in patients with severe liver disease because the entrance of ammonia into the cerebral circulation causes intoxication. This may be caused by portacaval shunting or by severe damage to the liver cells. Ammonia is produced in the gastrointestinal tract, probably from bacterial action.[57] Davidson reports that other toxic substances such as indoles and amines derived from tyrosine and tryptophan may also play a role in the pathogenesis. He suggests that these substances bypass the liver where they normally are detoxified and affect the brain tissue, perhaps causing the euphoria that commonly characterizes this condition.[58]

Altered sleep patterns may be present; patients sleep during the day and remain awake at night. Alternating states of depression and mania may occur.[58] Serum ammonia levels are elevated. Administration of protein to these patients will precipitate coma.

Treatment The usual treatment is the administration of antibiotics to decrease intestinal bacteria and thereby reduce ammonia production.[60] If this proves ineffective, reducing the dietary protein of high biological value to 30 g or less will be necessary. This protein restriction should be maintained for as short a time as possible since protein is needed for tissue regeneration. Foods which yield high amounts of ammonia and should be avoided are cheeses, meats, and vegetables.[61] Patients who are comatose must be nourished parenterally, with minimal protein intake and in some cases with protein completely eliminated. (See Chap. 24 for further discussion of parenteral nutrition.)

DISEASES OF THE PANCREAS

The pancreas is located in the upper abdomen, behind the stomach. This organ is responsible for the production of the hormone insulin and several important digestive enzymes (see Chap. 9) that aid in protein, fat, and carbohydrate digestion. The pancreatic duct allows the flow of pancreatic juices to join with bile in the common bile duct, from which they drain into the duodenum.

Pancreatitis

The presence of stones in the common bile duct or spasm of the sphincter may result in a backflow of pancreatic secretions and bile into the pancreas. Inflammation of pancreatic tissue, known as *pancreatitis,* may result. Pancreatitis brings bouts of moderate to severe pain in the upper abdomen that can last for hours or days. Jaundice is usually present. Weight loss, steatorrhea, malabsorption, diabetes mellitus, and pancreatic calcification may occur, depending on the degree of severity of the disease. Serum and urine amylase are increased and are used as diagnostic criteria for pancreatitis.

The acute form of pancreatitis may or may not progress to the chronic form. There are several theories accounting for the etiology of pancreatitis. Obstruction of the pancreatic duct, alcoholism leading to disease of the biliary tract, and reflux of duodenal contents into the pancreatic duct with regurgitation of bile from the common duct up the pancreatic duct have been proposed.

Duodenal intubation allows the collection of stimulated pancreatic juice for analysis of electrolytes and enzymes. The majority of patients with pancreatitis exhibit increased serum amylase.

Treatment   Pancreatic secretions are stimulated by the products of protein digestion and fat in the duodenum, and therefore these nutrients are restricted in the diet. In acute episodes of pancreatitis, intravenous feedings of fluids, electrolytes, and glucose are given. When oral feedings are tolerated clear liquids containing simple carbohydrates are started. The diet is

augmented progressively as tolerated, with the addition of protein and limited fat sources. Fat remains restricted until there is no evidence of steatorrhea (which results from decreased pancreatic lipase). Chronic pancreatitis is treated with a high-protein, high-carbohydrate, low-fat diet. Protein is necessary for optimal pancreatic function and should be encouraged. Simple carbohydrates are needed to provide energy and to prevent hypoglycemia. A diet low in fat may be initiated to inhibit pancreatic secretion.

Parenteral hyperalimentation may be started if the patient's intake is poor because of decreased appetite and constant pain. In all cases, alcohol should be restricted because the inflamed pancreas is unable to utilize it.

DISEASES OF THE GALLBLADDER

The gallbladder is a pear-shaped organ attached to the underside of the liver. The main function of the organ is to store and concentrate bile secreted by the liver. The gallbladder is usually full and relaxed between meals. Upon stimulation by secretion of the hormone cholecystokinin from the intestinal mucosa, the gallbladder contracts, releasing concentrated bile into the duodenum via the common bile duct.

Cholecystitis

The gallbladder may become infected by bacteria traveling from various parts of the body. Inflammation of the gallbladder is known as *cholecystitis.* Abnormal function of the organ may also result from pregnancy, overweight, constipation, or digestion upsets. Cholecystitis is accompanied by epigastric pain in the area of the gallbladder, vomiting, flatulence, and soreness in the upper right quadrant. Jaundice may appear in some cases.

Gallstones often develop as a result of infection or changes in bile composition. Diet, heredity, and female hormones are implicated in the disease. The formation of stones is called *cholelithiasis*. When stones occur in the presence of infection the condition is known as *cholecystolithiasis*. *Choledocholithiasis* develops when the stones slip into the common bile duct, resulting in obstruction. Ductal stones are found in 10 to 20 percent of all patients with stones in the gallbladder. Gallstones are composed of cholesterol, bile salt and pigment, or a combination of these.

Diagnosis can be made by means of oral cholecystography. Failure to visualize the contrast agent is definitive for gallbladder disease. Intravenous cholangiography gives visualization of the biliary tract and can reveal stones in the common bile duct.

Treatment Administration of chenodeoxycholic acid is effective in dissolving small gallstones. However, surgical removal of the gallbladder may be necessary in the presence of stones that are large in either number or size.

Nutritional therapy for gallbladder disease must be individualized. Patients soon learn their particular food intolerances. Generally, most gallbladder patients complain of distention and epigastric pain on ingestion of rich pastries, fatty foods, vegetables from the "gas-forming" group, and chocolate.

Fat stimulates the gallbladder and bile duct to contract; therefore, a low-fat diet is recommended. In acute attacks the use of a low-fat, clear liquid regimen is advisable, with parenteral supplementation if a state of malnutrition exists. Starches and lean meats may be added as soon as they are tolerated. It is advisable for the patient to follow a low-fat diet until surgical removal of the gallbladder.

If the patient is overweight, a low-caloric diet is recommended to achieve ideal weight. Protein sources should be relatively low in fat.

Gastrointestinal disease represents a major threat to the nutritional status of the patient. Disease affecting the esophagus interferes with the mechanics of feeding, requiring an alternate route for nutrition such as enteral (tube) or parenteral feedings.

Diseases of the stomach and bowel interfere with enzyme function and consequently result in malabsorption and the loss of nutrients through diarrhea or steatorrhea. Vitamin and mineral depletion often occurs. Elemental liquid diets or parenteral hyperalimentation may be used for nutritional support in conditions affecting the absorptive capacity of the gut.

Water losses and consequent fluid and electrolyte problems occur with diseases of the lower bowel. As with the small intestines, conditions affecting the colon and the rectum most often will improve with a diet modified in consistency and texture; in severe cases, intravenous hyperalimentation can help to meet the increased nutrient needs.

Liver and biliary diseases may require a diet modified in fat, while caloric requirements remain high in the period of stress. This increased energy need may be met with a special diet supplement of an elemental nature such as medium-chain triglycerides, glucose, or amino acids.

It is important for the student health professional to recognize and appreciate the significant impact on nutrient requirements that gastrointestinal diseases present, since nutritional status is an ultimate factor in the recovery from an acute or chronic gastrointestinal condition.

STUDY QUESTIONS

1 What is the rationale for a bland diet regimen in ulcer therapy? List those foods that should be eliminated from the diet of an ulcer patient.

2 Compare and contrast the malabsorption that is seen in celiac disease with that seen in cystic fibrosis.

3 What enzymes may be affected in ulcerative colitis? Why?

4 Explain the rationale for a high-fiber diet in the treatment of diverticulitis.

5 Why is protein restricted in the patient with hepatic coma?

CASE STUDY 18-1

S. is a 12-year-old white male admitted to the Children's Hospital after a 1-month episode of diarrhea, crampy abdominal pain, and bloody stools. The intake interview revealed a history of a 6- to 8-kg weight loss over the last year, complicated by acute attacks of abdominal cramps relieved by bowel movements numbering 6 to 20 loose stools daily. Physical examination revealed a pale, thin, hyperkinetic young boy. The abdomen was soft, with guarding on the right and mid quadrant. The spleen was palpable to 6 cm. Height and weight on admission were 152 cm and 35.7 kg respectively. An upper gastrointestinal x-ray study showed normal findings but a barium enema revealed a loss of haustration from the transverse colon to the rectum with diffuse small ulcerations, findings consistent with a diagnosis of colitis. Sigmoidoscopy findings were consistent with a diagnosis of ulcerative colitis, and a rectal biopsy revealed an inflamed, edematous mucosa with dilated crypts filled with polymorphonuclea leukocytes. Significant laboratory data on admission were as follows:

Blood pressure 108/76 mmHg

Temperature 98.2°F

Blood urea nitrogen, sugar, electrolytes normal

Serum calcium 9.8 mg/100 ml

Serum magnesium 2.0 meq/"l

Serum phosphorus 4.4 mg/100 ml

Serum alkaline phosphatase 6.3 units

Serum vitamin B_{12} 925 pg/ml

Serum folic acid 24 ng/ml

Serum iron 22 µg/100 ml

Total iron-binding capacity 344 mg/100 ml

Prothrombin time 12.4 s

Hemoglobin 10.4 g/100 ml

Hematocrit 32.6%

Mean corpuscular volume (MCV) 24 pg

Platelets 630,000/mm^3

The diagnosis was ulcerative colitis, with iron-deficiency anemia secondary to chronic blood loss.

Orders were to start S. on prednisone 20 mg twice daily; multivitamins once daily; ferrous sulfate 300 mg TID; folate 1 mg daily; and Tums 3 tablets TID. A dietary prescription for a 6-meal bland, low-residue, high-protein, limited-dairy-product (480 ml of whole milk or equivalent daily) diet was ordered.

S. progressed during the following several weeks of hospitalization. The number of bowel movements decreased significantly to 3 or 4 daily and were described as blood-free and loosely formed. Significant laboratory data after 3 weeks of hospital treatment were as follows:

Height 152.25 cm

Weight 37 kg

Hemoglobin 13.9 g/100 ml

Hematocrit 43.3%

MCV 82 µ3

MCH 26.5 pg

Serum calcium 10 mg/100 ml

S. was discharged with orders to continue taking multivitamins, ferrous sulfate, folate, Tums, and prednisone, and to follow a 6-meal bland, low-residue, restricted-dairy-products (480 ml whole milk or equivalent) dietary plan.

Case Study Questions

1 *How does ulcerative colitis affect absorption of key nutrients? What are the implications of this malabsorption?*

2 *With ulceration of the small bowel, what enzyme secretions might be affected? Relate this problem to the absorption of the associated nutrients.*

3 *Explain the rationale for the elimination of roughage, spices, and dairy products and the inclusion of a 6-meal dietary regimen in the treatment of ulcerative colitis.*

REFERENCES

1 F. Alexander, "Psychological Factors in Gastrointestinal disturbances," in F. Alexander and T. M. French (eds.), *Studies in Psychosomatic Medicine,* The Ronald Press Company, New York, 1948.

2 M. Sleisenger, and J. Fordtran, *Gastrointestinal Disease,* W. B. Saunders Company, Philadelphia, 1973, p. 7.

3 Ibid., p. 8.

4 Ibid., p. 9.

5 Ian Gillespie and T. J. Thompson, *Gastroenterology, an Integrated Course,* Churchill Livingston, London, 1972, pp. 12–32.

6 Ibid.

7 W. Gangon, *Review of Medical Physiology,* Lange Medical Publications, Los Altos, Calif., 1969, p. 292.

8 Gillepsie and Thompson, op. cit., p. 14.

9 Sleisenger and Fordtran, op. cit., p. 94.

10 Ibid.

11 W. J. Hogan, S. R. V. de Andrade, D. H. Winship, "Ethanol-Induced Human Esophageal Motor Dysfunction," *Journal of Applied Physiology,* 32:755–760, 1972.

12 D. Q. Castell, "Hormonal Control of the Gastroesophageal Sphincter Strength," *New England Journal of Medicine,* 282:886–889, 1970.

13 C. Cohen, and W. Lipslutz, "Hormonal Regulation of Human Lower Esophageal Sphincter Competence," *Journal of Clininical Investigation,* 50:449–454, 1971.

14 J. Babka, and D. O. Costell, "Effects of Specific Foods on the Lower Esophageal Sphincter," *Digestive Disease,* 18:391, 1973.

15 M. Paulson, *Gastroenterologic Medicine,* Lea and Fabiger, Philadelphia, 1969, pp. 662–663.

16 M. Greenberger, D. Winship, *Gastrointestinal Disorders; A Pathophysiologic Yearbook,* Medical Publications Inc., Chicago, 1976, p. 24.

17 Paulson, op. cit., p. 663.

18 P. B. Beeson and W. McDermott, *Cecil-Loeb Textbook of Medicine,* 13th ed., W. B. Saunders Company, Philadelphia, 1971, p. 1274.

19 Ibid.

20 B. W. Sippy, "Gastric and Duodenal Ulcers; Medical Care by an Efficient Removal of Gastric Juice Erosion, *Journal of The American Medical Association,* 64:1625, 1915.

21 J. S. Laurence, "Dietetic and Other Methods in Treatment of Peptic Ulcer," *Lancet,* 1:482, 1952.

22 J. W. Todd, "Treatment of Peptic Ulcer," *Lancer,* 1:291, 1952.

23 R. Dall, R. T. Friedland, and F. Puggott, "Dietetic Treatment of Peptic Ulcer," *Lancet,* 1:5, 1956.

24 "Position Paper on Bland Diet in the Treatment of Chronic Duodenal Ulcer Disease," *Journal of The American Dietetic Association,* 60:306, 1971.

25 J. A. Rothm and A. Ivy, "Effect of Caffeine upon Gastric Secretion in the Dog, Cat, and Man," *American Journal of Physiology,* 141:454, 1944.

26 S. Cohen and G. H. Booth, "Gastric Acid Secretion and Lower Esophageal Sphincter Pressure in Response to Coffee and Caffeine, *New England Journal of Medicine,* 293:897, 1975.

27 M. E. Ament, "Malabsorption syndromes in infancy and childhood," *Journal of Pediatrics,* 81:685—697, 867–884, 1972.

28 W. K. Dicke, "Coeliac Disease: Investigation of Harmful Effects of Certain Types of Cereal on Patients with Coeliac Disease," thesis, University of Utrecht, Netherlands, 1950.

29 R. R. W. Taconley, "Celiac Disease. An Inborn Error of Metabolism," *Digestive Disease,* 18:797, 1973.

30 K. G. Kenrick and J. A. Walker-Smith, "Immunoglobulins and Dietary Protein Antibodies in Childhood Coeliac Disease," *Gut,* 11:635, 1970.

31 P. A. Green and E. D. Wollanger, "Clinical Behavior of Sprue in the United States," *Gastroenterology,* 38:399, 1960.

32 Ibid.

33 M. E. Ament, op. cit., p. 875.

34 J. D. Kirschmann, "Nutrition Research," in *Nutrition Almanac,* South Minneapolis, Minn. 1974.

35 G. M. Gray, "Carbohydrate Digestion and Absorption," *New England Journal of Medicine,* **292:**1225, 1975.

36 A. Holzel, "Sugar Malabsorption and Sugar Intolerance in Childhood," *Proceedings of the Royal Society of Medicine,* **61:**1095, 1968.

37 A. D. Newcomer, "Disaccharidase Deficiencies," *Mayo Clinic Proceedings,* **48:**648–652, 1973.

38 A. Dahlquist, "Method for Assay of Intestinal Disaccharidases," *Analytical Biochemistry,* **7:**18, 1964.

39 S. J. Birge, H. T. Kautman, P. Cuatresas, and G. D. Whedon, "Osteoporosis, Intestinal Lactase Deficiency and Low Dietary Calcium Intake, *New England Journal of Medicine,* **276:**445, 1969.

40 C. Gallagher, Molleson, and J. H. Caldwell, "Lactose Intolerance and Fermented Dairy Products," *Journal of the American Society of Agronomy,* **65:**18–19, 1974.

41 H. Shwachman, "Gastrointestinal Manifestations of Cystic Fibrosis," *Pediatric Clinics of North America,* vol. 22, November 1975.

42 J. D. Allan, A. Mason, and A. Moss, "Nutritional Supplementation in Treatment of Cystic Fibrosis of the Pancreas," *American Journal of Diseases of Children,* vol. 126, July 1973.

43 R. B. Elliot, "Therapeutic Trial of Fatty Acid Supplementation in Cystic Fibrosis," *Pediatrics,* **57:** 474–479 1976.

44 K. Fried and E. Vare, "Lethal Autosomal Recessive Enterocolitis of Early Infancy," *Clinical Genetics,* **6:**418–419.

45 A. B. Cady, J. B. Rhodes, A. Littman, and R. K. Kane, "Significance of Lactase Deficit in Ulcerative Colitis," *Journal of Laboratory and Clinical Medicine,* **70:**279, 1976.

46 K. Zetzel, "Granulomatous (Ileo) Colitis," *New England Journal of Medicine,* **282:**600–605, 1970.

47 P. Plumey and B. Francis, "Dietary Management of Diverticular Disease," *Journal of The American Dietetic Association,* **63:**527–530, 1973.

48 W. O. Kirwan, A. N. Smith, A. A. McConnell, W. D. Mitchell, and M. A. Eastwood, "Action of Different Bran Preparations on Colonic Function," *British Medical Journal,* **4:**187–189, 1974.

49 D. P. Burkitt, A. R. P. Walker, and N. S. Painter, *Lancet,* **2:**1408, 1972.

50 J. M. Findlay, et al., "Effects of Unprocessed Bran on Colon Function in Normal Subjects and in Diverticular Disease," *Lancet,* **1:**146–149, 1974.

51 J. A. Benson, "Simple Chronic Constipation," *Postgraduate Medicine,* vol. 57, no., 1, January 1975.

52 C. Lieber, "Liver Disease and Alcohol: Fatty Liver Alcoholic Hepatitis, Cirrhosis and Their Interrelationships," *Annals of the New York Academy of Sciences,* vol. 252, April 1975.

53 C. Davidson, "Dietary Treatment of Hepatic Disease," *Journal of The American Dietetic Association,* May, 1976, p. 517.

54 Ibid.

55 G. Sereny, L. Endrenyi, and P. Denenyi, "Glucose Intolerance in Alcoholics," *Journal of Studies in Alcohol,* **36:**359–364, 1975.

56 H. O. Conn, W. M. Schrlilier, S. G. Elkington, and T. R. Johnson, "Cirrhosis and Diabetes. I: Increased Incidence of Diabetes in Patients with Laennec's Cirrhosis," *American Journal of Digestive Diseases,* 1969, p. 837–852.

57 G. J. Gabuzda, "Ammonium Metabolism and Hepatic Coma," *Gastroenterology,* **53:**806, 1967.

58 Davidson, op. cit. p. 518.

59 Ibid.

60 C. J. Fischer and W. W. Faloon, "Blood Ammonia Levels in Hepatic Cirrhosis. Their Control By the Oral Administration of Neomycin," *New England Journal of Medicine,* **256:**1030, 1957.

61 D. Rudman, R. Smith, A. Solom, D. Warren, J. Galambas, and J. Wenger, "Ammonia Content of Food," *American Journal of Clinical Nutrition,* **26:**487–490, 1973.

CHAPTER 19

THE KIDNEYS AND
URINARY TRACT

Roberta Ruhf Henry

KEY WORDS
Nephron
Blood Urea Nitrogen
Creatinine
Oliguric
Anuric
Acute Renal Failure
Chronic Renal Failure
Uremia
Azotemia
End-Stage Renal Disease
Dialysis

INTRODUCTION

If your physician does not think it wise for you to sleep, to take wine with such and such meat, do not be troubled, I will find you another who will not be of his opinion, the diversity of medical arguments and opinions includes every variety of form.
Michael de Montague 1533–1592

During the past thirty years, much progress has been made in the field of nephrology. Great advances have been made in the understanding of both normal renal physiology and the treatment of renal diseases. However, even with the development of artificial kidney machines and improved methods of kidney transplantation, nutritional support and diet therapy continue to be an extremely important aspect of the management of the individual with malfunctioning kidneys.

The primary focus of this chapter is on the nutritional management of renal disease. Included also is a brief review of normal kidney anatomy and physiology, to better enable the student to appreciate the effect of disease on kidney function.

NORMAL RENAL FUNCTION

Physiology

Normally, the two bean-shaped kidneys are located behind the peritoneum, one on each side of the spinal column. Each kidney, about the size of an adult fist, weighs approximately 150 g, or 5 oz, which is only 2 to 4 percent of the total body weight. The kidney is a very vascular organ, with its primary blood supply being the renal artery, a large branch of the aorta. Ordinarily, 180 l of blood, a full 20 to 25 percent of the total cardiac output, perfuses the kidneys each day. This perfusion results in an average daily urine volume of 1 to 2 l for an 80-kg adult male.

Each kidney contains approximately 1,000,000 microscopic functioning units called *nephrons*, and each nephron, although quite

Description	Primary Functions
Glomerulus The glomerulus is a capillary tuft, freely permeable to metabolic end products, other potentially toxic substances in the blood, and almost all other constituents of plasma except for most plasma proteins.	*Filtration* Initial site of plasma filtration where the so-called "ultrafiltrate" of plasma is created. (This glomerular filtrate contains no cells or proteins.)
Proximal tubule A highly convoluted section, the proximal tubule is the first tubular section of the nephron and is found almost totally in the outer cortex of the kidney. It is one cell layer thick, however, these cells are highly specialized in their functions. (ADH is not required.)	*Reabsorption and secretion* The proximal tubule isotonically reabsorbs 60–80% of the glomular filtrate; 80–90% of the filtred Na^+, Cl^- and H_2O is reabsorbed. Glucose, amino acids, urate, potassium phosphate, bicarbonate and any remaining proteins are reabsorbed. NH_4 H, organic acids and bases are secreted.
Loop of henle The loop of henle is a U-shaped and therefore relatively straight segment, dipping into the inner portion of the kidney, the medulla.	*Reabsorption* Na^+ is reabsorbed by a complex mechanism that allows the kidney to control urine Na^+ (the countercurrent mechanism, see p. 144), and a hypotonic fluid is the result.
Distal tubule Anatomically similar to the proximal tubule, the distal tubule is predominantly in the renal cortex. (ADH from the pituitary makes this segment more permeable to water in the presence of dehydration.)	*Secretion and acidification* Acid-base balance is regulated; H^+ and NH_3 are secreted into the filtrate. Urine becomes isotonic. Remaining Na, Cl, and H_2O are reabsorbed according to the physiologic state of the body).
Collecting duct The distal-most portion of the distal tubule is the collecting duct. A specialized segment, where "fine tuning" takes place and formed urine passes into the pelvis of the kidney.	*Concentration of filtrate* The Remaining Na^+, Cl^- and H_2O are reabsorbed. Further H^+ and NH_4 are secreted (as required by the physiologic state of the body).

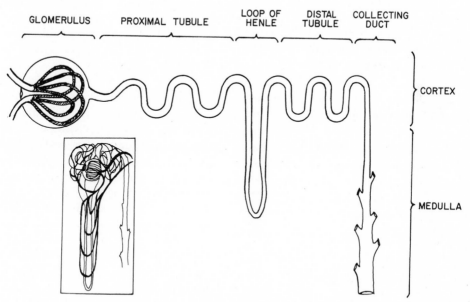

Figure 19-1

The functioning nephron. A description of each nephron segment and its primary function and a schematic view.

complex, can be looked at in its five basic segments. Figure 19-1 shows these segments and their respective functions. They are presented in the order found in the nephron unit, progressing from the first segment, which is intimately associated with its blood supply, to the end of the nephron where it ultimately elicits urine. This urine then passes into the renal pelvis, through the ureters, and into the bladder for excretion.

When the specific functions of the major segments of the nephron are examined (filtration, reabsorption, and secretion), the overall physiological activities of the kidneys should be readily apparent. These life-sustaining functions can be categorized according to role: those functions of the kidney which are related to homeostasis and those which can be related to the endocrine system.

Homeostatic Functions

1 *Waste excretion* The end products of metabolism, such as urea, creatinine, uric acid, and sulfates, as well as various drugs and potentially toxic substances, are excreted by the kidneys.
2 *Acid-base balance* (see Chap. 8) Hydrogen ions and bicarbonate are either excreted or retained to maintain the proper pH of the body's fluids.
3 *Water and electrolyte balance* (see Chap. 8) Water, sodium, potassium, and chloride, as well as electrolyte and solute levels of the body, are regulated by renal excretion when they are in excess and by retention when deficient.

Endocrine Functions

Another very important function is not readily apparent from review of the nephron structure. That is its vital role as an endocrine gland.

1 When oxygen delivery to the kidneys is diminished, the kidneys secrete, into the bloodstream, *erythropoietin*, a hormone which stimulates the bone marrow to produce red blood cells.
2 By secreting the hormone *renin*, the kidneys play an important role in blood pressure regulation. Renin has a dual role in blood pressure regulation (*a*) by directly splitting a plasma substrate into a smaller molecule known as *angiotensin I* which, in the presence of an enzyme, is converted to *angiotensin II*, a very potent vasopressor substance; and (*b*) indirectly by the action of angiotensin, which stimulates the adrenal cortex to secrete *aldosterone*, which in turn causes the kidneys to retain sodium. Renin, therefore, has a very profound effect upon the cardiovascular system.
3 The kidneys are influential in calcium and phosphate metabolism, bone structure, and parathyroid function by converting the inactive form of vitamin D, which is produced by the body (from the skin) or found in food, to its effective form, $1,25\text{-}(OH)_2D\text{-}_3$ or 1,25-dihydroxycholecalciferol. This *active form of Vitamin D* is essential for normal calcium absorption from the gastrointestinal tract and is now considered to be a hormone.[1,2]

With the homeostatic and endocrine functions of the kidneys intact in almost all of its nephrons, the kidneys will perform with efficiency to regulate the body's physiological state. Therefore, at any age, under normal conditions, the variety and amounts of nutrients that can be safely consumed are limitless. Normally, the kidneys easily dispose of the excess or waste produced by a full and varied diet.

RENAL FAILURE

Renal failure denotes the loss of nephron function severe enough to interfere with homeostatic and endocrine functions of the kidneys. This failure may occur rapidly or progressively but as the number of functioning nephrons

TABLE 19-1 BIOCHEMICAL INDICES OF KIDNEY FUNCTION

Increased	Decreased	Altered (distribution)
Serum creatinine	Glomerular filtration rate	Sodium
		Potassium
Blood urea nitrogen	Creatinine clearance	Calcium/phosphorus ratio
Serum uric acid	Urea clearance	Glucose metabolism
	Urine concentrating ability (but not necessarily urine volume)	Acid-base balance
		Fluid balance
	Hematocrit	

decreases, regardless of the cause, the kidneys become less able to eliminate the multitude of wastes produced from an unrestricted diet.

When the number of functioning nephrons decreases significantly, certain laboratory tests will detect this change in renal function. The biochemical indices are either increased, decreased, or altered by the disease state (see Table 19-1).

When greater than 60 to 75 percent of the total nephron mass is destroyed by disease (see Table 19-2 for the etiology of kidney diseases), and kidney function has decreased as evidenced by changes in the biochemical indices, dietary intervention and nutritional support become an essential part of the patient's care.

Nutritional Considerations

The primary nutritional goal is to maintain or achieve optimal nutritional status. Within the framework of renal disease, the minimization of protein catabolism, the maintenance of fluid balance, and the maintenance of electroyte balance are the goals of treatment. These are achieved by altering the intake of water, protein, calories, sodium, potassium, phosphorus, or calcium (see Table 19-3). From these goals, and from individualized assessment of the patient, an appropriate diet can be prescribed.

The control of protein, calories, sodium,

water (fluids), potassium, and phosphorus is extremely important in the nutritional management of adults and children with renal disease. However, it is incorrect to assume that every patient with renal disease needs diet modification of all of these nutrients. Diet therapy for patients with renal failure should be individualized.

We will now consider the relevance of the dietary constituents—protein, carbohydrate, fat, sodium, potassium, phosphorus, and water—to the diet of the patient with renal disease.

Protein

The three major constituents of food—carbohydrates, proteins, and fats—contain carbon, hydrogen and oxygen, and are metabolized to carbon dioxide and water, but *only* the proteins contain nitrogen. Protein is 16 percent nitrogen; i.e., 1 g of nitrogen is found in each 6.25 g of protein.

The metabolism of the amino acids in dietary protein produces nitrogenous waste products. Of these, approximately 70 percent are normally excreted in the urine and the remainder in the feces and through skin losses.[3] Furthermore, 80 to 90 percent of these amino acid catabolites, or breakdown products, are excreted in the urine as urea, with approximately 4 to 5 percent as creatinine, 3 percent as ammonia, and 1 to 2 percent as uric acid.

TABLE 19-2 ETIOLOGY AND CLINICAL MANIFESTATIONS OF CHRONIC RENAL FAILURE

Condition	Etiology	Clinical manifestations
Acute glomerulonephritis	Usually follows an infection such as streptoccocal pneumonia.	Headache, fever, anorexia, nausea and vomiting; hematuria and albuminuria. Edema of face and eyelids is common, later becoming more generalized
Chronic glomerulonephritis	May occur after acute nephritis. Role of infection is not clear	Albuminuria, massive edema; *may have* hypertension and associated headache; anemia. As disease progresses, creatinine and blood urea nitrogen are elevated
Nephrotic syndrome	Symptom complex which may occur during glomerulonephritis	Massive edema; proteinuria with decreased serum albumin and increased cholesterol
Polycystic kidney disease	Familial disease in which cysts develop in the parenchyma of both kidneys. Progressive renal insufficiency develops	Hypertension may be present; albuminuria, hematuria
Pyelonephritis	Bacterial infection reaching the kidney pelvis via the blood or lymphatics from other sites. Infection may be due to obstruction	Chills, fever, abdominal pain, backache, nausea, vomiting, urinary frequency, dysuria
Fanconi's syndrome	May be inherited or acquired. Proximal renal tubular transport function is impaired. Substances usually absorbed by the proximal tubule are lost	Failure to reabsorb phosphate, potassium and water; renal rickets; glycosuria; albuminuria; aminoaciduria

(continued)

When the kidneys fail, the urea and other nitrogenous wastes produced from the normal diet cannot be properly excreted. The inability of the kidneys to excrete urea is most evident by an elevation of the blood urea nitrogen (BUN). (Average range for BUN is 8 to 25 mg/100 ml). However, because of the great influence of dietary protein intake on BUN, and the fact that abnormal physiological states such as gastrointestinal bleeding, dehydration, and others, alter this measurement, BUN is not always considered a reliable tool for assessing kidney function.

A more accurate assessment of renal function is a measurement of urine creatinine clearance or of serum creatinine, since these are less influenced by dietary protein. Serum creatinine measures the kidney's ability to filter this product of muscle metabolism. (Average serum creatinine is relatively constant and is in the range of 0.5 to 1.4 mg/100 ml. Average creatinine clearance is 120 ml/min.)

Since one of the goals of the nutritional management of renal disease is to prevent catabolism and promote anabolism while maintaining or achieving nitrogen balance, dietary

TABLE 19-2   (continued)

Condition	Etiology	Clinical manifestations
Cystinosis	Genetic metabolic anomaly affecting renal transport. Cystine is deposited in organs	Similar to Fanconi's syndrome
Renal tubular acidosis	Defective urinary acidification or reabsorption of bicarbonate. Cause is unknown	Hypokalemia; osteomalacia may be present; hypophosphatemia, hypercalciuria
Chronic potassium depletion	May result from renal tubular disorders, Cushing's syndrome, aldosteronism. Most common abnormality is the kidney's inability to concentrate urine	Nocturia, polyuria, polydypsia, slight proteinuria
Tuberculosis of the kidney	Bacterial infection of the kidney via the bloodstream Can result in renal scarring and destruction	Frequently there are no clinical manifestations. However, there may be dysuria and intermittent hematuria

protein restriction is not usually imposed until the patient begins to develop the signs and symptoms related to a high protein intake. These may include any of the following: a BUN Greater than 100 mg/100 ml, nausea,

TABLE 19-3   GOALS OF NUTRITIONAL MANAGEMENT OF THE RENAL PATIENT

Nutritional goal	Nutrients altered to achieve goal
To minimize protein catabolism (adults and children)	Protein
To promote anabolism, i.e., growth (children)	Calories (joules): Carbohydrates Fats
To maintain fluid balance (adults and children)	Sodium Water (fluids)
To maintain electrolyte balance (adults and children)	Sodium Potassium Phosphorus (and calcium) Water (fluids)

vomiting, lethargy, anorexia, severe acidosis, or a creatinine clearance below 30 ml/min. Protein restriction should not be arbitrary; the quantity of protein allowed should be individualized according to kidney function as indicated by laboratory data and clinical condition. This fairly liberal philosophy is relatively new and can be related to the availability of hemodialysis and transplantation.

The quality as well as quantity of protein in the diets of patients with renal disease is also important. When protein is restricted, approximately 70 to 75 percent of the total protein intake should be from foods of high biological value, such as milk, eggs, and meats, which contain the essential amino acids. (See Chap. 3.)

Of interest to note is the fact that a remarkable number of patients automatically reduce their own dietary protein intake prior to any formal diet instruction. In so doing, they may be affecting the quality of protein and the total energy intake. Therefore nutrition counseling is directed toward the proteins and calories joules needed to prevent unwanted weight loss or breakdown of muscle mass. (For more specific recommendations on protein intake, see the discussion of "Stages of Chronic Renal Failure," below.)

Calories (joules)

Energy intake is a necesary component of the meal plans for renal patients. Efforts should be made to maintain or achieve ideal body weight. Although no current standard for energy requirements exists, 65 to 75 kcal (273 to 315 kJ)/kg of ideal weight is frequently used for adults with renal failure. Children and adolescents require as much as 100 to 150 kcal (420 to 630 kJ)/kg in order to support or enhance growth. The energy needs will vary according to age, sex, activity, height, and weight.

Nonprotein calories (joules) are especially important when patients are on a protein-restricted diet. Calories (joules) from concentrated carbohydrates (sugar, honey, sour balls or other hard candies, jelly, etc.) and fats (oils, margarine, butter) may be encouraged in order to spare endogenous protein breakdown and enable the body to utilize the dietary protein for anabolism. (See Table 19-4.)

Carbohydrates and Fats

In addition to protein, the patient with renal disease may also have difficulty in tolerating carbohydrate and fat because of abnormal metabolism.

Carbohydrate metabolism   In renal patients without any previous history of diabetes, glucose intolerance frequently occurs. This abnormality is not totally understood and is rarely of clinical significance. Fasting blood sugars are usually slightly elevated, as reflected by an abnormal glucose tolerance curve. In most instances this alteration in carbohydrate metabolism is not a contraindication to encouraging a high dietary intake of carbohydrate calories (joules). This abnormal state may be corrected by dialysis.

Patients with overt diabetes mellitus who were receiving hypoglycemic agents or insulin prior to the onset of renal disease frequently display a decreased need for insulin. However, this does allow more liberal amounts of carbohydrate calories (joules) in the diet. A liberal carbohydrate diet without concentrated sweets is usually tolerated.

TABLE 19-4 HIGH-ENERGY, LOW-ELECTROLYTE, LOW-PROTEIN SUPPLEMENTS

Product	Manufacturer	Composition and form	Approximate calories (joules)
Cal Power	General Mills	Deionized glucose; liquid (fruit-flavored)	2 kcal/ml (8.4 kJ/ml) (295 kcal/240 ml; 1239 kJ/240 ml)
Polycose	Ross laboratories	Glucose polymers (from hydrolysis of cornstarch); liquid or powder	Liquid: 2 kcal/ml (8.4 kJ/ml) Powder: 4 kcal/g (16.8 kJ/g)
Controlyte	Doyle Pharmaceutical Co.	Polysaccharides and vegetable oil; powder	5 kcal/g (21 kJ/g)
HyCal	Beecham-Massengill Pharmaceuticals	Demineralized glucose; liquid (fruit-flavored)	2 kcal/ml (8.4 kJ/ml)
Lipomul Oral	Upjohn Co.	Corn oil; liquid	3 kcal/ml (12.6 kJ/ml)

Fat metabolism Fat metabolism is also altered in renal failure. While cholesterol levels usually are normal (except in nephrotic syndrome—see discussion below), triglyceride levels are elevated in a majority of these patients. This phenomenon is not generally improved with dialytic therapy and a significant percentage of these patients show a type IV hyperlipoproteinemia pattern (see Chap. 17). This hypertriglyceridemia may be related to the insulin and glucose abnormality.

At this time, much controversy exists about the effectiveness of dietary treatment for these abnormalities of fat metabolism in patients with renal failure. When the patient is stable medically, weight reduction to ideal weight should be encouraged in an attempt to improve the hyperlipoproteinemia.

Sodium

Normal renal function permits the urinary sodium output to approximate the dietary sodium intake. While renal dysfunction does limit the ability of the kidneys to properly handle sodium, not every patient with renal failure requires a sodium-restricted diet. Ideally, the amount of sodium a patient requires is that amount which will prevent or control hypertension and heart failure and concurrently maintain a state of normal hydration.

An excellent method for determining a patient's hydration status is daily measurement of the weight. When a patient is receiving sufficient sodium, this should be reflected by a stable body weight. An excessive intake of sodium will lead to excessive fluid retention and weight gain, while a low intake of sodium will lead to an abnormal weight loss. Daily weights should routinely be recorded for all renal patients. Patients with fluid balance problems weigh themselves daily, chart these weights, and adjust their sodium and fluid intake accordingly.

Restricting the sodium in the diets of some patients with renal failure can lead to sodium depletion, as manifested by dehydration, with symptoms of orthostatic hypotension and leg cramps, as well as by worsening renal function. (The state of dehydration is accompanied by low blood pressure, caused by the diminished blood volume, and results in diminished renal function and a decrease in the glomerular filtration rate.) Unfortunately, sodium depletion, as a result of vigorous sodium restriction, is quite common in patients with renal failure. This is especially true in patients with polycystic kidney disease, medullary cystic kidney disease, and pyelonephritis (see Table 19-2). Since these disease states tend to cause polyuria and excessive urinary sodium loss, patients may be referred to as "salt wasters" or "salt losers."

Another common, preventable cause of sodium depletion and its resultant deterioration of renal function is the concurrent use of diuretic therapy and a diet that is severely restricted in sodium. The deleterious effect can be prevented if sodium losses are carefully monitored and dietary sodium intake is individualized.

Sodium-restricted diets are useful in preventing fluid retention, and thereby controlling blood pressure and preventing heart failure. Since the sodium needs of patients with decreasing renal function are not static but variable, the need for sodium restriction changes. Even patients with salt-losing nephropathy may develop edema and circulatory congestion and require some degree of sodium restriction.

Patients with advanced renal disease who are prone to sodium retention seem to have difficulty with extremes of sodium intake (too high or too low) and appear to do well with an intake in the range of 800 mg (35 meq) to 1600 mg (70 meq) per day;[4] however, sodium modification may vary from as little as 500 mg (22 meq) per day to as much as 4000 mg (173 meq) or more per day.

Sodium and food Certain canned or processed foods must be avoided in most sodium-restricted diets (see Table 19-5). Whether or

TABLE 19-5 HIGH-SODIUM SOURCES
(Usually avoided on a modified sodium diet)

Seasonings

Salt	Worcestershire sauce
Garlic salt	Salt brine
Onion salt	Baking soda
Celery salt	Baking powder
Catsup	Monosodium glutamate
Prepared mustard	Meat tenderizers
Chili sauce	Soy sauce

Meats and Fish (*smoked, cured or dried*)

Ham	Canned corned beef hash
Canadian bacon	Dried beef (chipped)
Regular bacon	Frankfurters
Sausage	Caviar
Cold cuts (luncheon meats)	Sardines
Corned beef	Tuna (packed in oil)
Pastrami	Anchovies
Salt pork	TV dinners

Cheese

American, cheddar	Cheese spreads
American, processed	Parmesan

Snack Foods (all those with obvious salt on them)

Potato chips	Party mixes
Pretzels	Salted nuts
Crackers	Salted popcorn
Corn chips and corn curls	

Miscellaneous

Bouillon	Relishes
Sauerkraut	Ethnic foods: Chinese,
Soups—all canned, frozen, dried	Italian, and koshered,
Olives	for example
Pickles	
Salad dressings	

not special dietetic low-sodium food products (e.g., low-sodium bread, margarine, etc.) are required depends on the level of sodium restriction. There are herbs, spices, and seasonings which can help to lend palatability to the patient's diet (see Table 19-6).

Sodium and medications Certain medications contribute a significant amount of sodium to a patient's total daily intake (see Table 19-7). When these medications are prescribed, the sodium content of the patient's diet should be altered accordingly. For example, if a patient requires a 2-g sodium diet (2000 mg or 87 meq sodium) and 2 g of sodium bicarbonate ($NaHCO_3$) is required to treat acidosis, the sodium content of the $NaHCO_3$, which is approximately 550 mg (24 meq sodium), must

TABLE 19-6 LOW-SODIUM HERBS, SPICES, AND SEASONINGS

Allspice	Wine
Almond extract	Wine vinegar (without salt added)
Basil	Mace
Bay leaf	Maple extract
Cardamom	Marjoram
Caraway seed*	Meat extract, low-sodium
Catsup, salt-free*	Meat tenderizer, low-sodium
Chili powder*	Mustard, dried or seed
Chives	Mint
Cinnamon	Nutmeg
Cloves*	Oregano
Cumin	Onion (fresh, juice, powder)
Curry powder*	Parsley (fresh, flaked, dried)*
Bouillon, low-sodium	Paprika
Dill	Pepper, black, red, white*
Fennel	Pepper, fresh, red or green
Horseradish (without added salt)	Peppermint extract
Honey	Pimento peppers
Juniper	Poppy seeds
Lemon juice	Purslane
Saccharin	Rosemary
Saffron	Sage
Savory	Sesame seed
Sorrel	Sugar, white or brown
Thyme	Sugar syrups
Turmeric	Vanilla extract
Garlic (fresh, juice, powder)	Vinegar

* These are known to contribute a significant amount of potassium per ½ tsp and might be avoided if a potassium-restricted meal plan is prescribed.

be subtracted from the dietary allowance. This patient, therefore, should be receiving a diet containing approximately 1500 mg (65 meq) sodium per day. Instructions should be given to the patient and family members regarding the sodium content of both the diet and drugs.

Sodium (Na) conversion:
$$1 \text{ meq Na} = 23 \text{ mg Na}$$
$$1 \text{ g NaCl (table salt)} = 400 \text{ mg Na}$$
$$1 \text{ teaspoon table salt} = 2300 \text{ mg Na}$$
$$= 100 \text{ meq Na}$$

$$1 \text{ g Na} = 1000 \text{ mg Na}$$
$$\text{Na} = 43 \text{ meq Na}$$
$$\text{Na} = \text{approximately 40\% of NaCl}$$

Potassium

Most patients with renal failure and adequate urine volumes (1000 ml or more per day) are able to eliminate a "normal" intake of dietary potassium of 2 to 6 g of 51 to 154 meq per day without difficulty. Normal serum potassium levels are 3.5 to 5.0 meq/l, and in the early stages of renal failure *hypokalemia,* a serum

TABLE 19-7   SELECTED MEDICATIONS WITH THEIR SODIUM CONTENT

Medication	Dosage	Sodium content, mg
Fleet's Enema	1 container	5092
Citrocarbonates	1 tsp	4550
Kayexalate, powder	15 g	1400–1700
Phospho-soda, unflavored	1 tbsp	1697
Sal Hepatica	Rounded tsp	1000
Eno Salts	1 tsp	738
Fizrin	1 packet	673
Pluto water	30 ml	612
Alka-Seltzer	1 tablet	532
Bromo-Seltzer	1 tsp	480
Bisodol, powder	1 tsp	471
Metamucil, Instant Mix	Packet	250
Effergyl, powder	Rounded tsp	200
Sodium bicarbonate	600 mg tablet	177
Glucola	210 ml	109
Shohl's Solution	10 ml	230
Antacids*		
Rolaids	1 tablet	53
Phosphogel	15 ml	39
Robalate	15 ml	28
Amphojel, suspension	15 ml	25
Basaljel	15 ml	18

* Although the sodium content of these antacids does not seem appreciable, if they are taken frequently or in large quantities, the sodium from this source could be significant.

Source: Sodium in Medicinals, Tables of Sodium Values, San Francisco Heart Association, Inc., 1966.

potassium level of less than 3.5 meq/l, may develop especially if "potassium-losing" diuretics are prescribed. In these instances a relatively high-potassium diet may be prescribed. Even so, a high load of potassium, whether given orally or intravenously, may be poorly tolerated by any patient with deteriorating renal function. For this reason, serum potassium levels and dietary intake of potassium should be cautiously monitored.

It is interesting to note that patients with *advanced* renal failure seem to tolerate *hyperkalemia,* a serum potassium level greater than 5.0 meq/l, better than normal, healthy people. In fact, these patients seem to encounter few problems with chronic potassium levels in the 5.0 to 6.5 meq/l range for prolonged periods of time. However, if the serum potassium level rises too rapidly or reaches an extremely high level, even in these patients, potassium intoxication and its associated side effects of cardiac arrhythmia, abnormal electrocardiogram, and ultimate cardiac arrest can occur. The exact level at which these side effects occur cannot be defined, since it is extremely variable from patient to patient. Therefore, the more limited potassium restrictions of 1.5 to 2.5 g (38 to 64 meq) per day may be prescribed.

Potassium and food   Essentially all foods contain potassium (except pure sugar and pure fat) and a potassium-restricted diet can be calculated to include almost any food in certain amounts; however, generally, to promote the patient's understanding, only certain foods that are very high in potassium are eliminated when potassium-restricted diets are prescribed. (See Table 19-8.)

High-protein foods, such as meat, fish, poultry, and milk, contribute a significant amount of potassium. For example, 1 oz of meat, fish, or poultry contains approximately 100 mg of potassium and if an individual consumes 1 lb of meat, fish, or poultry (approximately 1600 mg of potassium), a significant quantity of potassium would be obtained from meat alone. As a result, if a protein restriction is imposed, the potassium intake will simultaneously be reduced. When a patient's protein intake is not limited and a potassium-restricted diet is required, special food allowances (exchanges, portion sizes, etc.) should be stated.

Other sources of potassium   Potassium from food is not the only source of potassium which will influence the patient's serum potassium level. Other contributory factors must be assessed when an elevated serum potassium level exists. There are both endogenous and exogenous factors requiring careful consideration. They are as follows:

TABLE 19-8 SELECTED HIGH-POTASSIUM FOODS
(Usually avoided or limited on potassium-restricted diets)

Fruits [Containing 200 mg or more potassium per 100 g (3½-oz) portion]

Apricots, fresh or canned	Nectarines
Avocado	Papayas
Banana	Peaches, fresh
Cantaloupe	Prunes, dried (*all* dried fruit)
Casaba melon	Prune juice
Currants, black, red, white	Raisins
Dates	Rhubarb
Elderberries	Oranges
Honeydew	Orange juice

Vegetables [Containing 300 mg or more potassium per 100 g (3½-oz) portion]

Artichokes	Dark green, leafy vegetables:
Acorn squash	Beet greens
Butternut squash	Chicory
Carrots, raw	Collards
Celery, raw	Dandelion greens
Cowpeas	Kale
Lima beans	Mustard greens
Parsnips	Parsley
Potato, baked or French fried	Spinach
Potato chips	Swiss chard
Winter squash	Watercress

Miscellaneous	*Amount, portion size*	*Potassium content, mg*
Pumpernickel bread	1 slice	113
Bran	¾ oz	214
Coffee	5-oz cup	80–169 (depending upon strength and brand)
Molasses	3½ oz	1000–2000 (depending upon type)
Peanuts and other nuts	3½ oz	600
Salt substitute	¼ tsp	400
Chocolate and cocoa		variable
Coconut, dried, sweetened dried, unsweetened fresh	3½ oz	250–590
Low-sodium milk	8 oz	600
Milk, whole or skim	8 oz	350
Meat, fish, poultry	1 oz	100 (average)

Source: Based on figures from U.S. Dept. of Agriculture Handbook No. 8, Revised, 1963, and Handbook No. 456, 1976.

Exogenous Factors

1 Blood transfusions

2 Potassium salts, e.g., potassium chloride per se, or salt substitutes which are intentionally prescribed in anticipation of potassium loss when diuretics are used

3 Medications

4 Severely restricted sodium intake (see endogenous factor #2)

Endogenous Factors

1 Catabolism (potassium "leakage" from cell breakdown)

2 Severe vomiting and diarrhea (causing salt depletion, which in turn causes decreased glomerular filtration and retention of potassium)

3 Metabolic acidosis (presumably due to potassium leaving cells and hydrogen entering)

While dietary contol of potassium is an extremely important consideration in maintaining or achieving a normal serum potassium level, these other factors must also be well controlled or hyperkalemia will persist.

Potassium (K) conversion:

1 meq K = 39 mg K

40 meq K = 1500 mg K

51 meq K = 2000 mg K

1 g kCl = 507 mg K

= 13 meq K

K = approximately 50% of KCl

Phosphorus and Calcium

Altered calcium and phosphorus metabolism in renal failure causes secondary hyperparathyroidism and bone disease (renal osteodystrophy).[5] The condition is seen in children and adults. Recently the complex mechanisms involved have become more clearly understood, although they have not yet been fully elucidated. The condition evolves in the following steps:

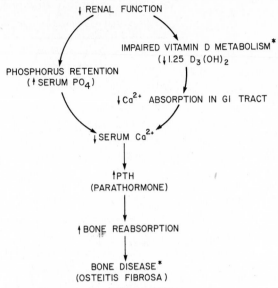

Figure 19-2

Secondary hyperparathyroidism and bone disease occur in acute renal failure when there is retention of phosphorus, a decreased absorption of calcium, and impaired vitamin D metabolism.

1 *Phosphorus is retained.* Normally, 60 percent of the phosphorus ingested from food is excreted by the kidneys and 40 percent is excreted via the gastrointestinal tract. When the kidneys begin to fail, phosphorus retention occurs and a process which can lead to secondary hyperparathyroidism begins. A homeostasis naturally exists between serum calcium and phosphorus (see Chap. 7). Therefore, when phosphorus is retained and the serum phosphate rises, the serum calcium falls in an attempt to maintain their equilibrium. (The reverse is also true as seen in tetany.) This reduction in serum calcium, coupled with the high serum phosphate, triggers the parathyroid glands to elaborate parathyroid hormone. This hormone raises the serum calcium by mobilizing calcium and phosphate from bone. Because phosphate is also liberated from bone by the action of parathyroid hormone, the serum phos-

phate level rises again and a vicious cycle develops.

Initially, blood tests detect this process, rather than overt symptoms. If this process is allowed to continue for a prolonged period of time, demineralization of bone (evident on radiological examination) can occur to the extent that the patient does become symptomatic, suffering from severe bone pain, and may experience spontaneous fractures and irreversible bone disease.

2 *Calcium absorption is decreased and vitamin D metabolism is impaired.* Patients with renal insufficiency require a much higher than normal amount of vitamin D to enhance calcium absorption. (Vitamin D is found in natural and fortified foods and is made in the skin on exposure to sunlight. See Chap. 6.) Without the active form of vitamin D, which is normally formed in the kidney, the calcium from food or medication will be poorly absorbed and instead will be excreted via the gastrointestinal tract. This results in a low serum calcium and again parathyroid hormone is elaborated by the parathyroid glands. Eventually because of phosphorus retention and impaired vitamin D metabolism, the parathyroid glands hypertrophy, producing excessive amounts of parathyroid hormone even if serum calcium and phosphate level become normal.

When serum phosphate and calcium are not well controlled, a situation can arise in which calcium and phosphate precipitate to form calcium phosphate, which is deposited at sites other than bone, such as soft tissue and blood vessels, a condition known as metastatic calcification.

Control of serum phosphate Both medications and diet are employed to control serum phosphate levels:

1 Phosphate binders, in the form of aluminum-containing antacids (e.g., Amphogel, Basaljel, Alucaps, Dialume), are prescribed. These are taken immediately after meals, since the aluminum in these preparations binds the phosphorus from the ingested food in the gastrointestinal tract. Too frequently the hospitalized patient experiences a rise in serum phosphate simply because the phosphate binders were not given in conjunction with meals.

Magnesium-containing antacids, such as Maalox or Mylanta, which are more palatable, are not generally prescribed for patients with renal failure, since magnesium cannot be excreted by the abnormal kidneys and an elevated serum magnesium can be toxic to the central nervous system. The medical team should be aware of the contents of any antacids the patient receives. The quantity of antacids prescribed will vary according to the patient's serum phosphate level. (Average serum phosphate is 2.3 to 4.3 mg/100 ml)

2 Calcium supplements and vitamin D preparations might be prescribed, if serum phosphate is appropriately controlled.

The serum phosphate level is influenced by diet as well as by the efficacy of the phosphate binders. The patient may be advised to avoid or limit high-phosphorus foods such as milk (and all milk products), organ meats, nuts (and nut products), cocoa, chocolate, whole grains, dried beans, and dried fruits. Meats, fish, poultry, and eggs, in large quantities, can also contribute a significant amount of phosphorus to the patient's diet.

Problems encountered with phosphate control It must be noted that constipation is a frequent side effect of the phosphate-binding agents prescribed to control serum phosphate. Stool softeners or laxatives are used to correct this problem, since the often necessary multirestricted diets (fluid and potassium in particular) interefere with the usual dietary treatment of constipation. The patient should be cautioned against home remedies for constipation.

Milk of magnesia, for example, contains a significant amount of magnesium, which can be harmful to the patient with renal failure.

Children frequently (and adults on occasion) have difficulty taking their prescribed phosphate binders. It therefore is often necessary to crush the medications and add them to foods or dissolve them in small amounts of their favorite (permitted) beverage. Special cookies containing these antacids can also be prepared and used in lieu of the large pills or capsules.

Patients need to be reminded to carry their phosphate binders with them at all times, for they are to be taken after *all* meals or large snacks, even if the patient is dining out.

Fluid (Water)

Normally a person's fluid intake and output are in equilibrium.

Sources of fluid intake include:

1 Overt fluids
2 Water content of solid foods (see Table 19-9)
3 Water of oxidation of solid foods [approximately (100 ml for every 1000 kcal (4200 kJ)]

Modes of fluid output include:

1 Respiration
2 Perspiration
3 Gastrointestinal (emesis, stool, drainage, etc.)
4 Urine
5 Breast milk (not usually present in patients with renal failure)

A person with kidney disease has precisely the same methods of fluid gain or loss (except as noted above) as a healthy person does; however, some patients with renal disease lose their ability to produce urine volumes sufficient to maintain fluid balance when a normal fluid intake is continued. When urine volume decreases, attempts should be made to adjust the fluid intake to ensure that fluid intake equals fluid output, thereby preventing overhydration and dehydration.

An *oliguric* (diminished urine volumes) or *anuric* (without urine) adult patient is usually advised to decrease fluid intake to 500 to 800 ml per day, to replace insensible loss. Children will be more severely restricted (200 to 500 ml per day), because of their smaller total body volume.

Patients should be carefully taught how to measure their fluid intake and output. Encouraging patients to record their own fluid intake and output records while in the hospital, with the close supervision of a staff person, is a very helpful teaching tool. All of the following factors need to be considered as part of fluid control.

Considerations for fluid control

1 Fluids have weight. *Weigh hospitalized patients daily.*
(1 l = 1000 ml = 2.2 lb = 1 kg)
(1 lb = 16 oz = 2 cups = 480 ml = 1 pt)
2 Fluid weight gains or losses occur at a much more rapid rate than solid weight changes do.
3 If fluid intake equals fluid output, there will be little or no change in weight from day to day, providing the patient is receiving sufficient calories (joules) to maintain solid weight.
4 For patient teaching purposes, and for accurate intake and output records, fluids are generally considered to be anything which is liquid at room temperature:
Ice
Water (including that taken with medications)
Sherbets
Popsicles
Ice cream
Tonics (sodas)
Soups and broths
All liquid medications including intravenous ones

TABLE 19-9   APPROXIMATE WATER CONTENT OF FOODS

Food	Amount of water per 100-g portion
Fruits, vegetables	
Cooked cereal	
Cooked rice, noodles,	80–90 ml
macaroni, other cereal products	
Meat, fish, poultry, eggs	50–75 ml
Breads, cheese	30–40 ml
Butter, margarine	15–20 ml
Dry cereal, crackers, sugars, oils	0–14 ml

Gelatin
Other beverages (tea, coffee, juice)
Milk
Syrups or water from
canned fruits and vegetables

5   The water content of solid foods must be borne in mind (see Table 19-9).

Renal Failure and Other Disease States

Occasionally a patient with renal failure has other disease entities requiring diet therapy, such as cardiovascular disease, ulcer disease, or diabetes mellitus. In these cases, the priorities have to be set according to the immediate needs of the patient. For example, if a patient with diabetes mellitus develops markedly elevated blood levels of urea nitrogen and creatinine, and has associated nausea, vomiting, and gastrointestinal distress, a decreased protein intake and a high-energy diet would be prescribed. The dietetic priority would be the renal failure and its associated symptoms, rather than the diabetes mellitus. In this example, the protein intake would be decreased and energy intake encouraged, using carbohydrates and fats. The patient's blood sugar would then be controlled by insulin therapy.

Acute Renal Failure

Acute renal failure is generally considered to be the sudden loss of renal function with a consequent decrease in urine volumes to oliguric levels (200 to 600 ml per day), usually without a previous history of renal impairment. (Acute renal failure on occasion does occur without oliguria, and in fact with urine volumes of 1500 ml or more. However, oliguric acute renal failure is most common. Also, acute renal failure can develop in patients with chronic renal impairment.) A continuation of the oliguric state for more than 24 to 48 h without treatment will result in the rapid accumulation of metabolic waste products (urea, uric acid, sulfates, creatinine, organic acids), and the rapid development of the symptoms of uremia. (See "Uremia," p. 401.) Therefore, if oliguria persists and serum creatinine continues to rise above normal levels, peritoneal dialysis or hemodialysis is usually instituted (see pp. 403–404.)

Causes of Acute Renal Failure

The causes of acute renal failure are numerous, but include damage due to hypotension, nephrotoxins, or obstructions:

1   Hypotension may be secondary to hemorrhage, severe dehydration, postoperative shock, septic abortion, crushing injury, or any other trauma causing shock. (See Fig. 19-3.)

2   Nephrotoxins are substances with a direct toxic effect on the kidneys. Examples are gold, mercuric chloride, carbon tetrachloride, a variety of medications, and ethylene glycol (antifreeze).

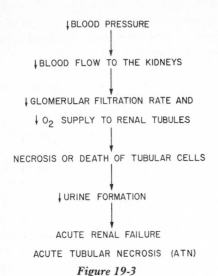

↓ BLOOD PRESSURE

↓ BLOOD FLOW TO THE KIDNEYS

↓ GLOMERULAR FILTRATION RATE AND
↓ O_2 SUPPLY TO RENAL TUBULES

NECROSIS OR DEATH OF TUBULAR CELLS

↓ URINE FORMATION

ACUTE RENAL FAILURE

ACUTE TUBULAR NECROSIS (ATN)

Figure 19-3

The physiological sequelae of acute renal failure as caused by hypotension.

3   Obstruction to the outflow of urine from the kidney is usually secondary to renal stones or prostate enlargement.

4   Obstruction of blood supply to the kidneys is usually secondary to renal artery thrombosis.

Obstruction renal failure is frequently totally correctable with surgical intervention.

Acute renal failure is seen more frequently in adults than in infants or children and is usually a self-limiting, potentially reversible disease entity, since the renal tubular cells are capable of regeneration. The length of time needed for total resolution of the renal failure is, however, variable and unpredictable and the primary cause of the renal failure does often conceal and interfere with its clinical course.

Nutritional Considerations in Patients with Acute Renal Failure

Calories (joules)   Inasmuch as acute renal failure is usually seen in conjunction with another major medical problem, most patients suffering from this type of renal failure are critically ill, severely catabolic, and unable to take oral

nourishment. At the same time, the energy needs of these patients are increased. This is related to the rate and degree of catabolism which accompanies the major predisposing insult. Therefore, the energy intake is increased either intravenously or orally, as soon as possible. Estimates of the energy requirements of these patients range from 2000 to 5000 kcal (8.4 to 21 MJ) per day.

In the initial anuric or oliguric phase of acute renal failure, when fluid intake must be severely limited, intravenous glucose is administered to supply sufficient calories (joules) to:

1   Support basal metabolic needs
2   Lessen endogenous protein breakdown
3   Prevent ketosis from fat catabolism

Hypertonic glucose solutions, 25 to 50 percent glucose, may be administered through large cannulated major vessels to supply needed calories (joules) (see Chap. 24).

When the patient is able to tolerate oral feedings, calories (joules) can be increased markedly by the addition of concentrated carbohydrates, fats, or both. In addition to butterballs (a butter and sugar mixture which can be flavored for somewhat improved palatability) and hard sugar candies, an increasing number of protein-free, high-energy, low-electrolyte food supplements and additives are currently available. (See Table 19-4 for examples of these supplements.)

Protein   The protein intake of patients in acute renal failure is severely limited if they are unable to take oral feedings. Indeed, in an anuric or oliguric patient with a rapidly rising blood urea nitrogen this might be considered advantageous, since protein or protein-containing foods will contribute to the urea nitrogen pool, thus enhancing the onset of uremia. However, malnutrition will develop after prolonged deficit of protein.

Fluids and sodium   An important priority is the restoration of proper fluid and sodium balance, since dehydration may be a causative factor in oliguric acute renal failure. Once normal fluid balance has been restored, additional intravenous fluids may be administered in quantities sufficient to maintain balance. Maintenance is best accomplished by allowing the patient quantities of fluid equal to basal requirements (300 to 500 ml per day) *plus* amounts sufficient to replace urine volumes, gastrointestinal losses, increased respiratory losses, or losses from excessive perspiration. The patient must be monitored for dehydration and overhydration. (See Chap. 8.)

Assessment of proper fluid balance should be made by charted daily weights. It is important to realize that when caloric intake is severely limited, a weight loss of 0.2 to 0.3 kg per day should be expected.[6] In these instances, if this loss is not obvious on the daily weight chart, or if in fact the patient gains weight, one may assume that the patient's fluid intake has been excessive.

Potassium hyperkalemia (a serum potassium of greater than 5 meq/l is a problem in acute renal failure and exists because (1) potassium excretion is severely limited by the decreased urine volumes, and (2) potassium is being released from cells at a fairly rapid rate by tissue breakdown. The presence of undrained blood or infection also contributes additional potassium. The hyperkalemia of acute renal failure is more life-threatening, because of its rapid onset, than that seen in chronic disease. Under these conditions potassium intake must be kept as low as possible, and a patient who is receiving intravenous feedings should not have potassium added. When the patient is able to tolerate oral feedings, the diet should be limited to practical levels of 1 to 1.5 g (maximum) per day until urine volumes begin to increase and the serum potassium levels are maintained within normal limits. At that time the potassium content of the diet can be liberalized.

Peritoneal dialysis or hemodialysis controls serum potassium levels and allows for a more liberal intake of dietary potassium; however, the patient's serum potassium levels need to be monitored frequently, with the food adjusted accordingly.

Phosphorus   In acute renal failure, phosphorus levels should also be carefully monitored and steps should be taken to keep the serum phosphate level as close to normal as possible.

The Diuretic Phase of Acute Renal Failure

As kidney function begins to improve, the patient enters what is commonly called the *diuretic* or *high-output phase* of the renal failure. During this recovery phase, fluids should be increased to equal the daily urine volumes, plus gastrointestinal, respiratory, and other losses. Serum sodium and potassium levels are closely monitored and help to determine the dietary needs of these minerals, but generally if the patient is alert and able to tolerate food and fluids, salt and water are permitted as desired. (Allowing the patient to determine fluid intake by thirst is the guide.) Potassium can be liberalized at this time, and frequently high-potassium intakes are required to replace the quantities lost and prevent depletion.

As blood urea nitrogen and creatinine begin their downward trend (which does not necessarily occur at the same time as or immediately following diuresis), dietary protein intake can gradually be increased, eventually returning to unlimited quantities.

Hyperalimentation in Acute Renal Failure

Despite the increased availability of hemodialysis, as well as the use of improved antibiotics, diuretics, anesthesia, and modern intensive care units, the mortality in acute renal failure remains quite high. Recent research suggests that the mortality rate can be decreased if adequate nutritional support is provided. To this end, the use of intravenous solutions containing the eight essential amino acids plus histidine and other essential nutrients in hypertonic glucose solution, administered by catheterization of the superior vena cava, has been tried successfully.[7-9] The mortality rate decreases and patients' general nutritional status, electrolyte balance, uremic symptoms, and wound healing improve. This type of hyperalimentation uses the rationale of the Giordano–Giovannetti diet (see p. 401) and provides proteins of high biological value with sufficient energy to permit the body to utilize urea for synthesis of the nonessential amino acids. (See "Uremia," p. 401.)

This method has not been widely used because of inherent problems of hyperalimentation (i.e., sepsis, solutions mixtures); however, it does have merit for patients who are unable to eat for prolonged periods of time. (See Chap. 24 for more specific details about parenteral nutrition.)

Chronic Renal Failure

Chronic renal failure is the term used to describe the gradual progressive deterioration of the functioning nephron mass. There are a wide variety of diverse etiologies associated with chronic renal failure (see Table 19-2). The many disease processes which can cause renal disease and ultimate failure differ in their clinical course, but all eventually cause regulatory and excretory dysfunction of the kidneys which can result in the uremic syndrome if permitted to progress without appropriate treatment. Specifically, treatment with the artificial kidney (hemodialysis) is usually indicated just prior to the onset of frank uremia.

In addition to the numerous causes of chronic renal failure, unlike the case in acute renal failure, there are various levels or stages of chronic renal failure which may or may not develop, depending upon the nature of the primary cause. As the disease state changes, compensatory changes in diet are made.

Stages of Chronic Renal Disease with Guidelines for Diet Modifications*

Chronic renal failure is categorized, according to decreasing kidney function, into four stages:

* Adapted from Peter Bent Brigham Hospital, *Diet Manual*, Boston, Mass.

1 Decreased renal reserve in renal impairment
2 Renal insufficiency (mild azotemia)
3 Renal failure (moderate to severe azotemia)
4 End stage

In the first stage of *decreased renal reserve* there is a loss of up to 50 to 60 percent of nephron function without significant loss of homeostatic function or easily detected abnormalities. There is usually no diet restriction except that for the hypertensive patient calories are adjusted to attain ideal body weight.

In the second stage of renal insufficiency, known as *mild azotemia,* a decrease in homeostatic function is noted, and an accumulation of nitrogenous waste products as indicated by slight elevations of BUN, creatinine, and uric acid, as well as an ensuing mild anemia. Only under conditions of marked metabolic stress of dietary excess is there a derangement of body fluids with associated symptoms. Dietary modifications of sodium are made, depending on the degree of hydration and the presence of hypertension. Potassium is restricted in accordance with serum levels, and phosphorus modification is dependent upon serum phosphate levels and the efficacy of phosphate binders. Fluid control is regulated according to urine output and the degree of hydration. There is usually no protein restriction and calories (joules) are adjusted to weight.

In the next progressive stage of renal failure, known as *moderate severe azotemia,* there is a significant decrease in the homeostatic functions of the kidneys, with a decrease in concentrating ability, markedly elevated BUN and creatinine, and a striking anemia. However, symptoms of uremia are not present. There is usually no immediate need for hemodialysis.

The following diet modifications are made:

Protein: Restricted to 0.6 to 1.0 g/kg ideal weight (40 to 60 g average), with at least 70 to 75 percent of the total allowance from high-biological-value proteins.

Sodium: Restriction depends upon the degree of hydration and blood pressure.

Potassium: Restriction depends upon serum potassium levels.

Phosphorus: Restriction depends upon serum phosphate levels (these are frequently elevated and 1.5 to 1 g or less of dietary phosphorus is usually recommended).

Fluid: When weight is stable (the patient is neither dehydrated nor overloaded) fluid intake should be either (1) 300 to 500 ml; or (2) a quantity sufficient to replace insensible loss *plus* fluid equivalent to the urine volume from the previous day; or (3) the quantity sufficient to maintain the desired stable daily weight.

Energy: Sufficient to prevent catabolism [Average for adults: 30 to 40 kcal/kg of body weight (126 to 168 kJ/kg); average for children: 100 to 150 kcal/kg (420 to 630 kJ/kg)].

Multivitamins: Usually prescribed.

In the last or *terminal stage* of renal failure, which is permanent and irreversible, there is a severe decrease in homeostasis, with the clinical picture of uremia developing if hemodialysis (or peritoneal dialysis) is not initiated. (See Table 19-10.)

Uremia (End-Stage Renal Disease Without Dialysis Intervention)

Uremia or the *uremic syndrome*, per se, is not a renal disease, but rather the complex of symptoms associated with untreated end-stage renal disease. It is characterized by numerous symptoms which can include any or all of the following, in addition to the biochemical abnormalities previously mentioned: anemia (secondary to decreased production of erythropoietin—B_{12} and folate levels are usually within normal limits); hypertension; gastrointestinal symptoms of anorexia, nausea, vomiting, hiccups, and bleeding; neuromuscular disorders such as twitching and seizures; coma; and eventual death. In fact, uremia has

appropriately been called "the total body disease."[10]

Diet Modification

Diets low in protein, but high in essential amino acids, e.g., the selected protein diet[11] or the Giordano–Giovannetti diet (G–G Diet),[12,13] are used.

The rationale for this low protein is that the small quantities of high-biological-value (HBV) proteins, with sufficient calories (joules), will allow the excess urea in the blood to be used for synthesis of the nonessential amino acids, thus reducing the BUN and utilizing the essential amino acids from the permitted HBV protein foods. Today, this type of diet is less frequently required, with the increased availability of hemodialysis. Patients rarely reach the stage at which this diet would be needed, since dialysis is usually initiated prior to the onset of the full-blown uremic syndrome.

It is very important to realize that this diet does not improve the function of the kidneys. It merely serves to reduce the BUN and decrease the gastrointestinal symptoms of uremia. A patient can maintain a positive nitrogen balance while following this diet, provided the permitted HBV protein foods and sufficient calories (joules) are ingested. The diet is a very stringent one, and is expensive, because of the need for the special low-protein products. Patients compliance is also frequently a problem.

Table 19-11 gives a sample meal plan for this type of diet. The following nutrients are restricted accordingly:

Protein: 0.26 g/kg of body weight (average, 18 to 25 g total protein per day). Almost the entire protein allowance is from HBV protein, as 6½ oz of milk and 1 egg. This contains approximately 14 g of HBV protein. The remaining 4 to 6 g is obtained from the low-biological-value proteins in fruits, vegetables, and starches. Special low-protein products are necessary.

Sodium: Amount depends upon the state

TABLE 19-10 GUIDELINES FOR DIET MODIFICATIONS DURING THE STAGES OF CHRONIC RENAL FAILURE

Renal stage	Diet treatment						
	Energy	Protein (Pro)	Sodium (Na)	Potassium (K)	Phosphorus (P)	Fluids	Vitamins
First stage (decreasing renal reserve)	Sufficient to maintain ideal body weight	Usually no restrictions	Usually no restrictions	Usually no restrictions		Usually no restrictions	
Renal insufficiency (mild azotemia)	Sufficient to maintain ideal body weight		Dependent upon degree of hydration & presence of hypertension	Dependent upon serum levels	Dependent upon serum levels & efficacy of phosphate binders	Dependent upon urine volumes & degree of hydration	
Renal failure (moderate–severe azotemia)	Sufficient to prevent catabolism. Average: adults 30–40 kcal (126–168 kJ)/kg; children 100–150 kcal (420–630 kJ)/kg	0.6–1.0 g/kg ideal weight. Average 40–60 g (70–75% from HBV* protein)	As for mild azotemia	As for mild azotemia	Dependent upon serum levels (frequently elevated); 1–1.5 g is recommended	With stable weight, no dehydration or overload: 300–500 ml or amount sufficient to replace insensible loss & fluid equivalent to urine volume from previous day	
End-stage renal disease	Sufficient to prevent catabolism. Average: 30–40 kcal (126–168 kJ)/kg	18–20 g; almost entire allowance is from HBV* protein	Dependent upon state of hydration & blood pressure. Average: 1000 mg (43 meq)	Dependent upon serum levels. Average: 1500–1800 mg/kg (38–46 meq)	Dependent upon serum levels & efficacy of phosphate binders	Dependent upon state of hydration; manipulated according to daily weight	
Peritoneal dialysis	35–45 kcal (147–189 kJ)/kg	Liberal or unrestricted	Liberal	Dependent upon serum levels	Dependent upon serum levels	Dependent upon state of hydration	
Hemodialysis: Children	100–150 kcal(420–630 kJ)/kg (Cal are encouraged to enhance growth, which is usually stunted with renal disease)	3–4 g/kg to encourage growth permitted amount is limited by the need for K & P modification since both of these are elevated in protein foods)	Dependent upon state of hydration & blood pressure. Average: 2000 mg (87 meq)	Dependent upon serum levels. Average: 2000 mg (51 meq)	As low as possible, with dairy products and milk limited to 120 ml/day. Dependent upon serum levels & efficacy of phosphate binders	20 ml/kg of body weight & fluid equivalent to previous day's urine volume	
Hemodialysis: adults	30–45 kcal (126–189 kJ)/kg of ideal weight or "dry weight"	1–1½ g/kg of ideal body weight; ⅔–¾ from HBV* protein	1500–2000 mg (65–87 meq) unless patient is producing large volume of urine containing Na; then regulated accordingly	Dependent upon serum levels. Average: 2000–2500 mg (52–64 meq)	1500 mg or less/day, dependent upon serum levels and efficacy of phosphate binders	Quantity to allow for 1–1½ kg fluid weight gain between treatments; 800–1000 ml & fluid equivalent to urine volume from previous day	Routinely prescribed, with addition of folic acid

402

TABLE 19-11 SAMPLE MENU FOR LOW-PROTEIN DIET

Breakfast
100 ml cranberry juice
1 ounce cream of rice cereal
2 teaspoons margarine (salt-free, if necessary)
2 teaspoons brown sugar
1 slice low-protein bread
1 teaspoon jelly
120 ml milk
1 teaspoon regular sugar
100 ml tea

Lunch
Fruit plate:
    1 medium apple
    2 canned peach halves
    2 canned pear halves
1 slice low-protein bread
1 teaspoon margarine (salt-free, if necessary)
1 teaspoon jelly
Water ice, sherbet, or special low-protein dessert
210 ml ginger ale with Karo syrup
100 ml tea
30 ml milk

Dinner
Vegetable plate:
    1 medium egg, any style
    ½ cup cooked green peas
    ½ cup cooked wax beans
    1 medium boiled potato
1 slice low-protein bread
2 teaspoons margarine (salt-free, if necessary)
1 teaspoon jelly
210 ml ginger ale with Karo syrup
100 ml decaffeinated coffee
30 ml milk
1 teaspoon sugar
Total calories (joules): approximately 2100 to 2200 (8820 to 9240 kJ)
Total protein: approximately 23 g

Notes: 1 Energy can be increased by adding additional sugar and salt-free margarine or oil or by incorporating the supplements listed in Table 19–4.

2 Desired potassium levels can be attained in this meal plan by altering the type of fruits and vegetables permitted.

3 Desired sodium levels can be attained by the addition of salt, per se, and/or sodium-containing foods.

4 The calcium and phosphorus content of this meal plan is low.

5 Multivitamins are recommended.

of hydration and the blood pressure (average, 1 g sodium per day)

Potassium: Amount depends upon serum potassium levels (average, 1500 to 1800 mg potassium)

Phosphorus: Amount depends upon serum phosphate levels and efficacy of phosphate binders

Fluid: Amount depends upon the state of hydration and is manipulated according to daily needs

Energy: In excess of 2000 kcal (8400 kJ) per day [35 to 45 kcal(147 to 189 kJ)/kg of body weight]

Multivitamins: Routinely prescribed

End-Stage Renal Disease (Treatment with Dialysis)

Dialysis can be defined as the removal of the toxic substances contained in body fluids by diffusion and osmosis across a semipermeable membrane. This is accomplished by using a dialysis solution (dialysate) that is similar in composition to normal blood plasma. Two types of dialysis therapy currently exist: peritoneal dialysis (intracorporeal dialysis, using the peritoneal membrane as the semipermeable membrane) and hemodialysis (extracorporeal dialysis, using an artificial kidney machine with synthetic semipermeable membranes).

Peritoneal Dialysis

Diet modifications A patient on peritoneal dialysis may experience the following dietary restrictions:

Protein: During the procedure, which can last from 24 to 72 h, protein is usually liberalized or unrestricted since large amounts of protein and amino acids are lost into the dialysis solution and must be replaced.

Sodium: The amount allowed depends upon the degree of hydration at the time of peritoneal dialysis, the rate of sodium and fluid removal during the treatment, and the blood pressure response to the treatment; again, allowance is frequently quite liberal during the procedure.

Potassium: Amount depends upon serum potassium levels.

Phosphorus: Amount depends upon serum phosphate levels.

Fluid: Amount depends upon the patient's state of hydration, as per sodium above.

Energy: In excess of 2000 kcal (8400 kJ) per day [35 to 45 kcal (147 to 189 kJ)/kg of body weight].

Vitamin supplements: Multivitamins are routinely prescribed.

While the basic diet for a patient receiving peritoneal dialysis can be fairly liberal during the procedure, patients may be uncomfortable and unable to consume the desired quantities of protein and calories (joules). Energy and protein supplementation may be required.

After the peritoneal dialysis is discontinued, or between treatments, patients usually require diet modifications similar to those outlined above for the third and fourth stages of chronic renal failure.

Hemodialysis

Hemodialysis is now a common treatment for patients with end-stage renal disease and is usually performed three times per week. The length of each treatment varies from 4 to 6 h, depending upon the institution, its philosophy, the type of equipment used, the patient's body size, existing biochemical abnormalities, and the patient's general state of well-being. Similarly, standards of diet modification for the hemodialysis patient are controversial and vary from institution to institution. Most would agree, however, that diet modifications should be individualized according to each patient's specific needs at any given time.

Diet modifications for adults receiving hemodialysis[14]

Protein: 1 to 1½ g/kg of ideal body weight; ⅔ to ¾ of total protein obtained from high-biological-value protein foods.

Sodium: Usually limited to 1500 to 2000 mg (65 to 87 meq) per day, unless the patient is still producing large volumes of urine containing significant amounts of sodium, in which case sodium should be regulated accordingly.

Potassium: Usually limited to 2000 to 2500 mg (52 to 64 meq) per day, but quantity depends upon serum potassium levels.*

Phosphorus: Quantity depends upon serum phosphate levels and effectiveness of phosphate binders. Usually limited to 1 g or less per day.

Fluid: Quantity sufficient to allow for a 1- to 1½-kg fluid weight gain between dialysis treatments. Most frequently the range for adults is 500 to 1000 ml *plus* an amount equivalent to the urine volume.

Energy: 30 to 45 kcal (126 to 189 kJ)/kg of ideal body weight or the quantity sufficient to attain ideal "dry" body weight. (*Dry weight* is generally considered to be the weight at which there is little or no excess fluid available for removal by dialysis. This is usually evident by a severe drop in blood pressure during the dialysis treatment.)

Vitamin supplements: Routinely prescribed, with emphasis on the water-soluble vitamins, which are partially removed during dialysis therapy.[15] Folic acid is also usually prescribed.

Diet modifications for children receiving hemodialysis.[16,17]

---

* Predialysis potassium levels are the reference levels that should be used, since postdialysis potassium levels are an unreliable reference. Dialysis very effectively removes potassium from serum, which is reflected in an abnormally low potassium level immediately postdialysis. After dialytic treatment there is a shift of potassium from the intracellular compartments where it normally is predominantly found to the extracellular compartments where it can be measured, thus effectively raising the serum potassium level in a relatively short period of time.

Protein: 3 to 4 g/kg of body weight, to encourage growth. (The amount of protein permitted the pediatric patient receiving hemodialysis is limited by the need for restriction of potassium and phosphorus, since both of these are plentiful in high-protein foods.)

Sodium: Average 2000 mg (87 meq) per day. Quantity depends upon the patient's state of hydration and blood pressure.

Potassium: Average 2000 mg (51 meq) per day. Quantity depends upon predialysis serum potassium levels, as for adults.

Phosphorus: As low as possible, with dairy products and milk limited to 120 ml per day. Quantity depends upon serum phosphate levels and effectiveness of phosphate binders.

Fluid: 20 ml/kg of body weight plus fluid equivalent to the previous day's urine volume.

Energy: 100 to 150 kcal (420 to 630 kJ/kg. (Calories (joules) are encouraged in effort to enhance growth, which is usually stunted in children with renal disease.)

Vitamin supplements: Routinely prescribed, with the addition of folic acid.

The hemodialysis patient—a total person The guidelines and recommendations for diet modification as outlined above are certainly necessary for most patients receiving hemodialysis treatments; however, there is one other extremely important consideration, namely, that the patient is undergoing a significant psychological adjustment further complicated by the prescribed multi-restricted diet.

The psychological impact of a chronic, irreversible, and potentially terminal disease, especially one which makes the individual "machine dependent," is understandably overwhelming.[18] Indeed, the patient requiring dialysis treatments has been called a "marginal man."[19]

In the case of children, this is particularly disruptive to development since both child and parents must now adjust to the trauma of a chronic life-threatening disease. Also, children are greatly restricted in their customary motor and exploratory activities which normally help them to gain mastery over their bodies and establish psychosocial independence. (See Table 19-12.)

Prior to any diet instruction, a thorough

TABLE 19-12 ISSUES OF MANAGEMENT OF PEDIATRIC RENAL PATIENTS*

I. Pediatric dialysis patients
    A. Fear of death
    B. Limited activity
        1. Access—fistula vs. shunt
        2. Chronically anemic
        3. Time—dialysis takes 4 to 6 h, 3 times/week
    C. Dependency vs. denial
    D. Limited peer contact
        1. Time of dialysis plus travel time—lost school days
        2. Hospitalizations
        3. Illness may cause below-average school achievement, resulting in need to repeat grades or semesters (classmates not the same age)
    E. Appearance
        1. Short stature (bone disease)
        2. Fistula/shunt
        3. Pale, less energy
        4. Delayed puberty, immature emotionally
    F. Home management
        1. Control of fluid intake—weight charts, prizes for best weights
        2. Dietary acceptance and compliance
        3. Care of access
    G. Medical crises leading to hospitalizations
II. Pediatric transplant patients†
    A. Reintegration—of a presumably healthy child who had been chronically ill
        1. Into family
        2. Return to school and peers—identity and body image problems
    B. Dependency leading to behavior problems
        1. Relationship of donor and patient
        2. Acute rejection leading to anxiety reactions
    C. Complications leading to fear of return to dialysis

---

* Contributed by Nancy Spinozzi, R.D., Renal Dietitian, Children's Hospital Medical Center, Boston, Mass.

† *Source:* D. M. Bernstein, "After Transplantation—The Child's Emotional Reactions," *American Journal of Psychiatry,* **127:**9, 1971.

diet history should be obtained and meals should be calculated to allow for as many of the patient's preferred foods as possible. Both the patient and the family should receive thorough diet instruction, with information on how the diet relates to the kidney. On special, rare occasions, e.g., holidays, birthdays, or anniversaries, a *moderate intake* of a restricted food should be permitted and allowances made.

Transplantation

Transplantation is a possible treatment for chronic renal failure but, unlike dialysis, a successful transplant can restore normal renal function. However, not every dialysis patient is a candidate for kidney transplantation. There are several reasons, which include the following:

1   The patient, having been given all pertinent information about transplantation and its associated problems, decides that dialysis is an acceptable way of life, and does not wish to have a transplant.
2   Medical reasons deem the patient unsuitable for transplantation (e.g., age, other concurrent illness, presensitization to donor antibodies).
3   A suitable donor may not be available.

On the other hand, because of the bone and growth problems associated with renal failure, attempts are made to perform a transplant in pediatric patients as soon as possible. Growth does seem to improve if transplantation is performed prior to the onset of puberty, when the epiphyses have not yet closed. This is not to imply that transplantation in children is without its complications, for the complications are quite similar to those seen in adults.[21,22]

Nutritional Considerations

The nutritional management of patients with transplants—children and adults—primarily depends upon how well the transplanted kidney functions; i.e., if the kidney functions perfectly, an ad lib. diet is usually permitted, but if the kidney does not function well, the diet is adjusted as it would be for renal failure or dialysis.

In addition to adjusting the diet according to the status of the new kidney, there are other extremely important factors which influence the patient's nutritional needs. All patients receiving a kidney transplant (except for identical twins) are routinely required to take immunosuppressive medications such as azathioprine (Imuran) and corticosteroids such as prednisone, to reduce the risk of the body's rejection of the transplanted kidney. These medications, unfortunately, have potential adverse side effects which can affect the patient's nutritional status. Some of these and their consequent nutritional considerations are listed in Table 19-13.

Obesity and a "cushingoid" appearance are frequently seen side effects of the steroid therapy, especially when very high doses are used to treat a rejection episode. Since obesity is a common problem, patients should be given anticipatory guidance. They should be advised to use much common sense and discretion in food selection and portion size. (This concept is frustrating to the patient who has always been thin; however, eventually, in most cases even thin patients taking steroids will gain a substantial amount of weight when not watching their diet.) "Preventive dietetics" is strongly recommended since the psychological stress of an altered body image can become problematic to both children and adults.

Another important nutritional consideration is that, since dialysis does impose some inconvenience to the patient (usually including a modified diet), many patients view transplantation as the only means of achieving a "normal" life and a normal diet. After transplantation, if complications arise and a modified diet is prescribed, depression, anger, and anxiety may result. Patients need the continuing support of the health care team to achieve a realistic expectation of kidney function following transplantation. Diet modifications

TABLE 19-13 IMMUNOSUPPRESSION: SOME ASSOCIATED SIDE EFFECTS AND POSSIBLE NUTRITIONAL IMPLICATIONS*

Side effects† Azathioprine (Imuran)	Common dietetic considerations
Severe bone marrow depression Infection (fungal, protozoal, viral, and uncommon bacteria)	All foods served by reverse precaution or precaution technique
	Small frequent feedings—high-energy, high-protein foods
Toxic hepatitis or biliary stasis	Modified fat diet
Nausea, anorexia	Small frequent feedings
Diarrhea, vomiting	Fluid and electrolyte replacement
Steatorrhea	Low-fat diet
Negative nitrogen balance	High-protein, high-energy foods
Prednisone	
Sodium retention	Moderate to low sodium intake
Potassium loss	High-potassium foods
Peptic ulcer	Liberal bland diet, unless actively bleeding
Pancreatitis	Moderate to low fat intake
Abdominal distention	Small frequent feedings
Ulcerative esophagitis	Modified food consistency
Altered carbohydrate metabolism, manifestation of latent diabetes mellitus, higher insulin needs in patients with previous diabetes	Decreased concentrated sweets or American Diabetes Association diets
Negative nitrogen balance (secondary to protein catabolism)	High-energy, high-protein foods
Altered fat metabolism	Low-cholesterol or appropriate diet for specific type of hyperlipidemia

* The nutritional considerations stated here are quite general. As always, diets should be modified on an individual basis. Kidney function will, of course, also influence the diet prescribed.

† *Source: Physicians' Desk Reference,* 30th ed., Medical Economics Company, Oradell, N.J., 1976, pp. 674, 1234–5.

might be necessary even after the transplant is performed and patients should be prepared for this.

NEPHROTIC SYNDROME

The nephrotic syndrome is not a disease, but rather a group of symptoms—biochemical and clinical—which can result from a variety of disease states. Glomerulonephritis is the most common cause of nephrotic syndrome, but it is also seen in metabolic diseases, systemic sensitivity diseases, circulatory disease, allergic states, and infective processes. The major symptoms include edema, massive proteinuria, hypoalbuminemia, and hyperlipidemia (as hypercholesterolemia). These symptoms occur primarily because of glomerular injury, which causes the loss of plasma protein in the urine while, at least initially, other blood chemistries such as BUN and creatinine are within normal limits.

Depending upon the cause and the patient's response to medical treatment (usually steroids) some patients with nephrotic syndrome can develop end-stage renal disease and require dialysis treatments or transplantation.

Diet Modifications

Protein: Normal or high intake, unless the patient is azotemic. (The exact amount of protein needed is still controversial. Certain physicians prescribe 150 g or more of protein per day and others suggest, on the premise that the more protein ingested, the greater the protein loss in the urine, that an ad lib. protein intake is sufficient. Since the edema seen in nephrotic syndrome is primarily due to the change in oncotic pressure occurring because of the large quantities of protein lost in the urine, the patient is usually encouraged to consume a well-balanced "high" protein diet.)

Sodium: An intake of 1000 to 2000 mg per day is frequently prescribed. (Once again, the philosophy of the primary physician is an important factor, as is the patient's clinical response to medical therapy.)

Potassium: Usually not restricted, but individualized according to each patient's serum levels.

Phosphate: Usually not restricted, but quantity depends upon serum levels.

Energy: Ad lib., or the quantity sufficient to achieve ideal weight. (Because of the edematous state, the patient's actual weight is difficult to determine.)

Cholesterol: Low-cholesterol diet, if serum level is elevated.

Vitamin supplements: Might be prescribed.

Childhood Nephrosis (Childhood Nephrotic Syndrome)

Childhood nephrosis is a primary renal disease which usually occurs in children between the ages of 1½ and 5 but is on occasion, seen in older children and adults. It is not common and affects females more frequently than males. The cause is unknown and it does develop without other concurrent renal disease. The symptoms are very similar to those of nephrotic syndrome, although perhaps more pronounced. Basically the same dietary management outlined for nephrotic syndrome is utilized for childhood nephrosis.

URINARY TRACT INFECTIONS

The most common kidney-related diseases are urinary tract infections. These infections are common in women, because of their anatomy, but on occasion are seen in men and in children.

Urinary tract infections can be potentially damaging to the kidneys, and if allowed to go untreated can possibly lead to chronic pyelonephritis, which is potentially irreversible and can lead to end-stage renal failure. Causes of urinary tract infection include congenital obstructions or other obstructive processes such as kidney stones, injury to the urinary tract, or chronic inflammation from bacteria.

Nutritional Considerations

Nutritional management usually involves:

1 Push fluids—2 l or more per day
2 Acid-ash diet: High- protein foods, such as meats, fish, eggs, and gelatin products, are encouraged. Only specific fruits—cranberries, plums, and prunes—are permitted. (This diet increases the acidity of the urine*)

or

Alkali-ash diet: High intake of milk and milk products, most vegetables, citrus fruits (and their juices), and all other juices or fruits which are not permitted on the acid-ash diet. (This diet decreases the acidity of the urine and thereby produces a more alkaline urine*)

* Normal urine pH is 6 (range, 4.8 to 8.5).

NEPHROLITHIASIS (RENAL STONES OR CALCULI)

Nephrolithiasis is quite common in the United States, primarily affecting people 20 to 55 years of age, although children and older adults can develop renal stone disease. Calculi can occur as either single or multiple stones and can develop anywhere along the urinary tract. They are usually caused by the precipitation of urine salts, although the details of the mechanisms of stone formation are quite complex and not fully understood.[23] Factors which may promote the formation of renal calculi are numerous but generally are those conditions which increase the concentration of the urine, the quantity of urine excreted, or both. Examples of these conditions include dehydration, which increases urine concentration; excessive intake of vitamin D; milk-alkali syndrome; primary hyperparathyroidism and prolonged immobilization, which cause calcium loss from bone and thus increase calcium excretion; and the other metabolic diseases which characteristically increase the excretion of uric acid, oxalate, glycine, or cystine. In addition, anatomic factors such as infection, obstruction, and other abnormalities of the urinary tract may play a role in renal stone formation.

Of the major constituents of renal calculi—calcium, uric acid, oxalate, cystine, and glycine—calcium stones are by far the most common, with the largest percentage of these stones consisting of calcium oxalate. A slightly smaller percentage are a combination of calcium oxalate and calcium phosphate. (These can occur with or without excessive calcium excretion.) Uric acid stones are less common than calcium-containing stones, and cystine or glycine stones are rare.

Nephrolithiasis, per se, can damage the kidneys by causing either a pressure necrosis, an obstruction, or a predisposition to infection. For this reason, removal or passage of renal stones is extremely important. The three most common methods of treating nephrolithiasis and preventing it from causing permanent damage to the kidneys are:

1 Encouraging spontaneous passage
2 Surgical or urological removal
3 Medications; examples for specific types of stones are:
   a Calcium stones—phosphate preparations or cellulose phosphate[24]
   b Uric acid stones—allopurinol, which prevents uric acid synthesis and lowers serum and urine uric acid levels
   c Cystine stones—D-penicillamine, which combines with cystine to form a soluble product

Nutritional Considerations

Diet modification was not listed above as a means of preventing or treating renal calculi, even though various diets have been used through the years, since much controversy exists about this mode of therapy. The efficacy of these diets has been less than optimal. However, there is agreement that there are instances when changes in a person's eating patterns will be helpful, regardless of the etiology of the renal calculi. For example, all patients should be encouraged to maintain or achieve a nutritionally well-balanced diet and all patients with a history of renal stone disease should *force fluids* to 3 to 4 l per day. (Since calculi are caused by precipitation of urine salts, increasing the fluid intake will increase urine volume and therefore dilute the precipitating salts.)

In specific instances, diet modifications based on the etiology of the stone formation may be somewhat helpful. Examples of such diet modifications include the following:

1 Calcium stones with idiopathic (of unknown cause hypercalciuria: Low-calcium diets or avoidance of dairy products; acid-ash diet* (see p. 408), since calcium stones tend to be insoluble in alkaline urine.

2 Oxalate stones with hyperoxaluria (as in

---

* Acid- and alkali-ash diets are used less frequently today, apparently because medications which are relatively harmless serve the same or better purpose; however, on occasion, these diets might be prescribed.

ileal disease): Low-oxalate diet. (Foods commonly avoided include rhubarb, spinach, dandelion greens, asparagus, cranberries, almonds, cashew nuts, chocolate, cocoa, and tea)

3 Uric acid stones with hyperuricosuria: Low-purine diet (rarely used today since medications are quite effective; (foods which would be avoided include all organ meats, anchovies, meat extracts, gravies, and alcoholic beverages); alkali-ash diet (see p. 408), since uric acid stones tend to be insoluble in acid urine.

4 Cystine stones with cystinuria: Low-methionine diet (Foods frequently avoided include milk and milk products, eggs, cheese, fish, and certain fruits and vegetables); alkali-ash diet, since cystine stones tend to be insoluble in acid urine.

Although there is no general agreement about the efficacy of diet modifications for renal stones, all seem to concur that *forcing fluids* and a well-balanced diet is essential and beneficial.

STUDY QUESTIONS

1 Describe the nutritional goals which should be achieved by diet therapy for individuals with renal failure.
2 What nutrients are frequently controlled in the food intake of the patient with kidney failure?
3 What biochemical and clinical information would you use to monitor kidney function?
4 Why is the protein intake decreased in end-stage renal disease when the patient is not being treated by chronic hemodialysis?
5 Differentiate between the diets of a post-transplant patient and a patient being maintained on chronic hemodialysis.

CASE STUDY 19-1

Sara is a 20-year-old student with end-stage renal disease secondary to chronic glomerulonephritis. She has been receiving hemodialysis treatments 3 times per week, 5 h per treatment, for approximately 6 months, and is essentially anuric. She has resumed her status as a full-time student and is maintaining above-average grades. She is 5 ft 2 in tall, and normally weighs 52 kg. Her average fluid weight gains between Dialysis treatments have been 2 to 2½ kg. However, on occasion she has had weight gains of up to 3 kg between dialysis treatments. She was recently hospitalized with shortness of breath and a preliminary diagnosis of fluid overload. Her weight on admission was 60 kg and her blood pressure was 220/120. Her admission followed an extended weekend trip to her hometown for a class reunion. Laboratory values were as follows:

> BUN—40 mg/100 ml
> Serum creatinine 1.8/100 ml
> Serum potassium—4.0 meq/l
> Serum phosphorus—4.3 Bodansky units
> Serum sodium—150 meq/l

CASE STUDY QUESTIONS

1 How much fluid should Sara be allowed?
2 What energy level would be appropriate? How much protein should be planned in Sara's diet?
3 Should dietary sodium be restricted? If so, how much?

REFERENCES

1 A. J. Vander, *Renal Physiology,* McGraw-Hill Book Company, New York, 1975, pp. 128–129.

2 H. F. DeLuca, "The Kidney as an Endocrine Organ Involved in The Function of Vitamin D," *American Journal of Medicine,* **58:**39–47, 1975.

3 C. F. Anderson, R. A. Nelson, J. D. Margie, W. J. Johnson, and J. D. Hunt, "Nutritional Therapy for Adults with Renal Disease," *Journal of the American Medical Association,* **222:**69, 1973.

4 D. W. Seldin, N. W. Carter, and F. C. Rector, Jr., "Consequences of Renal Failure and Their Management," in M. B. Strauss and L. G. Welt (eds.), *Diseases of the Kidney,* 2d ed. Little, Brown & Co., Boston, 1971, p. 654.

5 A. C. Schoolwerth, and J. E. Engle, "Calcium and Phosphorus in Diet Therapy of Uremia," *Journal of The American Dietetic Association,* **66:**460–464, 1975.

6 J. P. Merrill, "Acute Renal Failure," in M. B. Strauss and L. G. Welt, op. cit., p. 654.

7 R. M. Abel, C. H. Beck, W. M. Abbott, J. A. Ryan, Jr., C. O. Barnett, and J. E. Fischer, "Improved Survival from Acute Renal Failure After Treatment with Intravenous Essential L-Amino Acids and Glucose; Results of a Prospective, Double Blind Study," *New England Journal of Medicine,* **288:**695–699, 1973.

8 S. J. Dudrick, E. Steiger, and J. M. Long, "Renal Failure in Surgical Patients. Treatment with Essential Amino Acids and Hypertonic Glucose," *Surgery,* **68:**180–186, 1970.

9 R. M. Abel, W. M. Abbott, C. H. Beck, Jr., J. A. Ryan, and J. E. Fischer, "Essential L-Amino Acids for Hyperalimentation in Patients with Disordered Nitrogen Metabolism," *American Journal of Surgery,* **128:**314–323, 1974.

10 G. L. Bailey, *Hemodialysis Principles and Practice,* Academic Press, Inc., New York, 1972, Chap. 1.

11 G. L. Bailey, and N. R. Sullivan, "Selected Protein Diet in Terminal Uremia," *Journal of The American Dietetic Association,* **52:**125–259, 1968.

12 C. Giordano, "Use of Exogenous and Endogenous Urea for Protein Synthesis in Normal and Uremic Subjects," *Journal of Laboratory and Clinical Medicine,* **62:**231.

13 S. Giovannetti, and Q. Maggiore, "A Low Nitrogen Diet with Protein of High Biological Value for Severe Chronic Uremia," *Lancet,* **1:**1000, 1964.

14 B. T. Burton, "Current Concepts of Nutrition and Diet in Diseases of the Kidney. Part II, Dietary Regimen in Specific Kidney Disorders," *Journal of the American Dietetic Association,* **65:**631, 1974.

15 J. Burge, "Vitamin Requirements of Hemodialysis Patients," *Dialysis and Transplantation,* October/November 1974.

16 N. S. Spinozzi, Personal communication, 1976. (Renal Dietitian, Children's Hospital Medical Center, Boston, Mass.)

17 C. Chantler and M. A. Holliday, "Growth in Children with Renal Disease with Particular Reference to the Effects of Calorie Malnutrition: A Review," *Clinical Nephrology,* **1:**230–242, 1975.

18 N. B. Levy, (ed.), *Living or Dying, Adaptation to Hemodialysis,* Charles C Thomas, Publisher Springfield, Ill., 1974.

19 M. K. Landsman, "The Patient with Chronic Renal Failure: A Marginal Man," *Annals of Internal Medicine,* **82:**268–270, 1975.

20 P. G. Stein and J. J. Winn, "Diet Control in Sodium, Potassium, Protein, and Fluid: Use of Points for Dietary Calculation," *Journal of The American Dietetic Association,* **62:**538–551, 1972.

21 F. N. Fine and B. M. Korsch, "Renal Transplantation in Children," *Hospital Practice,* March 1974, pp. 61–69.

22 M. A. Topor, "Kidney Transplantation, Especially in Pediatric Patients," *Nursing Clinics of North America,* **10:**503–516, 1975.

23 H. E. Williams, "Nephrolithiasis; Physiology in Medicine," *New England Journal of Medicine,* **290:**33, 1974.

24 C. Y. C. Pak, C. S. Delea, and F. C. Bartter, "Successful Treatment of Recurrent Nephrolithiasis (Calcium Stones) with Cellulose Phosphate," *New England Journal of Medicine,* **290:**175–180, 1974.

CHAPTER 20

THE ENDOCRINE SYSTEM AND SKELETAL DISORDERS

Susan K. Golovin

KEY WORDS
Hyperthyroidism
Goiter
Myxedema
Addisonian Crisis
Growth Hormone
Polyuria
Cortisol
Corticosteroids
Polyuria
Polyphagia
Polydipsia
Ketosis
Hypoglycemia
Gouty Attack

INTRODUCTION

The endocrine system consists of a series of ductless glands scattered throughout the body: thyroid, parathyroids, pituitary, adrenals, and pancreas, the reproductive organs, (with some dispute) the thymus. The pineal body is also recognized as an endocrine gland, acting as a neuroendocrine modulator of hypothalamic function. The endocrine system is one of the two major control systems of the body. The other system, the nervous system, is functionally interrelated, for the level of hormone secretion is under the control of the nervous system and the level of hormones affects the nervous system directly or indirectly. The endocrine system and its glands primarily control metabolic processes, growth, maturation, and reproduction; and integrate the body's response to stress.

The hormones secreted by the endocrine glands either follow a rhythmic pattern or are secreted in response to blood levels of a specific substance, such as sodium, water, sugar, calcium, or another hormone. In health, the blood levels of each hormone are maintained at specific levels. Disease of any of the endocrine glands may cause an increase or decrease in hormone secretion, and the resultant symptoms of dysfunction are those of increased or decreased regulation of the bodily processes that are normally controlled by the gland and its specific hormone.

This chapter will consider the physiology and the malfunction of those glands of the endocrine system where diet therapy is involved, with particular focus on the pancreas, since the treatment of the disease process diabetes mellitus primarily involves diet therapy. In addition, the role of diet therapy in diseases of the bones and joints will be considered.

THYROID

Physiology

The thyroid gland is located below the larynx on both sides, and anterior to the trachea. The

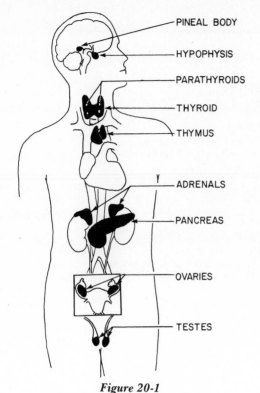

PINEAL BODY

HYPOPHYSIS

PARATHYROIDS

THYROID

THYMUS

ADRENALS

PANCREAS

OVARIES

TESTES

Figure 20-1
The glands of the endocrine system.

function of the thyroid gland is twofold: (1) It maintains an optimal metabolic level in the tissues by stimulating the oxygen consumption of most body cells and by helping to regulate lipid and carbohydrate metabolism, and (2) it establishes or permits the long-term functions of growth and promotes skeletal maturation.

In order to accomplish these functions, the thyroid secretes three hormones, thyroxine (T_4), triiodothyronine (T_3), and thyrocalcitonin. The raw material essential for thyroid hormone synthesis is iodine. Iodine, once ingested, is converted to iodide and is absorbed, remaining chiefly in the extracellular fluids except for that portion taken up by the thyroid gland. Small amounts of excess iodide not taken up by the thyroid gland are excreted in the urine. A minimum daily intake of 100 to 150 μg of iodine is needed to maintain normal thyroid function.

The thyroid gland collects and concentrates iodide from the blood, converts iodide to thyroid hormone, and stores some of these hormones and secretes the remainder into the blood for distribution to all cells of the body. The function of the thyroid gland is controlled by a secretion of the anterior lobe of the pituitary known as thyroid-stimulating hormone or TSH. TSH secretion is regulated in part by the pituitary, which is sensitive to high levels of circulating thyroid hormone, and in part by neural mechanisms mediated through the hypothalamus.

Thyroid hormone has an effect on many of the biochemical processes within the body:

1 *Metabolic rate* Increases oxygen consumption by tissues that are metabolically active.
2 *Metabolism of protein, lipids, and carbohydrates*
   a *Protein* Favors protein anabolism; however, in large doses thyroid hormone stimulates protein catabolism, leading to negative nitrogen balance.
   b *Lipids* Increases the oxidative processes of fat metabolism and increases the rate of both the biosynthesis and catabolism of cholesterol in the liver and extrahepatic tissue.
   c *Carbohydrates* Increases the rate of glucose absorption from the gastrointestinal tract and increases utilization of glucose by the cells.
3 *Cardiovascular function* Increases the blood flow, cardiac output, and heart rate, stimulates myocardial metabolism, and maintains hematopoiesis.
4 *Central nervous system* Increases mental acuity.
5 *Growth and tissue differentiation* Essential for normal growth.
6 *Vitamin metabolism* Increases the quantity of enzymes and, since vitamins are an essential part of enzymes or coenzymes, thyroid hormone causes an increased need for vitamins.

The consequence of thyroid dysfunction is reflected in the secretion of too much or too little thyroid hormone, which in turn affects all or some of the above functions. Table 20-1

TABLE 20-1   THYROID FUNCTION TESTS

Test	Description	Average values*
Radioactive iodine uptake (RAI)	Tracer doses of ^{131}I are given orally and thyroid uptake is measured by a gamma ray counter. Used in diagnosing hyperthyroidism.	10–50% 24 h
Thyroxine (T$_4$)	Measures free thyroxine which determines metabolic status. Used in diagnosing both hyper- and hypothyroidism.	4–11% (resin sponge uptake)
Triiodothyronine (T$_3$)	Measures triiodothyronine. Used in diagnosing hyper- and hypothyroidism.	24–36% (resin sponge uptake)
Thyroid-stimulating hormone (TSH)	TSH blood levels are valuable in providing a differential diagnosis. Elevated TSH levels are seen in hypothroidism due to primary thyroid failure. Decreased TSH levels are seen in secondary hypothyroidism due to hypothalamic or pituitary disease.	up to 0.2 mU/ml

* *Source:* J. Wallach, *Interpretation of Diagnostic Tests,* 2d ed., Little, Brown and Company, Boston, 1974.

summarizes the most commonly used tests to evaluate thyroid function.

Hypothyroidism

Hypothyroidism is an endocrine disorder manifested by a decrease in thyroxine activity. Thyroxine (T$_4$) may be suppressed by a number of factors:

1 Inadequate consumption of iodine
2 High intake of goitrogens
3 An inborn error of metabolism

The first few months of life constitute a critical period at which time T$_4$ and T$_3$ must be present for normal cerebral development, and the lack of hormone results in defective myelinization and severely retarded mental development.

Cretinism is a condition resulting from early hypothyroidism. Cretinous children are dwarfed, with large protruding tongues and bellies. They are the product of a prolonged pregnancy and at birth have an above-normal birth weight and length, are puffy and cyanotic, and show retarded prenatal osseous development and prolonged neonatal jaundice. Treatment begun after the first few months of life for the most part is ineffective and results in mental retardation.

Those who develop hypothyroidism as children grow slowly and show delayed epiphyseal closure. Hypothyroid children may exhibit the following: lack of energy, respiratory infection, constipation due to decreased peristalsis, decreased linear growth, thick scaly skin with a yellow tinge and some mottling, cardiac enlargement, bradycardia, and depressed thyroid function tests [T_3, T_4, and radioactive iodine (RAI) uptake].

Also, because of an abnormality in nitrogen metabolism there is deposition of mucoprotein in subcutaneous and extracellular spaces. This material is osmotically active and results in fluid retention. This watery, mucus-like substance is responsible for dry swelling with abnormal mucin deposits in the skin, giving a puffy look to the face.

Since thyroid hormones must be present for heat production, hypothyroid individuals usually experience cold intolerance. Also, T_4 and T_3 promote catabolism of carbohydrate and fat; therefore, hypothyroidism results in a decreased rate of cholesterol breakdown, causing an increase in serum cholesterol to over 300 mg/100 ml in a large proportion of patients.

Obesity is not a problem related to the condition, for even though catabolism is low, appetite also becomes depressed. There may be moderate anemia as a result of decreased bone marrow metabolism and poor vitamin B_{12} absorption from the intestine.

Hormone therapy is used for treatment. In children a delicate balance must be maintained in order to provide sufficient hormones to maintain positive nitrogen balance without precipitating protein catabolism and growth deficits.

Endemic Goiter

When exogenous iodine intake falls below 10 μg per day, thyroxine levels are insufficient. This results in increased TSH secretion and ultimately in thyroid hypertrophy. This condition, known as *iodine-deficiency goiter,* was common in the United States, in the Great Lakes area, before the advent of iodized salt. The classic cases of these endemic goiters occur in regions where iodine is lacking (and therefore iodine intake is low) because of low

environmental soil and water resources. Another cause of endemic goiter is attributed to goitrogens. *Goitrogens* are vegetables of the Brassicaceae family, notably cabbage, rutabagas, and turnips, which contain progoitrin, as well as a substance which converts progoitrin into goitrin, an active antithyroid agent. Progoitrin activator is heat-labile, yet some activators remain even if the vegetables are cooked. Usually, these goitrins present no problems. However, large consumption by those with low iodine intake could possibly result in the so-called "cabbage goiter."

Goiter, for some unknown reason, will sometimes develop in people with normal thyroid function (euthyroids) who take cough medicines that are high in iodine. There is some possibility that goiter can be induced by a high iodine intake since large surveys in the United States found high urinary iodine and high iodine intake in people with goiters living in goiter-prevalent areas. This is of interest, since the average American diet often consists of such high-iodine foods as seafood, iodized salt, milk, bread made with iodate dough conditioners, and foods with iodine-containing dyes, not to mention iodine residues from compounds used to sterilize commercial processing equipment. A varied United States diet, containing 2 to 6 g of iodized salt, provides approximately 500 μg of iodine per day.

Hypothyroidism sometimes accompanies endemic goiter, while hyperthyroidism is rarely identified with the condition. If the goiter is progressive and multinodular, iodine will be of little help. However, in the early hyperplastic state, endemic goiter will regress with iodine intake.

A daily intake of 100 μg of iodine is recommended for adults, with somewhat higher levels for adolescents and pregnant and lactating women.

Graves' Disease

Graves' disease is a combination of goiter, hyperthyroidism, and exophthalmos (protruding eyeballs). The occurrence of the disease is rare before age 10 and unlikely in the elderly. The condition is more prevalent among females than males (seven to one).

General symptoms include nervousness, exophthalmos, hyperexcitability, irritability, restlessness, emotional instability, weight loss, increased bowel motility, tremor, sweating, and heat intolerance. T_4, T_3, and RAI uptake are increased. When the metabolic rate increases, the need for all vitamins increases. Despite this, documentation of actual vitamin deficiencies is infrequent. However, endogenous protein and fat stores are catabolized, and weight loss persists even though the patient has an excessive appetite.

The excess of T_4 and T_3 results in bone demineralization, and therefore high urinary and fecal loss of calcium and phosphorus. Also, hyperthyroidism puts a heavy load on the cardiovascular system. Cardiac output increases, as does pulse rate, while circulation time decreases, thus producing tachycardia and tremor, and a rise in body temperature. In addition, the excess of T_4 and T_3 increases carbohydrate absorption from the intestine, causing a rise in blood sugar after a carbohydrate meal and possibly glycosuria if the renal threshold is exceeded.

Treatment

Diet therapy Until the hyperthyroidism is controlled, ample energy intake is necessary to protect body tissues and to prevent weight loss. Mild hyperthyroidism calls for a 15 to 25 percent increase above the normal recommended dietary energy allowance, and severe hyperthyroidism, a 50 to 75 percent increase, which may mean a diet containing 4500 to 5000 kcal (18.9 to 21 MJ). In addition, protein allowance should be liberal: approximately 1 to 2 g/kg of ideal body weight. Carbohydrate intake should be increased to compensate for disturbed carbohydrate metabolism, to provide energy, and to spare protein; the increased carbohydrate intake necessitates an increased thiamine intake, which is essential for energy metabolism. Water should be adequate to compensate for losses incurred by the increased metabolic rate, sweating, and heavy breathing. The mineral and vitamin requirements—especially calcium, phosphorus, and the B vitamins—may have to be supplemented. One quart of milk per day can help to enhance calcium balance and will provide protein.

Stimulants, such as coffee, tea, and tobacco, should be eliminated, as they further aggravate symptoms of nervousness, etc. Alcohol should receive a doctor's clearance before being incorporated into the diet, as individual tolerances differ.

It is necessary to counsel the patient to be conscious of the fact that once hyperthyroidism is treated, obesity could be a problem if the excessive intake established during the hyperthyroid period continues.

Drug therapy Drug therapy consists of agents which block the iodine uptake by the thyroid and therefore prevent thyroid hormone synthesis. PTU (propylthiouracil) a synthetic goitrogen, is one such drug.

Exogenous thyroid hormone has not been documented to have any general usefulness for weight reduction. In fact, it can make one nervous and heat-intolerant; i.e., it can cause symptoms similar to hyperthyroidism. Short-term weight loss may occur if the individual's activity level increases in response to these symptoms. Exogenous thyroid hormone is contraindicated for those with cardiovascular disorders. Further, the hypermetabolism caused by excess thyroid hormone increases the body's demand for adrenal hormones. Thus, thyroid hormone administration may result in an acute adrenal insufficiency, especially if the patient already has adrenal insufficiency or hypopituitarism. Also, thyroid hormone may increase appetite.

THYMUS

The thymus gland, located in the chest cavity just above the heart, is large in infancy, and undergoes progressive atrophy after puberty. It is primarily a lymphoid organ, producing the antibodies necessary for the body's immune response. (See Chap. 16)

PARATHYROID

Physiology

Although location and number may vary, in general, humans have four parathyroids, two located in the superior poles and two in the inferior poles of the thyroid. The main function of the glands, is maintenance of a constant ionized calcium level in the extracellular fluid, which is necessary for blood coagulation, normal cardiac and skeletal muscle contraction, and nerve function. The circulating level of ionized calcium acts directly on the parathyroid glands in feedback fashion to regulate parathyroid hormone excretion. When plasma calcium is high, hormone secretion falls, and calcium is absorbed by the bones. When plasma calcium falls, parathyroid hormone increases, and calcium is mobilized from the bone. Further, the parathyroid stimulates the intestinal mucosa to increase calcium absorption and excrete phosphate. This mechanism is yet to be clearly defined. Also, the serum phosphorus is maintained via a homeostatic mechanism controlled by the parathyroid gland. As the serum phosphorus increases, the parathyroid hormone acts to inhibit the kidney from reabsorbing phosphorus. Phosphorus excretion (in the urine) increases, and the normal serum calcium/phosphorus ratio returns.

Tetany

Tetany is a condition caused by a disturbance of calcium and phosphorus metabolism, or by inadvertent parathyroidectomy during thyroid surgery. Tetany can be classified as:

1 Alkalotic tetany, usually due to hyperventilation or vomiting
2 Hypocalcemic tetany, associated with rickets, osteomalacia, steatorrhea, and renal insufficiency; in newborns, temporary hypofunction of the parathyroid, causing tetany, may be precipitated by feeding an overload of phosphate, in the form of cow's milk

Symptoms of tetany include convulsions, cramps, and muscle twitching. Total plasma calcium may fall as low as 4 mg/100 ml (normal 8.5 to 10.5 mg/100 ml).

The major goal of treatment is to restore plasma calcium without precipitating marked hypercalcemia or hypercalciuria. Dietary recommendation is for a high-calcium (1800 to 2400 mg), low-phosphorus diet. This is difficult to achieve, however, since most foods high in calcium, for example, milk, also contain high levels of phosphorus. Aluminum salts are used to decrease the absorption of dietary phosphorus.

A vitamin D supplement of 100,000 units is recommended (to enhance calcium absorption); however, the patient must be carefully monitored to avoid hypervitaminosis D (see Chap. 6). A more practical approach is to limit the intake of milk and milk products, and to supplement the diet with calcium compounds. (see Table 20-2). This allows a normal complement of calcium, yet avoids increasing the phosphorus levels.

ADRENALS

The adrenals are small, paired structures lying on either side of the midline of the abdominal cavity, above the kidneys. Each gland consists of an outer cortex and inner medulla. The cortex secretes the following steroids (analogs,

TABLE 20-2 CALCIUM SUPPLEMENTS

Compound	Calcium content	Possible route	Oral dose
Calcium gluconate	9%	Oral, IV, IM	15 g daily in divided doses
Calcium lactate	13%	Oral	5 g 3 times a day
Calcium chloride	27%	Oral, IV	6–8 g in divided doses; best with milk
Calcium levulinate	13%	Oral, IV	4–5 g 3 times a day with meals
Calcium carbonate	40%	Oral	1 g 4 times a day

IV = intravenous; IM = intramuscular.

known as *corticosteroids*): cortisol and corticosterone, which are referred to as *glucocorticoids;* secreted in response to physical and emotional stress; and aldosterone, a *mineralocorticoid,* which maintains sodium balance and extracellular fluid volume. The adrenal medulla secretes the catecholamines epinephrine and norepinephrine, which, although not life-sustaining, help to integrate the body's reaction to stress.

Cushing's Syndrome

Cushing's syndrome (or disease) is glucocorticoid excess caused by lesions in the hypothalamus; adrenocorticotropic hormone (ACTH)-secreting tumors of the pituitary, lung, or elsewhere; tumors of the adrenal cortex; idiopathic adrenal hyperplasia; or excess corticosteroid therapy.

Since glucocorticoids increase protein catabolism, the patient with uncontrolled Cushing's syndrome is protein-depleted. The amino acids from catabolism are converted into glucose by the liver, causing blood sugar to rise. This, coupled with the anti-insulin effect of glucocorticoids on the peripheral tissues, causes a decrease in the body's use of glucose, and diabetes mellitus may develop. Of those with Cushing's disease 80 percent have an ab-

normal glucose tolerance test and 20 percent have overt diabetes mellitus. Other symptoms include thin skin and subcutaneous tissues, poorly developed muscles, and thin, scraggly hair. Minor injuries result in bruises and ecchymoses, wounds heal poorly, and growth is inhibited in children.

Significant mineralocorticoid excess is responsible for the characteristic "moon face," as it causes considerable sodium and water retention. Potassium depletion and weakness are also part of the pathology. Eighty-five percent of these patients have high blood pressure, which can be attributed to the glucocorticoid effect on blood vessels.

There is not necessarily a weight gain, but there is a redistribution of fat to the back of the neck ("buffalo hump") and supraclavicular regions. Relatively thin extremities accentuate an enlarged abdomen. Purple striae are common, and are located over the abdomen, thighs, and upper arms.

A high-protein diet (1 g/kg of body weight) is recommended to prevent or correct negative nitrogen balance. Sodium restriction may be useful in decreasing fluid retention.

The steroid used to treat Cushing's syndrome can result in osteoporosis (a softening and demineralization of the bone). The osteoporosis is caused by protein catabolism which inhibits new bone formation and breaks down existing bone matrix. Further, glucocorticoids not only have an anti-vitamin D action, but also increase the glomerular filtration rate, thus increasing calcium secretion.

Total adrenalectomy is the treatment of choice for progressive Cushing's disease. Partial adrenalectomy does not eliminate the possible recurrence of the syndrome. Of course, a total adrenalectomy results in adrenocortical insufficiency, or Addison's disease, which is far easier to treat.

Addison's Disease

Addison's disease, or adrenocortical insufficiency, can be due to destruction of the adrenal by tuberculosis (now a rare cause), adrenal atrophy due to unknown (probably immunological) damage, corticosteroid withdrawal after long-term treatment, or surgical removal of the adrenals to treat Cushing's syndrome. Currently, metastatic malignancy is increasingly the cause.

In normal individuals, aldosterone maintains extracellular fluid volume. With adrenal insufficiency, there is decreased sodium absorption, and increased sodium ion excretion by the kidneys as a result of insufficient secretion of aldosterone by the adrenals. Chloride ions and water are secreted into the urine in large quantities, causing decreased extracellular volume and low blood pressure. The body responds by retaining potassium, causing high serum potassium levels. If the disease is untreated, blood volume falls, precipitating the *Addisonian crisis.*

Classic symptoms of Addisonian crisis include shock, low serum sodium, high serum potassium, and low serum glucose. Other symptoms, precrisis, include poor heat tolerance from high levels of sodium in the perspiration, and abdominal discomfort and diarrhea, because of the inability to reabsorb fluid from the intestinal lumen at normal rates. Also, there may be a low serum glucose, anorexia, vomiting, weight loss, and dermal

pigmentation due to high levels of certain hormones, namely melanocyte-stimulating hormone (MSH) and adrenocorticotropic hormone (ACTH).

Treatment consists of replacement of adrenocortical hormones. This is accomplished with cortisol, which should be taken with meals to minimize gastric irritation. Weight gain is a complication of this therapy.

Patients taking cortisol should be monitored for a high salt intake. The salt intake should approximate 10 g/day. High-salt foods (such as condiments, potato chips, and cold cuts) plus 3 or 4 salt tablets with meals are recommended to achieve this level. Nevertheless, about 70 percent of patients require a sodium-retaining hormone, such as the mineralocorticoid desoxycorticosterone, to prevent orthostatic hypotension. In a few cases only salt therapy is required.

The low blood sugar necessitates small, frequent high-protein, low-carbohydrate meals, as well as a bedtime snack. Fasting can lead to hypoglycemic episodes. A high fluid intake will help to alleviate the threat of dehydration. Foods extremely high in potassium, such as bananas and orange juice, should be avoided, but there is no reason for severe restriction. If mineralocorticoid therapy is prolonged, symptoms such as cardiac arrhythmias and headaches can occur because of potassium depletion. In this case, the patient requires supplemental potassium, and salt intake should be decreased until sodium balance is achieved.

Corticosteroid Therapy

Since glucocorticoids have an antiinflammatory and antiallergenic effect, they are used to treat a host of diseases or conditions that have an allergic or autoimmune component (e.g., hives, rheumatoid arthritis.) With such therapy, it is important to consider diet-drug interrelationships.

An adjunct of corticosteroid therapy is weight gain due to appetite stimulation and fluid retention. If there is no need to increase sodium intake (as there is with Addison's disease), sodium should be restricted (some recommend less than 500 mg/day).

Therapeutic cortisone may result in negative nitrogen balance. Therefore the diet for patients taking this medication should be high in protein, and high in carbohydrate to spare protein. Cortisone therapy can also precipitate hypokalemia, in which case supplemental potassium must be taken with meals.

Adrenocortical steroid therapy, including ACTH and glucocorticoids, increases gastric acid and pepsin secretion, and may alter the resistance of the mucosa to these secretions and cause irritation. This may induce peptic ulcers which could ultimately hemorrhage. Therefore, patients on this therapy must be advised to take frequent (small) meals.

The diet for someone on prolonged ACTH therapy is high in protein (100 g), high in carbohydrate (200 to 300 g), and low in sodium (1000 mg), is divided into frequent small feedings, and includes a vitamin C supplement, since ACTH depletes the adrenal tissue of vitamin C.

PITUITARY

The pituitary gland (also called the hypophysis) is about the size of a large pea, and lies just beneath the hypothalamus of the brain, to which it is connected by the pituitary or hypophyseal stalk. Although small, it is a complex structure composed of 2 lobes, the anterior lobe and the posterior lobe, each separately responsible for the secretion of hormones (see Table 20-3).

These hormones are released from the an-

TABLE 20-3 PITUITARY HORMONES AND THEIR FUNCTION

Hormone	Function
Anterior pituitary hormones	
Growth hormone (Somatotropin)	Promotes growth by influencing metabolic functions, especially protein formation
	Decreases the rate of carbohydrate utilization throughout the body
	Increases the mobilization of fats and the use of fats for energy
Corticotropin (Adrenocorticotropic hormone, ACTH)	Affects the secretion of the adrenocortical hormones which affect metabolism of protein, carbohydrate, and fat
Thyrotropin	Controls the amount of thyroxine secreted by the thyroid gland
Gonadotropins	Influences reproductive activities
Posterior pituitary hormones	
Antidiuretic hormone (Vaso Pressin)	Affects the rate of water excretion
Oxytocin	Helps to mobilize milk from the glands to the nipple during lactation upon suckling

terior pituitary in response to *neurohormones* (formerly called *releasing factors*) which are produced in the hypothalamus in response to nervous, hormonal, and other influences. In certain disease states or conditions, this feedback mechanism between the hypothalamus and the pituitary becomes altered. This fact has caused some authorities to relate this mechanism to the etiology of nonorganic failure to thrive, a condition in which the child, despite adequate food intake, fails to grow. They regard these children as having clinical findings suggestive of idiopathic hypopituitarism, and raise the question of whether these children respond to an adverse family environment and emotional deprivation by an altered release of growth hormone from the pituitary. These children present with a perverted or voracious appetite and are either excessively passive or aggressive in behavior. Improvement is noted with changes in parental management or placement in a stimulating environment. (See Chap. 11.)

Growth hormone (somatotropic hormone or somatotropin) plays a significant role in the normal growth and development of the human body by promoting protein synthesis in all body organs through the transport of amino acids into the cell; it thus aids in determining the rate of organ enlargement. Also, growth hormone controls growth in bone length by controlling cartilage production in the ends of long bones, a process known as *chondrogenesis.*

The secretion of growth hormone is related to a person's nutritional status. Growth hormone increases during the hypoglycemia that is seen in states of starvation and fasting as protein stores are depleted. During these periods, an inverse relationship is noted, with growth hormone secretion increasing as protein stores decrease. This has clinical application in the treatment of kwashiorkor: when adequate protein is provided, a reversal in growth hormone secretion occurs, thereby normalizing carbohydrate and fat metabolism. Adequate calories (joules) alone are not sufficient to cor-

rect the excess production of growth hormone.

The conditions resulting from altered pituitary function are summarized in Table 20-4; for the most part these do not necessitate dietary intervention.

PANCREAS

The pancreas is a carrot-shaped gland located along the greater curvature of the stomach. It is a double gland with an *exocrine portion* producing the digestive enzymes (amylase, lipase, trypsin) and an *endocrine portion* producing the hormones glucagon and insulin, on which we will focus. (The role of the pancreas in digestion is discussed in Chap. 9.)

Small islets of endocrine tissue known as the islets of Langerhans (islets are small masses of one type of tissue within another) are found in the pancreas. Their numbers have been estimated to be between 500,000 and 2 million. Each islet is well supplied with blood vessels and contains two types of cells, *alpha cells* and *beta cells,* each responsible for hormone production:

> *Alpha cells* Secrete *glucagon,* a hormone that speeds the conversion of glycogen to glucose and thereby raises blood glucose level; thus, glucagon has a *hyperglycemic effect.*
>
> *Beta cells* Secrete *insulin,* a hormone that is necessary for cellular uptake of glucose and also speeds the synthesis of glycogen in the liver—both actions draw sugar from the blood; therefore, insulin has a *hypoglycemic effect.*

The secretion of both glucagon and insulin is controlled by the blood glucose level. When blood sugar falls, glucagon is secreted; when blood sugar rises, insulin is secreted, causing blood sugar to be maintained within the narrow limits of 80 to 100 mg/100 ml.

Presently, there is no named disease associated with glucagon secretion, although there

TABLE 20-4 CONDITIONS RESULTING FROM ALTERED PITUITARY FUNCTION

Condition	Mechanism	Diet commentary
Acromegaly	↑ Growth hormone	Diabetes is a complication and diet is part of the treatment
Pituitary dwarfism	↓ Overall pituitary hormones ↓ Thyroid function ↓ Adrenal function	
Diabetes insipidus	↓ Antidiuretic hormone	Weight loss can be a problem because of patient's fear of drinking fluids and a lack of sleep due to increased urination
Precocious puberty	The hypothalamic mechanism which initiates puberty is activated earlier than usual, and stimulates pituitary to release gonadotropic hormones	

↑ = increased; ↓ = decreased.

are reports of patients with chronic low blood sugar associated with a lack or deficiency of alpha cells, an apparently hereditary disorder. The disease impairing insulin secretion, diabetes mellitus, we will consider in detail, since this disease now affects 5 percent of the population in the United States (also a decline in glucose tolerance is now a recognized phenomenon of aging) and diet is the cornerstone of treatment.

Diabetes Mellitus

Diabetes was first noted by the Egyptians in the year 1500 B.C. During the first century a Greek physician described a condition in which the body excreted large quantities of urine. He called this phenomenon *diabetes* from the Greek word meaning "to flow through." Centuries later the Latin word *mellitus,* "honeyed," was added to describe the glucose-laden urine.

In 1952 F. G. Banting and C. H. Best discovered insulin. Although its exact action is not clear it is believed to serve in the following functions:

1 Transportation of glucose through cell membranes

2 Conversion of glucose to glycogen and storage in the liver (glycogenesis)

3 Conversion of glucose to fat (lipogenesis)

4 Oxidation of glucose via the glycolytic pathway by phosphorylation catalyzed by glucokinase

The symptoms of diabetes mellitus show how these metabolic processes are affected by insulin deficiency. The sequence of symptoms is as follows:

Hyperglycemia An abnormally high blood sugar. The blood sugar may reach between

300 and 1200 mg/100 ml from failure of the liver to synthesize glycogen and failure of the cells throughout the body to utilize glucose. This causes the blood sugar to rise and the kidneys to exceed their capacity to reabsorb glucose (i.e. glucose levels reach the renal threshold), which means that glucose spills into the urine. When blood sugar exceeds 180 mg/100 ml, sugar spills into the urine, causing *glycosuria*.

↓

Glycosuria Sugar in the urine. The excretion of large amounts of glucose, which is osmotically attracted to water, means that large amounts of water are excreted (osmotic diuresis), along with the loss of urinary sodium and potassium. Glycosuria causes *polyuria*.

↓

Polyuria The secretion of large amounts of urine. The excessive water loss, along with excretion of electrolytes from the extracellular fluid, affect the intracellular fluid, with the net effect of intracellular and extracellular dehydration, stimulating *polydipsia*.

↓

Polydipsia Increased or excessive thirst due to water loss.

Because of the body's inability to utilize glucose for energy and the loss of glucose in the urine (every gram of glucose lost represents 4.1 kcal or 17.2 kJ), the body is left in a state of starvation manifested by an excessive appetite and excessive food intake, known as *polyphagia*.

Polyphagia Excessive food intake. Despite excessive food intake, the body's inability to utilize glucose causes protein and fat stores to be mobilized for energy, resulting in muscle wasting and *weight loss*. The body's reliance on fat stores for an energy source causes an accumulation of ketones and the state of *ketosis* develops.

↓

Ketosis During the body's accelerated lipolysis of fats, an increase of fatty acids is sent to the liver, resulting in an accelerated formation of ketone bodies (β-hydroxybutyric acid, acetoacetic acid, acetone). These ketone bodies are released into the bloodstream and are metabolized to some extent but are then excreted in the urine as a result of overproduction. (The presence of ketone bodies in the urine is detected by a positive Acetest reaction.) Since these ketoacids have a low threshold for excretion and about one-half need sodium for excretion, sodium is drawn from the extracellular fluid. As a result, the sodium concentration in the extracellular fluid usually decreases, and the loss of this basic ion adds to the acidosis already caused by the excessive ketoacids in the extracellular fluid. Subsequently, all the reactions that take place in metabolic acidosis take place in diabetic acidosis (see Chap 8). These include *Kussmaul respiration* (rapid and deep breathing), causing excessive expiration of carbon dioxide; a marked decrease in the bicarbonate content of the extracellular fluids; and excretion of chloride ions by the kidneys. The resultant shift in the fluid compartment causes hypovolemia (low blood pressure) leading to *diabetic coma* and death. These extreme effects occur only in the most severe degrees of untreated diabetes.

(Note: The breath of poorly controlled diabetics smells fruity because of the expired ketone bodies. This helps to differentiate between diabetic coma and insulin reaction.)

Polyuria (excessive elimination of urine), *polydipsia* (excessive thirst, *Polyphagia* (excessive eating), *weight loss*, and *asthenia* (lack of energy) are the earliest symptoms of diabetes. The diagnosis of diabetes is established by the following procedures.

Diagnosis of diabetes mellitus If a physician suspects that a patient is manifesting symptoms characteristic of diabetes, an oral glucose tolerance test (GTT) may be ordered to confirm the

TABLE 20-5 ADMINISTRATION OF THE ORAL GLUCOSE TOLERANCE TEST

Glucose dose		Diet	Special considerations
Child	Adult		
1 g/kg of body weight; under the age of 18 months, 3 g/kg.	1.75 g/kg of body weight or approximately 75–100 g of glucose	150-g carbohydrate diet for 3 days prior to the test. Patient fasts overnight. No caffeine or nicotine for 12 h prior to the test	The following medications may influence results: Dilantin Thiazide diuretics Glucocorticoids Oral contraceptives

diagnosis. (See Table 20-5.) When a diabetic is given a glucose load, the blood sugar will rise higher and return to normal more slowly than occurs in a nondiabetic. (See Fig. 20-2.) If a patient has experienced symptoms of diabetes and has had an elevated 2-h postprandial blood sugar determination (postprandial = after meals), it is not necessary to tax the body further with a glucose load. It is not recommended that one administer a glucose tolerance test while a person is hospitalized, as the imposed sedentary life results in a blood sugar level that is higher than normal because of the lack of activity.

The nurse or nutritionist can assist by explaining the diet preceding the test, the administration of the glucose, and the collection of blood samples. With children, commercially prepared glucose solutions might be more acceptable if given in their own cup or through a straw, and special games or some entertainment should be planned to amuse the child during the period of blood sample collection. Blood sugar values are taken when the patient is fasting and at 1, 2, and 3 h after glucose administration (see U.S. Public Health Service Criteria, Fig. 20-2), and urine samples are collected for sugar determinations.

Another possible future diagnostic tool is the determination of hemoglobin A_{1C}, a glycoprotein which is the most abundant minor hemoglobin component in human erythrocytes. Research interest was sparked by the finding that hemoglobin A_{1C} levels are twice as high in diabetics as in nondiabetics and research further indicates that the diabetics' level

of hemoglobin A_{1C}, if measured over a sufficient time span, may reflect adequacy of control of the disease.

Classification of diabetes mellitus Diabetes mellitus can be classified according to onset into

Figure 20-2
(1) U.S. Public Health Service criteria for diagnosing diabetes after administration of an oral glucose tolerance test. (2) Normal and abnormal glycose curves after administration of a glucose tolerance test.

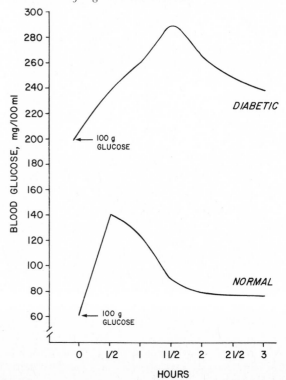

juvenile-onset type or *ketosis-prone* and *adult-onset type* or *non-ketosis-prone.*

Juvenile-onset type This type of diabetes mellitus generally manifests itself when the patient is young. Onset is sudden with a presentation of the full spectrum of symptoms. The body's total dependence on an exogenous supply of insulin causes the juvenile-type diabetic to be ketosis-prone.

Adult-onset type The maturity-onset type becomes manifest in patients generally over 40 years of age; however, some adults do develop juvenile-type diabetes and must depend on an exogenous source of insulin. Because patients with adult-type diabetes continue to produce some of their own insulin, they are not prone to ketosis. Characteristically, the patient is obese, and presents with one or two mild symptoms such as nocturnal polyuria and fatigue.

As a clinical entity, diabetes mellitus progresses according to certain stages: the *prediabetic*, the *chemical*, and the *overt stages, and chronic diabetes.* This so-called natural history or stage of disease development may progress rapidly or slowly or not at all and in some cases the diabetes may temporarily disappear. The following is a generalized schema and does not represent a definite pattern.

Prediabetes The stage that exists prior to identifiable diabetes mellitus. It includes the time from conception to the time of impaired glucose tolerance. During this period, a glucose tolerance test is normal; however, the thickening of basement membranes of some tissues, a characteristic diabetic lesion, is present.

Chemical diabetes During this stage the patient does not have symptoms, and fasting glucose and glucose tolerance tests are normal. However, the glucose tolerance test, if administered during pregnancy or under stress, would be abnormal.

Overt diabetes During this stage the diagnosis is facilitated by abnormal test results or symptoms, or both.

Chronic diabetes The final stage of the disease, with progression marked by vascular lesions.

Juvenile-Onset Type or Ketosis-Prone Diabetes Mellitus*

For the most part, the symptoms of diabetes mellitus in children are similar to those in adults. The differences are that the onset is sudden and that the child is more likely to be underweight than the overweight adult diabetic. Also, the child is unresponsive to oral hypoglycemic drugs and requires insulin.

The child is frequently brought to medical attention because of growth failure in spite of a voracious appetite. Bedwetting in a previously trained child may be noted. The diagnosis is confirmed by laboratory data. (See "Diagnosis of Diabetes Mellitus," above.)

The high incidence of vascular changes is considered to be the most important problem in juvenile diabetes. Eighty-five percent of patients are reported to show such changes after 20 years, with the onset of these complications occurring within 12 to 13 years from the date of diagnosis.

The overall growth of diabetic children appears to be related to the control of diabetes; however, to what extent the degree of control should approximate normoglycemia is not known. Slight delays of growth in stature have been noted but the tendency is to approximate adult height after a prolonged growth period. The onset of diabetes just prior to a growth spurt has been noted to interfere with adult height.

Since the onset of vascular changes and life expectancy have been considered to be independent of clinical control, many different opinions have evolved as to whether strict clinical control and strict adherence to the prescribed diet should even be a consideration for

* Contributed by Rosanne B. Howard

a growing child, whose psychosocial development may be thwarted by such treatment. However, the facts that poor control seems to intensify vascular disorders and interferes with growth, and that good control necessitates a balance of food and insulin, leads us to consider that diet is an essential component of treatment. The goals of treatment are as follows:

Insulin to approximate glycemic equilibrium

Diet for normal growth and activity (based on a child's likes and dislikes, with allowances made for self-expression and independence)

Restoration of the diabetic child to average physical and emotional well-being, which necessitates an acceptance on the part of the child and family that he or she is a "normal child" who happens to have diabetes, not a "diabetic child" constricted by the disease

Since diabetes in children is often first manifested as the state of ketoacidosis, initial treatment is a medical emergency requiring constant attention. A sample of blood is immediately drawn for determination of a blood glucose, pH, carbon dioxide, blood urea nitrogen, and total and differential white blood cell count, and urine is taken (by catheterization if necessary) for sugar and acetone tests. On the basis of the results a plan for fluid and electrolyte and insulin therapy is initiated.

After this period, the long-term establishment of glycemic equilibrium begins through diet and insulin control. This control is often brittle because of the variation in physical activity, emotional stresses at home and school, and the effects of maturation and growth.

As the child grows, he or she will need more insulin. This concept is somewhat confusing to parent and child alike, who sometimes think that the increase in insulin means that the disease state is worsening. Insulin requirements are based on body size and approx-

imate 0.5 to 1 unit/kg of body weight. However, initially, the insulin requirement may be low because the pancreas is still capable of producing insulin. This period is known as the "honeymoon period" and could last 6 to 18 months. During this period the insulin is continued in homeopathic doses because of the problem encountered in reintroducing insulin. Usually, a combination of two types of insulin is used: an intermediate-acting insulin such as NPH and a short-term or regular crystalline insulin. *Two-thirds* of the required dose is administered in the form of intermediate insulin, given before breakfast, and *one-third* of the dose in the form of regular insulin, given before dinner. A rotation of insulin injection sites between the upper arm, the thigh, buttocks, back, and abdomen is necessary to prevent signs of induration or lipoatrophy at the sites of injection.

The use of a combination of insulins with different periods of onset and peak action (see Table 20-6) helps to approximate glycemic equilibrium throughout the day. However, food must be given in amounts to match these same periods of insulin activity. The *balance of food to insulin and exercise* is the goal of diet therapy. This is accomplished by a weighed diet or by the "middle of the road approach," in which the child is given an exchange diet based on age and energy needs. A helpful analogy in understanding this approach is that of a baseball game: this diet places the child in the right ball park but allows the child the freedom to move from base to base. The child, by learning the food groups comprising the exchange system—milk, meat, bread, fruit, vegetables, fat—learns to choose the foods in the amounts that can be effectively utilized by the body. For the most part, all foods that contain sugar are eliminated. Although some physicians do allow the limited use of ice cream or cookies on a once-per-week basis, this practice is generally not agreed upon. Others contend that if the child had an allergy to sugar, producing allergic symptoms, sugar would be avoided, and that this same principle should follow for the

TABLE 20-6 COMMERCIALLY AVAILABLE INSULINS*

Type	Duration of blood sugar–lowering effect	Peak of action
Regular†	5–7 h	2–3 h
Semilente	12–16 h	1–2 h
NPH†	24–28 h	8–12 h
Lente†	24–28 h	8–12 h
PZI‡	36–48 h	14–20 h
Ultralente	36 h	8–14 h

* Insulins are available in different units of strength per ml, e.g., U-80, U-100. The syringe used must be calibrated to the strength of insulin. There is a trend toward using only U-100 insulin.

† Most popular.

‡ Rarely used today.

diabetic child. Furthermore, it is argued that allowing sugar foods on a once-per-week basis places special significance on the sugar-containing food, reinforcing the child's feeling of being deprived at other times. It is felt that the emphasis should be on a natural food diet without sugar.

A preschool-age child is capable of understanding the foods good for his or her body. On the average, children are taught to give their own insulin injections around the age of 7 or 8 years. As they approach school age they are capable of daily urine testing which, along with an occasional blood sugar determination, forms the basis for determining diabetic control. (See Table 20-10 "Urine Tests for Glucose," below.)

It should be noted that certain drugs can cause false-negative and false-positive reactions in various tests for glycosuria. Large quantities of ascorbic acid can also cause a false-positive test.

Urine tests are taken before meals. Before breakfast a second voided urine is taken because the accumulation of sugar in the bladder from the night causes the urine sample to be misleading. Periodically, fractional (or block) urine specimens are collected over a 24-h period, which represents the amount of glucose excreted in the urine at different periods during the day. The amount of carbohydrate lost in the urine—the total grams of glucose—should not exceed 20 percent of the total carbohydrate intake and some diabetologists consider control good only at 10 percent. (For example, a 5-year-old child consuming 150 g of carbohydrate per day would be allowed to spill 10 to 15 g of glucose in the urine, depending on the physician's definition of good control.)

Spilling some sugar, or 1+ on a urine test, is considered essential in order to prevent hypoglycemic periods resulting from too much insulin or too much exercise, which cause a lack of available glucose, especially to the brain, which is dependent on a continuous source of glucose. These periods are upsetting to the child and frequent occurrences can cause damage to the central nervous system. When the blood sugar falls to 50 mg/100 ml, headaches, nervousness, sweating, trembling, confusion, and incoordination result, known as an *insulin reaction*. Immediate treatment by giving a readily available source of glucose—sugar in water, or fruit juices—is essential. If the child is unconscious, glucagon is administered. (A glucagon emergency kit is available and some physicians suggest keeping one in the home.) Candy or sugar should be carried by the child so that it can be taken when the first symptoms appear. Children who participate in sports activities or vigorous play should learn to increase their food intake in anticipation of a busy day. However, a meal taken just prior to an event can cause discomfort in the best of athletes, and the diabetic child who has not prepared in advance would be better advised to eat a source of concentrated carbohydrate than to eat or drink a lot in preparation for the event.

In interpreting the period of hypoglycemia, the *Somogyi effect* must be considered. This effect consists of subclinical hypoglycemia (subclinical = too mild to cause symptoms), followed by a reactive hyperglycemia and ketonuria despite high levels of circulating insulin. The explanation is probably that the subclinical low blood sugar stimulates the secretion of insulin antagonists, such as catecholamines and glucagon, whereby insulin is made ineffective. The condition is recognized when, despite an increasing dose of insulin, there is a concomitant rise in blood sugar and a continued spillage of sugar in the urine. Treatment consists of splitting the insulin dose or reducing the total dose, or both.

Another problem encountered in interpreting hypoglycemic periods is presented by the adolescent patient who has a low blood sugar and yet has a urine that is positive for acetone. This biochemical profile is one of a teenager who is attempting to lose weight by severe food reduction. As a child approaches adolescence, the problem of weight control is one of many issues. This concern with body image, and the peer pressure to smoke and drink, is often reflected in poor diabetic control. The natural tendency to rebel appears heightened in adolescent diabetics, whose anger and denial are interpreted as a subconscious mourning process for the intact bodies they do not have. The problem-age period is between the ages of 12 and 15 years and is exhibited in the following vignette.

Betty

Betty is a 14½-year-old black ninth grader from the inner city whose diabetes was diagnosed at age 11 years, 2 months. At that time she was admitted to the hospital in mild acidosis following a 3-week history of lethargy, polydipsia, and polyuria. Discharged 1 week later taking 30 units of NPH and 10 units of regular insulin, her requirement fell to 4 units of NPB 4 months later. During the second year of her diabetes, she became increasingly resentful, particularly over the lipoatrophy in her thighs. She has been reluctant to discuss her condition with anyone but her closest friends. On several occasions she has admitted to not taking her insulin at all but has, so far, escaped severe ketoacidosis. While she tests her urine erratically and makes little attempt to adhere to a pre-

scribed diet, she has become more conscientious about her clinic visits and has been able to discuss her problems with the social worker and the nurse in the Diabetes Clinic.*

The management of the adolescent just described has begun to be facilitated by the nurse and social worker who have obviously been able to develop a helping relationship. (See Chap. 10.) During adolescence, youths must consolidate their own identity by integrating their own sexuality and separating from parents; the diabetic adolescent must also integrate the disease into his or her identity formation. The adolescent is concerned with the here and now and cannot be prodded into diet adherence by the threat of long-term complications.

The parents of both the young child and the adolescent need support incorporated into the diet counseling session, to deal with the anxiety experienced in having a child with a potentially life-threatening disease. The differences in child-rearing practices must be considered, as there is a continuum ranging from restrictive to permissive. Some ordinarily permissive parents will find it difficult to set limits, feeling sorry for the child. This easily leads to the child's using food as a tool with which to manipulate parents. Restrictive parents may find it difficult to foster independence in diabetic management. It is important to widen the angle of dietary vision to include the needs of both the child and parents, as described by Stitt.†

In dealing with chronic illness, we must think of special dietary requirements for the particular chronically ill child at his particular age, and then consider to what extent those requirements can be derived from

* Norman Spacks, Case Presentation, Grand Rounds, Children's Hospital Medical Center, Boston, Mass., Spring, 1975.
† Stitt, Pauline, "The Family Approach To Feeding Chronically Ill Children," *Children*, vol. 5, November–December 1958, p. 215.

family care that would be suitable for the whole family. Additions, deletions, and modifications may then have to be made for the child—or perhaps for the rest of the family—but the part of food which they can all share needs to be clearly established, for that becomes the foundation on which salutary influences can be built.

Maturity-Onset Type or Non-Ketosis-Prone Diabetes Mellitus

The maturity-onset type of diabetic has beta cells with a normal morphology and a normal insulin content but the beta cells are "sluggish" and therefore cannot produce an adequate amount of insulin for the body, especially when the person is overweight, a common condition among adult-onset diabetics.

The most important goal in the treatment of the maturity-onset type of diabetic is to achieve ideal body weight while maintaining optimum nutrition.

Achievement of this goal [weight reduction] may be associated with the reduction or disappearance of the requirements for exogenous insulin, improvement or correction of fasting hyperglycemia and glucose intolerance, and reduction of known risk factors for atherosclerotic vascular disease such as obesity, hypertension, hyperlipidemia and hyperglycemia.*

It is desirable for patients to be slightly leaner than their ideal body weight since insulin requirements are based on body size. A second goal of treatment is to prevent excessive glycosuria and hyperglycemia, while the final goal is to prevent the secondary complications of retinopathy, neuropathy, and nephropathy.

Peripheral vascular disease and coronary artery disease occur much more frequently in the diabetic. Nearly 75 percent of diabetic deaths in the United States are attributable to vascular disease. The onset and progression of vascular disease may be independent of dia-

betic control. However, it is generally agreed that lack of control may intensify vascular disorders. Atherosclerosis may be accelerated by high circulating fat levels and the deposition of fat in the walls of blood vessels. This clogging of the blood vessels can cause a decrease of blood flow to tissues. If this happens tissue may die and gangrene can develop.

Treatment

The first treatment of choice for maturity-onset type diabetics is control by diet. However, if this proves ineffective an oral antidiabetic agent may be prescribed.

The oral antidiabetic agents are not insulin (insulin is a protein, and if ingested would be digested) but consist of two classes of drugs:

1 *Sulfonylureas* These sensitize the beta cells to glucose. For any given blood sugar level, the rate of insulin release is greater; thus, blood sugar is lowered. These drugs are effective only if the pancreas functions and are therefore prescribed only for maturity-type diabetics. Examples: Orinase (tolbutamide), Diabinese (chlorpropamide).

2 *Biguanides* These do not depend on endogenous insulin, but cannot replace insulin. Their mode of action is not clear. They were most often prescribed for non-insulin-dependent patients, but because of the lactic acidosis side effect they have been removed from the market.

There has been much debate regarding the use of oral agents, since one study (University Group Diabetes Program) found a higher cardiovascular mortality rate in the groups treated with tolbutamide a sulfonylurea) or with phenformin (a biguanide) than in the placebo- and insulin-treated groups. However, the results of the study are as yet unconfirmed and the U.S. Food and Drug Administration is closely monitoring the use of these agents.

* Committee on Food and Nutrition American Diabetics Association: *Diabetes*, 20:633, 1971.

Type of Diet

There are several different philosophies regarding the type of diabetic diet prescribed: the weighed diet, the measured diet, and the unmeasured or "free" diet. Whatever the philosophy, the nutritional care plan should always be individualized to meet the needs of each patient.

The *weighed diet* consists of weighing all food to comply with gram specifications. It is rigid and allows little flexibility in life style.

The *unmeasured diet* for young juvenile-onset diabetics entails flexibility of daily caloric intake to match energy demands. Meals and snacks are geared to appetite, with close attention paid to timing, so as to avoid drastic swings in blood sugar. Considering the unpredictability of a youngster's energy requirements (growth, activity, etc.) plus the beneficial psychological aspects of a less rigid regimen, the benefits of the unmeasured diet are impressive.

The *measured diet* is probably advisable for the majority of maturity-onset, obese diabetics, who require a fixed caloric intake. Once the patient's energy and other nutrient requirements have been calculated, the food allowance is divided into "exchanges," depending on its carbohydrate, protein, and fat content. All exchanges within a food group contain approximately the same caloric content, and the patient is allowed a certain number of exchanges per day within each group. The patient is taught to exchange within, and not between, groups; for example, a starch exchange and a meat exchange are not of similar nutrient composition and therefore cannot be exchanged or substituted for one another. The American Diabetic and Dietetic Associations have compiled a list of food exchanges (see Table 20-7).

Diet Therapy

The nutritional requirements of diabetics are, in general, the same as for all individuals. Diet therapy is one of the most important factors in the management of the diabetic patient. The major aim of diet therapy for the adult-onset type of diabetic is to achieve or maintain ideal body weight; for the juvenile diabetic, the aim is to balance food intake with insulin action, while providing adequate food energy for activity and growth.

Exercise should be an integral part of diabetic management, since activity facilitates glucose entry into the cells, and therefore lowers blood sugar, as well as insulin requirements.

We will now consider in more detail some of the significant nutrients and their relationship to the diet of a diabetic patient.

Calories (kilojoules) The decision regarding a patient's energy requirement should be based on the patient's age, height, weight, sex, activity level, and growth. A careful nutritional history should take all of these factors into account. To aid in establishing an appropriate energy level some general guidelines are provided. (See Table 20-8.) It must be remembered that these general guidelines are an aid in planning energy levels; however, patients can adapt to them and subsequently waste or conserve energy. Therefore, it is an important part of treatment to monitor weight and diet, and to make adjustments accordingly.

Carbohydrate The amount of carbohydrate allowed in a diabetic's diet has been the target of much debate. Recent evidence shows that as long as total calories (joules) are not increased, increasing the total carbohydrate allowance does not seem to affect the insulin requirements of insulin-dependent diabetics. In the less severe, typically obese diabetic, substitution of *complex* carbohydrate (starches—breads, cereal, grains) for fat does not seem to increase blood sugar or affect glucose tolerance. Furthermore, if carbohydrate is severely restricted, dietary protein and fat containing saturated fat and cholesterol will be increased to maintain the appropriate energy level of the diet. Considering the relationship between diabetes and

TABLE 20-7 DIABETIC EXCHANGE LISTS

List 1: Milk exchanges (includes non-fat, low-fat, and whole milk)

This list shows the kinds and amounts of milk or milk products to use for one milk exchange. Those appearing in **bold type** are **non-fat.** Low-fat and whole milk contain saturated fat. One exchange of milk contains 12 g of carbohydrate, 8 g of protein, a trace of fat, and 80 kcal (336 kJ).

Non-fat fortified milk:

Skim or non-fat milk	1 cup (8 oz)
Powdered (non-fat dry, before adding liquid)	⅓ cup
Canned evaporated skim milk	½ cup
Buttermilk made from skim milk	1 cup
Yogurt made from skim milk (plain, unflavored)	1 cup

Low-fat fortified milk:

1%-fat milk (omit ½ fat exchange)	1 cup
2%-fat milk (omit 1 fat exchange)	1 cup
Yogurt made from 2% fat milk (plain, unflavored) (omit 1 fat exchange)	1 cup

Whole milk (omit 2 fat exchanges)

Whole milk	1 cup
Canned evaporated whole milk	½ cup
Buttermilk made from whole milk	1 cup
Yogurt made from whole milk (plain, unflavored)	1 cup

List 2: Vegetable exchanges

This list shows the kinds of vegetables to use for one vegetable exchange. One exchange is ½ cup and contains about 5 g of carbohydrate, 2 g of protein, and 25 kcal (105 kJ).

Asparagus	Green pepper	Okra
Bean sprouts	Greens:	Onions
Beets	Beet	Rhubarb
Broccoli	Chards	Rutabaga
Brussels sprouts	Collards	Sauerkraut
Cabbage	Dandelion	String beans, green or yellow
Carrots	Kale	Summer squash
Cauliflower	Mustard	Tomatoes
Celery	Spinach	Tomato juice
Cucumbers	Turnip	Turnips
Eggplant	Mushrooms	Vegetable juice cocktail
		Zucchini

The following raw vegetables may be used as desired:

Chicory	Endive	Lettuce	Radishes
Chinese cabbage	Escarole	Parsley	Watercress

(Starchy vegetables are found in the bread exchange list)

List 3: Fruit exchanges

This list shows the kinds and amounts of fruits to use for one fruit exchange. One exchange of fruit contains 10 g of carbohydrate and 40 kcal (168 kJ).

Apple	1 small
Apple juice	⅓ cup
Applesauce (unsweetened)	½ cup
Apricots (fresh)	2 medium
Apricots (dried)	4 halves
Banana	½ small

(continued)

TABLE 20–7 (continued)

Berries:
    Blackberries   ½ cup
    Blueberries   ½ cup
    Raspberries   ½ cup
    Strawberries   ¾ cup

Berries:	
Blackberries	½ cup
Blueberries	½ cup
Raspberries	½ cup
Strawberries	¾ cup
Cherries	10 large
Cider	⅓ cup
Dates	2
Figs (fresh)	1
Figs (dried)	1
Grapefruit	½
Grapefruit juice	½ cup
Grapes	12
Grape juice	¼ cup
Mango	½ small
Melon:	
Cantaloupe	¼ small
Honeydew	⅛ medium
Watermelon	1 cup
Nectarine	1 small
Orange	1 small
Orange juice	½ cup
Papaya	¾ cup
Peach	1 medium
Pear	1 small
Persimmon, native	1 medium
Pineapple	½ cup
Pineapple juice	⅓ cup
Plums	2 medium
Prunes	2 medium
Prune juice	¼ cup
Raisns	2 tbsp
Tangerine	1 medium

(Cranberries may be used as desired if no sugar is added)

List 4: Bread exchanges (Includes bread, cereal and starchy vegetables)

This list shows the kinds and amounts of breads, cereals, starchy vegetables and prepared foods to use for one bread exchange. Those appearing in **bold type** are **low-fat**. One exchange of bread contains 15 g of carbohydrate, 2 g of protein, and 70 kcal (294 kJ).

Bread:

White (including French and Italian)	1 slice
Whole wheat	1 slice
Rye or pumpernickel	1 slice
Raisin	1 slice
Bagel, small	½
English muffin, small	½
Plain roll, bread	1
Frankfurter roll	½
Hamburger bun	½
Dried bread crumbs	3 tbsp
Tortilla, 6 in	1

Cereal:

Bran flakes	½ cup
Other ready-to-eat unsweetened cereal	¾ cup

(continued)

TABLE 20–7 (continued)

Puffed cereal (unfrosted)	1 cup
Cereal (cooked)	½ cup
Grits (cooked)	½ cup
Rice or barley (cooked)	½ cup
Pasta (cooked)	½ cup
Spaghetti, noodles, macaroni	
Popcorn (popped, no fat added)	3 cups
Cornmeal (dry)	2 tbsp
Flour	2½ tbsp
Wheat germ	¼ cup

Crackers:

Arrowroot	3
Graham, 2½ in 2 sq.	2
Matzo, 4 x 6 in	½
Oyster	20
Pretzels, 3⅛ in long by ⅛ in diameter	25
Rye wafers, 2 x 3½	3
Saltines	6
Soda, 2½ s in 2	4

Dried beans, peas, and lentils:

Beans, peas, lentils (dried and cooked)	½ cup
Baked beans, no pork (canned)	¼ cup

Starchy vegetables:

Corn	⅓ cup
Corn on the cob	1 small
Lima beans	½ cup
Parsnips	⅔ cup
Peas, green (canned or frozen)	½ cup
Potato, white	1 small
Potato (mashed)	½ cup
Pumpkin	¾ cup
Winter squash, acorn or butternut	½ cup
Yam or sweet potato	¼ cup

Prepared foods:

Biscuit, 2 in diameter (omit 1 fat exchange)	1
Corn bread, 2 x 2 x 1 in (omit 1 fat exchange)	1
Corn muffin, 2 in diameter (omit 1 fat exchange)	1
Crackers, round, butter type (omit 1 fat exchange)	5
Muffin, plain small (omit 1 fat exchange)	1
Potatoes, french fried, length 2 to 3½ in (omit 1 fat exchange)	8
Potato or corn chips (omit 2 fat exchanges)	15
Pancake, 5 x ½ in (omit 1 fat exchange)	1
Waffle, 5 x ½ in (omit 1 fat exchange)	1

List 5: Meat exchanges (Lean meat)

This list shows the kinds and amounts of lean meat and other protein-rich foods to use for one low-fat meat exchange. One exchange of lean meat (1 oz) contains 7 g of protein, 3 g of fat, and 55 kcal (231 kJ).

Beef:

baby beef (very lean), chipped beef, chuck, flank steak, tenderloin, plate ribs, plate skirt steak, round (bottom, top), all cuts rump, spare ribs, tripe	1 oz

Lamb:

leg, rib, sirloin, loin (roast and chops), shank, shoulder	1 oz

(continued)

TABLE 20-7 (continued)

Pork:	
leg (whole rump, center shank), ham, smoked (center slices)	1 oz
Veal:	
leg, loin, rib, shank, shoulder, cutlets	1 oz
Poultry:	
meat without skin of chicken, turkey, cornish hen, guinea hen, pheasant	1 oz
Fish:	
any fresh or frozen	1 oz
canned salmon, tuna, mackerel, crab, lobster	¼ cup
clams, oysters, scallops, shrimp	5 or 1 oz
sardines, drained	3
Cheeses:	
Cheeses containing less than 5% butterfat	1 oz
Cottage cheese, dry, 2% butterfat	¼ cup
Legumes:	
Dried beans and peas (omit 1 bread exchange)	½ cup

List 5: Meat exchanges (Medium-fat meat)

This list shows the kinds and amounts of medium-fat meat and other protein-rich foods to use for one medium-fat meat exchange. For each exchange of medium-fat meat omit ½ fat exchange.

Beef:	
ground (15% fat), corned beef (canned), rib eye, round (ground commercial)	1 oz
Pork:	
loin (all cuts tenderloin), shoulder arm (picnic), shoulder blade, Boston butt, Canadian bacon, boiled ham	1 oz
Liver:	
heart, kidney, sweetbreads (these are high in cholesterol)	1 oz
Cheeses:	
Cottage cheese, creamed	¼ cup
mozzarella, ricotta, farmer's, neufchatel, parmesan	3 tbsp
Eggs and Peanuts:	
Egg (high in cholesterol)	1
Peanut butter (omit 2 additonal fat exchanges)	2 tbsp

List 5: Meat exchanges (High-fat meat)

This list shows the kinds and amounts of high-fat meat and other protein-rich foods to use for one high-fat meat exchange. For each exchange of high-fat meat omit 1 fat exchange

Beef:	
brisket, corned beef (brisket), ground beef (more than 20% fat), hamburger (commercial), chuck (ground commercial), roasts (rib), steaks (club and rib.)	1 oz
Lamb:	
breast	1 oz

(continued)

TABLE 20-7 (continued)

Pork:
spare ribs, loin (back ribs), pork (ground), country
style ham, deviled ham | 1 oz

Veal:
breast | 1 oz

Poultry:
capon, duck (domestic), goose | 1 oz

Cheese:
cheddar types | 1 oz

Processed meats:
Cold cuts | 4½ x ⅛ in slice
Frankfurter | 1 small

List 6: Fat exchanges

This list shows the kinds and amounts of fat-containing foods to use
for one fat exchange. To plan a diet low in saturated fat select only
those exchanges which appear in **bold type.** They are **polyunsaturated.**
One exchange of fat contains 5 g of fat and 45 kcal (189 kJ).

Margarine, tub or stick*	1 tsp
Avocado (4 in diameter)†	⅛
Oil:	
Corn, cottonseed, safflower, soy, or sunflower	1 tsp
Olive†	1 tsp
Peanut†	1 tsp
Olives†	5 small
Almonds†	10 whole
Pecans†	2 large whole
Peanuts†	
Spanish	20 whole
Virginia	10 whole
Walnuts	6 small
Nuts, other†	6 small
Butter	1 tsp
Bacon, fat	1 tsp
Bacon, crisp	1 strip
Cream, light	2 tbsp
Cream, sour	2 tbsp
Cream, heavy	1 tbsp
Cream cheese	1 tbsp
French dressing‡	1 tbsp
Italian dressing‡	1 tbsp
Lard	1 tsp
Mayonnaise‡	1 tsp
Salad dressing, mayonnaise type‡	2 tsp
Salt pork	¾ in cube

---

* Made with corn, cottonseed, safflower, soy, or sunflower oil only.

† Fat content is primarily monounsaturated.

‡ If made with corn, cottonseed, safflower, soy, or sunflower oil can be used on
fat-modified diet.

Source: These *exchange lists* are based on material in "Exchange Lists for Meal
Planning" prepared by Committees of the American Diabetes Association, Inc., and
the American Dietetic Association in cooperation with the National Institute of
Arthritis, Metabolism and Digestive Diseases and the National Heart and Lung
Institute, National Institutes of Health, Public Health Service, U.S. Department
of Health, Education, and Welfare.

TABLE 20-8 CALORIES AND KILOJOULES PER KILOGRAM OF IDEAL BODY WEIGHT CONSIDERING ACTIVITY LEVEL AND PRESENT WEIGHT

	Sedentary		Moderate activity		High activity	
	kcal	kJ	kcal	kJ	kcal	kJ
Overweight	20–25	84–105	30	126	35	147
Normal	30	126	35	147	40	168
Underweight	35	147	40	168	45–50	189–210

Source: Adapted from Robert S. Goodhart and Maurice E. Shils, *Modern Nutrition in Health and Disease,* 5th ed., Lea & Febiger, Philadelphia, 1973, p. 849.

cardiovascular disease this is not recommended. Thus, the latest recommendation for carbohydrate is that it comprise between 45 and 55 percent of the total calories (kilojoules). Habitual use of simple sugars (table sugar, candy, soft drinks, etc.) should be eliminated, but they may be allowed under certain circumstances, such as prior to athletic competition or periods of vigorous exercise, or on sick days, in order to maintain the body's glucose insulin ratio.

Protein Fifteen to twenty percent of the total food intake should be provided as protein. The diets of children and adolescents need careful supervision to ensure protein intakes of high biological value in the range of 1.5 to 2 g protein/kg of body weight. Patients with renal or hepatic complications may require protein restriction.

Fat Approximately 35 percent of the total food intake is recommended as fat. Emphasis is placed on the substitution of polyunsaturated fat for saturated fat and on the limitation of cholesterol intake. (See Chap. 17.)

Food servings Once the total energy (kilocalories, kilojoules), carbohydrate, fat, and protein requirements have been determined, the amount must be converted into food servings for the day, which are then spread throughout the day into 3 meals and either 2 or 3 snacks depending on the type of management: in-

sulin, oral hypoglycemic agents, or diet alone. With insulin therapy, the food is divided so as to match insulin activity. Current practice no longer distributes food between meals and snacks as rigidly as in the past. In the past, the total carbohydrate was calculated into very specific amounts to be consumed at certain times. The carbohydrate was divided into thirds, fifths, or sevenths at meal and snack times to match insulin activity. This often imposed hardships since it meant that a patient consumed one-half of a serving or exchange. The new system allows a more normalized meal pattern. Table 20-9 summarizes the calculation of a diabetic diet.

Alcohol Including alcohol in the diabetic diet is at the physician's discretion. Of course, sweet mixed drinks, sweet wines, and aperitifs should be avoided. In making the decision as to how much to include, the high caloric content of alcohol (7 kcal/g of alcohol) is a consideration. Also, since alcohol lowers blood sugar, a combination of alcohol and insulin can potentiate hypoglycemia, so alcohol when taken should be consumed with food. Alcohol with sulfonylureas can produce a harmless but disconcerting reaction (flushing, tingling of the face, etc.) and the patient should be forewarned.

Sick-day diet On sick days, patients should be encouraged to eat in order to prevent hypoglycemia. Food should be distributed throughout

TABLE 20-9 CALCULATION OF A DIABETIC DIET

Diet calculations are based on energy needs of an overweight, sedentary diabetic weighing 72 kg.

Calories

1 Determine total energy needs according to age, weight, and activity level and patient's need to lose weight.

25 kcal or 105 kJ/kg is the recommended level

$$25 \times 72 \text{ kg} = 1800 \text{ kcal}$$
$$105 \text{ kJ} \times 72 \text{ kg} = 7560 \text{ kJ}$$

Total Energy = 1800 kcal or 7560 kJ

Carbohydrate

2 Determine the total carbohydrate allowance by taking 50% of the calories or kilojoules determined above, since 50% of the energy needs may be allotted as carbohydrate in the diabetic diet.

$$1800 \text{ kcal} \times 50\% = 900 \text{ kcal of carbohydrate}$$
$$7560 \text{ kJ } 50\% = 3780 \text{ kJ of carbohydrate}$$

Next, determine the total grams of carbohydrate by dividing the total carbohydrate calories by 4 or dividing the total kilojoules by 17.

$$\frac{900 \text{ kcal}}{4} = 225 \text{ g carbohydrate}$$

$$\frac{3780 \text{ kJ}}{17} = 225 \text{ g carbohydrate}$$

Total Carbohydrate = 225 g

Protein

3 Determine the total protein allowance by taking 15% of the calories or kilojoules determined above, since at least 15% of the total energy requirement must be allotted as protein to supply body needs.

$$1800 \text{ kcal} \times 15\% = 270 \text{ kcal of protein}$$
$$7560 \text{ kJ} \times 15\% = 1134 \text{ kJ of protein}$$

Next, determine the total grams of protein by dividing the total protein calories by 4 or dividing the total kilojoules by 17.

$$\frac{270 \text{ kcal}}{4} = 68 \text{ g protein}$$

$$\frac{1134 \text{ kJ}}{17} = 68 \text{ g protein}$$

(continued)

TABLE 20-9 (continued)

Total Protein = 68 g

Fat

4 Determine the total fat allowance by taking 35% of the calories of kilojoules determined above, since 35% the level recommended to control dietary fat, yet supply energy needs.

$$1800 \text{ kcal} \times 35\% = 630 \text{ kcal of fat}$$
$$7560 \text{ kJ} \times 35\% = 2646 \text{ kJ of fat}$$

Next, determine the total grams of fat by dividing the total fat calories by 9 or dividing the total kilojoules by 38.

$$\frac{630 \text{ kcal}}{9} = 70 \text{ g fat}$$

$$\frac{2646 \text{ kJ}}{38} = 70 \text{ g fat}$$

Total Fat = 70

---

the day to prevent peaks and valleys of blood sugar. Sweet liquids, such as Jello or ginger ale, or soups are easy to tolerate and provide a ready source of carbohydrate. In the case of vomiting or diarrhea the patient should contact his or her physician immediately so as to avoid electrolyte imbalance and dehydration.

Travel When traveling, a diabetic should carry food along, as traveling could mean delayed meals. Such portable foods as cheese and crackers or peanut butter and crackers, or any other snack providing protein plus carbohydrate, are recommended.

Special dietetic products Reading labels carefully will guide the patient in food shopping. Dietetic and diabetic foods may be costly and are often inappropriate—some "dietetic" foods are low in sodium, not sucrose. Many other "dietetic" foods may be low in sucrose but high in fat and therefore not low in calories (joules)—for example, dietetic chocolate bars.

In addition, many over-the-counter drugs contain sugar (e.g., cough syrups), and the diabetic must be taught to recognize potential sources of sugar.

A sufficiently cordial relationship should exist between the patient and the nutrition educator so that the patient does not hesitate to call before buying.

Artificial sweeteners (e.g., saccharin) may be used in the diabetic's diet; however, discretion is encouraged due to the unknown long-term effect on the body. Some artificial sweeteners use sorbitol plus mannitol as the sweetening agents. These substances are sugar alcohols that are metabolized more slowly than sucrose and enter the bloodstream at a reduced rate. They provide a small amount of calories (joules) but not enough to cause concern.

Nutrition Education

The treatment of diabetes mellitus requires diet as part of the integral treatment; thus, the nutrition education of the diabetic patient is paramount in care.

The ability of the nutritionist to help the patient to change a lifetime of eating experiences revolves around the personal meaning that the patient derives from the counseling sessions. (See Chap. 10.)

After diagnosis the patient must learn to cope with the threat of a long-term chronic illness and is not usually ready to hear new information, let alone integrate the information in order to make the behavioral change that is necessary. Therefore, the nutrition educator must focus first on the patient's level of need. This will vary depending upon:

Age
Socioeconomic status
Education
Culture

The nutrition educator will need to explain the following concepts during the learning program:

How food acts in the body

How food and insulin act in the body

How food and insulin act in the diabetic condition

How food, insulin, and activity are regulated in the diabetic condition

Urine testing for glucose   The diabetic patient is routinely instructed as to how and when to test the urine for glucose. There are two methods for doing this, chemical and enzymatic. (See Table 20-10.)

The chemical methods (of which Clinitest tablets are perhaps the most widely used) are based on the fact that glucose is a reducing sugar. Copper is commonly used in the reaction—if it is reduced, there is a color change, and the amount of glucose present will determine the degree of change. Thus, these tests are quantitative. However, since other sugars within the aldehyde group are also reducing sugars, the reaction is not specific for glucose.

Testape is the popular example of the enzymatic reaction. These methods employ the enzyme glucose oxidase. Hydrogen peroxide produces the color change indicative of the presence of glucose. These methods are highly specific for glucose, but are not quantitative.

Whatever the method employed, the patient should be instructed to record the results of tests, and to bring the records when making regular visits to the physician. The accuracy of the tests depends not only on the test itself, but also upon the skill of the tester.

New Concepts in Diabetes

Somatostatin is a polypeptide hormone that inhibits alpha-cell production of glucagon (as well as beta-cell insulin secretion) and inhibits growth hormone release. Since growth hormone has anti-insulin effects, current research is aimed at the possibility of developing somatostatin into a pharmacologic agent for treating diabetics.

TABLE 20-10 URINE TESTS FOR GLUCOSE

Test	Results
Benedict's solution	blue (negative) → dark orange (2% glucose)
Clinitest tablets	blue (negative) → orange (4+ or 2% glucose)
Testape	yellow (negative) → blue (4+)
Clinistix	Red (negative) → purple (positive)

Similar tests are available for testing the urine for acetone and albumin

Research in virology has suggested several model systems in which diabetes is produced in animals via viruses. Epidemiologists have likewise underlined the possible link between viruses and the onset of diabetes.

Sorbitol is a sugar alcohol produced when glucose is reduced in mammalian tissues. In certain tissues (lens of the eye, liver, peripheral nerves, Schwann cell of the peripheral nerves, aorta), glucose can enter cells without the aid of insulin. Once in, it is acted on by an enzyme and converted to sorbitol. Since the sorbitol cannot leave the cell and has osmotic properties, it holds water in the cell, causing swelling and damage. Thus, sorbitol is now being considered as the cause for diabetic cataracts and a possible causative agent in diabetic neuropathy. Research is now being directed toward blocking the enzyme that allows sorbitol formation. (Dietary sorbitol is not metabolized in this fashion and has no role in cataract formation.)

Current technological and clinical research is geared toward developing methods which would provide insulin in a more continuous and need-oriented way through pancreas transplantation, islets of Langerhans transplantation, and artificial pancreas development and implantation. Work is also being conducted on cultured beta cells. Although research is not yet clinically applicable, it does offer the hope for future implementation.

Adult Hypoglycemia

Adult hypoglycemia, defined as a plasma glucose level less than or equal to 40 mg/100 ml,

produces vague symptoms which occur several hours after meals. These include sweating, nausea, and dizziness. This reactive hypoglycemia is due to a delay in insulin secretion (as a result, the blood sugar, upon testing, is initially higher), causing insulin to be high at an inappropriate time. This is confirmed with a 5-h oral glucose tolerance test, and can be indicative of early diabetes. However, the condition also occurs after a gastrectomy, because glucose enters the intestine more rapidly, and is absorbed very quickly. In a large category of patients, symptoms are related to functional, or nonorganic, causes. A high-protein diet, low in carbohydrate and divided into frequent small feedings, is recommended.

BONE AND JOINT DISORDERS

Gout

As yet, the pathogenesis of gout is uncertain but the disorder is characterized by a derangement of purine metabolism. Uric acid is the end product of the metabolism of purine compounds such as nucleic acids and xanthines.

Gout, a metabolic disease with a familial tendency, is seen predominantly in men over 35 years old and occasionally in postmenopausal women. The condition is manifested by the following symptoms:

1 Hyperuricemia
2 Acute attacks of arthritis

TABLE 20-11 PURINE CONTENT OF FOOD

Range of purine content	Food
High (150–1000 mg/100 g)	Liver, kidneys, sweetbreads, brains, heart, mussels, anchovies, sardines, meat extract, consommé, gravies, fish roes, herring
Moderate (50–150 mg/100 g)	Meat, fowl, fish (except as noted above), other seafoods, lentils, yeast, whole-grain cereals, beans, peas, asparagus, cauliflower, mushrooms, spinach
Negligible	Vegetables, fruits, milk, cheese, eggs, refined cereals, cereal products, butter and fats (in moderation only), sugar, sweets, vegetable soups

3 Eventual degenerative and destructive changes in the joints

4 A tendency to form deposits of sodium monourate, either nodular deposits known as *tophi,* or diffuse deposits in cartilage, in tissues around joints, and around the helix of the ears

Normal serum uric acid is 2 to 6 mg/100 ml. With gout there is an increase in serum levels to 6 to 10 mg/100 ml; in rare cases values to 20 mg/100 ml have been observed. High levels of uric acid are suggestive of gout but may also be attributable to renal failure, leukemia, polycythemia, multiple myeloma, or toxemia of pregnancy.

In the past it was thought that uric acid was derived solely from purines ingested in food and from the body's own tissue proteins. It is now known that metabolic precursors of urates are formed not only from endogenous and exogenous preformed purines but also from simple available compounds in the body such as carbon dioxide, glycine, and ammonia, which can be synthesized into uric acid. This information makes the dietary treatment of gout less significant. However, some authorities continue to recommend diets low in purines as they feel that this influences the total metabolic pool of uric acid. Table 20-11 lists the purine content in various foods.

A high fluid intake is one dietary measure that *has* proved helpful in the treatment of gout. This increase in fluids is necessary to help eliminate uric acid, slow progressive kidney involvement, and prevent renal calculi.

Coffee, tea, and chocolate contain methyl xanthines which are metabolized to methyl urates and at one time were eliminated from the diet of gouty patients. It has since been learned that these methyl urates are not deposited in the tissues and therefore the beverages are now allowed.

A high-carbohydrate diet tends to increase uric acid excretion, while a high-fat diet not only decreases excretion but actually can precipitate a gouty attack. A diet high in protein and fat is therefore avoided. Weight control is extremely important. Preferably, the patient should be 10 to 15 percent below his calculated normal weight. However, sudden weight reduction and fasting can exacerbate the condition.

During an *acute* gouty attack the dietary purines should be kept to a minimum (100 mg/day) to avoid adding uric acid to the metabolic pool. A diet high in carbohydrate and low in protein and fat is recommended. Fluids should be forced.

The diet for the interval between attacks should be a well-balanced diet adjusted to the energy level needed to maintain the patient at his or her desired weight. Between attacks a high fluid intake, 2 qt/day, is recommended. Alcohol inclusion in the diet is controversial; it will not necessarily precipitate an attack but the usual recommendation is either to eliminate or to dilute it. Gouty patients should check with their physicians regarding the use of alcohol.

Benemid (probenecid), a drug which promotes uric acid excretion into the urine, is used to treat gout. Fluids plus sufficient alkalies to maintain an alkaline urine are necessary to prevent the precipitation of uric acid crystals when Benemid or other uricosuric agents are used. Alkalies have replaced the alkali-ash diet that was once used to maintain an alkaline urine.

Allopurinol, a drug which inhibits uric acid production, is another agent of choice in the treatment of gout. Fluids should be encouraged when this drug is being administered.

Rheumatoid Arthritis

Rheumatoid arthritis is a chronic progressive inflammatory tissue disorder of unknown etiology, resulting in stiff, sore joints, usually in the fingers, wrists, knees, ankles, or toes. The average age at onset is 35, and the incidence doubles as one nears 60. The female to male incidence rate is 3 to 1.

Negative nitrogen and calcium balance, muscle atrophy, and bone decalcification are part of the disease process. Some authorities have observed changes in carbohydrate metabolism during the active stage of the inflammatory process; however, this has not been a universal finding.

Due to a catabolic response, the patient may be underweight, and this may be further complicated by a poor food intake, especially when the disease process in the hands and the finger joints interferes with the patients' ability to feed themselves.

The anemia observed is not related to iron deficiency, but rather to a hemolytic process and as such is not amenable to iron therapy.

The dietary treatment revolves around the drugs used to control the inflammatory process, namely aspirin and, in some cases, corticosteroid therapy. The latter may necessitate a moderate sodium restriction to minimize edema. With aspirin administration, frequent small feedings are recommended to minimize gastric irritation. Aspirin should be administered after meals and in some instances a bland diet may be needed to further guard against gastric distress.

The same dietary and drug treatment is initiated with osteoarthritis.

Juvenile Arthritis

The peak age of onset in juvenile arthritis is the preschool years, and more girls are affected than boys. The clinical course of the disease is variable. Growth disturbances sometimes occur as a result of abnormal influences on the epiphyseal plate. This is an important consideration for the nutritionist monitoring diet and growth in these children. Over one-half of the children afflicted with juvenile arthritis recover completely within 1 or 2 years.

Normal nutrition, based on age, body size, and activity needs, should be considered. (Activity may be decreased substantially, thereby altering energy needs) The child's frustration and anxiety may negatively affect food behavior, and this requires supportive management. Food may be only one area of control that the child has during an acute episode of inflammation. During this period of stress and inflammation, fever may occur, increasing basal energy needs.

STUDY QUESTIONS

1 The states of hyperthyroidism and hypothyroidism have different effect on the body's metabolism and subsequent diet therapy. Explain.
2 Differentiate between adult-onset and juvenile-onset diabetes
3 Describe the progressive symptomatology of diabetes from hyperglycemia to ketosis.

CASE STUDY 20-1

R. G. is a 59-year-old sedentary male executive currently undergoing his annual physical examination, which is positive for hypertension, angina, obesity, and abnormal glucose tolerance. His present height is 5 ft 10 in and his weight is 205 lb (ideal weight 154 lbs).

The dietary history reveals a food intake high in cholesterol and saturated fat, and containing approximately 2800 kcal (11.76 mJ) per day. He eats frequently in restaurants, and when at home enjoys his wife's gourmet meals. He has 1 or 2 cocktails before his meals; however, he is not a dessert eater.

The diagnosis of adult-onset diabetes was made. He was started on Orinase and referred to the nutritionist for dietary counseling.

Case Study Questions

1   What is the major aim of therapy?

2   Calculate R. G.'s caloric requirement with the proper proportions of carbohydrate, protein, and fat.

3   What life-style factors should be considered in planning his dietary regimen?

BIBLIOGRAPHY

Ballin, J. C., and P. L. White: "Fallacy and Hazard, Human Chorionic Gonadotoprin, 500 Calorie Diet and Weight Reduction," *Journal of the American Medical Association, 230:* 693, 1974.

Bunn, H. F. et al.: "The Biosynthesis of Human Hemoglobin A" *The Journal of Clinical Investigation, 57:* 1652, 1976.

Cornblath, E.: "Diabetes in Childhood," *Pediatric Annals, 4:* 1975.

"Diabetes, Epidemology Suggests a Viral Connection," *Science,* **188:** 347, 1975.

Drash, A.: "Diabetes in Childhood, a Review," *Journal of Pediatrics, 78:* 919, 1971.

Eaton, R. P.: Evolving Role of Glucagon in Human Diabetes Mellitus, *Diabetes, 24:* 523, 1975.

Jirani, S. K. M.: "Does Control Influence the Growth of Diabetic Children?," *Archives of Diseases of Children, 48:* 109, 1973.

Kempe, C. H. et al. (eds.): *Current Pediatric Diagnosis and Treatment,* 3d ed., Lange Medical Publishers, Los Altos, Cal., 1974.

Meissner, C. et al.: "Antidiabetic Action of Somatostatin Assesed by Artificial Pancreas," *Diabetes, 24:* 988, 1975.

Paz-Guevara, A. T. et al.: Juvenile Diabetes Mellitus after forty years," *Diabetes, 24:* 559, 1975.

Powell, G. F., and Blizzard Brasel: "Emotional Deprivation and Growth Retardation Stimulating Idiopathic Hypopituitarism," *New England Journal of Medicine, 23:* 1271, 1967.

Schmitt, B. D.: "An Argument for the Unmeasured Diet in Juvenile Diabetes Mellitus," *Clinical Pediatrics,* **14:** 68, 1975.

Silver, H. K. et al.: *Pediatrics,* 10th ed., Lange Medical Publishers, Los Altos, Cal., 1973.

"University Group Diabetes Program: V, Evaluation of Phenformin Therapy," *Diabetes, 24:* (Supplement 1), 1975.

Weininger, J., and G. M. Briggs: Nutrition Update, *Journal of Nutrition Education,* **7:** 141, 1975.

CHAPTER 21

THE OVERWEIGHT CONDITION

Patricia A. Kreutler
Nancie H. Herbold
Rosanne B. Howard
Peggy L. Pipes

KEY WORDS
Overweight
Obesity
Adipocyte
Prevention

INTRODUCTION

Obesity is an overriding concern, a perplexing problem of our society. We ride to school or to the office and sit at our desks or in front of television with plenty to eat. The net result is an overweight nation imbued with anxiety about weight but doing little to prevent the problem.

The American attitude toward obesity assumes a moralistic stance, with the condition viewed as indicative of gluttony, weakness, and self-indulgence, and thinness as a visible virtue. This Puritan and simplistic notion pervades even the medical community, and treatment is often handicapped by this distorted cultural value. The obese individual, especially the obese child, may be ostracized from the group and must bear the fat as a social stigma and receive the censure of all.

Society's rejection can further enhance the obese individual's use of the eating function as a pseudosolution of a personality problem. It is often difficult to differentiate between the psychological problems that play a role in the development of obesity and those that are a product of the obese state. Based on observations of the obese patient's ability to adjust to life stresses, Bruche has divided the population into three main groups.[1] The first group is composed of competent people who are probably heavy in accordance with their constitutional make-up, whose weight excess is not related to abnormal psychological functioning. The weight excess in this group is moderate and fairly stable; weight reduction regimens are successful or body image is accepted. In the remainder of the population, obesity is related to psychological problems. Individuals are subdivided into two groups: those with *developmental obesity,* in whom obesity is intrinsically interwoven with their whole development, which is characterized by many features of personality disturbance and disturbed patterns of family transactions; and those with *reactive obesity,* whose weight gain follows some traumatic emotional experience. In the latter two groups, overeating may serve as a defense against deeper depression. Their control over underlying anxieties may be so precarious that a "scare approach" to noncompliance with a reducing regimen can add to their difficulties, rendering them unable to maintain their fragile emotional balance and forcing them further into the obese state and deeper depression.[2]

Thus, an oversimplistic approach that ignores the diversity of clinical pictures presented by obese individuals can be extremely detrimental and can actually precipitate conflicts, imposing even a heavier burden than the weight. A multidisciplinary approach (doctor, nurse, nutritionist, social worker, psychologist, psychiatrist, exercise physiologist) may offer more hope for this intricate problem. However, the cure for obesity lies in its *prevention*.

Prevention of obesity calls for social acceptance of human diversity and fostering freedom and initiative in the individual. It repudiates manufactured, stereotyped ways of life and demands instead respect for human individuality.[3]

With the admonition to all future clinical practitioners of nutrition that their role is in *prevention,* this chapter in the first part will explore the known causes and treatment of obesity. The second part will examine the obese state as a clinical manifestation of Prader-Willi syndrome.

THE OVERWEIGHT CONDITION— THE OBESE STATE

Patricia A. Kreutler

Nancie H. Herbold

Rosanne B. Howard

DEFINITION

Obesity may be defined as a condition in which there is an accumulation of body fat in excessive proportion to total body mass. This concept should be contrasted with that of *overweight,* which merely indicates a weight which is greater than that assumed to be ideal or desirable, without any specific reference to body composition. Since the body is composed of several types of tissues, including muscle, fat, and bone, each of which contributes weight to the organism, a muscular athlete may in fact be overweight yet not obese. Thus, a person who is obese is generally overweight, but someone who is overweight may or may not be obese. Most clinicians identify a person as obese, however, when he or she is 15 to 20 percent above the age-, sex- and height-related weight norm (see below).

DIAGNOSIS

There are several methods used to determine if, in fact, an overweight condition is caused by an accumulation of adipose tissue; that is, by obesity.

Physical appearance.   Inspection of one's nude body in front of a mirror is often the simplest and most direct way to recognize obesity; similarly, buttons that won't button, zippers that won't zip, and steadily increasing clothes size in adults over 25 years of age indicate a weight increase that is probably caused by the accumulation of adipose tissue.

Skinfold thickness.   The "pinch test," in which a fold of skin and its underlying subcutaneous fat is picked up from the side of the lower chest or the back of the arm and pinched between thumb and forefinger, can also be used to assess obesity. If the fold is greater than an inch in thickness, the individual is probably obese.

A more sophisticated and accurate pinch test has been developed, using a calibrated device called a caliper. This is a standardized instrument which should be used by a trained professional to ensure accurate and consistent results. Using the caliper, skinfold thickness is routinely measured at the back of the right upper arm (triceps skinfold thickness) at a point halfway between the shoulder bone and the elbow, although other sites have been used as well. The minimum skinfold thickness measurements that are indicative of obesity in Caucasian Americans are shown in the Appendix, Table A-4. Note that girls and women have greater values than do boys and men, and that skinfold thickness increases with age. Norms have not yet been established for persons older than 50 years, and data for children under 5 years of age are few. Investigators in Sweden have defined skinfold norms for Swedish children under 3 years of age.[4]

It should be remembered that the data in the table are based on average measurements from a specific population, and also that reproducibility of measurement is extremely important yet difficult to achieve.

Height-weight tables Charts compiled from life insurance statistics have traditionally been used in the assessment of body weight. The tables originally indicated average weights for age and height, and demonstrated an increase with age. Thus, the "recommended" or "ideal" weight increased for each age group, continuing through adulthood. We now recognize that this rate of increase is not desirable, and that average weights of an increasingly sedentary (and overweight) population are not standards consistent with overall good health. In light of these considerations, the revised tables are based on weights associated with lowest mortality rates, and reflect the philosophy that adults should maintain their weight at a level appropriate for a 25-year-old individual. The newer tables (see Appendix, Table A-3) list a range of desirable weights for adults, allowing for differences in body frame. Unfortunately, there are no clear-cut criteria for determining whether an individual has a small, medium, or large frame; this fact imposes a limitation upon the use of these tables as an absolute guideline for an individual's desirable body weight. Nevertheless, the new tables are

an improvement over the original standards, and provide a rough estimate of whether a person's weight is consistent with his or her height and body frame.

Growth charts for children and adolescents. The presence of obesity in children, from infancy through 18 years of age, can be estimated by the use of growth charts. Rates of linear growth and weight gain are expressed in percentiles. An infant may be in the 30th percentile for length but in the 95th percentile for weight; the nutritionist should suspect that the child is being overfed, and conversation with the mother about the child's diet will probably confirm the suspicion. Similarly, feeding practices should be questioned if the child who has consistently been in the 50th percentile for weight shows a steady increase up to the 90th percentile. As with the height-weight tables used for adults, these norms do not consider factors of bone structure or body composition, but discrepancies or inconsistencies in growth patterns should be investigated.

In the past, growth charts based on data collected in Boston and Iowa about 30 years ago were used to evaluate growth patterns in children. Recently, new charts have been prepared under the supervision of the National Center for Health Statistics.[5] The revised charts are based on large, nationally representative samples of children, and are divided into ages 0 to 36 months, and 2 to 18 years; each age group is further subdivided by sex. The more extensive population groups used to compile these charts should give a better approximation of "normal" growth and development for children from all sectors of the country.

Data based on body composition. Several methods of estimating body fat content (in contrast to total body mass) are available, but because of the time and expense involved in their use, these sophisticated techniques are generally used only in a research laboratory rather than in a clinic or screening center. Determination of body density indicates the degree of fatness: since fat has a specific gravity less than that of bone or muscle (0.92 vs 1.1), a measurement of body density (mass per unit volume) which approximates 0.92 indicates an abnormal accumulation of fat in proportion to muscle and bone. An estimation of lean body mass related to total body weight is also an indication of "fatness." Lean body mass can be measured by counting the amount of ^{40}K (a radioactive isotope of potassium) present in the nonfat cells in the body.

The best estimates of obesity are those which consider fat accumulation rather than total weight; however, many clinical situations, generally modified by time, cost, and personnel, permit only the use of tables or growth charts. If the limitations of these data are kept in mind, they are valuable to the clinician in determining whether a patient is overfat.

ETIOLOGY

Although the overall mechanism in the development of obesity is an imbalance in energy intake versus energy expenditure, obesity is a multifactorial condition; its underlying cause is complex and not completely understood in all cases. Much research has been undertaken to assess the importance of several factors which are thought to contribute to the imbalance, and a discussion of a few of these is in order.

Heredity
Although there are several animal strains in which obesity is an inherited trait, no such pattern has been established in humans. While it is true that obese parents often have obese children,[6] factors of life style and attitudes toward food undoubtedly play a role in the etiology of the observed familial pattern. Some additional evidence linking obesity with genetics is provided by studies showing that identical twins, even when raised in different homes, tend to show more similar weights than do fraternal twins, even if the latter are raised together in

the same environment. These types of data imply that genetic factors play a role in the development of obesity, but both the mechanism and relative importance are unknown.

One factor in the development of obesity that has been related to heredity is the body type (somatotype) passed down from parents to children. An *ectomorph* is a lean, thin person, with delicate bones and long thin fingers; an *endomorph* is a round, "soft" individual in whom the abdominal area tends to be larger than the chest. Someone classified as a *mesomorph* has a muscular chest which is larger than the abdomen. It is very unusual for an ectomorph to become obese, and while it is not inevitable than an endomorph will be fat, the probability is quite high that this will happen unless positive steps are taken to avoid it.

Endocrine and Metabolic Status
While attempts have been made in the past to associate obesity with disturbances of the endocrine system, especially the thyroid, very few cases of obesity are caused by an underactive thyroid; moreover, hypothyroidism responds to hormone replacement therapy. Most endocrine abnormalities associated with obesity, including the hyperinsulinism observed in many patients, appear to be a consequence, rather than a cause, of the overfat condition, for they diminish or disappear following weight loss. Some researchers have suggested that the activities of certain enzymes associated with lipid metabolism are altered in some persons, but there is little concrete evidence to support this theory as a primary causative factor of obesity.

Adipose Cell Theory
Shortly after Winick demonstrated that availability of food during growth and development affected the number and size of cells in various organs of both rats and humans,[7] Hirsch and Knittle presented evidence that both the number and size of adipose tissue cells were greater in obese than in nonobese children.[8] Studies with rats confirmed that over-

feeding early in life caused hyperplasia of adipose tissue, producing an increase in the number of adipocytes which persisted throughout life.

Additional studies with obese adults indicated that the number of cells, as well as the amount of lipid contained in each cell, was increased in comparison with findings in those who were nonobese. Moreover, weight reduction decreased the amount of lipid per cell, but did not affect the number of adipose cells. Further, studies by Sims et al.[9] suggested that adult-onset obesity represents an increase in the size, but not the number, of adipocytes.

The theory that has developed from these observations is as follows: Overfeeding in early life will cause excessive hyperplastic growth of adipose tissue, as well as an increased lipid accumulation within each cell. Thus, there is more *lipid* contained in more *cells*. The increased cell number persists throughout life; even though weight reduction may occur later, resulting in a loss of lipid from the cells, the adipocytes remain, waiting to be refilled with fat as soon as energy intake exceeds energy output.

Although the theory has not been universally accepted by researchers, it has prompted several investigators to examine the question "Do chubby infants become obese adults?" Evidence has been presented which indicates that infant obesity is correlated with obesity in childhood[10,11] and that childhood obesity predisposes to obesity in adult life.[12] A recent report describes a retrospective study which suggests that infants' weights during the first 6 months of life correlate with their adult weights (at 20 to 30 years of age). Of those adults who were above the 90th percentile for weight as infants, 36 percent were overweight; 14 percent of the subjects who were below the 75th percentile as infants were obese as adults. Many other factors presumably were involved in this outcome, as social class, education, and parental weight were also related to adult weight.[13] It is therefore apparent that while infant obesity may predispose to adult obesity, there are several other considerations to be examined, and the question remains far from resolved.

The apparent increasing incidence of obesity among infants has led clinicians to examine infant feeding practices in order to determine if these can be associated with the increased weights observed in the population. Several studies, both in the United States and Great Britain, have demonstrated a high prevalence of infant overfeeding, associated with the early introduction of solid foods and also with the practice of bottle feeding rather than breast feeding. Nutrition education programs should be undertaken to inform new mothers that, while it is important to make sure that their baby's nutritional requirements are met, excessive energy intake is undesirable because it can lead to obesity, with its attendant complications, both medical and social.

Environmental and Social Factors

Several environmental factors are conducive to excessive weight gain. First and foremost is the availability of food products to which we are exposed in our affluent society. Closely associated with this is the role of socioeconomic status in defining population groups in which obesity is common. As socioeconomic status improves, the prevalence of obesity tends to decrease.

Cultural and ethnic considerations also influence attitudes toward body size. In some cultures, especially those of the Mediterranean countries, a plump and rounded woman is preferred to a thin and angular one. Being overweight is considered a sign of prosperity and contentment in many cultures as well. The ingestion of certain types of foods, specific for a particular culture, also increases the probability of becoming obese (see Chap. 14). Another overriding attitude, seemingly unrelated to ethnic origin, is that a chubby baby is a healthy one.

Social customs also contribute to the positive energy balance that precedes weight gain. Most occasions, be they weddings, funerals, holidays, or sporting events, are associated with food. In fact, it is considered rude not to offer a guest in your home something to eat or drink. This custom was perfectly acceptable, and necessary as well, when visitors arrived after a long trip; riding down the street in an automobile to visit a neighbor is hardly a trip, but the ritual of offering food as a sign of hospitality still persists.

Occupational hazards also abound in our present-day society. Business meetings over cocktails and dinner, coffee breaks, and office parties are no small part of our daily lives. Students have a difficult time concentrating on homework without a snack, and study breaks invariably include food.

A significant change in our daily activity patterns is also responsible for the development of obesity. Not only do we alter our habits as we age, from being a star on the high school or college athletic team to working at a predominantly "sit-down" job, but those activities in which we do engage have been modified by the introduction of energy-saving machines. Labor-saving devices have been installed in most homes and offices, the use of automobiles and public transportation has modified our mode of travel, and vertical motion is generally accomplished by escalators and elevators rather than stairs. Spectator sports include a greater portion of the population than do the participatory sports.

It has been suggested that this relative lack of exercise in comparison to energy intake is the major factor contributing to the prevalence of obesity in the United States.

Regardless of its specific etiology, obesity is the result of an energy intake that exceeds energy utilization. A very fine balance between input and output must be maintained when we consider that theoretically an intake that exceeds expenditure by even 100 kcal (420 kJ) per day will result in an annual weight gain of about 10 lb (4.5 kg), since it is generally accepted that a pound of adipose tissue contains approximately 3500 kcal (14.7 MJ). Efforts at maintaining body weight at a stable level must

focus on monitoring both food intake and activity patterns. Fig. 21-1 indicates some of the factors related to the development of human obesity.

Psychological and Emotional Factors

Because food is so strongly associated with our life styles, people sometimes tend to use food as a type of weapon. A mother who rewards her child for good behavior or a good report card with a piece of candy or chocolate cake is instilling an attitude toward food which may have far-reaching implications. Similarly, if a child's failure to eat a particular food that mother has prepared is interpreted as "I don't love you," the child might be made to feel guilty, and may soon learn to eat in order to please others. Thus, a child can be influenced to view food as a way to manipulate, and be manipulated by, other people.

Physiological Factors

For many years there has been interest in the physiological control of hunger and satiety. Various models have been proposed to explain the signals which cause us to start and stop eating. The glucostat theory proposed by Mayer[14] states that a center in the hypothalamus is sensitive to the rate of glucose utilization. When food is ingested, blood glucose levels rise and glucose utilization increases; hypothalamic receptors are stimulated and send a signal to stop eating. Conversely, when glucose utilization decreases several hours after a meal, the hunger center responds and tells us to eat again.

Because the theory does not explain all the observations related to eating behavior, other models involving plasma amino acid levels, lipid stores, prostaglandins, endocrine signals, and nervous impulses have been proposed. Moreover, several studies indicate that hunger and feeding behavior are dissociated in the obese person. Schacter observed that obese subjects respond to external cues of sight, smell, and taste rather than to true feelings of hunger.[15] It is apparent that the regulation of

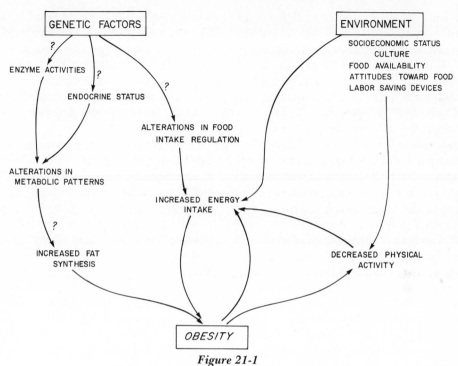

Figure 21-1
Factors related to the development of obesity.

food intake is indeed a complex phenomenon, and that its complexities are far from being understood.

TREATMENT

Energy-Restricted Diets

Adults An energy-restricted diet can be planned that is nutritionally adequate and that reflects the life style of an individual while producing a 1- to 2-lb weight loss per week. The diet should accommodate for cultural and religious preferences, socioeconomic level, physical activity, and age, and should meet nutrient needs for energy, protein, vitamins, and minerals. The amount of energy (that) the adult patient must consume to achieve this weight loss can be determined by multiplying the individual's ideal body weight (in kg) by:

20 to 25 kcal (84 to 105 kJ) for a sedentary individual

30 kcal (126 kJ) for a moderately active individual

35 kcal (147 kJ) for a markedly active individual[16]

For example, a woman whose ideal body weight should be 55 kg and who is moderately active should consume approximately 1650 kcal (6930 kJ) (55 kg × 30 or 55 kg × 126). Since 1 lb of body fat has the energy content of 3500 kcal (14.7 MJ), a 500-kcal (2.1-MJ) deficit per day will produce a 1-lb weight loss at the end of 1 week.

Children Like adults, each child has its own individual energy requirements based on body size, age, and level of activity, all of which must be considered in planning the child's weight-reducing diet. Severe restriction of food can interfere with growth potential and a weight loss of no more than 1 lb per week is recommended. An energy requirement based on height can help to provide an estimate of actual needs.[17] On this basis, a child's requirement between the ages of 7 and 11 approximates 36 kcal (151.2 kJ) per inch, or 14.1 kcal (59.5 kJ) per cm, of body height. Once the child's energy requirement is established, 500 kcal (2100 kJ) [or 600 to 800 kcal (2500 to 3360 kJ) if inactive] can be subtracted from that requirement to obtain the energy intake needed to produce a 1-lb weight loss per week.

Diet control is difficult to establish in children and requires the cooperation of all family members. The child is especially isolated when food must be restricted. Food has its own special meanings (see Chap. 10) and often a large void is caused in the child's life when the diet is imposed and special foods (cakes, candy, cookies) are removed. Activities must be planned to fill this gap. Parents must learn to establish a helping rather than a controlling relationship; they must learn to foster the control within the child rather than to control the food. They must adopt a consistent approach that utilizes some of the techniques of behavior modification and must exert patience with the child even when compliance is poor.

Activity is another important component of the weight control program which is often resisted by the passive, withdrawn obese child. The child will need understanding and a gentle exercise program based on incorporating movement into the daily life style; e.g., walking instead of riding to school, using stairs instead of elevators, playing with toys and in games that encourage body movement. Eventually as body image improves the child may be ready for a community- or school-based swimming program, scouting, or Little League. Recommendations must be realistic and must be based on the family's life style.

Nutrient distribution The recommended dietary allowance for protein is 0.8 g/kg of ideal body weight for an adult and 1 g/kg for the school-aged child (see Appendix, Table A-1, for other age groups). This can be increased in accordance with age (for growth needs) and patient preferences without exceeding the given energy restriction. Lean beef, chicken, fish, and skim milk are utilized for protein sources, since protein is often accompanied by fat.

Fat and carbohydrate provide 40 to 50 percent of the total energy content of the diet. Fat is incorporated into the diet to provide satiety but in limited amounts because of its high energy value. Carbohydrate foods are needed for proper protein utilization and to provide vitamins, minerals, and fiber. Baking and broiling are the suggested methods of food preparation.

An energy-restricted diet can usually be planned to meet vitamin and mineral requirements. However, if an individual is following a diet of 1000 kcal (4200 kJ) or less, and in energy-restricted diets for growing children, a vitamin supplement is advisable.

Total nutrient needs can be accommodated by utilizing the food exchange system as presented under Diabetes Mellitus" in Chap. 20. This system provides variety in the foods from the basic food groups while controlling daily intake. (See Table 21-1.)

Role of Exercise

Exercise should be an adjunct of all weight-reducing programs. The type and amount of exercise should be determined by the individual's previous activity patterns and current physical condition. Exercise aids in toning muscles and increases cardiopulmonary efficiency. Table 21-2 summarizes energy expenditure for various activities.

Approach to Dieting by Behavioral Control

Since treatment of obesity has generally been a failure, new methods of treatment are continually being sought. Behavior modification is a technique which has been introduced into the treatment of obesity. The goal of behavior modification in this context is to change learned eating behaviors. This is accomplished by establishing an individualized program which attempts to modify eating practices. (See Chap. 10.)

The program starts with a description of the behavior to be controlled. For this purpose, the individual keeps daily records of the following: time of eating, place of eating, physical position when eating, social aspects of the situation, activities associated with eating, perceived degree of hunger, perceived mood, food selected, and amount consumed—both by volume and by calories (or kilojoules).[18]

Next, antecedent conditions (also known as discriminatory stimuli) must be assessed.[19,20] These antecedent conditions are also determined by food records which the patient is asked to keep for several weeks.

It must be noted that therapy does not actually begin until after the completion of these records, which are carefully scrutinized. Intervention is then based on the type of maladaptive behavior. For example, the individual who eats rapidly is instructed to put the fork down between each bite of food; for the individual who eats when bored, activities are substituted to fill the void.[21] In all behavior modification programs small changes are initially instituted and then incorporated slowly into the individual's life style.

Reinforcement for appropriate behavior is the final component of the behavior modification program and is carried out in a number of ways. One, known as a contingency contract, establishes a system of rewards for the appropriate behavior. Family participation is used, especially with children, and each member is instructed on how to respond to the individual. Responses must be consistent so that changes can be incorporated into the individual's life style. For long-term success, behavioral change is essential and must be associated with weight loss.[22] Ultimately, the patient should assume responsibility for his or her own behavior.[23]

Studies seem to indicate that there is a role for the use of behavior modification techniques in the treatment of obesity.[24,25] Penick et al. compared behavior modification with group psychotherapy.[26] Therapy was conducted for 3 months with 32 obese patients. The group treated with behavior modification lost more weight than the matched control group treated with psychotherapy. These data may indicate the benefits of conducting behavior modification in a group rather than individually as had traditionally been done. The results of this study also showed that there is a range of success with behavior modification, as shown by the patients' weight losses, which ranged from minimal to maximal. On the basis of such studies nutritionists are currently being trained in behavior modification and are learning to conduct successful treatment groups.[27] Further research is needed to adequately assess the efficacy of behavior modification as a mode of treatment in weight reduction.

Starvation Regimens

Starvation regimens have been used for the treatment of obesity; they usually require hospitalization. During this time (30 days or longer) the patient is given only water (a minimum of 2 qt per day to maintain homeostasis) and a vitamin and mineral supplement (including potassium and calcium) in order to produce a state of ketosis. With starvation, the body's first physiological need is to supply the brain with adequate fuel and all available sources of glucose are utilized. When this supply has been depleted, muscle protein and adipose tissue are metabolized to meet the body's energy requirements. Amino acids from the lean body muscle mass are deaminated and converted in the liver to glucose for use by the liver. Gradually, the body makes a metabolic adaptation to starvation and triglycerides from adipose tissue are hydrolyzed, yielding glycerol and free fatty acids. Glycerol is converted in the liver to glucose (gluconeogenesis) but the net yield of glucose is small. The body must then rely on free fatty acids for energy. Because of the excessive rate of metabolism, these are incompletely oxidized in the liver,

TABLE 21-1 SAMPLE WEIGHT CONTROL DIET

Food group	Servings	Carbohydrate	Protein	Fat	Energy, kcal	Energy, kJ
Milk (skim)	2	24	16	—	160	672
Vegetables	3	15	6		75	315
Fruit	5	50			200	840
Breads	8	120	16		560	2352
Lean meat	8		56	24	440	1848
Fat	5			25	225	945
Total					1660	7917

Foods to use freely:	Foods to avoid:*
Diet beverages†	Sugar
Coffee	Candy, gum
Tea	Honey
Bouillon	Jam, jelly
Unsweetened pickles	Cookies, cake, pie
Lettuce	Syrup
Radishes	Soft drinks
Sugarless gum	Condensed milk
	Fried foods, gravies
	Sauces
	Alcohol

1600 kcal (6720 kJ) Menu plan

Breakfast:

8 oz	Skim milk
4 oz	Orange juice
½ cup	Bran flakes
1 slice	Whole wheat toast
1 tsp	Margarine
	Coffee

Snack

½ Grapefruit

Lunch:

8 oz	Skim milk
½ cup	Tuna with 2 teaspoons mayonnaise
2 slices	Rye bread
	Lettuce & tomatoes
1	Peach

Snack

1 Apple

Supper:

5 oz	Broiled chicken (without skin)
1 small	Potato, baked, with 1 tsp margarine
½ cup	Carrots
½ cup	String beans
1	Roll with 1 tsp margarine

TABLE 21-1 *(continued)*

½ cup	fresh fruit cocktail
	Tea
Snack	
4	Graham crackers
	Tea

* On occasion, to meet an individualized need, one or more of these foods may be planned into an energy-restricted diet.

† To be used with Discretion.

producing ketone bodies, water, and carbon dioxide. The ketone bodies become the major source of energy for the body, as well as for the brain, and weight loss is rapid, e.g., 1 lb per day.[28] Side effects which may accompany this

TABLE 21-2 ENERGY EXPENDITURE FOR VARIOUS ACTIVITIES

	Energy expended,	
Activity	*kcal/(kg·h)*	*kJ/(kg·h)*
Bicycling (moderate speed)	2.5	10.5
Crocheting	0.4	1.7
Dishwashing	1.0	4.2
Dressing and undressing	0.7	2.91
Driving car	0.9	3.8
Eating	0.4	1.7
Exercise		
Light	1.4	5.9
Moderate	3.1	13.0
Severe	5.4	22.7
Ironing (5-lb iron)	1.0	4.2
Painting furniture	1.5	6.3
Running	7.0	29.0
Sawing wood	5.7	23.9
Skating	3.5	14.7
Skiing (moderate speed)	10.3	43.3
Sweeping	1.4	5.9
Vacuuming	2.7	11.3
Swimming (2 mph)	7.9	33.2
Walking (3 mph)	2.0	8.4
Walking (5.3 mph)	8.3	34.9

Source: Adapted from F. J. Stare and M. McWilliams, *Living Nutrition,* 2d ed., John Wiley and Sons, Inc., New York, 1977, p. 101.

type of regimen include headaches, nausea, and constipation. Biochemical alterations include elevated serum lipids and uric acid, and electrolyte abnormalities. Loss of hair, loss of muscle mass, and interference with growth in children have also been noted.

The quick weight loss and reduced hunger induced by the state of ketosis make starvation regimens useful in the treatment of the massively obese patient. However, the major metabolic consequence associated with starvation is the loss of muscle protein.[29] To prevent this condition, Blackburn advocates the addition of protein to prevent muscle loss while maintaining a state of ketosis.[30] This is accomplished by adding 3 to 6 oz of lean meat two times per day to the diet, which otherwise consists of noncaloric liquids and a vitamin and mineral supplement.

Weight loss during either a starvation regimen or a protein-sparing fast is rapid; but whether this weight loss can be maintained is questionable. Because of the poor success in maintaining weight loss after completing a starvation regimen, more is being done to transfer the patient from a protein-sparing fast to an energy-restricted diet and finally to a weight maintenance plan. Behavior modification is being used in conjunction with diet to aid in weight maintenance. However, until long-term follow-up studies are done the success of this type of treatment remains questionable.

For many, the medically oriented approach has lost appeal and many individuals

TABLE 21-3 OTHER APPROACHES TO WEIGHT CONTROL

Diet	Description	Comment
Formula	Liquid formula containing carbohydrate, protein, fat, vitamins, and minerals, usually made from skim milk. Contains approximately 225 kcal (945 kJ) per 8-oz serving. Recommended intake is four 8-oz servings per day providing 900 kcal (3780 kJ), in place of ordinary foods	Contains no fiber, is an artificial method of eating, and is monotonous. Patients generally regain weight when they cease taking formula
Weight groups [Weight Watchers, Diet Workshop, Take Off Pounds Sensibly (TOPS)]	Standardized energy-restricted diet is given to all participants. Weekly group meetings for encouragement and support	Well-balanced diet but does not allow for individual differences and growth needs
The Stillman Diet The Atkins Diet The Mayo Clinic Diet	See Chap. 14	

have turned to community-based programs [Weight Watchers, TOPS (Take Off Pounds Sensibly)—see Table 21-3]. Situated in neighborhood locales, these draw interest and evoke peer pressure.

Drugs

Because weight loss is difficult to achieve, and even more difficult to maintain, pharmaceutical agents have been used to promote weight reduction. It should be stated at the outset that these drugs are generally unsatisfactory in the long run, and they should be used only under the supervision of a physician.

Several drugs have been introduced to produce anorexia, or loss of appetite. The classic compounds that have been used for this purpose are the amphetamines. While they do cause appetite depression, their anorectic effect is relatively short-lived, and more importantly, they produce serious side effects, generally associated with their stimulatory action on the central nervous system. Among the side effects noted are addiction, insomnia, constipation, and excitability. The Food and Drug Administration has stated that amphetamines are of limited value (they often become a crutch for obese patients in their attempt to lose weight),

and should be prescribed by physicians only for a short period of time and in conjunction with an energy-restricted diet.[31]

Because the amphetamines produce several debilitating side effects, new anorectic agents have been developed. Fenfluramine appears to exert a depressive effect on the central nervous system, producing drowsiness rather than excitability in its users. This fact will presumably reduce its potential for abuse. Studies are under way to determine its mechanism of action; it has been shown to have hypoglycemic activity and appears to be an effective appetite suppressant; when used in conjunction with an energy-deficient diet, fenfluramine may prove to be a useful adjunct to weight reduction therapy for certain patients.

Many overweight people have turned to the use of laxatives and diuretics to promote decreased absorption of ingested food and to increase water loss, respectively. Their use should be discouraged, because serious fluid and electrolyte imbalances may result from their indiscriminate use. In addition, a patient who experiments with these preparations will experience a false sense of security and accomplishment when he or she steps on the scales. Although weight loss will have been achieved, good food habits which encourage mainte-nance of a real and continued weight loss (i.e., a reduction of adipose tissue) will not have been established, with the inevitable result of another weight gain.

Even though most obese people are not hy-pothyroid, thyroxine and triiodothyronine have been prescribed to effect a weight loss. A weight loss does often occur; however, it is transient and the weight tends to be regained when therapy is discontinued. Importantly, severe cardiovascular effects and negative cal-cium and nitrogen balance have been observed in patients receiving thyroid hormones for the treatment of obesity.

Because human growth hormone is known to mobilize free fatty acids without depleting nitrogen stores, some researchers have suggested that it might be a good candidate for use in treating patients who have been unsuc-cessful in losing weight by dietary means. How-ever, the quantity of the hormone that is avail-able is insufficient for adequate and conclusive testing.

Human chorionic gonadotropin (HCG) is a placental hormone that has been used in con-junction with a 500-kcal (2.1 MJ) diet for the treatment of obesity. Simeons introduced this regimen in 1954 and reported that the use of HCG reduced appetite and improved the mood of his patients.[32] However, Simeons could not dissociate the weight loss attributed to HCG from that caused by the severe dietary energy restriction.

Several studies have been carried out since Simeons' report to verify his results. Asher and Harper[33] did a double-blind study in 1973 and reported a significant weight loss in the hormone-treated group. Recently, however, Stein et al. reported that there was no statisti-cally significant effect of HCG on weight loss over and above that related to the low-caloric diet.[34] The controversy over the effectiveness of this drug in weight reduction will undoubt-edly continue. It should be remembered that hormones have been shown to be relatively in-effective in precipitating a weight loss, and their use is usually contraindicated.[35]

Surgery

An increasingly common approach to weight loss is intestinal bypass surgery. Because this procedure is not without risk, the careful selec-tion of suitable patients is an important consid-eration. The procedure should be reserved for patients who are morbidly obese, which implies a life-threatening situation if obesity is allowed to continue, and who have been unable to lose weight by more traditional means. Weight cri-teria for the procedure have generally been set at more than 100 lb overweight, or double the ideal body weight. The rationale for this ad-mittedly drastic procedure is to decrease the intestinal absorptive area so that ingested food (energy) does not gain entrance to the body.

In the original procedure, a short section of the jejunum was anastomosed to the colon, thereby bypassing the entire ileum and most of the jejunum. Extremely severe diarrhea with electrolyte depletion was an almost universal side effect, and that procedure has been aban-doned. One of two procedures is now gener-ally performed. The first is called an "end-to-side" bypass, in which approximately 14 in of proximal jejunum is anastomosed to the distal ileum, leaving only 4 in of the terminal ileum above the ileocecal valve and the ascending colon. The second procedure, in which the proximal jejunum is joined to the cut end of the ileum, is called an "end-to-end" bypass. Either of these operations results in a 16- to 22-ft-long loop of intestine which is sutured closed or anastomosed to the transverse section of the colon in the respective procedures.

The effectiveness of the surgical proce-dure can be assessed in several ways. In addi-tion to the observed weight loss, various clinical findings are seen: a flat oral glucose tolerance curve; steatorrhea; decreased urinary xylose; decreased serum carotene, tryglyceride, and cholesterol levels; and a decreased absorption of vitamin B_{12} (necessitating vitamin B_{12} ther-apy in postoperative patients).

For most patients steady weight loss occurs for 1 or 2 years after the surgery, and then a plateau is reached. This has commonly been attributed to reactive hypertrophy of the functional bowel segment, resulting in an increase in absorptive capacity.

Some of the unwanted effects of jejuno-ileal bypass should be mentioned. First, there is a 3 to 6 percent mortality rate associated with the surgical procedure itself. In addition, nausea and diarrhea are major problems. Negative calcium, potassium, and magnesium balances have also been reported. A serious side effect is hepatic steatosis (fat deposition in the liver). The observation that plasma amino acid patterns closely resemble those found in kwashiorkor, a condition in which fatty liver is also present, has led some clinicians to supplement the dietary intake of bypass patients with amino acids. Only limited success has been achieved, and other factors which may contribute to the pathogenesis of liver disease in these patients (accumulation of bile acids or of toxic substances produced by intestinal bacteria) have been considered.[36]

Renal stones, which have been identified as calcium oxalate, are also common in bypass patients. Hyperabsorption of dietary oxalate occurs in these individuals, and has been related to intestinal and mucosal abnormalities associated with altered calcium and bile salt metabolism. Prevention of renal calculi can be enhanced when several measures are employed: restriction of dietary fat and oxalate, plus calcium supplementation. Additional benefit in some patients may be derived from the use of cholestyramine, a resin that binds bile salts and dietary oxalate.[37]

A recent report suggests that decreased food intake and altered taste preferences accompany the weight loss in postsurgical patients.[38]

On the positive side, Solow et al. have reported psychological benefits associated with the surgery. Following weight loss, patients showed an improvement in mood, self-esteem, body image, and activity levels, and an increased effectiveness in interpersonal and vocational endeavors.[39] Much more information is needed to evaluate the long-term benefits of this drastic procedure, particularly in light of the consequential side effects. The selection of patients must be a primary consideration. In addition to the patients' being physically and psychologically able to withstand the surgical procedure and its metabolic and physiological consequences, they must be prepared to undergo a second operation if it becomes necessary to either revise or take down the bypass. A comprehensive symposium on jejunoileostomy for obesity has been published recently.[40]

STUDY QUESTIONS

1 Differentiate between the terms obesity and overweight.

2 Discuss the various etiological theories proposed to explain the obese state.

3 Describe the methods of weight reduction that would be contraindicated in the treatment of obesity.

4 What type of surgical intervention may be offered to the morbidly obese patient?

5 What are the presently accepted treatment methods for obesity?

CASE STUDY 21-1

Christopher is a 7½-year-old who was brought to the school nurse by his second grade teacher who noted that the boy was short of breath while playing during the recess period.

The nurse recorded his height at 132 cm and weight at 64.9 kg, which represented a weight gain of 4 kg since school had begun. On the suggestion of the school nurse the child was brought by his parents to the Children's Hospital Weight Control Clinic.

The history revealed a child of a normal pregnancy and delivery with a birth weight of

3.5 kg. Weight increments were normal until about age 4. The family history was negative for obesity. The parents were professors at a local college and extremely academically oriented. Chris's mother had returned to teaching and continued her Ph.D. program when Chris began attending preschool.

After school Chris is left in the care of a baby-sitter except for two afternoons per week when he goes to religious classes and music lessons. He is an extremely bright boy who enjoys reading and has little time for or interest in physical activity.

On physical examination adiposity in the mammary region was noted. His abdomen was pendulous, with white and purple striae, and his penis was submerged in pubic fat. Blood pressure was 130/85, taken with a normal-size sphygmomanometer. Anthropometric data showed Christopher's height to be at the 90th percentile and his weight to be off the Stuart-Meridith growth grid for 7-year-olds. He was approximately 34 kg overweight. Skinfold measurement was 30 mm (at the 95th percentile for 13-year-olds). Laboratory tests included thyroid function tests; a complete blood count; blood glucose; serum cholesterol, potassium, chloride,

sodium, pH, carbon dioxide, alkaline phosphatase, and 17-ketosteroids; urine sugar; blood urea nitrogen; and wrist x-ray for bone age determination. All tests were within normal limits.

A diet history was difficult to obtain since Chris often gets himself off to school and is left in the care of the baby-sitter after school. A diary kept by his mother showed his total food intake to approximate 1700 kcal (7140 kJ).

The diagnosis of exogenous obesity, causing slight hypertension, was made on the basis of anthropometric data, blood pressure, and normal laboratory findings. The parents' attitude was one of resistance and denial, and they repeatedly inquired about the possibility of endocrine disturbance.

CASE STUDY QUESTIONS

1 What influences do you think have prompted the development of the child's obese state?

2 What type of program would you recommend?

3 Could this problem have been prevented? How?

THE CHILD WITH PRADER-WILLI SYNDROME

Peggy L. Pipes

INTRODUCTION

Prader-Willi syndrome, described by Prader, Labhart, and Willi in 1956, is a condition in which feeding difficulties such as poor sucking ability and failure to thrive in infancy are usually followed by a very rapid weight gain, resulting in obesity in early childhood.[41] The etiology of the syndrome is unknown. It is generally thought to be due to a prenatal developmental defect in the hypothalamus, the appetite control center of the body.

Other significant symptoms include hypotonia, hypogenitalism, very small hands and feet, and behavioral problems which become apparent during the school-age and adolescent years. Intelligence ranges from severely retarded to near-normal. Because of the hypotonia and delays in motor development, young children with the disorder engage in limited activity and, with increasing obesity, sedentary activities become preferred.[42]

The rate of weight gain and the degree of obesity increase with age, usually beginning as the children learn to walk and obtain their own food. Linear growth commonly proceeds at a very slow rate. Most individuals with Prader-Willi syndrome are short and grossly obese. Diabetes, secondary to obesity, commonly develops during adolescence. It is characeristically nonketotic and non-insulin-dependent, and responds to weight reduction.

Affected individuals, because of their lack of satiety awareness, usually exhibit peculiar food behavior, such as gorging and stealing food. (One child has been reported to eat twelve pies at one sitting and continue to be hungry.) There are other reports of bizarre food consumption and pica, involving such foods as pet foods, garbage, and frozen foods. A combination of learning problems or mental retardation along with the obesity may lead these children to have a poor self-image, manifested in trantrums, outbursts of rage, and disobedience. A successful treatment program is based on environmental control, diet, and the consideration that each child will manifest the syndrome in varying degrees and that treatment should be highly individualized.

ENVIRONMENTAL CONTROL

A successful program for weight control or reduction demands that all who have contact with affected individuals understand both the need to restrict energy intake and the behavioral aspect of the syndrome. The preoccupation that affected individuals have with food and their continuous effort to secure food must be viewed as a component of the syndrome and not as misbehavior. In addition, efforts to transfer the responsibility for dietary control to the individual have never been successful. Parents or caretakers must assume this responsibility, providing foods with appropriate numbers of calories, (joules) monitoring the sneaking of food, and managing any inappropriate behavior. It is important for schools, workshops, and merchants to understand that stealing food and money to buy food is common among individuals with this syndrome and that sack lunches and snacks must be locked and unavailable. The person with Prader-Willi syndrome should not enter a grocery store, enroll in cooking classes, or drop by the candy counter of the drugstore.

The family or caretakers and school or workshops must be highly motivated, willing to control the food environment by making food unavailable to these persons and knowledgeable in and willing to apply principles of behavior modification. Both parents and affected individuals require constant supervision and support as they learn to conform to an energy-restricted diet.

School personnel and relatives may have difficulties in recognizing a potential problem when a child does not appear overweight, and they must be included in the program to control weight. They will have to restrict the use of foods as reinforcers and carefully plan food experiences within the dietary plan for the child. Food for special occasions such as birthday parties and halloween must be included as part of the energy intake which has been planned. Methods which have proved effective are to delete 50 kcal/day (210 kJ/day) from the intake for 1 or 2 weeks prior to the festivities, or to plan special low-caloric foods for these activities.

An effective weight control program will require that families make food unavailable by locking refrigerators and cupboards or even putting locks on the kitchen door. It is imperative that the table be cleaned off immediately after each meal and that food remain out of reach and out of sight. The person responsible for implementation of the diet plan needs to be knowledgeable in energy values of stolen foods and accommodate for these by making equal reductions in meal patterns.

DIET

When the syndrome is diagnosed in infancy it is possible to prevent obesity. Careful monitoring of the child's energy intakes and growth pattern can provide baseline data that can be used to design diets to prevent the very rapid rate of weight gain which usually occurs in the preschool years. If obesity is manifest then a program to effect reduction in weight is important.

It has been suggested from carefully controlled studies which monitored food intake in relation to weight gain and linear growth that energy intake per centimeter of height is a useful reference in establishing the energy needs of children with Prader-Willi syndrome in the preadolescent years. Data from these studies have indicated that most children maintain an approximate weight and growth by consuming 10 to 11 kcal (42 to 46 kJ)/cm of height.[43,44] Variations in energy needs have, however, been noted among children; diets should be individually designed and adjustments in energy intakes made as children grow taller.

If attempts to prevent obesity have been unsuccessful, a goal for a slow but continuing weight loss should be established. Intakes of 8.5 kcal (36 kJ)/cm of height have effected losses of approximately 1 kg per month. This distribution of fat is kept in the range of 20 to 25 percent calories/kilojoules, protein 20 to 30 percent calories/kilojoules in 2 to 3 g/kg protein, and the remainder of the calories (joules) as carbohydrate.[45] In some centers, a protein-sparing diet has been used with success.

STUDY QUESTIONS

1 Why is control of the environment essential in planning the weight reduction diet of the child with Prader-Willi syndrome?

2 What suggestion would you offer to parents to help facilitate environmental control?

3 Based on the recommendations given in this section, plan a diet for Andrea (Fig. 21-2). She is 8 years old, weighs 34.4 kg, and is 129.6 cm tall.

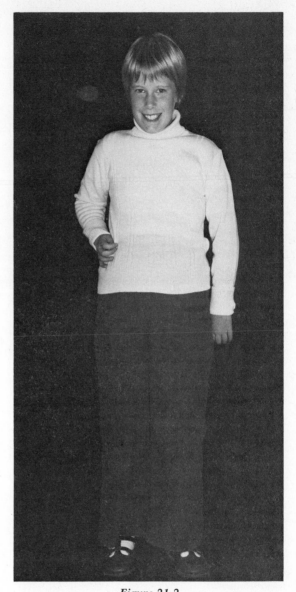

Figure 21-2

An 8-year-old child with Prader-Willi syndrome controlled within 18 lb of her appropriate weight for her height, as a result of a positive reinforcing controlled environment, and a "total family approach."

REFERENCES

1 H. Bruche, *Eating Disorders: Obesity, Anorexia Nervosa and the Person Within,* Basic Books, Inc., Publishers, New York, 1973, p. 124.

2 Ibid., p. 128.

3 Ibid., p. 387.

4 P. Karlberg, I. Engstrom, H. Lichtenstein, et al., "Development of Children in a Swedish Urban Community. A Prospective Longitudinal Study. III.

Physical Growth During the First Three Years of Life," *Acta Paediatrica Scandinavica Supplement,* **187**:48–66, 1968.

5   National Center for Health Statistics, "NCHS Growth Charts, 1976," *Monthly Vital Statistics Report,* vol. 25, no. 3, suppl. (HRA) 76-1120, Health Resources Administration, Rockville, Maryland, 1976.

6   J. Mayer, "Obesity: Causes and Treatment," *American Journal of Nursing,* **59**:1732–1736, 1959.

7   M. Winick, J. A. Brasel, and P. Rosso, "Nutrition and Cell Growth," in M. Winick (ed.), *Current Concepts in Nutrition,* vol. 1, *Nutrition and Development.* John Wiley and Sons, Inc., New York, 1972, pp. 49–97.

8   J. Hirsch and J. L. Knittle, "Cellularity of Obese and Nonobese Human Adipose Tissue," *Federation Proceedings,* **29**:1516–1521, 1970.

9   E. A. Sims, E. S. Horton, and L. B. Salans, "Inducible Metabolic Abnormalities During Development of Obesity," *Annual Review of Medicine,* **22**:235–250, 1971.

10   E. E. Eid, "Follow-up Study of Physical Growth of Children Who Had Excessive Weight Gain in the First Six Months of Life," *British Medical Journal,* **2**:74–76, 1970.

11   P. Asher, "Fat Babies and Fat Children," *Archives of Disease in Childhood,* **41**:672–673, 1966.

12   J. K. Lloyd, O. H. Wolf, and W. S. Whelan, "Childhood Obesity: A Long-Term Study of Height and Weight," *British Medical Journal,* **2**:145–148, 1961.

13   E. Charney, H. C. Goodman, M. McBride, B. Lyon, and R. Pratt, "Childhood Antecedents of Adult Obesity. Do Chubby Infants Become Obese Adults?" *New England Journal of Medicine,* **295**:6–9, 1976.

14   J. Mayer, *Overweight.* Prentice Hall, Inc., Englewood Cliffs, N.J., 1968, pp. 20–21.

15   S. Schacter, "Obesity and Eating. Internal and External Cues Differentially Affect the Eating Behavior of Obese and Normal Subjects," *Science,* **161**:751–756, 1968.

16   R. Goodhart and M. Shils, *Nutrition in Health and Disease,* 5th ed., Lea and Febiger, Philadelphia, 1973, p. 849.

17   V. Beal, "Nutritional Intake," in R. W. McGammon, *Human Growth and Development,* Charles C Thomas, Publisher, Springfield, Ill., 1970, pp. 77–78.

18   H. A. Jordan, "A Behavioral Approach to the Problem of Obesity," Paper presented at the Behavior Modification Workshop, Philadelphia, October 1974.

19   Ibid.

20   L. S. Levitz, "Behavior Therapy in Treating Obesity," *Journal of the American Dietetic Association,* **62**:2, 1973.

21   Ibid.

22   H. A. Jordan, op. cit.

23   R. B. Stuart and B. Davis, *Slim Chance in a Fat World: Behavioral Control of Overeating,* Research Press, Champaign, Ill., 1972.

24   H. A. Jordan and L. S. Levitz, "Behavior Modification in a Self-Help Group," *Journal of the American Dietetic Association,* **62**:27, 1973.

25   L. S. Levitz and A. J. Stundard, "A Theraputic Coalition for Obesity: Behavior Modification and Patient Self-Help," *American Journal of Psychiatry,* **131**:4, 1974.

26   S. B. Penick et al., "Behavioral Modification in the Treatment of Obesity," *Psychosomatic Medicine,* **23**:49, 1971.

27   B. Paulson et al.,"Behavior Therapy for Weight Control: Long Term Results of Two Programs with Nutritionists as Therapists," *American Journal of Clinical Nutrition,* August 1976, pp. 880–888.

28   G. F. Cahill, "Physiology of Insulin in Man. The Banting Memorial Lecture 1971," *Diabetes,* **20**:785–799, 1971.

29   G. Blackburn, "Adaptation to Starvation," in *Intake: Perspectives in Clinical Nutrition,* Eaton Laboratories, 1973, p. 5–6.

30   Ibid. pp. 7–10.

31   *FDA Drug Bulletin,* U.S. Food and Drug Administration, Rockville, Maryland, December 1972.

32   A. T. W. Simeons, "The Action of Chorionic Gonadotrophin in the Obese," *Lancet,* **2**:946, 1954.

33   W. L. Asher and H. W. Harper, "Effects of Human Chorionic Gonadotrophin on Weight Loss, Hunger, and Feeling of Well-Being," *American Journal of Clinical Nutrition,* **26**:211–218, 1973.

34   M. R. Stein, R. E. Julis, C. C. Peck, W. Hinshaw, J. E. Sawicki, and J. J. Deller, "Ineffectiveness of Human Chorionic Gonadotropin on Weight Reduction: A Double-Blind Study," *American Journal of Clinical Nutrition,* **29**:940–948, 1976.

35   R. S. Rivlin, "Therapy of Obesity with Hormones," *New England Journal of Medicine,* **292**:26–29, 1975.

36   D. H. Lockwood, J. M. Amatruda, R. T. Moxley, T. Pozefsky, and J. K. Boitnott, "Effect of Oral Amino Acid Supplementation on Liver Disease After Jejunoileal Bypass for Morbid Obesity," *American Journal of Clinical Nutrition,* **30**:58–63, 1977.

37   J. Q. Stauffer, "Hyperoxaluria and Calcium Oxalate Nephrolithiasis After Jejunoileal Bypass," *American Journal of Clinical Nutrition,* **30**:64–71, 1977.

38   G. A. Bray, R. E. Barry, J. R. Benfield, P. Castelnuovo-Tedesco, and J. Rodin, "Intestinal Bypass Surgery for Obesity Decreases Food Intake and Taste Preferences," *American Journal of Clinical Nutrition,* **29**:779–783, 1976.

39   C. Solow, P. M. Silberfarb, and K. Swift, "Psychosocial Effects of Intestinal Bypass Surgery for Severe Obesity," *New England Journal of Medicine,* **290**:300–304, 1974.

40 W. W. Faloon (Chairman), "Symposium on Jejuno-ileostomy for Obesity," *American Journal of Clinical Nutrition,* **30**:1–129, 1977.

41 A. Prader, A. Labhart, and H. Willi, "Ein Syndrome Von Adipositas, Kleinwucks, Kryptorchismus und Oligophrenie nach Maytonieartigen zustand in Neugeborenenalter," *Schweizerische Medizinische Wochenschrift,* **86**:1260, 1956.

42 B. D. Hall and D. W. Smith, "Prader-Willi Syndrome," *Journal of Pediatrics,* **81**:286, 1972.

43 P. L. Pipes and V. A. Holm, "Weight Control of Chil-ican Dietetic Association,* **62**:520–524, 1973.

44 V. A. Holm P. L. Pipes, "Food and Children with Prader-Willi Syndrome," *American Journal of Diseases of Children,* **130**:1063, 1976.

45 P. L. Pipes and V. A. Holm, op. cit., p. 522.

CHAPTER 22

THE NERVOUS SYSTEM AND HANDICAPPING CONDITIONS

Rosanne B. Howard
Linda Fetters
Dorothy M. MacDonald

KEY WORDS
Neurotransmitter
Failure to Thrive (FTT)
Anorexia Nervosa
Handicapped Child
Handicapped Adult
Postural Control
Prone
Supine
Aspiration
Primitive Oral Reflexes
Proximal
Distal
Breck Feeder
Beniflex Feeder

NUTRITION IN THE TREATMENT OF DISORDERS AND DISEASES OF THE NERVOUS SYSTEM

Rosanne B. Howard

INTRODUCTION

The nervous system organizes, integrates, monitors, and controls all of the activities of the body. Vital to body function, the system is afforded protection by bone structure, meninges, cerebrospinal fluid, and the blood-brain barrier, which prevents foreign substances from entering the cerebrospinal fluid. However, the high degree of specificity of the nervous system makes it more vulnerable to alterations in metabolism, especially to changes in levels of oxygen and glucose. The finding that minerals (calcium, magnesium, sodium) and vitamins (thiamine, pyridoxine, nicotinic acid, ascorbic acid, and vitamin B_{12}) are needed for adequate nerve cell function established the relationship between diet and the nervous system. This relationship was reinforced by research on the effects of early malnutrition on the brain (see Chap. 12) and more recently by accumulating evidence of the effects of a normal diet on brain biochemistry.

Of prime concern, early in this chapter, is the response of the nervous system to the normal diet and the use of diet in the comprehensive treatment and rehabilitation of individuals with diseases or conditions affecting the nervous system. Later sections discuss motor control and its relationship to feeding, and present special feeding techniques for use with the handicapped individual.

THE NERVOUS SYSTEM

Function

The nervous system is divided anatomically into two primary components: the central and the peripheral parts. The *central nervous system* is composed of the *brain* and the *spinal cord*. The *peripheral nervous system* lies outside of the skull and the vertebral column and is composed of the spinal and the cranial nerves. The peripheral nervous system is subdivided further into the *somatic system,* which supplies the skin and skeletal muscles, and the *autonomic system,* which supplies impulses to smooth muscle, cardiac muscle, and the glands of the body, which functionally interrelate closely with the nervous system. (For example, at least two glands, the adrenal medulla and the pituitary, secrete their hormones in response to nerve stimuli.) Overall, the autonomic nervous system helps to control arterial pressure, gastrointestinal motility and secretion, urinary output, sweating, body temperature, and other body functions. In turn, the hypothalamus, one of the major areas of the brain, controls the autonomic nervous system, and also regulates body weight, fluid intake, and food intake. The role of the hypothalamus, as one of the neural centers for the control of the quantity of food intake, is considered in Chap. 21.

The nervous system is formed by two types of cells:

Neurons   The excitable, conductile units

Glia   The connective, supportive, and nutritive units

Neurons are present throughout the nervous system, with 90 percent located in the brain. It is estimated that 10 billion neurons comprise the system, and that the glia outnumber the neurons 10 to 1. The number of functioning units increases during development, peaking at maturity. With age, nerve cells grow old and die, and the population of neurons irrevocably declines.

The neurons are varied in size and shape but possess certain common characteristics. Each neuron contains a cell body or soma, which gives rise to one or more extensions or processes that serve to connect the cell body to other neurons and the central nervous

system or to an organ. These processes are structurally and functionally of two types: the *axon,* extending from the cell body into the peripheral nerve (which conducts impulses away from the cell body), and the *dendrites,* relatively short projections of the soma serving as the receiving portions (which conduct impulses toward the cell body).

The glia cells occupy the space between neurons and are considered to have a connective, supportive, and nutritive role for the neurons they enclose. Some glia cells, known as the *oligodendrocytes,* form myelin, which comprises the sheath that may surround the axons and dendrites. (Both types of processes may develop a sheath or may remain without one). The myelin sheath is composed of layers of fat, protein, polysaccharides, water, and salt, and increases the speed of impulse along the axon or dendrite. These cells that form the myelin are particularly sensitive to a variety of diseases, which are known as the demyelinating diseases, e.g., multiple sclerosis. The major lipids in myelin are cholesterol, cerebrosides, cephalins, and sphingolipids. The lipid component of the sheath is also subject to change in those genetic disorders known as the lipidoses.

Whole neurons (cell body, axon, dendrite) may be *afferent,* conducting impulses toward the brain (as in the sensory portion of the brain), or *efferent,* conducting impulses away from the brain (as in the motor portion of the system), or *internuncial* or *associative* neurons found between afferent and efferent neurons. The junction between neurons is known as the *synapse,* which is the site of impulse transmission. These areas of connection are functional, not an anatomical continuity. The passage of an impulse across a synapse is chemically mediated by substances, called *neurotransmitters,* that are present in the neurons. When the neurotransmitters are released, the neuron transmits signals across synapses or to muscle cells, or secretory cells outside the brain transmit impulses to efferent neurons within the brain. Each neuron is thought to release only a single type of neurotransmitter which either excites or inhibits the impulse, depending upon its biochemical effect on the postsynaptic neurons, or those with which it makes contact. When the impulse arrives at the axon ending, the chemical substance is released from small vesicles located in the branched ends of the axon (telodendria). Once released, the chemical diffuses across the space between the two neurons (synaptic cleft) and either depolarizes the next neuron or inhibits depolarization. The chemical is then destroyed by an enzyme or by oxidation.

In the brain there are six compounds that are fairly well established as brain neurotransmitters: *acetylcholine; gamma-amino butyric acid;* the three catecholamines *epinephrine* (or *adrenalin*), *norepinephrine,* and *dopamine;* and *serotonin.* These transmitter substances, with the exception of acetylcholine, are derived from amino acids or are amino acids themselves and as such are closely dependent on nutrient intake. Recent evidence indicates that at least three major kinds of neurotransmitters are affected by diet: acetylcholine, serotonin, and the catecholamines, such as dopamine and norepinephrine.

The Effect of Diet on Brain Neurotransmitters

Research by Wurtman and Fernstrom on rats has indicated that following a meal high in carbohydrate, there is an increase in the rate of synthesis of serotonin (5-hydroxytryptamine), the best studied of all the brain products.[1,2] Serotonin is produced in the body tissues (the major loci are the brain and the gastrointestinal system). In the brain all the serotonin present is confined to a group of neurons known as the raphe nuclei, whose cell bodies are located in the brainstem, and whose nerve fibers ascend into the rest of the brain and descend down through the spinal column. It has been proposed that serotonin is involved in avoidance learning, the effects of hallucinogenic drugs, sleep, sensitivity to pain, the con-

trol of food intake, and the release of pituitary hormones.

Serotonin is produced from the amino acid tryptophan, which is carried to the brain through the bloodstream by a transport protein. Tryptophan has difficulty in competing with the other neutral amino acids for a transport protein. However, the insulin secreted by the pancreas in response to a high-carbohydrate diet assures tryptophan of a carrier protein, for it facilitates the uptake of all the neural amino acids except tryptophan, thus increasing the relative concentration of tryptophan in the blood and allowing it access to a transport protein and passage into the brain. The increased concentration of brain tryptophan then accelerates the synthesis of serotonin in the brain.

It is hypothesized that diet-induced changes in the concentration of serotonin in the raphe nuclei neurons would be paralleled by changes in the amount of serotonin released into the synapses when the neurons transmit impulses. These serotoniergic neurons would therefore function as sensors, converting a signal that is circulating in the bloodstream into a statement in brain language, thereby conveying messages about peripheral metabolism. The long-term and the short-term consequences of diet changes are manifested by the plasma amino acid pattern, and also, since the serotoninergic neurons are known to be associated with a number of neuromechanisms, messages about growth, development, and stress are transmitted.

In addition to its effect on serotonin, the diet also influences the rates of synthesis of acetylcholine, produced in the brain from choline, and of the catecholamines, which are synthesized from the neutral amino acid tyrosine.

It is now becoming more established that normal diets can affect brain metabolism, opening a new era in understanding and possible treatment of neurologic and even psychiatric disorders.

Disturbances in food intake have been characteristic of psychiatric patients, and the use of pharmacologic doses (called orthomolec-ular therapy) of vitamins (e.g., niacin and vi-tamin C) to treat depressive anxiety and schizo-phrenia first gained popularity during the 1920s and 1930s when frank niacin deficiency states and the dementia of pellagra actually ex-isted in the institutionalized mental patient. Since that time there have been no well-controlled studies to support the use of large doses of vitamins, and their use raises ques-tions concerning safety and side effects. Al-though the role of diet in the treatment of mental illness awaits further elucidation, the diet of all patients suffering from psychiatric disturbances should be reviewed for adequacy, since anorexia or bizarre food preferences may be interfering with the body's need for essen-tial nutrients, further complicating mental status.

The Effect of Emotions on Neurohormonal Function

In addition to the effects of the normal diet on brain function and of malnutrition on the developing brain (see Chap. 12), the effect of the emotions on neurohormonal function has been subject to debate centering around two conditions with major nutritional implications: nonorganic failure to thrive, which is observed in the young child, and anorexia nervosa, which usually appears during adolescence or the young adult years.

Nonorganic Failure to Thrive (FTT)

Growth and development are dependent on the fulfillment of the physical, emotional, and sensory needs of the child. The effects of each of these determinants are closely interrelated with one another. Deprivation of the child, whether deliberate, as with child abuse, or oth-erwise, as through ignorance, manifests in growth failure, malnutrition, and delays in motor and social development. Spitz and Wolf first noted this deleterious effect in their study of institutionalized infants.[3] In describing the anaclitic depression suffered by these children,

they noted loss of appetite and weight, in-somnia, greater susceptibility to infection, and gradual decline in developmental quotient. Whether the failure to thrive is related pri-marily to the caloric deprivation, as proposed by Whitten,[4] or is due to the psychic effects upon pituitary function,[5] is hard to determine.

The disorder becomes apparent some-where between the ages of 9 and 18 months. The infant is usually withdrawn and anorexic, and may be involved in self-stimulatory behav-ior, including rumination. The toddler has a shallow emotional response and solemn aspect. A voracious appetite, pica, or proclivity to fluids, and a protuberant abdomen further characterize these children.

Upon hospitalization or transfer to a dif-ferent home environment, most children begin to thrive. Again, is it the food or is it the pres-ence of tactile, vestibular, and emotional stimu-lation? This underlying question has yet to be answered but in clinical practice failure to thrive exists as a mixed entity. A treatment plan which considers all aspects—the child's nutritional, emotional, and physical needs—must be devised.

Intervention poses a threat to parents, who fear condemnation or adverse judgment, sometimes causing them to react in a defensive or hostile manner, especially when asked about the child's daily food intake.

With hospitalization, the child's weight may make immediate increments or accrue only after a prolonged period. A regular daily caloric intake should be maintained during this period, as well as a diet based on age, with en-ergy and protein needs related to expected height and weight. These children initially may not recognize satiety and will need to have limits set.

Many of these children had problems in the neonatal period with sucking, stooling, or sleep patterns. Recognition of these early signs and providing the parents with practical and emotional support during this period can help to establish an enduring parental-infant bond and possibly ameliorate or prevent this syndrome. Some infants are difficult to feed because of subtleties inherent in their own make-up, and parents need the assurance that it is not necessarily their fault. Also, anticipatory guidance directed to the period after hospital discharge helps parents to understand that feeding problems may continue because of the child's negative perceptions of food, and that time, consistency of approach, and understanding are needed on their part to work out these problems. Data suggest that stress in the household and lack of familial and social ties in the family of the child with nonorganic failure to thrive make social programming critical to ensuring nutritional well-being. Parents are often as needy as the child, and health professionals should direct care accordingly.

Anorexia Nervosa

Since the classic descriptions of Gull[6] and Lasegue[7] over 100 years ago, the attempts to explain anorexia nervosa with one psychoanalytic theory have imposed stereotyped images on a vastly complex picture. The concept that the condition was an expression of repudiation of sexuality dominated earlier clinical thinking. The modern psychoanalytical approach has turned from this symbolic concept and now focuses on the nature of the parent-child relationship from its beginning and on behavior and attitudes not directly related to food, although the preoccupations with food and weight are the characteristic manifestations of this condition.

The disorder mainly afflicts teenage girls from middle- to upper-class families who show an obsession to avoid overeating, hyperactivity, and denial of fatigue. The eating disturbance has two phases: the absence or denial of the desire for food, and uncontrollable impulses to gorge, usually without hunger awareness and followed by self-induced vomiting. Electrolyte imbalances and malnutrition resulting from the compounded effect of starvation, self-induced vomiting, and the abuse of laxatives has led to fatality in a small percentage of cases.

Weight loss, amenorrhea, constipation, abdominal pain, and unusual growth of hair on the body are physical symptoms which have led some researchers to consider the syndrome primarily as a malfunction of the neuroendocrine system localized in the hypothalamus. This has led to the exploration of the role of neurotransmitters and the catecholamine, dopamine, to explain the combined changes in anorexia nervosa,[8] and to subsequent trials of antidepressants such as amitriptyline, which has been found to produce short-term success in some patients.[9] However, that a psychological origin of the illness causes the secondary physiological disturbances is the theory that presently continues to prevail.

In attempts to comprehend the behavior problems of the patient and to reconstruct the patterns of family interaction, Bruch identifies the major issue as a struggle for control and for a sense of identity, competence, and effectiveness.[10] The early history usually reveals an exceptionally healthy, cooperative, academically successful, model child. There is usually a recognizable time of onset, commensurate with an event that makes the patient feel "too fat" and prompts the self-imposed diet.

Owing to distorted body images, these individuals continue to see themselves as fat. Nutritional rehabilitation of the malnourished state is a difficult task that is wholly dependent on the psychological treatment of the illness to overcome these negative perceptions and normalize food intake. The recovery period is a long and arduous process, sometimes requiring hospitalization for 6 months to a year. Management issues are complex, as these patients are knowledgeable about food and are extremely manipulative of their energy intake and expenditure. The dietitian's role is dependent on the treatment approach used. Different modes of treatment, using psychoanalysis, behavior modification, and drugs, singly or in combinations, are employed in various centers around the country. Bruch warns that despite transient weight increases with behavior modification techniques, an approach that focuses on this treatment method without attention to the severe underlying psychological problems is potentially damaging.[11]

THE HANDICAPPED CHILD

At any point in the life cycle, the brain is vulnerable to insult, but never more so than during the course of development. Problems due to gene abnormalities (e.g., hereditary diseases such as inborn errors of metabolism) or those occurring during embryogenesis which are related to sporadic preconception changes in germ cells (e.g., Down's syndrome, multiple congenital anomalies) or later during pregnancy (e.g., fetal malnutrition, plasma insufficiency, toxemia, drug addiction) or at birth (e.g., prematurity, trauma, hypoglycemia, hyperbilirubinemia) or during early childhood (e.g., complications of infection, tumors, cranial trauma) may result in physical handicaps accompanied in many instances by mental retardation. The following section will highlight areas that are important to the nutrition, care, and treatment of the handicapped child.

Although the causes of handicapping conditions are numerous and varied, the growth and developmental milestones of childhood can act as common denominators to help parents and professionals recognize behavior apart from the handicapping condition, set appropriate goals, and develop a consistent instead of an overbenevolent approach to feeding.

Feeding these children often requires special remediation techniques (see "Feeding the Handicapped Child," and "Feeding the Child with a Cleft Lip and Palate" later in this chapter) and always requires an understanding that food to this child might not necessarily symbolize love. Because of prolonged hospitalizations, and gavage feedings or forced feedings, food may possibly come to symbolize frustration or conflict to the child, an attitude around which a whole host of feeding behavior

problems may develop. These must be separated from the organically based feeding problems. For example, rumination is a finding in many of the severely retarded children; it involves the regurgitation of previously swallowed food and then the reswallowing of it, providing a form of self-stimulation. It is often initiated by placing the fingers in the mouth or throwing the head back with the tongue extended, causing the child to ruminate and perpetually exude a sour odor. Treatment involves programmed brief social behavior reinforcers[12] and the thickening of feedings.

Growth

To the clinician working with an organically handicapped or mentally retarded child, the understanding of somatic growth is difficult. There is much confusion over the relationship between brain damage and growth. An anthropometric study of 678 handicapped children by Pryor and Thelander somewhat helps to elucidate an understanding of the growth deviations that can occur.[13] They found that growth was most adversely affected in children with Down's syndrome that was caused by a chromosomal aberration, next in those with multiple congenital anomalies that were apparently due to prenatal environmental insults during embryogenesis, and less in those with cerebral palsy due to birth injury or severe hypoxia at birth. To further elucidate growth deviations, they propose a helpful analogy, namely that of a time clock. This time clock sets off a chain reaction that encompasses implantation, differentiation of tissues, growth, and development in both prenatal and postnatal life. It seems that interference with the time clock distorts growth specifically and according to when the interference occurs. Thus, the growth of a child with Down's syndrome, caused by a chromosomal aberration which has occurred early on the time clock, is more adversely affected than the growth of a child with cerebral palsy, which represents a later period after normal gestation.

In the majority of cases, the basis for poor physical growth will not be clearly known. However, the clinician must not be satisfied with assuming that poor physical growth is completely due to the brain damage of the child. A detailed evaluation of the present and past food intake may provide additional clues to the poor physical growth. For example, a vitamin or trace mineral (e.g., zinc) deficiency may be compromising growth in a child with a limited food intake. Severely handicapped children receiving maintenance tube feeding require particularly careful diet supervision.

Energy Needs

Energy needs for this population of children should be determined according to body size (calories per centimeter of body height) and motor status. With regard to motor status, one study by Culley and Middleton surprisingly showed that the type of motor dysfunction did not noticeably affect the caloric needs of these children except as a factor interfering in their ability to walk. Children whose motor dysfunction was severe enough to prevent ambulation required approximately 75 percent as many calories as ambulatory children of comparable height. In this study, whether the child had hypotonia, ataxia, spasticity, or choreoathetosis (see definition p. 471), energy needs were the same per centimeter of body height and were related to the degree of ambulation.[14] A detailed food diary that is kept for a 2-week period, with the energy intake compared to the weight lost or gained, can begin to give a clue to the child's caloric needs, providing the child is not edematous. Underweight and overweight are the two conditions which most demand nutritional intervention.

Feeding Problems

Besides altering growth and energy needs, the handicapping condition can pose obstacles to accomplishing the developmental tasks of childhood. A child needs head support, trunk support, and sitting balance, eye-hand coordination, and the ability to grasp, hold, and release objects before feeding independence can be established. If parents are helped to recognize their child's readiness to progress, the handicapped child is given the opportunity to achieve some level of feeding independence. The following areas can be commonly identified as problems for which an individualized solution must be sought:

Sitting balance

Head and neck control

Lip control

Tongue control

Sucking, swallowing, chewing, drinking

Mouth sensation (lack of mouth sensation or hypersensitivity to temperature changes or tactile stimulation)

Startle reflex (a child with cerebral palsy may respond to a loud noise by a startle reflex)

This is further discussed under "Feeding the Handicapped Child," below.

Pain and fatigue may present additional obstacles to feeding. A brief period of relaxation before meals may be helpful and small frequent feedings rather than large meals may impose less stress in some instances. A weak, lethargic infant who is sleeping for long periods should be awakened at appropriate intervals for feeding; otherwise, important energy needs will not be met. Initially the child might be fed earlier than other family members until he or she is ready to join the family meal without demanding too much attention. All family members should be shown the special feeding techniques so that the responsibility does not fall always to one member. Everybody concerned with feeding the child should adopt the same approach, using the *same words* at the *same time* in the *same place* with the *same utensils*. All will need the discipline to maintain a calm, friendly attitude, for overreacting to negative behavior by shouting, forcing, or cajoling only serves to reinforce the behavior.

Drugs

The use of drugs may also interefere with feeding, causing drowsiness, altering taste, interfering with appetite (amphetamines), or promoting an insatiable appetite (steroids). Drugs also affect nutritional status by their influence on nutrient absorption, gastrointestinal flora, electrolyte balance, and metabolism. Anticonvulsant drugs, which are commonly used in this population, are known to produce folate deficiency and may increase a child's need for vitamin D. Low serum folate levels and megaloblastic anemia have been associated with diphenylhydantoin therapy and also with phenobarbital and primidone.[15] Children taking these medications should be monitored by periodic complete blood counts (CBC). Rickets has been reported in mentally retarded children receiving long-term anticonvulsant therapy. Factors influencing this state are related to the number of anticonvulsants taken, the size of dosage, the child's mobility, and exposure to sunlight.[16] It is postulated that these drugs induce hepatic enzymes which degrade vitamin D.[17] Children who are receiving long-term anticonvulsant drug therapy should therefore have periodic determinations of serum calcium, phosphorus, and alkaline phosphatase.

Ketogenic Diets

When anticonvulsant medications prove ineffective, ketogenic diets have been used successfully in controlling intractable myoclonic and akinetic seizures in some patients.[18] A ketogenic diet is one which promotes the formation of ketones in the body (see Chap. 5) and is formulated with fat as the major energy source, with protein to meet the recommended allowances, and with carbohydrate severely restricted. Traditionally, to induce ketosis, a 3:1 ratio of fat to carbohydrate and protein was planned. Since the advent of medium-chain triglycerides (MCT), a greater ketogenic effect has been induced by providing 50 to 70 percent of the calories (kilojoules) as MCT Oil.[19] The rapid absorption and metabolism of MCT is the explanation give of this effect.

The need for strict compliance makes this diet easier to facilitate in the very young or severely retarded child.[20] Food must be weighed or measured accurately to control the proper proportions of carbohydrate, protein, fat, and MCT Oil, and urine must be tested daily to monitor the degree of ketosis.

Additional Concerns

Increased metabolic demands from stress, fever, or underlying disease states are further nutrient considerations along with the need to monitor fluid balance closely, a particular problem in patients with mechanical feeding difficulties or an inability to respond to thirst or to express needs. Bowel and bladder problems related to neuromuscular deficits and leading to constipation and urinary tract infections are prevalent and in many instances can be ameliorated by diet intervention. For example, a child with myelomeningocele (a congenital defect in the closure of the vertebral column) who has impaired bladder and bowel control may derive benefit from a high-fiber diet for constipation, along with fluids and an acid-ash diet or medications to control urinary tract infections. Vitamin-mineral supplementation is often advisable to ensure nutrition in many handicapped children, whose food intake is somewhat unsure.

We will now specifically consider two conditions that are representative of the spectrum of this population of handicapped children and the types of nutritional intervention that should be offered; namely, Down's syndrome and cerebral palsy. This discussion should serve as a conceptual basis for evaluating the nutritional needs of other children with handicaps or developmental disabilities. By analyzing the effect of the condition on growth, feeding ability, nutrient effectiveness, and motor activity, a nutritional care plan can be determined for every handicapped child.

Down's Syndrome

Down's syndrome (Trisomy 21) is a chromosomal aberration involving the presence of an extra chromosome 21. (When chromosomes are examined, they are sorted and numbered from 1 to 22, plus the sex chromosomes X and Y.) Moderate to mild mental retardation, growth retardation, hypotonicity, bridged palate, and a narrow nasal passage are characteristic symptoms with feeding implications. The incidence of other congenital defects (e.g., heart defects, pyloric stenosis, tracheoesophageal fistula) is high in this population, further complicating management.

Growth deficits are marked, with the rate of gain in stature being deficient during all intervals between birth and 36 months of age, and most notably between 2 and 24 months of age, when it is as much as 24 percent less than normal.[21]

Hypotonicity of the muscles is a finding in all of the children; however, the degree of involvement varies considerably among the children. Some children may have difficulty with sucking or later with chewing because of muscle weakness and will need remediation techniques (see "Feeding the Handicapped Child" below), while others have no problems at all. A narrow palate also may hinder feeding as it can interfere with a proper seal for sucking and it provides an easy catchment area for food to accumulate in. The tongue of the child with Down's syndrome is normal in size; however, it projects and appears larger because the hypotonicity affects control of the tongue muscles, and the small premaxillar area makes the tongue seem larger when protruding. Many children are mouth breathers because of a narrow nasal passage and have heavy nasal secretions, a condition to which the children seem prone. Children must be trained to clear the nose of exudate and to keep the mouth closed during eating. Although tooth eruption is delayed, food progressions can be established on the basis of developmental readiness.

The hypotonicity, which affects activity, and the growth deficits of children with Down's syndrome, makes the incidence of obesity quite high, and energy needs are better expressed in terms of body height (calories or kilojoules per cm of body height) than in terms of the recommended dietary allowances for children according to age group.[22] Parental concerns about weight can lead them to strict dietary control and the child to nutrient deficits. Counseling must be directed to appropriate amounts of food based on height. Also, with these children food can easily be used as a social reinforcer, and since some children do not recognize their own satiety, they can be easily overfed.

Hypotonicity also affects muscle control of the bowel, and impaired peristalsis and constipation are frequent findings. Another consistent finding in Down's syndrome has been a markedly reduced serotonin level in the peripheral blood, prompting investigation to find a suitable etiological explanation. Attempts to alter this metabolic pathway by treatment with 5-hydroxytryptophan and pyridoxine have resulted in conflicting and contradictory interpretations which await further research.

Early intervention programs with a nutritional and nursing component direct attention to normalization of the feeding experience. Parents who are overwhelmed by the birth of a child with Down's syndrome need help to recognize the normal developmental aspects of feeding so that as their child achieves one developmental level, they can foster progression to the next, from baby foods to table foods to meal-time independence. Table 22-1 summarizes the guidelines used for feeding stimulation of the infant with Down's syndrome between birth and 6 months in the Early Intervention Program of the Developmental Evaluation Clinic at Children's Hospital Medical Center, Boston. One interesting observation made in the Early Intervention Program at Children's Hospital Medical Center was that parents were not able to encourage independ-

TABLE 22-1 GUIDELINES FOR AN EARLY FEEDING STIMULATION PROGRAM

For children with Down's syndrome from birth to 6 months

Positioning	Hold the child upright, head well supported, slightly downward (never back) Bottle should be tilted so that the neck of the bottle is filled with milk		by placing them around the bottle; as the infant develops, holding the bottle independently can be encouraged (normal skill at 9 months). When the child is ready to take over, use a small 4-oz clear plastic bottle which will be easier for the child to manipulate
Equipment	Nipples should be appropriate to the child. There is a range of shapes and degrees of softness to suit the child; however, nipples should remain firm Bottles also vary from the standard 8-oz glass bottle to nursing systems such as the one put out by Playtex with a plastic pouch that can be squeezed gently during feeding to encourage intake. The type of bottle should be determined by the needs of the child	Baby food	As the child begins to suck the fingers, place a small amount of strained fruit on the fingers occasionally during the feeding to let the child begin to learn that fingers come to the mouth with food When feeding baby foods, place small amounts on the end of the baby spoon (small bowl, teflon-coated) and insert it toward the center of the tongue with a slight downward pressure. Allow the child to swallow before presenting another mouthful. Do not rush. Bring the spoon from different sides during the feeding, encouraging the child to follow with its eyes
Stimulation	Cue into the infant's behavior and feed accordingly: 　1　when the infant is hungry 　2　when the infant is full Cuddling, comforting, and talking to the infant should be part of all feeding situations. As the child develops awareness, naming foods and the food color, size, and shape can help to provide meaningful stimulation Encourage the infant to use the hands		As the child develops head control and can lateralize the tongue (move it from side to side), gradual increments in texture can begin

Source: Developmental Evaluation Clinic, Children's Hospital Medical Center, Boston, Mass.

ence in feeding skills as readily as in other areas of development and appeared to be hesitant to relinquish this dependency.[23]

Cerebral Palsy

The term *cerebral palsy* designates neurologic disorders created by damage to the motor centers of the brain that occurs before, during, or shortly after birth. Physical handicaps range from mild to severe and intelligence from normal to subnormal. Various types of neuromuscular problems characterize this condition, and children may have spasticity (hyperactive muscle stretch reflexes) choreoathetosis (involuntary movements), ataxia (incoordination and balance problems), or flaccidity (decreased muscle tone). The child's ability to see, hear, or speak may also be impaired.

Owing to motor involvement of the cranial nerves that control the infant's ability to suck and swallow, it is during initial feedings that neurologic deficits may first become manifest. Early intervention with remediation techniques (see "Feeding the Handicapped Child") can help facilitate feeding and prevent behavior problems from evolving around the organically based ones.

Feeding difficulties due to neuromuscular impairment and persistence of primitive reflexes make nutrient deficiencies a common finding,[24–26] and demand the attention of all health professionals to help these children meet their recommended allowances for essential nutrients. Hammond et al. found that the degree of mental retardation impeding self-help skills influenced dietary intake more than the motor handicaps imposed by the cerebral

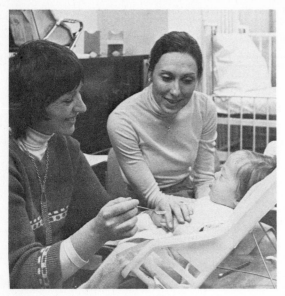

Figure 22-1

Early Intervention Program for children with Down's syndrome at Children's Hospital Medical Center, Boston, Mass. Intervention program consists of pediatrics, physical therapy, psychology, speech therapy, nursing, and nutritional guidance. The nursing-nutritional component is directed toward helping parents to recognize the normal developmental aspects of feeding so that they can foster independent feeding in their child.

palsy.[27] The degree to which the mouth area is involved has been closely associated with poor intake, and the extent of mouth involvement and general growth have been observed to closely parallel one another.[28] Time, fatigue, and loss of food from the mouth are the implicated factors. Growth deficits are marked in these children, and athetotic children are smaller than spastic children. Berg and Isaksson reported in a survey of 23 children with cerebral palsy that all were short for their age and heavy for height. In an earlier study, Berg reported finding an abnormal body composition, with body cell mass that was reduced for height and an excess of extracellular water, and in this case inactivity and malnutrition were considered relevant.[29]

Energy needs should be tailored to the size of the child, with the type of motor dysfunc-

tion considered as well. Nonambulatory, spastic children are at risk of becoming overweight, especially as they approach adolescence. It is questionable whether children with athetotic motions require additional energy intake to support their constant muscular activity when their energy needs are compared to those of normal active children. Energy expenditure in children with cerebral palsy has been found to be lower.[30] However, there is a great range of variation which must be considered in dietary planning. Since the total food intake may be small, the quality is important. Incorporating powdered milk, evaporated milk, wheat germ, and bran into foods can help to enrich the mixture, and thickening fluids slightly with yogurt or baby cereal can facilitate drinking. Fluid intake is a particular concern in this population and must be closely watched, as much fluid is dribbled from the mouth during feeding.

Constipation is another problem that is encountered and is due to decreased peristaltic activity and abnormal muscle tone. Treatment includes stool softeners, fluids, high-laxative foods (see "Constipation" in Chap. 18), and gentle abdominal massage.

Hyperkinesis and Diet

The hyperkinetic child is significantly handicapped by intrinsic or constitutional inefficiencies. The ambiguous nature of the handicap has caused much confusion in the diagnosis of the syndrome, which in many instances is based solely on anecdotal observations of the child's behavior. The Council on Child Health of the American Academy of Pediatrics describes the hyperkinetic child as one of normal intelligence who fails to learn at a normal rate even though given the same educational opportunities as other children with equal intelligence. In addition, the child is noted to exhibit, to some degree: (1) short attention span, (2) easy distractibility, (3) impulsive behavior, and (4) overactivity.[31] At present, the drug treatment of hyperkinesis involves the use of dextroamphetamine and methylphenidate, which are known to produce anorexia and are reported to suppress growth.[32,33]

In 1973 Feingold proposed that hyperkinesis was associated primarily with the ingestion of low-molecular-weight chemicals and suggested dietary treatment. The diet is low in salicylates and food additives and consists of homemade products, and fresh meats, milk, and vegetables. Foods and beverages containing natural salicylates, food flavorings, and food colors, and drugs with salicylates, are avoided.[34] His findings have prompted much controversy in the lay press as well as in professional circles. The National Advisory Committee on Hyperkinesis and Food Additives of the Nutrition Foundation[35] convened in 1975 to review evidence on this subject and concluded that the nutritional qualities of the diet may not meet the long-term nutrient needs of children. Since that time a study by Conners et al. concluded that the K-P diet may reduce hyperkinetic symptoms; however, the problems inherent in the study design leave the conclusion open to question.[36] The Feingold hypothesis bears further investigation, for it remains open to speculation that one of the many ingested foods may be one of several factors aggravating the dysfunction of children with attentional disorders.

THE HANDICAPPED ADULT

The handicapped adult with limbs compromised by injury, arthritis, amputations, progressive neurologic disease (e.g., multiple sclerosis, Parkinson's disease, muscular dystrophy), or brain and spinal cord damage faces the same problems as the handicapped child but in addition must learn to reintegrate the adult need for self-fulfillment and productivity into a compromised life style. Feelings of frustration, boredom, embarrassment, anger, isolation, and exclusion may set up a host of defenses that can interfere with the rehabilitative process. The dysphagia of the stroke (cerebrovascular accident) patient makes swallowing difficult and the often accompanying aphasia can make it impossible for the patient to communicate needs.

The need for a diet that is high in nutrient density becomes paramount in the care of the individual who can tolerate only small feedings, and vitamin-mineral supplementation may be required. Protein is especially important in recovery from the stress of the acute phase, and fiber and fluid must be incorporated into the diet to promote peristalsis and maintain fluid balance (for the patient who cannot tolerate roughage, bran, soaked in milk and mixed into foods, can be a solution). Special therapeutic diets may also be used to treat the disease or condition precipitating the handicap; e.g., a low-fat, low-cholesterol diet for the patient recovering from a cerebrovascular accident. Also low-fat diets have been used with mixed success in some patients with multiple sclerosis.[37] Drug-diet interactions present complications, especially for those patients with Parkinson's disease who are being treated with levodopa. The protein in the diet should be controlled to maximize clinical benefits from the drug. Also, excessive amounts of pyridoxine taken as a vitamin supplement can interfere with the effect of levodopa.

Variations in texture need to be individualized according to the patient's tolerance and degree of motor impairment. The edentulous patient may find that dentures are loose-fitting during the recuperative phase and will require their adjustment to facilitate feeding.[36]

Spinal cord injuries that affect bladder control make urinary tract infections a common problem. Many patients are maintained on an acid-ash diet (see Chap. 19) or on high dosages of vitamin C to acidify the urine. Prolonged immobility can lead to calcium mobilization from bones and to renal calculi, for which an acid-ash diet or a low-calcium diet may be used. Obesity may be an overriding problem in the handicapped adult, who may find eating the outlet for frustration or boredom.

The occupational therapist, physical therapist, and home economist become integral members in the nutritional rehabilitation as patients relearn activities of daily living. Careful selection of feeding utensils and home appliances is necessary in allowing full independence. The kitchen represents many hazards and especially to the handicapped. Simplifying tasks, and encouraging carefully planned tasks with lists to expedite the process, can help to ameliorate the frustration that is especially felt during the early stages of rehabilitation and readjustment.

The development and function of the nervous system and the treatment of its disorders is dependent on nutritional status. An evaluation that acknowledges the biological and psychological characteristics of the individual and that reconciles the growth and developmental needs to the altered demands of the handicapping condition is essential. The complexities of management and the continuing aspects of care require the sevice of an interdisciplinary team: doctor, nurse, nutritionist, dietitian, speech pathologist, physical therapist, occupational therapist, dentist, psychologist, working together in an atmosphere of mutual respect to formulate a treatment program that addresses each individual need.

FEEDING THE HANDICAPPED CHILD

Linda Fetters

THE RELATIONSHIP OF MOTOR CONTROL AND FEEDING

The development of independent movement in a child allows the child freedom. This development of independent movement proceeds systematically. The sequence is the same in all children; however, the *rate* and *quality* of this sequence may vary. Control of the body (postural control) develops as the central nervous system matures and as the baby is stimulated by the environment.

Postural control develops from head to toe, and proximally to distally. Control begins with the child in the horizontal position and gradually increases and improves, enabling the child to assume the upright or vertical position. Until the upright position is attained and the infant has developed skill in the use of the upper extremities, the infant must be fed by another person. This dependent feeding usually occurs with the infant in a semirecumbent position. Full support is given to the infant's body and head. In response to the acquisition of independent abilities by the infant, parents begin to remove their support. The child who is beginning to sit independently (4 to 6 months old) can be placed in a high chair for feeding rather than being cradled in the parent's arms. The infant who is developing skill in hand-to-mouth activities (3 to 4 months onward) will want to self-feed and less parental help will be necessary. This move toward independent feeding is contingent upon the acquisition of normal patterns of movement. The child must acquire *head, trunk,* and *upper extremity control* in order to make independent feeding possible.

The acquisition of postural control is in part contingent upon two aspects of development; normal muscle tone and the integration of primitive reflexes. Abnormal muscle tone and the persistence of primitive reflexes are two characteristics of the child with central nervous system dysfunction that are usually associated with abnormal feeding behavior. The importance of muscle tone and the integration of primitive reflexes for normal feeding abilities will now be considered.

Muscle Tonus

Normal muscle tone is a prerequisite for normal movement. Muscle tone (or tonus) is a state of tension in the body musculature that indicates it is ready to perform its function of movement and postural control. Normal muscle tone is increased enough to permit stability and decreased enough to permit movement. Muscle tonus is controlled by the central nervous system and abnormalities in muscle tone reflect problems with the normal neural control of tonus. In the child with central nervous system dysfunction—for example, the child with cerebral palsy—muscle tonus may be abnormally increased, decreased, or fluctuating between these two extremes. Hypertonic, spastic, and stiff are all terms used to describe muscle tone that is abnormally increased. Hypotonic, flaccid, and floppy are terms used to describe tone that is abnormally decreased.

Normal muscle tone is important for independent feeding abilities. The state of tonus in the body affects the acquisition of independent feeding postures and arm and head movements. The child with increased tonus may not be able to bend at the hips to enable sitting. When placed in a sitting posture, the child may not be able to control its head or trunk to maintain this position. If a child has decreased tone, the ability to assume and maintain a sitting posture may also be difficult or impossible. Normal tonus is also important in the oral musculature used for feeding. Tonus may be decreased, preventing jaw control and lip closure, or it may be increased, preventing movement of the tongue, lips, and jaws for chewing. Feeding problems encountered by children with central nervous system dysfunction may vary, in part because their muscle tonus may be different. As a consequence, the treatment of their problems needs to be individualized.

Primitive Reflexes

During the maturation of the central nervous system, primitive reflexive responses become integrated at appropriate times so that more purposeful, voluntary activity can develop. An example of this development is the integration of the asymmetrical tonic neck reflex (ATNR). This reflexive posture, sometimes called the "fencing position," is normally present in infants from birth to around 4 months of age.

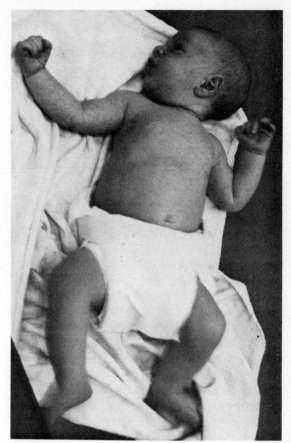

Figure 22-2

Normal asymmetrical tonic reflex posture in a 6-week-old infant. The asymmetrical tonic neck reflex is more evident in the arms than in the legs. This posture is never an obligatory position in the normal infant.

The posture is shown in Fig. 22-2. The arm and leg on the side to which the face is turned show increased extension; the opposite arm and leg show increased flexion. The normal infant's activities are not dominated by this response. Movement away from this position occurs easily so that the infant can suck on its fingers regardless of the position of the head. The infant with central nervous system dysfunction may be dominated by this reflex as a result of the lack of the normal maturation of the central nervous system (see Fig. 22-3). The position of the infant's head may dictate the

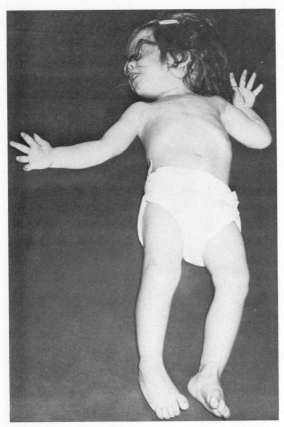

Figure 22-3
Abnormal persistence of the asymmetrical tonic neck reflex in a 3-year-old child. The retention of this reflex has interfered with the child's sitting balance and with hand-to-mouth activities.

lated by placing a nipple or finger into the mouth. Stimulation can be enhanced by touching the hard or soft palate. The infant will suck vigorously on the stimulant. The *rooting reflex* enables the child to find the breast or bottle. If the corners of the infant's mouth or the upper or lower lips are gently touched with a finger or nipple, the mouth will turn toward the stimulation and the head will follow. The rooting response is present from birth on, gradually becoming weaker until it disappears at around 3 months of age. In breast-fed children the rooting response may persist for a longer period.

The *biting reflex* is normally present from birth on, becoming weaker and disappearing at about 3 to 5 months.[38] It is elicited by pressure on the gums, and consists of a phasic bite and release in response to the stimulation. This response is usually not strong. The more sustained bite develops later.

Normally, the *gag reflex* is present from birth on to adulthood. It becomes weaker as chewing begins.[38] The gag reflex is protective in nature and allows return of food from the back to the front of the mouth. It can be elicited by placing a finger at the back of the oral cavity and pressing down on the tongue.

These four infantile oral reflexes—suckle-swallow, rooting, biting, and gag—may be evaluated separately; however, their importance for function lies in their sequential action as the child eats.[39] The dependent infant relies on reflexive responses to find and properly ingest food. The infant performs this feeding repertoire on a background of normal respiration. The infant must be able to nose-breathe in a relaxed manner. In order to do this the infant needs an unobstructed airway from nose to lungs and the ability to coordinate breathing with swallowing. This coordination reflects the nature of control within the central nervous system.

As the primitive oral reflexes are being integrated, the infant is gaining head and trunk control, allowing an independent sitting posture. As independent sitting improves, the in-

position of the limbs. The child may not be able to bring food to the mouth while looking at the food. The lack of normal integration of this response may prevent the child from gaining head and trunk control and prevent the normal acquisition of arm and head movement to allow the child to self-feed.

Organization of Oral Reflexes for Feeding

The *suckle-swallow reflex* appears in the normal baby within the first day or second day of life and remains until 3 to 5 months.[38] It is stimu-

TABLE 22-2 NORMAL ORAL REFLEXES

Reflex	*Description*
Moro reflex	A proprioceptive response elicited by dropping the head back suddenly; the response includes a rapid extension and abduction of the limbs, followed by flexion and adduction of the limbs Normal occurrence: Birth to 4 months Retention produces: Total body responses to stimuli Interferes with: Sitting balance; hand-to-mouth activities
Asymmetrical tonic neck reflex	A proprioceptive response elicited by turning the head from side to side; increased extension is seen on the side to which the face is turned and increased flexion in the opposite limbs Normal occurrence: Birth to 4 months Retention produces: Asymmetrical postures Interferes with: Sitting balance; hand-to-mouth activities
Hand grasp	A stimulus to the palm of the hand (from the ulnar side) elicits finger flexing and grasping of the object Normal occurrence: Birth to 3 or 4 months Retention produces: Fisted hands; difficulty in opening hands Interferes with: Holding utensils
Suckle-swallow	A stimulus introduced into the mouth elicits vigorous sucking followed by a swallow if liquid is present Normal occurrence: 1 or 2 days after birth to 3–5 months Retention produces: Suckling response to any oral stimuli Interferes with: Taking food from spoon with lips; cup drinking; chewing
Rooting	A stimulus to the oral area (corners of the mouth, upper and lower lip) causes lips, tongue, and finally head to turn toward the stimulus Normal occurrence: Birth to 3–5 months Retention produces: Asymmetrical oral response to stimuli; head turning to oral stimuli Interferes with: Maintaining head position for appropriate feeding
Gag	A stimulus to the posterior tongue or soft palate causes constriction of the posterior oral musculature to bring stimulating substance forward Normal occurrence: Birth to adulthood Retention produces: Increased oral sensitivity Interferes with: *Hyperactive gag*—Food is constantly pushed forward and out of the mouth *Hypoactive gag*—Food can passively enter the esophagus or trachea
Bite	Pressure on the gums elicits a phasic bite and release Normal occurrence: Birth to 3–5 months Retention produces: Biting all objects placed in the mouth Inteferes with: Mouthing activities; ingesting food; more mature biting; chewing

fant gains ability in upper extremity functions, including hand-to-mouth behavior. All of these sensory motor abilities indicate that the child is moving toward independence, including independent feeding.

Summary

The development of postural control and independent movement proceeds from head to toe, proximally to distally. The development of normal movement is contingent upon normal muscle tonus and the integration of primitive reflexive responses. The acquisition of independent postural control and movement allows the child to be independent in activities such as feeding. Just as primitive reflexes must be inhibited for independent postural control to develop, primitive oral reflexes must be integrated so that more purposeful oral reflexes may occur. (See Table 22-2.)

The child with central nervous system dysfunction may not be developing independent sensorimotor abilities. Abnormal muscle tone may be preventing head and trunk control and the child may be dominated by primitive reflexive behavior in the body and oral areas, causing feeding problems. The potential problems need thorough evaluation.

EVALUATION OF A CHILD WITH A FEEDING PROBLEM

The habitual feeding behavior of the child with central nervous system dysfunction may show abnormalities from birth. Reviewing the early histories of children with various handicapping conditions frequently reveals early feeding difficulties (e.g., poor sucking ability, taking only small amounts of liquid per feeding, prolonged feeding time, or choking and aspirating liquid). Abnormalities in early coordinated feeding behavior may be the first sign of central nervous system dysfunction. Infants with early feeding difficulties should be monitored in order to rule out long-term difficulties. Feeding problems may also become evident when spoon-feeding and solid foods are introduced.

The evaluation of a child with a feeding problem is best accomplished with an interdisciplinary team of professionals who are experienced in the area of feeding. The team may consist of a nutritionist, a nurse, and physical, occupational, and speech therapists. The consulting services of a dentist and psychologist may also be helpful and are often necessary. Anecdotal information regarding past and present problems can be collected by taking a history; however, it is essential for the team to observe the child during mealtime. Evaluation at mealtime in the home or another familiar surrounding is recommended, since fewer variables are introduced into the feeding situation.

Asking the parents about feeding does not always reveal problems because of the lack of parental objectivity. For example, the child may be ingesting the appropriate amount of calories (joules) in a well-balanced diet, but the parents may not be aware that the texture of blenderized food is inappropriate, or that they are positioning the child with the head tipped back in order to help the food slide down passively instead of allowing active swallowing with the child positioned upright.

When observing feeding, observe the total child. Questions concerning the child's motor development to be answered during the observation include:

Does the child have normal muscle tone?

Does the child have head and trunk control that is appropriate for age level; if the child has not achieved head and trunk control, has control been provided with the use of an appropriate chair or other support?

Are the child's movements spontaneous and in normal patterns; can the child isolate movements of the hands to bring food or objects into the mouth?

What are the child's facial movements and expressions; can the child isolate mouth, tongue, and jaw movements to drink, chew, and swallow?

The normal child has a relaxed face at rest and fine facial control is exhibited during interaction with people and during feeding. The child with abnormal muscle tone may have an expressionless face because of hypotonia, or exaggerated grimacing because of hypertonia (sometimes termed the "spastic grin). Isolated fine facial movements are often lacking in the child with abnormal muscle tone.

Along with general observations, specific evaluation must be given to the following specific categories.

Positioning

Positioning a child properly can facilitate good feeding patterns and prevent choking, gagging, and aspiration. The flexed forward position will encourage swallowing, while the extended position (particularly if the head and neck are extended) will make swallowing very difficult and promote gagging.

The child who has not achieved head and trunk control needs the support of an appropriate chair or should be held on the parent's lap during feeding. Feeding time is not a time for the child to have to struggle to keep the head up and trunk stable. These can be goals of therapy at a different time, although they can be reinforced during feeding time. Support should be provided so that the child can maintain the vertical position. With certain exceptions, feeding should not take place with the child in the supine position, because in this position choking and gagging may occur, increasing the risk of aspiration. (In the event of choking or gagging, try to remove the food from the child's mouth. Avoid pushing the food further into the throat. If needed, turn the child prone with the head hanging down so that gravity will assist in bringing the food forward into the mouth.) The child who is fed in the supine position also misses the visual experiences that can be gained in the upright position and the stimulation which the vertical position gives the body to facilitate postural control.

Oral Reflexes

The persistence of primitive oral reflexes prevents the child from developing more advanced patterns for feeding. It is not only the persistence of primitive reflexes that is abnormal but the *intensity* and *quality* of the reflexes are also frequently abnormal. The four oral reflexes should be evaluated separately and their coordination should be functionally evaluated.

Rooting The child with central nervous system dysfunction may show remnants of the rooting response much longer than the normal child and, as a consequence, when its mouth is stimulated the child's head turns toward the stimulus. This will cause unwanted head movements. In some children the rooting reflex may not be nor-

mally present; e.g., in infants with severe central nervous system problems or very premature infants.

Suckle-swallow This reflex may be retained for several years in severe cases. Stimulation in the mouth causes immediate suckling. This will prevent drinking from a cup and normal patterns of taking food from utensils such as a spoon.

Bite reflex This is particularly persistent in the child with hypertonicity. When this reflex is retained it is always stronger than normal. In severely handicapped children this reflex may persist for life if they have not been helped to overcome it.

Gag reflex This reflex is often exaggerated in children with hypertonicity so that even a minimal stimulus will cause the child to gag. The reflex may be diminished or absent in the child with hypotonia, which is dangerous since it increases the risk of choking or aspirating food.

These four oral reflexes tend to be increased in the child with hypertonia and decreased or absent in the child with hypotonia.

Oral Digital Stimulation

The child's response to stimulation around the mouth must be evaluated. Stimulation can be provided by touching the inside and outside of the mouth, the tongue, and the gums with a finger. This may be done while testing oral reflexes. To be primarily observed are muscle tone changes in response to this stimulation. Infants normally have a great deal of oral experience. The oral area is very sensitive and well utilized as the infant explores its environment. The handicapped child may have had very little or abnormal oral experience and as a consequence the face, mouth, and lips may be overly sensitive to stimulation. The child with abnormal muscle tone may become stiff when the oral area is stimulated. Muscle tonus in the oral area will feel tight and stiff in the child with hypertonia, just as the rest of the body does. In contrast, the oral area of the child with hypotonia may feel flaccid, and little response will be shown to stimulation. The same responses that are elicited with oral digital stimulation may be elicited when food is placed into the child's mouth.

Jaw Control

Normally the jaws are lightly closed at rest and in motion they can be held in any position and move freely. The handicapped child usually has poor control of the jaws. Frequently the jaws are halfway or totally open at rest. The jaws may fall open due to lack of tone or the jaw may be pulled open and retracted or protruded by hypertonicity. The normal development of rotary and horizontal jaw movements may be completely absent in the child with central nervous system dysfunction.

Lip Control

The lips should be observed at rest and while the child is eating. Muscle tonus affecting lip control can be felt during oral digital stimulation. In the normal child, the lips are lightly closed at rest, and in spontaneous motion show a full range of gross and fine movements.[40] In the child with hypertonicity the lips may be tense and slightly closed at rest. When movement occurs, the lips may follow the gross movements of the jaw and lose their fine control. The child with hypotonia may show slack or parted lips and also lacks fine control. Good control of the soft palate will be lacking.

The lack of fine lip control will affect the child's ability to handle some foods, even if the child is fed by another person. Cleaning food from a spoon with the upper lip may be difficult or impossible. Lip closure around a cup will also be difficult and liquid will dribble from the corners of the mouth. It is difficult to swallow normally with the lips parted or widely separated, and for some children it is impossible.

Tongue

Normally, the tongue is adaptive and flexible in its motions. It is capable of fine coordinated movements and only protrudes voluntarily.[40]

The tongue of the child with hypertonus may be rolled (cigar-shaped) and may protrude involuntarily from the mouth. In the primitive suckle-swallow reflex, the tongue normally protrudes from the mouth and then draws liquid back into the mouth. If this primitive response is not normally inhibited with maturtion of the central nervous system, tongue protrusion occurs in response to oral stimulation. As a consequence, food may be pushed out of the mouth as soon as it is introduced. The child with hypotonia may have a floppy, immobile tongue that passively protrudes from the mouth.

The child with any type of abnormal muscle tonus may have an inflexible tongue that tends to move with the gross movements of the jaws. The abnormal pressures that the tongue exerts on the teeth, gums, and jaw, coupled with abnormal muscle tension around the oral area, may cause malformations of teeth and jaws.

Breathing

Breathing patterns should be evaluated while the child is at rest and also while active because it may be difficult for the child to coordinate relaxed breathing with ingestion of food and the risk of aspiration may increase. Normally, breathing is regular and deep. Breathing will easily change with increased activity. The child with abnormal muscle tone may have shallow, irregular breathing patterns and frequently breathes through the mouth.

Hand-to-Mouth Activity

The newborn usually has the ability to bring the hand to the mouth for sucking activities. Reaching and voluntary grasp begins at 3 to 4 months. Reaching begins as gross flailing movements which eventually become directed and controlled. Hand and finger movements develop from gross motions to precise, fine muscular movements, with the child finally able to pick up very tiny objects with a pincer grasp by the age of 6 months.

The child with central nervous system dysfunction and resulting abnormalities in muscle tone may not be able to bring the hand to the mouth easily. The child may have a persistent primitive hand grasp reflex which will make handling of food and utensils difficult. Retention of the asymmetrical tonic neck reflex means that when the child attempts to bring the hand to the mouth the head turns away.

TREATMENT OF THE CHILD WITH FEEDING PROBLEMS

A thorough evaluation of the child's feeding problem provides insight into the major problems and helps to determine the best therapeutic intervention. A therapeutic plan should be established with the parents so that they understand the suggested treatment. The techniques that are chosen and suggested to the parents must be demonstrated to them and then given a period of trial. Not all techniques will show immediate success. Specific evaluation and program planning for a child with a neurologic disorder should be accomplished by a feeding team or at least by an individual with in-depth experience and training in feeding children with special needs. Some overall guidelines can be mentioned.

Positioning

Children should be fed in an upright posture. A chair may need to be adapted or built (Fig. 22-4) to enable a child with delayed or abnormal motor development to sit in the upright position. The chair should support those parts of the body that the child cannot control independently. Keeping the legs apart may add stability to the sitting posture of a

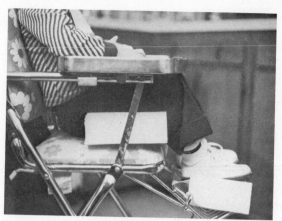

Figure 22-4

Proper positioning for a child with extensor hypertonicity throughout the body. Because of his extensor hypertonicity this child tends to thrust out of the chair without some adaptation of his sitting position. He is positioned with hip flexion, which will tend to reduce the extensor hypertonus. The hip flexion is maintained by securing his tray close to his body, and by placing a thick foam pad under his thighs. His feet are kept in good alignment by the use of another foam pad. The child is sitting in a symmetrical position, which is very important for him since he still exhibits an asymmetrical tonic neck reflex.

child with hypotonia and it may help to reduce hypertonicity. A well-controlled and comfortable sitting position is an important component of successful feeding. The prone position can be utilized for infants who are still sucking and for children in whom sucking should be encouraged.

Abnormal Muscle Tone

The quality and quantity of muscle tonus should be assessed by a therapist. A program intended to provide control for abnormalities in muscle tone may be designed by the therapist and may be carried out prior to feeding in order to help prepare the child for mealtime. For example, a child with extensor hypertonicity may benefit from being put on its side, with the physical therapist or parent rock-

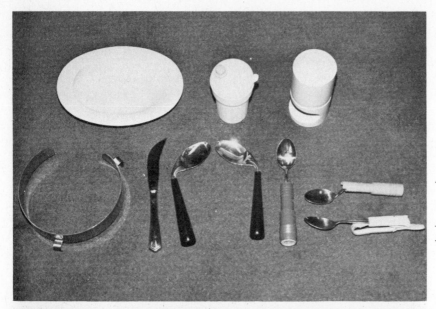

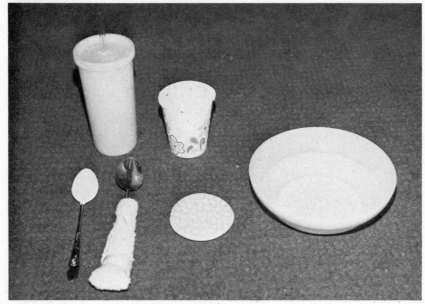

Figure 22-5
Adaptive feeding equipment. Top: Specialized utensils. Reading clockwise: Shallow Melmac bowl with sides to provide a scooping surface; Plastic feeding cup with lid, spout, and gravity device to control the flow; Melmac cup with indentation to facilitate grasp; Plate guard, attached to plate to provide a scooping surface; Curved knife to allow cutting with slight movement; Right-handed and left-handed spoons for pronation or supination difficulties; Spoon with built-up handle for easier grasp; Spoon with strap, placed over the back of hand to allow self-feeding by an individual who cannot grasp a spoon; Swivel spoon to help those without the arm flexion needed to change the direction of the spoon as it reaches the mouth. Bottom: Home adaptations and commonly available utensils utilized for special feeding. Reading clockwise: Teflon-coated baby spoon for the child with persistent bite reflex; Washcloth wrapped around spoon handle and taped, for those with a tight grasp or hypertonicity in the upper extremities; Rubber suction-cup soap holder, used to secure plates; Plastic bowl with shallow sides to allow scooping; Paper cup with cut-out nose opening; Tupperware cup with cover and straw—gentle squeezing on the sides facilitates straw drinking.

ing the child at the hips to encourage rotation in the trunk. This may help to inhibit hypertonicity in the total body, and as a result of the decreased extensor hypertonus the child may be able to flex the hips and assume a better sitting posture.

Feeding Environment

Mealtime can be noisy and overstimulating for a child who already may be having trouble with handling stimulation. The child with special needs may need to be fed separately, away from the family or other people, for one meal a day. At this time the parent may work with the therapeutic plan. At other mealtimes the child with special needs may join the family or group of children to participate in the socialization that mealtime provides and to benefit from modeling of good feeding habits by other members of the group.

It will be helpful to have all the food, utensils, and other equipment necessary for feeding the child easily accessible and available in one place. This will decrease the energy and time expenditure during the feeding period.

Adaptive Equipment

Various types of equipment are produced commercially to assist children with feeding. Many pieces are useful and often inexpensive. Simple adaptations of plates, cups, and utensils that are already available in the family kitchen, however, can be made by a parent at almost no cost. (See Fig. 22-5.) Each child's needs should be assessed individually, and recommendations for equipment should be made on this basis. However, some simple suggestions may be helpful.

Wrapping a washcloth around the handle of a spoon and securing it with tape may make it easier for a child to hold if the child has a very tight grasp or hypertonicity in the upper extremities. Securing the plate on the table with a rubber suction cup (the kind usually used to hold soap) will make it easier for the child to remove food from the plate with a utensil. Cutting out a side piece in a paper or plastic cup will allow the child's nose to fit into the cup without forcing his head into an extended position which may increase hypertonicity and also make it difficult for the child to control his head.[41]

In the child with central nervous system dysfunction, abnormal muscle tone and the persistence of primitive reflexes are associated with feeding problems and poor nutritional status. An evaluation which considers the child's oral-pharyngeal motor ability and head, trunk, and arm control, along with evaluation of the home environment, utensils used, and the daily food, fluid and drug intake, can help to alleviate the problem while affording the child the opportunity of a pleasant rather than a frustrating experience with food.

CASE STUDY 22-1

History

C. is a 10-month-old girl with cerebral palsy. She has hypertonicity throughout her body (spastic quadriparesis). C. has had four hospitalizations for aspiration pneumonia. Her parents have been feeding her in the supine position with her head tipped back because she had been choking, gagging, and pushing food from her mouth when she was fed in an upright position. In the supine position gravity could assist the swallowing process.

C.'s diet consisted of milk and baby cereals. All the food had a thin texture which was difficult for C. to handle. The food frequently dribbled from C.'s mouth.

Because of C.'s difficulties, parental anxiety surrounded the feeding situation, so that both the parents and the child reacted negatively to mealtime and C.'s food intake was poor. She consumed only 450 kcal (1890 kJ) per day.

Her height (66 cm) and weight (6 kg) fell below the third percentile on growth charts for infant girls. She was clearly failing to thrive.

During her last hospital admission the feeding team, consisting of a nurse, nutritionist, speech therapist, and physical therapist, were asked to evaluate C. and to make suggestions for improving her feeding, including a good position for feeding, ways to improve her ability to ingest food, and a plan for adequate calories and nutrition in her diet to ensure growth.

Main Problems

C.'s overwhelming problem was her extensor hypertonicity. In addition to extensor hypertonus, increased oral sensitivity, and tongue protrusion, C. retained an asymmetrical tonic neck reflex. She responded to all stimulation by thrusting her body into an extended position with head thrown back, legs stiff, and body arched. This dominant extensor thrusting was preventing C. from developing head and trunk control and the hypertonus was making lip closure and jaw control difficult. C. still retained remnants of a suckle-swallow reflex and this had developed into tongue protrusion. Stimulation of any type around her mouth elicited extensor thrusting with protrusion of the tongue. The thin texture of C.'s food added to the problems caused by her hypertonicity.

Case Study Question

1   On the basis of the information in this chapter, develop a treatment plan and list goals in order of priority.

FEEDING THE CHILD WITH A CLEFT LIP AND PALATE*

Dorothy M. MacDonald

DEVELOPMENTAL DEFECT

The precise cause of cleft lip and cleft palate is unknown. Although heredity appears to be a factor in one-third of the cases, the exact pathogenesis is elusive. It is a developmental defect, occurring in the first trimester of pregnancy. Most researchers feel that a complex combination of factors are involved in the etiology of clefts.

A cleft lip is a split in the upper lip. Normally, the lip is formed by the union of two tabs of tissue that grow in from the sides of the face and a central tab that grows down from the tip of the nose. This occurs during the fourth to the sixth week of fetal life. With a cleft lip, the maxillary and premaxillary processes forming the upper lip fail to fuse. The cleft lip may be unilateral incomplete, unilateral complete, bilateral complete, and, in rare instances, midline. These clefts vary in severity from a slight identation to a wide-open cleft.

This defect is often but not necessarily accompanied by a cleft palate. (See Fig. 22-6.)

The hard or primary palate consists of the premaxilla, the maxilla, and the palatine bone. The soft or secondary palate is a fibromuscular structure that divides the nasal from the oral pharynx, and is constantly modified in shape and position by the palatal musculature. The incisive foramen, with a bilateral suture extending to the interproximal space between maxillary lateral incisor and canine, is the dividing line between the primary and secondary palate. (See Fig. 22-7.)

In the seventh to twelfth week of fetal development, bone and tissue normally grow in from the sides of the upper jaw to join in the middle. Failure of this union results in an opening between the mouth and the nose. The palatal defect varies in width and length, depending on when and where the growth process stopped. There may be a cleft of the soft palate alone or a cleft of both the soft palate and part or all of the hard palate. There may also be a cleft in one or both sides of the upper gum. The last type is usually accompanied by a cleft lip. The various types of cleft palates mentioned can all cause feeding and respiratory problems.

FEEDING APPROACH

The child born with a cleft of the lip, palate, or both presents a challenge to those responsible for primary care. The practitioner must be

* The author of this section wishes to acknowledge the support of the Plastic Surgery Service of Children's Hospital Medical Center: Joseph E. Murray, M.D.; John B. Mulliken, M.D.; and George H. Gifford, M.D.

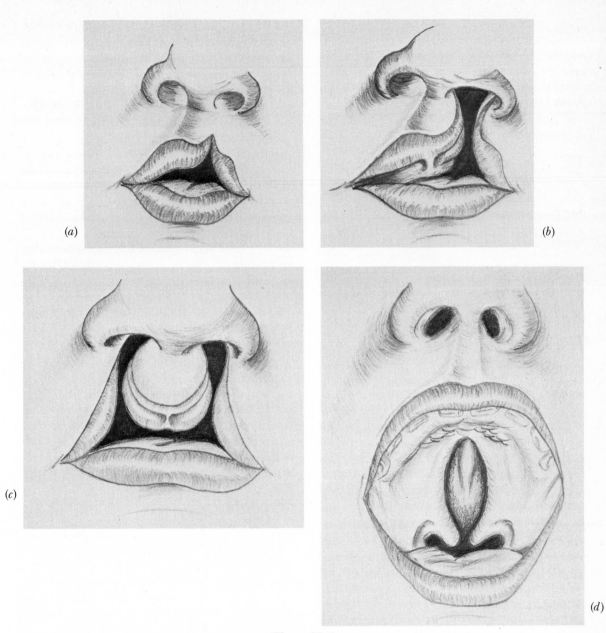

Figure 22-6
*Defects of the lip and palate: (a) Unilateral incomplete cleft, (b) Unilateral
complete cleft, (c) Bilateral complete cleft, and (d) Cleft palate. (Illustration by John B. Mulliken, M.D., Plastic Surgeon Children's Hospital Medical Center, Boston, Mass.)*

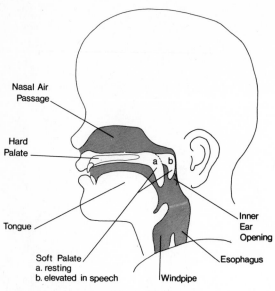

Nasal Air Passage

Hard Palate

Tongue

a b

Inner Ear Opening

Esophagus

Soft Palate
a. resting
b. elevated in speech

Windpipe

Figure 22-7
Normal physiology of the oropharynx.

Most infants with clefts are deprived of normal oral feedings. There is little documentation of the psychosocial impact on these infants, and although a positive feeding experience helps to foster development it is a positive parent-child relationship that is the important determinant. The approach to the care of the infant with a cleft should be to emphasize the positive (e.g., by telling the parents that the infant has beautiful eyes, is alert and responsive and nice to hold). Personal experience has shown that a supportive relationship with parents that encourages parent-child interaction (holding the infant, singing and talking to it) can help to ameliorate adjustment problems.

FEEDING TECHNIQUES

The methods of feeding an infant with a cleft vary, depending upon the philosophy of the medical center and the type of cleft.

In order to suck well an infant must be neurologically intact, with lip and tongue control and properly formed primary and secondary palates. Normal feeding can take place because most of the sucking action employs the hard palate. If the infant has only a cleft of the soft palate, he usually can be fed normally but in a sitting-up position. Reflux of fluids through the nose sometimes happens no matter what feeding procedure is being used; this occurs because fluids are forced through the cleft by the normal action of the tongue. If the infants were lying down, most of the feeding would enter the nose. All the other types of clefts usually require a special feeding device, unless the infant is breast-fed. (See below.)

At Children's Hospital Medical Center, Boston,[42] the device that is primarily used is called a Breck feeder; this is a bulb type of syringe with a rubber or plastic tip on the ends. Beniflex feeders (Mead Johnson) have also been used. These are soft plastic bags with a

able to respond to the intake needs of the child as well as provide the family with guidance.

Parents are often overwhelmed by the birth of their deformed infant and run the gamut of emotions from guilt, resentment, or anxiety, to depression, and in some instances even to withdrawal. They need constant support and opportunity to ventilate their feelings in order to provide the healthy parent-child relationship that is essential to a positive feeding experience.

It is very important to point out to the parents that most babies with clefts of the lip or palate do have feeding problems. Instead of giving assurance that might backfire and cause more anxiety, the practitioner can acknowledge the fact that these infants are difficult to feed but that for the most part by either patient or frantic trial and error parents do succeed and these children thrive and return for follow-up as sturdy and robust as other children. Parents as well as hospital staff can adjust more easily to special feeding techniques if they are at ease about the eventual outcome.

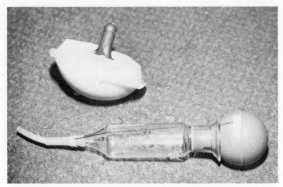

Figure 22-8
Feeding equipment. Top: Beniflex feeder; Bottom: Breck feeder.

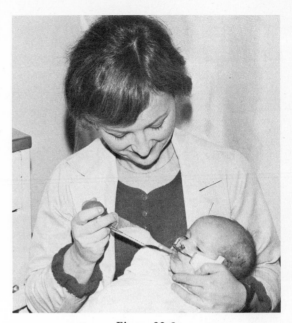

Figure 22-9
Proper positioning of the child, with feeding equipment within easy reach.

horizontal cross-cut nipple attached. The Beniflex feeders can work well with soft palate clefts or partial clefts of the hard palate. (See Fig. 22-8.)

Breck Feeder Method (Used with clefts of lip or palate)

1 Prepare the infant prior to feeding; i.e., change diapers, wrap in a blanket

2 The infant usually feeds better if its arms are restrained against the body by use of a special jacket or by wrapping tightly with a blanket

3 Prepare formula at room temperature or slightly warmer; also prepare a small amount of water

4 Choose a comfortable chair and have equipment set up on a table where it can easily be reached

5 Hold the infant close to you, in an upright position (see Fig. 22-9)

6 Fill the syringe with formula

7 Insert the tip of the syringe in the side of the infant's mouth, with the tip resting about halfway down the tongue

8 With one hand around the infant's head, stroke its cheek or gently move its chin up and down, which will stimulate the infant to make sucking motions

9 The infant will probably resist these attempts and may even start to choke and gag

10 Be patient. As the infant starts to swallow, place gentle pressure on the bulb to aid the infant in obtaining the formula

11 Stop feeding frequently to calm the infant and to bubble (a lot of air is swallowed with this type of feeding)

12 Experiment to find where best to place the tip of the syringe on the tongue. This depends on where the infant feels most comfortable

13 Continue the same technique until the infant has learned how to obtain nourishment

14 When the formula is finished, rinse the syringe and give the infant a small amount of water in order to clean the mouth

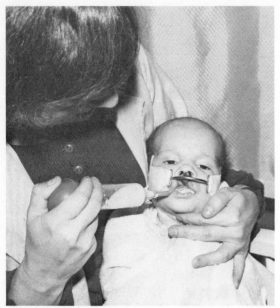

Figure 22-10
Placement of the tip of the Breck feeder. Tip of the syringe is inserted from the side of the mouth; tip rests about halfway down the tongue.

15 After feeding, continue to hold and calm the infant; also continue to bubble
16 Place the infant on his right side or in a sitting position after feeding

The ideal method of learning this feeding procedure is to have someone who is experienced demonstrate the technique.

Beniflex Feeder Method

1 Follow steps one through five as above
2 Prepare the feeder as directed on the package
3 Insert the nipple into the infant's mouth
4 Stimulate the infant to suck by stroking its cheeks or moving its chin
5 As the infant attempts to suck, apply gentle pressure on the feeder bag
6 Finish feeding with a small amount of water to clean the mouth

7 Bubble frequently
8 Place the infant on its right side or in an upright position after feeding

Solid foods should be introduced when the infant is the appropriate age. There is no reason why the infant cannot be taught to eat from a spoon, but if this is difficult, solids are added to the formula feeding in order to provide the added source of nutrients.

BREAST FEEDING

Some mothers desire to breast-feed and are often unreasonably discouraged by their physician. If the mother is knowledgeable and enthusiastic about breast feeding and realizes the inherent problems and the infant has the strength, breast feeding should be encouraged. It is a highly individualized process and much care must be given to ensure adequate nutrition, since an inadequate intake is often the cause for discontinuation.

There is information available to mothers of infants with clefts from La Leche League International.[43] Included are the following guidelines:

1 Breast feeding is much easier when the breast is full.
2 Have the mother place her index finger on the top edge of the areola of the nipple and her middle finger on the bottom—this presses the nipple out. Place the nipple in the infant's mouth.
3 The infant can now "milk" the nipple.
4 Rather than sucking, the infant uses its jaws, tongue, cheeks, and gums to press the milk from the breast.
5 The infant's head should be held close to the breast during the entire feeding.
6 In counseling the mother, explain that the technique of manually extending the nipple and the "milking" motion of the in-

fant's gums are more important than suctioning.

7 Most important, be very supportive toward the mother.

FEEDING BEFORE AND AFTER SURGICAL CORRECTION

Preoperative Feeding for Cleft Lip

The first repair is usually done when the infant weighs 10 lb or is 6 to 8 weeks old. The Breck feeder technique is the preferred method of feeding. If solid food has been started, it is best to mix it with the formula and give it through the feeder.

Postoperative Feeding for Cleft Lip

1 Follow instructions for the Breck feeder technique.

2 Take care not to exert pressure on the suture line.

3 Give clear liquids for the first two postoperative feedings (to prevent anesthesia reaction).

4 Gradually increase feedings as tolerated by the infant.

5 Follow the formula feeding with a small amount of water (to prevent contamination of the suture line).

6 "Suture line care" must be given after each feeding to prevent infection.

7 The infant will continue to use the Breck feeder for at least 1 month postoperatively, or longer if the physician desires.

Preoperative Feeding for Cleft Palate

1 The palatal repair does not take place until the child is 12 to 14 months old.

2 The infant should be weaned from the feeder at 4 to 6 months of age. A cup and spoon should be started at this time.

3 It is often helpful to use a small cup such as a whiskey jigger. If a plain cup is too difficult, one of the infant cups on the market may be used; e.g., a Tippy-Tom cup (one that has a covered cap with a lip attached).

4 Prior to surgery it is important for the child to become accustomed to clear fluids: broths, Jello, apple juice, water, and carbonated beverages that have been allowed to become flat. Carbonated beverages and sour fruit drinks are irritating to the nasal mucosa and should be avoided.

5 The child *must not* be taught the use of straws.

6 The child should be discouraged from putting the hands or other objects in the mouth. Using arm restraints periodically may be necessary to discourage this activity. Also, restraints are used postoperatively, so that this helps the child become accustomed to them.

Postoperative Feeding for Cleft Palate

Clear fluids are offered to the child frequently for the first 5 days postoperatively. It is important to push fluids in order to prevent infection and to keep the child well hydrated. After the first 5 days the diet progresses to full fluids, which are given for the next 10 days. These fluids can consist of high caloric, high-protein frappes, custards, blenderized diets, etc. On the second 10 days, the diet progresses to soft foods: finely mashed foods, chopped meats, strained vegetables and fruits. After 20 days of fluid and soft diet the child may resume a normal diet. Hard foods such as Zwieback, hard candy, lollipops, etc. should be avoided for at least 1 or 2 months postoperatively.

The first year of life is difficult for the child born with a cleft lip or palate. It is the health professional's responsibility to provide support and information to the parents. Frequent follow-ups through phone calls and hospital visits are imperative. Referring parents to other parents of children with a cleft also plays an important role. In Boston, there is a parents' group called "Prescription Parents."

The technique used for feeding children with clefts is very complex and must be individualized to suit each child. Health professionals must exhibit the confidence and patience needed in dealing with these children in order to set a positive feeding example for parents.

STUDY QUESTIONS

1 What is the effect of the normal diet on brain neurotransmitters?

2 The effect of emotions on neurohormonal function may possibly be related to the etiology of two clinical entities, nonorganic failure to thrive and anorexia nervosa. Explain.

3 Describe the eating disturbances that are characteristic of anorexia nervosa and those that are characteristic of failure to thrive.

4 What are the considerations in feeding the handicapped child? The handicapped adult?

5 By analyzing the effect of the condition on growth, feeding ability, nutrient effectiveness, and motor activity, conceptualize a nutritional care plan for a child with Down's syndrome and a child with cerebral palsy.

6 List all the normal oral reflexes and their usual times of occurrence.

7 How does the persistence of early primitive reflexes influence the feeding behavior of the child with central nervous system dysfunction?

8 What measures would you use to evaluate a feeding problem in a handicapped child?

9 What team members would you choose to have represented in the evaluation of a handicapped child?

10 Explain the developmental defect that is operative in cleft lip. In cleft palate.

11 Outline the feeding techniques for a child with a cleft lip and cleft palate, differentiating between the Breck feeder method and the Beniflex feeder method.

12 What are the differences in pre- and postoperative care for the child with a cleft lip and for the child with a cleft palate?

13 What type of anticipatory guidance would you give to the parents of a child with a cleft?

REFERENCES

1 J. D. Fernstrom, and R. J. Wurtman, "Brain Serotonin Content: Increase Following Ingestion of Carbohydrate Diet," *Science,* **174:**1023–1025, 1971.

2 R. J. Wurtman, and J. D. Fernstrom, "Effects of the Diet on Brain Transmitters," *Nutrition Reviews,* **32:**193–199, 1974.

3 R. Spitz, and K. M. Wolf, "Anaclitic Depression: An Inquiry into the Genesis of Psychiatric Conditions in Early Childhood," *Psychoanalytic Study of the Child,* **2:**313, 1946.

4 C. F. Whitten, "Evidence That Growth Failure from Malnutrition Is Secondary to Undereating," *Journal of The American Medical Association,* **209:**1675, 1969.

5 G. F. Powell et al., "Emotional Deprivation and Growth Retardation Stimulating Idiopathic Hypopituitarism. II. Endocrinologic Evaluation of the Syndrome," *New England Journal of Medicine,* **276:**1279–1283, 1967.

6 W. W. Gull, "Anorexia Nervosa," *Transactions of the Clinical Society* (London), **7:**22–28, 1874.

7 C. Lasegue, "On Hysterical Anorexia," *Medical Times & Gazette,* 1873, pp. 265–266, 367–369.

8 Travaglini et al., "Some Aspects of Hypothalamic

Pituitary Function in Patients with Anorexia Nervosa," *Acta Endocrinologica,* **81**:252–262, 1976.

9 H. Needleman et al., "Amitriptlyline Therapy in Patients with Anorexia," *Lancet,* **2**:580, 1976.

10 H. Bruch, *Eating Disorders: Obesity, Anorexia Nervosa and the Person Within,* Basic Books, Inc., Publishers, New York, 1973, p. 251.

11 H. Bruch, "Perils of Behavior Modification in Treatment of Anorexia," *Journal of The American Medical Association,* **230**:1419–1422, 1974.

12 Marc Shein, "Treatment for the Hospitalized Infantile Ruminator: Programmed Brief Social Behavior Reinforcers," *Clinical Pediatrics,* **14**:719–724, 1975.

13 H. Pryor and H. Thelander, "Growth Deviations in Handicapped Children: An Anthropometric Study," *Clinical Pediatrics,* **6**:501–512, 1967.

14 W. J. Culley and T. Middleton, "Caloric Requirements of Mentally Retarded Children with and without Motor Dysfunction," *Journal of Pediatrics,* **75**:380–384, 1969.

15 E. H. Reynolds, "Folate Metabolism and Anticonvulsant Therapy," *Proceedings of the Royal Society of Medicine,* **67**:6, 1974.

16 F. Lifshitz and N. Maclaren, "Vitamin D-dependent Rickets in Institutionalized, Mentally Retarded Children Receiving Long-Term Anticonvulsant Therapy. I. A survey of 288 Patients," *Journal of Pediatrics,* **83**:612–620, 1973.

17 K. De Luka, R. E. Masotti, and N. W. Partington, "Altered Calcium Metabolism Due to Anticonvulsant Drugs," *Developmental Medicine and Child Neurology,* **14**:318–321, 1973.

18 P. R. Huttenlocker, A. J. Wilbourn, and J. M. Signore, "Medium Chain Triglycerides As Therapy For Intractable Childhood Epilepsy," *Neurology,* **21**:1097–1103, 1971.

19 J. M. Signore, "Ketogenic Diet Containing Medium-Chain-Triglycerides," *Journal of The American Dietetic Association,* **62**:285–290, 1973.

20 Vera Pettaway, Nutrition Service of Dietary Department, Children's Hospital Medical Center, Boston, Mass., Personal communication.

21 Christine Cronk, "Growth in the Down's Syndrome Population. A Longitudinal Study Conducted in the Development Evaluation Clinic, Children's Hospital Medical Center, Boston, Mass." (in press).

22 W. J. Culley, et al., "Caloric Intake of Children with Down's Syndrome (Mongolism)," *Journal Pediatrics,* **60**:772–775, 1965.

23 Sue Cullen, "Toward Independence in Social Development and Self-Help Skills of Young Children with Down's Syndrome. A Study Conducted in the Developmental Evaluation Clinic, Children's Hospital Medical Center, Boston, Mass." (in press).

24 S. Peeks, and M. W. Lamb, "Comments on the Dietary Practices of Cerebral Palsied Children," *Journal of The American Dietetic Association,* **27**:870–876, 1951.

25 A. L. Gourge, and S. W. Ekvall, "Diets of Handicapped Children: Physical, Psychological and Socioeconomic Correlations," *American Journal of Mental Deficiency,* **80**:149, 1975.

26 M. I. Hammond, M. N. Lewis, and E. W. Johnson, "A Nutritional Study of Cerebral Palsied Children," *Journal of The American Dietetic Association,* **49**:196–201, 1966.

27 Ibid.

28 D. O. Ruby, and W. D. Matheny, "Comments on Growth of Cerebral Palsied Children," *Journal of The American Dietetic Association,* **40**:525, 1962.

29 K. Berg, and B. Isaksson, "Body Composition and Nutrition of School Children with Cerebral Palsy," *Acta Paediatrica Scandinavica Supplement,* **204**:41, 1970.

30 K. Berg, "Nutrition of Children with Reduced Physical Exercise Due to Cerebral Palsy," *Bibliotheca Nutritio Dieta,* **19**:12, 1973.

31 Council on Child Health of the American Academy of Pediatrics, "Medications for Hyperactive Children," *Pediatrics,* **55**:560, 1975.

32 D. J. Safer and R. P. Allen, "Factors Influencing the Suppressant Effects of Two Stimulant Drugs on the Growth of Hyperactive Children," *Pediatrics,* **5**:66, 1973.

33 D. J. Safer, R. P. Allen, and E. Barr, "Growth Rebound after Termination of Stimulant Drugs," *Journal of Pediatrics,* **86**:113, 1975.

34 B. Feingold, "Food Additives and Child Development," *Hospital Practice,* **8**:11, October, 1973.

35 National Advisory Committee on Hyperkinesis and Food Additives, *Report to the Nutrition Foundation,* Nutrition Foundation, New York, June 1, 1975.

36 C. K. Conners et al., "Food Additives and Hyperkinesis: A Controlled Double-Blind Experiment," *Pediatrics,* **58**:154, 1976.

37 R. L. Swank and R. D. Bourdillon, "Multiple Sclerosis: Assessment of Treatment with a Modified Low Fat Diet," *Journal of Nervous and Mental Diseases,* **131**:468–488, 1960.

38 Helen Mueller, "Facilitating Feeding and Prespeech", in P. Pearson and C. Williams, (eds.), *Physical Therapy in the Development Disabilities,* Charles C Thomas, Springfield, Ill., 1972, pp. 286–288.

39 Lorraine, Ogg, "Oral-Pharyngeal Development and Evaluation," *Journal of the American Physical Therapy Association,* **55**:237, 1975.

40 Helen Mueller, *Pre-Speech Evaluation and Therapy,* 16mm black and white film with written out-

line, University of California, Los Angeles, Cal., 1967.

41 Nancy Finnie, *Handling the Young Cerebral Palsied Child at Home,* E. P. Dutton, New York, 1975.

42 Children's Hospital Medical Center, *Cleft Lip and Cleft Palate—Questions and Answers for Parents,* Children's Hospital Medical Center Public Relations Department, Boston, Mass., 1976.

43 La Leche League International, Reprints: 9616 Minneapolis, Franklin Park, Ill. 60131.

CHAPTER 23

THE ORAL CAVITY AND DENTAL HEALTH

T. Howard Howell*

KEY WORDS
Odontogenesis
Plaque
Caries
Peridontal Disease
Fluoride
Calculus
"Bottle Caries" Syndrome

INTRODUCTION

The oral cavity is the initial segment of the gastrointestinal tract; there food is masticated, buffered, degluted (swallowed), and mechanically prepared for digestion. Thus, the covering tissues of the oral cavity are subjected to a wide spectrum of thermal, chemical, and mechanical stimuli. In order to perform their functions optimally and to maintain the structural integrity needed to withstand various insults, the tissues of the oral cavity must be given special care and adequate nourishment. Indeed, general health is dependent upon, as well as reflected in, the status of the oral mucosa and associated hard tissues. For this reason, it is necessary for the practicing health professional to understand the nutritional requirements for good general health and to be capable of recognizing pathological states derived from nutritional deficits.

STRUCTURE OF TEETH

Teeth develop as the result of several genetically determined, mutually inductive interactions of the embryonic ectoderm and mesoderm of the jaws. Fully differentiated teeth are composed of three calcified tissues: *enamel*, *dentin*, and *cementum*. Contained within and protected by these hard dental tissues is the delicate, highly vascular innervated connective tissue, the *dental pulp*. (See Fig. 23-1.)

The *crown* is that portion of the tooth covered by enamel. As the hardest calcified tissue, *enamel* serves as a resistant overcasing for the relatively resilient underlying dentin. Enamel contains a very small percentage of organic matter; it is derived from ectodermal cells, the ameloblasts, which persist until the teeth erupt into the oral cavity. Ameloblasts must be present in order for dentin to be laid down by

* The author wishes to acknowledge the editorial assistance of Ellen Eisenberg, D.D.S., Instructor in Oral Pathology.

493

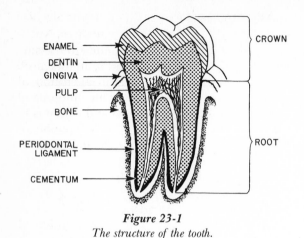

ENAMEL
DENTIN
GINGIVA
PULP
BONE
PERIODONTAL LIGAMENT
CEMENTUM

CROWN
ROOT

Figure 23-1
The structure of the tooth.

connective tissue, the *periodontal ligament.* Containing cells with multiple developmental potential, this ligament functions as a source of new cementum and alveolar bone, supports the tooth in its bony socket, and has proprioceptive nerve endings and an ample blood supply.

It is apparent that the structural and supporting dental tissues are in an interdependent, dynamic relationship to one another and as such are sensitive to alterations in their environment. They are, as are all tissues, dependent upon an intact and adequate blood supply which in turn is dependent upon well-balanced nutrition for maintenance of vitality.

the mesodermally derived odontoblasts. *Dentin* determines the morphology of the tooth and is its main calcified component. It is the natural boundary of the pulp, and is maintained by the persistent odontoblasts, located at the periphery of the pulp. Also of mesodermal origin is the *cementum,* a modified form of bone which is fabricated by the cementoblasts and deposited in layers which invest the dentin of the root. Cementum serves as the site of attachment for specialized fibers (the periodontal ligament) that anchor the teeth to the surrounding bone.

Giving vitality to these hard tissues is the *dental pulp.* Of mesodermal origin, it is a well-vascularized connective tissue which contains nerve endings with the capacity to transmit only the sensation of pain. Dental pulp houses the odontoblasts, the cells which secrete dentin matrix (the organic portion within which calcification takes place) and which have the propensity to do so continually as a protective response to minor tooth-directed insults of bacterial, mechanical, thermal, or chemical nature provided the tooth remains vital. As this "secondary" or "separative" dentin is laid down, the size of the pulp chamber and canal is progressively narrowed.

Communicating with the pulp and holding the teeth firmly in the alveolar processes of the maxilla and mandible is the specialized fibrous

GROWTH AND DEVELOPMENT OF TEETH (ODONTOGENESIS)

The development of the primary teeth begins at 6 weeks in utero and by 8 weeks in utero 20 tooth buds are evident. At birth, the established primary dentition continues to calcify, and development of the permanent first molars begins. By 6 months of age, odontogenesis and early calcification of all the permanent anterior teeth, except the upper lateral incisors, has taken place. The eruption of the incisors occurs between 6 months and 1 year of age. The age of eruption will vary with race, sex, nutritional status, and systemic conditions of the child. Slight deviation from the eruption dates are not cause for concern, since a broad time range is considered normal (see Table 23-1). However, a significant delay in tooth eruption may be indicative of a nutritional or endocrine disturbance. Hereditary disorders of tooth and bone development and Down's syndrome are among the other possible causes for delay.

The primary dentition is composed of 20 teeth and is fully erupted by approximately 2 years of age. At 6 years, the permanent teeth begin to erupt, and the full complement of permanent teeth is usually established by 18 to 21

TABLE 23-1 AGE AND STAGE OF TOOTH DEVELOPMENT

Age	Milestones
6 weeks in utero	Beginning of tooth development
8 weeks in utero	Twenty primary tooth buds present
20 weeks in utero	Beginning of permanent tooth development
16–24 weeks	Beginning of calcification of primary teeth
Birth–6 months	Development and calcification of the permanent first molars and anterior teeth (except the lateral incisors)
1–2 years	Eruption of the primary molars and cuspids
2–6 years	Gradual resorption of roots of primary teeth. Continued development and calcification of permanent first molars and anterior teeth. Beginning of development and calcification of crowns of permanent bicuspids and second molars
6–8 years	First permanent molars erupt; permanent incisors erupt
6–12 years	Roots or primary teeth are resorbed and crowns are shed
9–10 years	First bicuspids erupt; second bicuspids erupt
12–13 years	Permanent second molars erupt
18 years on	Permanent third molars erupt

Sources: M. Michael Cohen, *Pediatric Dentistry,* The C. V. Mosby Company, St. Louis, 1961; Tryphena Humphrey, *Pediatrics Digest,* December, 1969; Isaac Schour and M. Massler, "The Development of the Human Dentition," *Journal of The American Dental Association,* **28:**1153–1160, 1941.

years of age. Sixteen teeth are located in the maxilla and sixteen in the mandible.

NUTRITIONAL INFLUENCES ON ORAL HEALTH

The degree to which nutrition influences the oral structures is dependent on the type of tissue and its stage of development. Nutrition is particularly significant to the infant and young child, when most teeth are undergoing formation and calcification. Thereafter, nutritional factors assume a different role, in main-tenance and growth of the gingiva, the alveolar bone, and other periodontal structures. Nutritional deficiencies can affect the oral tissue, manifesting as frank deformities, an increased predisposition to disease, or an alteration of the response to disease. Adequate amounts of calcium, phosphorus, fluoride, and vitamins B, C, A, and D contribute to the formation of sound tooth structure and the maintenance of the oral tissues.

Calcium, Phosphorus, and Vitamin D

Vitamin D influences intestinal absorption of calcium and phosphorus, both components of the crystalline matrix of the teeth. Adequate amounts of these nutrients are therefore essential to tooth formation and calcification (see Chap. 7) However, once formed, teeth are not affected by the presence or absence of calcium or phosphorus in the diet.[1] Should the percentage of available calcium be lowered during development the result will be enamel hypoplasia and irregular formation of the dentin, despite the fact that dentin receives calcium preferentially over bone.[2] Irregular markings that can be observed in the dentin may document periods of stress and malnutrition. Altered eruption patterns and decreased calcification of alveolar bone are other manifestations of vitamin D deficiency.

Vitamin A

The function of vitamin A is to maintain the integrity of structures of ectodermal origin such as the skin and the cornea (see Chap. 6). In tooth development, vitamin A is necessary for the normal differentiation and function of the ameloblasts, the cells of ectodermal origin that are responsible for enamel formation. Enamel hypoplasia has been reported in severe and prolonged vitamin A deficiency in both experimental animals[3] and in malnourished children.[4] The eruption rate is retarded and, in states of prolonged deficiency, ceases. In addition, the alveolar bone formation is defective

Eruption and shedding of primary teeth

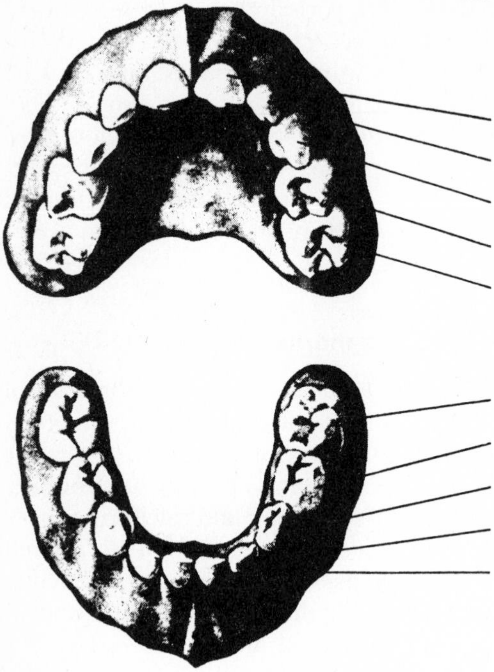

UPPER (MAXILLARY)	APPROXIMATE AGE OF ERUPTION	APPROXIMATE AGE OF SHEDDING
Central incisor	7½ mo.	7½ yr.
Lateral incisor	9 mo.	8 yr.
Cuspid	18 mo.	11½ yr.
First molar	14 mo.	10½ yr.
Second molar	24 mo.	10½ yr.
LOWER (MANDIBULAR)		
Second molar	20 mo.	11 yr.
First molar	12 mo.	10 yr.
Cuspid	16 mo.	9½ yr.
Lateral incisor	7 mo.	7 yr.
Central incisor	6 mo.	6 yr.

Figure 23-2

Eruption and shedding of primary teeth. (Photo courtesy of The New England Disabilities Communication Center.)

and the gingiva becomes hyperplastic and more susceptible to bacterial invasion.

Vitamin C

The promotion of collagen fibers and maintenance of odontoblastic function are among the basic roles of vitamin C (see Chap. 6). Since the deficiency of vitamin C affects the ability of connective tissue cells to elaborate their collagenous intracellular substances, formation of dentin by the odontoblasts is severly affected. In addition, weakness of the collagen fibers of supporting structures affects the ability of the teeth to withstand stress resulting in increased mobility and loss. Vitamin C–deficient patients frequently exhibit severe gingivitis with tissue hyperplasia and bleeding. This condition may be affected by an altered response to local irri-

tants. There appears to be an increase in capillary fragility and susceptibility to infection.

Protein

Since protein substances comprise the major organic components of enamel and dentin, states of protein malnutrition can affect the development of teeth. Kwashiorkor, a disease of protein deficiency, is associated with delayed eruption and hypoplasia of deciduous teeth.

B Complex Vitamins

Deficiencies in thiamine, pyriodoxine, pantothenic acid, folic acid, and vitamin B_{12} may result in glossitis and stomatitis. Severe deficiencies may present as erosive and ulcerative

Eruption of permanent teeth

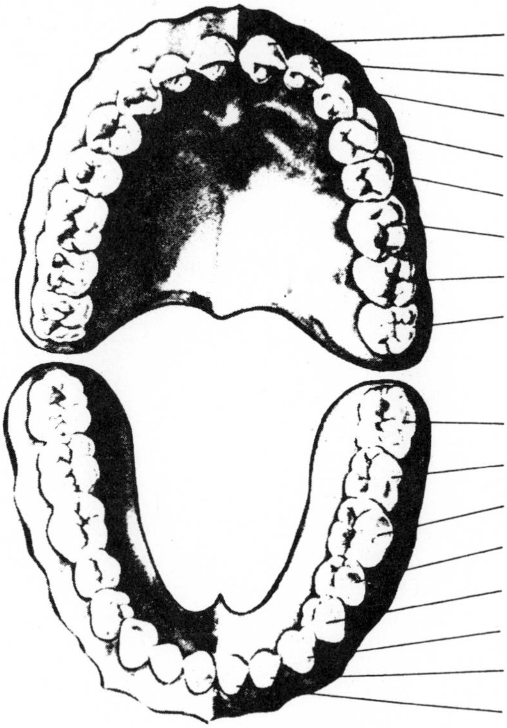

UPPER (MAXILLARY)

Central incisor . . . . .7-8 yr.

Lateral incisor . . . . .8-9 yr.

Cuspid . . . . .11-12 yr.

First bicuspid . . . . .10-11 yr.

Second bicuspid . . . . .10-12 yr.

First molar . . . . .6-7 yr.

Second molar . . . . .12-13 yr.

Third molar . . . . .17-21 yr.

LOWER (MANDIBULAR)

Third molar . . . . .17-21 yr.

Second molar . . . . .11-13 yr.

First molar . . . . .6-7 yr.

Second bicuspid . . . . .11-12 yr.

First bicuspid . . . . .10-12 yr.

Cuspid . . . . .9-10 yr.

Lateral incisor. . . . . .7-8 yr.

Central incisor . . . . .6-7 yr.

Figure 23-3

Eruption of permanent teeth. (Photo courtesy of The New England Disabilities Communication Center.)

lesions. Tongues affected by these deficiencies generally show enlargement due to edema and papillary atrophy. A deficiency of riboflavin may result in angular cheilitis, an irritation of the corners of the mouth that frequently leads to erosion, ulceration, and fissure formation. Vitamin B_{12} and folic acid deficiencies produce anemic states, reflected by the oral soft tissues as generalized pallor and atrophy. These tissues become more susceptible to injury.

Fluoride

The most widely accepted theory concerning the effectiveness of fluoride in decreasing dental caries is that fluoride is incorporated into calcium crystals of the enamel hydroxyapatite, forming fluorapatite. This exchange renders the enamel more resistant to solubility in acid.[5]

$$Ca_{10}(PO_4)_6(OH)_2 + 2F^- \longrightarrow$$
Hydroxyapatite fluoride ions

$$Ca_{10}F_2(PO_4)_6 + 2OH^-$$
Fluorapatite hydroxyl ions

Fluoride may also act to suppress the metabolic activity of the oral bacteria that are responsible for dental caries and periodontal disease. In addition, systemic fluoride at optimum levels (1 ppm) has been shown to alter the morphology of the teeth by reducing the depths of the pits and grooves on the occlusal surfaces of molar teeth, thereby reducing the area of mechanical retention of plaque. The use of fluoride is discussed further under "Fluoridation," below.

DENTAL CARIES

Dental caries is a disease characterized by destruction of the enamel, cementum, and dentin. The mechanism appears to be the demineralization of these calcified tissues by organic acid produced by bacteria in dental plaque.

Dental plaque is generally colorless and transparent unless it has absorbed pigment from foodstuff or is stained with disclosing solution. The plaque complex adheres to the tooth surface and can be detached only by mechanical cleaning. It is composed of mixed species of bacteria which are embedded in an intracellular matrix formed by bacterial and salivary polymers, epithelial cells, and leukocytes. Bacteria comprise 60 to 70 percent of the total plaque volume and this bacterial popula-

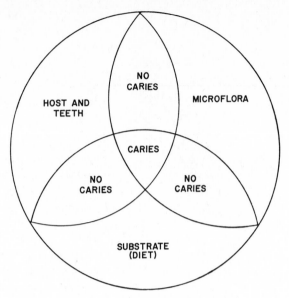

Figure 23-5

The interaction between host and environment in the production of dental caries. (Adapted from P. H. Keyes, "Present and Future Measures for Dental Caries Control," Journal of the American Dental Association, 79: 1395–1404, 1969.)

Figure 23-4

The progression of dental caries. (A) Into the enamel; (B) into the dentin; (C) into the pulp (nerve) of a tooth, resulting in an abscess. (Photo courtesy of The New England Disabilities Communication Center.)

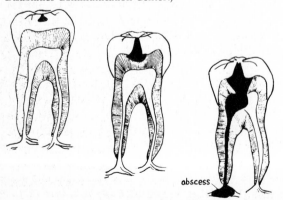

tion is in a constant state of flux as the plaque ages. The change in the bacterial population is due to alteration in the environment of the plaque and to the availability of factors necessary for the optimal growth of some bacterial species. Not only does the compostion of plaque change as it grows but plaque composition also differs depending on its location in the oral cavity. Thus, plaque found in the pits and fissures of the occlusal surfaces may differ greatly from plaque found at the gingival margins.

Certain acidogenic bacteria in dental plaque such as steptococci and lactobacilli act upon monosaccharides and disaccharides, producing lactic acid which decalcifies the enamel. A plaque pH of 5.5 or lower is necessary for the initiation of a carious lesion. Pits and fissures on the tooth surface are the most frequent sites of caries attack, while smooth surfaces are less susceptible. Should the caries progress through the enamel and into the dentin, pain may be felt. Further progression of the carious lesion may cause degeneration of the pulpal tissue. The bone surrounding the apex of the root may subsequently be affected.

Studies have shown that carbohydrates are an essential substrate for bacterial initiation of dental caries. The decreasing order of cariogenicity of carbohydrates has been demonstrated to be as follows: sucrose, glucose, maltose, lactose, fructose, and sorbitol.[6]

Dentists often measure the extent of dental caries by means of totaling the decayed (D), missing (M), and filled (F) teeth. This DMF score is useful as an epidemiologic tool to compare the incidence of dental caries in societies, groups, or individuals.

Prevalance

Dental caries appears to be a fairly recent disease. Studies of ancient human skulls reveal that dental caries was a relatively rare finding.[7] Indeed, in some parts of the world today dental caries is an uncommon disease.[8] Conversely, in the United States, dental caries is one of the most prevalent diseases of children. By 10 years of age, 80 percent of children in this country have dental caries, with the greatest carious activity in the primary teeth occurring between the ages of 4 and 8 years, and in the permanent teeth between 12 and 18 years. It has been estimated that the cost of treatment for dental caries in the United States exceeds the cost of treatment for any other single disease.[9]

During the past 10 years, three major surveys of our population have identified dental caries as a nutrition-influenced disease.[10–12]

Consumption of refined carbohydrates is the one significant factor directly correlated with the incidence of dental caries. In adolescent children of all races, the caries index rose progressively as refined carbohydrate in the diet increased. Present estimates now approximate sugar consumption at 100 lb per person per year.

Prevention

The key to treatment lies in the prevention of dental caries by a combined program of diet, oral hygiene, and fluoridation.

Diet

An adequate and sugar-free diet is paramount in the prevention of dental caries. Sucrose is the most cariogenic sugar and as such needs to be restricted.[13] This often presents problems of compliance due to the culturally ingrained use of sugar (see Chap. 10).

The more complex polysaccharides such as starch are less cariogenic and can be substituted in the diet for sugar. Starch is a very large molecule, relatively insoluble and practically nondiffusible through dental plaque; these physical and chemical properties of starch make it less caries-conducive.[14] In Guatemalan children fed a high-starch diet, a low caries rate was found. In contrast, neighboring children fed a diet containing sugar were found to have a higher caries rate.[15] The frequency of sugar intake is also considered a significant factor in caries formation since frequent between-meal snacks increase the length of time that teeth are exposed to sucrose. When consumed, the sugar-containing food should be part of the main meal, allowing time for tooth brushing and the use of dental floss ("flossing") afterwards. Snacks such as fresh fruits, nuts, breads, cheese, crackers, and vegetables may be substituted for between-meal snacks that are higher in sucrose content. Since the length of time that sugar remains on the teeth also influences caries formation, sticky or retentive foods should be avoided (see Table 23-2).

Fluoridation

The prophylactic effect of fluorides in the prevention of dental caries has been well established. This effect is greatest during the period

TABLE 23-2 DIET GUIDELINES TO HELP PREVENT DENTAL CARIES

Avoid foods with high concentrations of sugar, especially the chewy, sticky varieties:

Candy—especially caramels, gum drops, hard candy, lollipops, Life Savers, breath mints

Sugar, honey, syrups

Jams, jellies, preserves

Marshmallows, marshmallow fluff

Cookies, cake, pies

Sweet rolls, Danish pastry, sugar-coated doughnuts

Sugar-coated cereals

Dried fruits (raisins, prunes, and apricots)

Tonic, Kool-Aid, Zarex

Popsicles, ice cream on sticks

Caramel and taffy-coated apples, caramel-coated popcorn

Space Food Sticks, Breakfast Bars

Canned fruit

Eat a well-balanced diet (milk, bread, fruit and vegetables), especially emphasizing foods with detergent action (such as raw fruits and vegetables)

Snack foods:

Cold cuts, cold meats, hard-cooked eggs, cheese, cottage cheese, cheese spreads, raw vegetables (carrots, celery sticks), fresh or water-packed fruits, juices, pretzels, potato chips, popcorn, corn curls, crackers, nuts

Dessert:

Fresh or water packed fruit, yogurt plain or with added fresh fruit, cheese and crackers

Decrease the amount of sugar in the diet and the frequency of eating sugar-containing foods

Brush—floss—rinse mouth after eating

Source: Children's Hospital Medical Center, Boston, Mass.

of calcification and is best accomplished through the fluoridation of local water supplies. (The benefit of prenatal exposure to fluoride is, however, equivocal.) Consumption of fluoridated water results in a 50 to 65 percent decrease in caries when the fluoride is provided at the optimal level of 1 ppm (1 mg/l). Approximately 150 million people in more than 30 countries are drinking optimally fluoridated water; of these, 92 million live in the United States.[16]

Acute toxicity from fluorides in the drinking water is technically impossible because of the monitoring devices used in community water departments. One would have to consume 500 gallons of water containing 1 ppm fluoride to arrive at a toxic dose.

Dental fluorosis is caused by the ingestion of excessive amounts of fluorides (greater than 1 ppm of water) during the period of calcification of the developing teeth. It results in a mottled, opaque enamel which in some instances is chalky and crumbles easily. The fluorides usually come from artesian wells located in areas with a naturally high fluoride content.

Fluoride tablets or drops taken in amounts ranging from 0.5 to 1 mg daily provide both a preeruptive (endogenous) and posteruptive (topical) effect. Generally, a 30 percent reduction in tooth decay is produced.[17] Giving fluoride supplements to infants and children is raising concern over excessive intake. Fomon recommends no supplementation during the first 6 months of life, a maximum of 0.25 mg daily from 6 to 18 months, a maximum of 0.5 mg daily from 18 to 36 months, and a maximum of 0.75 mg daily from 3 to 6 years of age.[18]

Topical fluoride gels applied semiannually to children's teeth by dentists have repeatedly been demonstrated to produce a 30 to 40 percent reduction in caries. Fluoride mouth rinses are also gaining use as a preventative.

Noncariogenic Sweetener

Noncariogenic sweeteners offer promise for prevention of dental disease, but their long-term effect on the body is, as yet, unknown. Sugarless chewing gums commonly contain sorbitol, a nonnutritive sweetening agent, which appears to be less cariogenic than sucrose.

At present, xylitol is being investigated as a possible sweetening substitute for sucrose and fructose. In Scandinavia, marked caries reduction was observed in volunteers who substituted xylitol for sucrose over a period of 2 years as compared with subjects consuming foods containing sucrose and fructose.[19] The investigators concluded that xylitol was clearly noncariogenic. Further investigation concerning the relative cost and the acceptability of xylitol as a sucrose substitute is needed.

PERIODONTAL DISEASE

Periodontal disease is a disease which affects the gingiva, bone, and other supporting structures of the teeth.[20] The disease is primarily an inflammatory response to local irritants such as dental plaque, calculus, and food debris. Poor oral hygiene, which permits plaque and calculus to accumulate, is the major factor responsible for this destructive disease. Food impaction, faulty restorations, missing teeth, mouth-breathing, and the use of tobacco influence the severity of pathologic periodontal conditions. In addition, systemic illnesses such as diabetes, hyper- or hypoparathyroidism, and leukemia alter the response of the periodontal tissues to local irritants. The role of diet and nutrition in the causation of periodontal disease is ill-defined at present, although it has been demonstrated that the amount and composition of dental plaque and calculus are influenced by the diet.[21,22]

Calculus is a significant pathogenic factor which tends to perpetuate the inflammation of peridontal disease. There are many theories regarding calculus deposition but none are totally acceptable. According to the physiochemical theory, calculus is dental plaque which has undergone calcification and mineralization. Saliva and fluid from the gingival crevice serve as the mineral sources for calcification. Epidemiologic studies of periodontal disease around the world strongly suggest that there is a direct relationship between the amount of plaque and calculus on the tooth surface and the severity of periodontal disease.[23]

In the United States approximately 66 million adults are affected with periodontal disease and 20 million have lost all their natural teeth as a consequence of this disease.[24] Indeed, periodontal disease is the major cause of tooth loss in persons 35 years of age or older.[25] Although the adult population is the group most affected by periodontal disease, the onset may occur in childhood or puberty.

Prevention

Prevention of periodontal disease is accomplished by efficient removal of dental plaque. At present, the best method of controlling dental plaque formation is mechanical cleans-

Figure 23-6

Progression of periodontal disease. (A) Slight calculus deposit; (B) moderate calculus deposit and gingival inflammation; (C) heavy calculus deposit, gingival inflammation, and loss of bony support; (D) advanced disease state with loss of tooth. (Photo courtesy of The New England Disabilities Communication Center.)

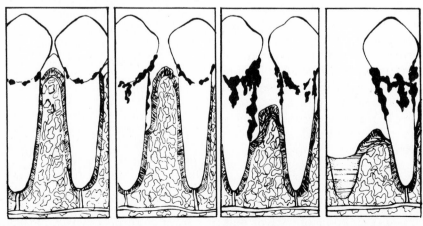

ing (flossing, brushing) by the patient. Alteration of the diet may be a necessary adjunct to plaque control.

Diet

The strong relationship of sucrose to plaque formation and consequent periodontal disease would necessitate reducing sucrose in the diet as part of any conscientious prevention program.

Studies have shown that firm or fibrous foods provide the following advantages in promoting good periodontal health:

1 They provide stimulation to the oral soft tissues
2 They decrease calculus formation
3 They promote keratinization (hardening of the epithelial tissue surrounding the tooth)

Firm foods (raw fruits, vegetables, and meats) require vigorous chewing, which prevents atrophy and degeneration of the oral hard and soft tissues. Detergent foods (raw fruits and vegetables) act as mechanical cleansers, helping to decrease plaque and calculus formation.[26] These foods promote keratinization by mechanically irritating the epithelium. Dietary treatment for the patient with periodontal disease involves:

1 Formulating a well-balanced diet with a reduction of sucrose-containing foods
2 Use of foods with firm consistency
3 Use of detergent foods at the end of a meal or as snacks

Successful prevention of periodontal disease is contigent upon the patient's following these fundamentals of food intake and oral hygiene.

SPECIAL CONCERNS

"Bottle Caries" Syndrome

Young children who habitually fall asleep while sucking a nursing bottle of juice or milk are candidates for "bottle caries." During sleep, the rates of sucking, swallowing, and salivary secretion decrease so that carbohydrates present in the juice or milk tend to pool in the oral cavity, remaining in contact with the teeth for a prolonged period of time and promoting the formation of lactic acid. Thus, the caries process is enhanced, and rampant decay of the primary teeth is the result.

To prevent this serious oral health problem, it is recommended that children not be put to bed with a bottle. Should a diagnosis of "bottle caries" be made, it is imperative that the child's parents be educated about the cause of the disease and given guidance in methods of nontraumatically weaning the child from the bottle. (See "Weaning" in Chap. 12.)

Oral Hygiene in the Sick and Handicapped

Systemic disease or debilitating conditions may alter the quality and quantity of saliva. Since saliva is normally bacteriostatic, decreased secretion or changes in its chemical composition may permit greater oral bacterial activity, promoting the caries process. The individual who is caring for a debilitated patient must take the responsibility for the patient's oral hygiene by digitally removing debris from the mouth, gently cleansing the oral mucosa and teeth with a moistened gauze sponge, and flushing the oral cavity with noncaustic mouth rinses.

Oral health requirements of the handicapped or mentally retarded child are often superseded by more urgent medical concerns or are neglected because the parents, guardians, or health professionals are reluctant to tackle management-complicating problems such as hypersensitive gag or bite reflexes during the course of dental care. Specialized pedodontic methods are necessary for children with congenital anomalies of the oral cavity and associated structures, or for children who have compromised function and coordination as a result of mental retardation syndromes.

Children who are physically incapable of carrying out personal oral hygiene techniques must be given daily custodial oral care. Parents or guardians must monitor the child's diet and must take charge of removing debris from the child's oral cavity by brushing and flossing the child's teeth for him. For those handicapped children who experience difficulty with a toothbrush, chewing on a cellulose sponge strip with toothpaste on both sides can facilitate cleansing. As the child chews, the sponge is forced around tooth surfaces. To ensure cleanliness, the sponge may be boiled following use.[27] Electric tooth brushing is also useful for those patients with inadequate dexterity.

Edentulous Patients

Although many elderly persons are fully or partially edentulous, it is apparent that tooth loss is *not* an age-related phenomenon. Proper nutrition and good oral hygiene, practiced throughout the lifetime of the individual, work in unison to maintain the health and integrity of the oral tissues.

Persons who are edentulous or who wear dentures may have problems with mastication and consequently with deglutition. Compensating for this difficulty, the individual may choose soft foods such as breads and cereals which lack essential nutrients and fiber. To avoid the risk of inadequate nutrition, vitamin and mineral supplements, bran, and wheat germ may be incorporated into the diet to replace missing nutrients and fiber until the individual seeks dental care.

STUDY QUESTIONS

1 At what age would you expect complete eruption of the primary dentition? Of the permanent dentition?

2 What nutrients affect tooth development and calcification?

3 What factors are necessary for the development of dental caries?

4 Describe the combined program of diet, oral hygiene, and fluoridation necessary to prevent dental caries and periodontal disease.

5 What are the special dental concerns for the sick, the handicapped, and the elderly patient?

CASE STUDY 23-1

Mary, a 2½-year-old child, was brought to the clinic by her mother with the complaint of food refusals and irritability.

The recent medical history revealed that aside from several colds, her overall health was good and she was up to date with her immunizations.

A diet history revealed that Mary was bottle-fed from birth. Baby and junior food additions were well tolerated. At the end of the first year, soft table foods were accepted but Mary made little progress in moving toward more textured table foods. Increasingly, she became more selective with foods, refusing all that required chewing. Foods taken from the refrigerator and ice cream caused immediate rejection. Milk had to be served at room temperature. Mary's total intake of milk was 40 oz per day. She refused all

meats, vegetables, and fruits except applesauce, preferring cereal, sugared cereal (nonfortified), spaghetti, and crackers.

The medical examination was normal except for a slight overweight condition, with height at the 50th percentile and weight at the 80th percentile on the Stuart-Meredith growth grids, and iron deficiency that was revealed by the laboratory report (hemoglobin, 9.69 g/100 ml; hematocrit, 31 percent). The upper and lower primary molars were decayed and a draining fistula above the central incisors was noted. Pain was elicited by touching the decayed teeth. Otherwise, the remaining teeth were noncarious and the oral mucosa of the lips, cheek, tongue, floor of the mouth, and palate were within normal limits.

The diagnoses of "bottle-caries" syndrome,

iron-deficiency anemia, and a slight overweight condition were made. The patient was referred to the dentist for extractions and restorative work and to the nutritionist for counseling and advice on weaning and on a diet suitable for Mary's age that would control weight and include proper foods.

CASE STUDY QUESTIONS

1 *What are the factors that have led to the development of "bottle caries" syndrome?*

2 *On the basis of the diet history, identify the missing nutrients. What are your recommendations for diet?*

3 *How could this problem have been prevented?*

REFERENCES

1 A. Nizel, *Nutrition in Preventive Dentistry: Science and Practice,* W. B. Saunders Company, Philadelphia, 1960, p. 103.

2 Ibid., p. 104.

3 M. Goodhart and R. Shils, *Modern Nutrition in Health and Disease,* Lea and Febiger, Philadelphia, 1973, p. 740.

4 E. A. Sweeney et al., "Linear Hypoplasia of Deciduous Incisor Teeth in Malnourished Children," *American Journal of Clinical Nutrition,* 24:29, 1971.

5 F. Brudevold et al., "The Chemistry of Caries Inhibition: Problems and Challenges in Topical Treatments," *Journal of Dental Research,* 46:37–45, 1967.

6 E. Newbrun, "Sucrose, the Arch Criminal of Dental Caries," *Journal of Dentistry for Children,* 35:239, 1969.

7 L. I. Falin, "Histological and Histochemical Studies of Human Teeth of the Bronze and Stone Age," *Archives of Oral Biology,* 5:5–13, September 1961.

8 A. L. Russell, "International Nutrition Surveys: A Summary of Preliminary Dental Findings," Journal of Dental Research, 42:233–244, 1963.

9 W. O. Young and D. F. Striffler, *The Dentist, His Practice and the Community,* W. B. Saunders Company, Philadelphia, 1969, p. 73.

10 U.S. Dept. Health, Education, and Welfare, Health Services and Mental Health Administration, *Ten State Nutrition Survey 1968-1970. V. Dietary,* Washington, D.C., Publ. no. (HMS) 72–8133, 1970.

11 G. Owen et al., "A Study of the Nutritional Status of Pre-School Children in the United States 1968–1970," *Pediatrics,* 54:597–646, 1974.

12 U.S. Dept. Health, Education, and Welfare, Public Health Service, "Plan and Operation of the HANES (Health and Nutrition Examination Survey)," *Vital and Health Statistics,* ser. 1, no. 10 A.B., February 1973.

13 Newbrun, op. cit., p. 239.

14 Nizel, op. cit., p. 36.

15 W. J. Loesche and C. A. Henry, "Intracellular Microbial Polysaccharide Production and Dental Caries in a Guatemalan Indian Village," *Archives of Oral Biology,* 12:189–194, 1967.

16 J. M. Dunning, "Current Status of Fluoridation," *New England Journal of Medicine,* 27:30–34, 84–88, 1965.

17 F. Brudevold et al., op. cit., pp. 37–45.

18 S. Foman, "Nutritional Disorders of Children: Prevention, Screening, and Follow-up, U.S. Dept. Health, Education, and Welfare, Washington, D.C., Publ. no. (HMS) 76-5612, 1976, p. 91.

19 A. Scheinin et al., "Turku Sugar Studies I. An Intermediate Report on the Effect of Sucrose, Fructose and Xylitol on the Caries Incidence in Man," *Acta Odontologica Scandinavica,* 32:383–412, 1974.

20 U.S. Dept. Health, Education, and Welfare, *Research Explores Pyorrhea and Other Gum Diseases: Periodontal Disease,* U.S. Public Health Service Publ. no. 1482, 1970.

21 J. Carlsson and J. Egelberg, "Effect of Diet on Early Plaque Formation in Man," *Odontologisk Revy,* 16:112, 1965.

22 Bernier and Muhler, *Improving Dental Practice Through Preventive Measures,* The C. V. Mosby Company, St. Louis, 1971.

23 H. Loe, E. Theelache, S. B. Jensen, "Experimental Gingivitis in Man," *Journal of Pedo.,* 36:177, 1965.

24 U.S. Dept. Health, Education, and Welfare, *Research Explores Pyorrhea,* op. cit.

25 H. M. Goldman, "Prevalance of Periodontal Disease in the United States," *International Dental Journal,* 5:458, 1955.

26 A. Nizel, op. cit., pp. 372–374.

27 The New England Developmental Disabilities Communication Center, *Home Dental Care for the Handicapped Child,* Children's Hospital Center, Boston, Mass., 1976, p. 10.

CHAPTER 24

SURGERY, STRESS, BURNS, AND NUTRITIONAL CARE

Shirley R. Goldstein

KEY WORDS
Ecosystem
Catabolic Response to Stress
Hyperalimentation
Elemental Diet
Iatrogenic Malnutrition

INTRODUCTION

The Individual and the Ecosystem

The ability to meet stress is the outcome of the human "ecosystem." This system is, in essence, the saga of people's interrelationship with the psychological, economic, environmental, and biological forces that govern their lives from conception to adulthood. Precluding genetic limitations (biological and intellectual), these forces impact on people, conditioning them to meet the daily demands of stress in order to achieve a state of emotional and physiological well-being.

Ability to deal with stress is a reflection of the integrity of this system—that is, the degree to which an adult or child is able to cope with stress is a measure of the strength or weakness of these interdependent, interreactive forces. There is no greater challenge to the system that when an individual copes with the stress of illness. Illness tests the dynamics of the system—with all forces amplified and affecting one's ability to overcome and survive.

This chapter focuses on the stress of surgery and burns, as well as on the physiological and psychological demands made on the human ecosystem. In addition to discussion of nutritional management and other support systems, it will help the student to focus on the human aspect of illness. It will reinforce the need for supportive measures of kindness, reassurance, and empathy, all as vital as any technical support system in helping the patient to overcome and survive.

PSYCHOLOGICAL RESPONSE TO SURGERY

Humans deal with serious stress, e.g., the trauma of surgery, by eliciting conditioned emotional responses and displaying patterns of behavior that constitute an aspect of their defense system.[1]

Surgery poses a life-threatening experience for many. It symbolizes fear of the

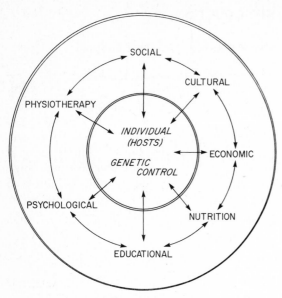

Figure 24-1

The human "ecosystem." The human "ecosystem" is the term used to designate the interaction of the physiological, economic, environmental, and biological forces that govern life. Homeostasis within the system helps to combat the inherent stresses of surgery, which may alter any or all of the forces impinging on the individual.

unknown, of possible mutilation, death, pain, loss of potency, etc. While some individuals may accept surgery with a degree of anxiety and fear, many exhibit symptoms of regression, depression, acute anxiety, or anger. They may deny the seriousness of their illness, and refuse to seek medical advice, or manifest their fear by frequent emotional outbursts. These patterns represent defense mechanisms by which human beings, conditioned from infancy, deal with stress and attempt to achieve emotional balance and strength.

The establishment of a trusting, helping relationship with patients by the health care team further assists them in reaching this goal. The patient who requires surgery is soon divested of autonomy—the control over his or her future will be entrusted to others. All need reassurance as to outcome, as well as opportu-

nities to verbalize concerns. Older patients fear physical and psychological abandonment. They frequently lose hope for the future, become depressed, and refuse to eat. In the past, burn patients were kept in special rooms, psychologically and physically removed from interaction with others. The effects of long-term isolation were greatly damaging.

Children especially need trusting relationships—a trusted parent present at all times, rooming in when possible. The continuity of the parent-child unit relieves the acute anxiety of separation and enables the child to remain secure in facing surgery. As part of preparation for surgery at Children's Hospital in Boston, teaching sessions are held by the nursing staff for children and their parents. Posters depicting specific pre- and postoperative procedures serve as the basis for discussion, and as objects of play, as well as the means of acting out feelings of anger, fear, and anxiety. The child is given insight into the procedure that will take place, and is better able to adjust to the surgery. The parent, when better informed and more confident, can further enhance the parent-child relationship by providing reassurance and support.

The need to provide psychological support and sympathetic understanding can be further demonstrated by the process of getting patients to resume eating. A system of psychological support must be incorporated into patient care management to encourage a return to positive eating habits. Refusal to eat, use of food as a tool of manipulation, chronic complaining as an attention-getting device are all expressions of human need. Prior to surgery, pain, vomiting, anorexia, and fear often interfere with meals, negatively conditioning the patient to food. Postoperatively, the patient must relearn to identify food and mealtimes as a pleasurable, nonpainful experience. With appropriate dietary management tailored to age and need, the patient again becomes confident in food and is reconditioned to a positive mealtime experience.

PHYSIOLOGICAL RESPONSE TO SURGERY

Each individual's metabolic response to surgery is determined by:

Extent of the surgery

Ability to digest and absorb nutrients after the surgery

Nutritional status

Nutrient Stores

It is well documented that a sound nutritional state is a critical factor in the body's defense system,[2] and that adequate stores of the following are necessary:

Protein

Liver glycogen

Tissues saturated with vitamin C

Adequate vitamin K

All nutrients are essential in meeting surgical trauma, in wound healing, in fighting infection, and in regaining health. A malnourished individual, depleted of such essential nutrients, is a major risk for surgery, and must, if time permits, be rehabilitated prior to surgical events. Clinical signs of weight loss and hypoproteinemia characterize the at-risk patient. Weight loss, an early sign, is often the unfortunate consequence of the disease process that fosters the anorexia that leads to inadequate food intake. Often the hemoglobin or hematocrit levels are low as a result of insidious blood loss caused by a yet-undetected neoplasm. Preoperative attempts are therefore directed at reversing these conditions so as to make an individual a safe candidate for surgery and reduce its risk (which is further compounded by the catabolic response to the stress).

Catabolism and Hormonal Response

In response to the severe stress of surgery, burns, hemorrhage, and other traumatic events, the body directs its physiological efforts toward adaptation for survival. It attempts to compensate for the accompanying catabolic, starvation-like state by converting to metabolic pathways that will provide glucose and energy to the cells, and preserve adequate blood volume.

The following responses are observed:

1 The catecholamines norepinephrine and epinephrine are released into the bloodstream, where they exert a hemodynamic, metabolic effect. The outcome is:
   - A *vasoconstrictive effect* on blood vessels which results in increased cardiac output, thus maintaining adequate blood pressure and volume.
   - An *increased production and release of glucagon*. Its hormonal action (on the liver and adipose stores) results in increased glycogen hydrolysis and increased gluconeogenic activity (with the net result of increased glucose release) in the liver, and lipolysis of fat stores (which results in release of free fatty acids for energy needs).
   - A *suppression of the peripheral action of insulin*. The alteration of the normal glucagon ratio (insulin levels are *higher* than glucagon levels during nonstressful times) results in the posttraumatic insulin resistance and mild glucose intolerance that characterize early trauma.
   - A *lipolytic effect*, whereby triglycerides are hydrolyzed, releasing glycerol and free fatty acids into the bloodstream to provide another source of energy.

2 In the event of hypovolemia, the *renin-angiotensin system* is activated, resulting in increased aldosterone secretion and sodium ion retention by the kidney.

3 *Antidiuretic hormone* (ADH) is released by

the pituitary. This antidiuretic effect, combined with sodium retention, serves to maintain adequate blood volume and flow, and temporarily to reduce urinary output following stress.

4 A *cortisol response* is elicited: increased adrenocorticotropic hormone (ACTH) is secreted by the pituitary, resulting in increased adrenal secretion of corticosteroids, especially cortisol. These stimulate the following gluconeogenic reactions:

- Amino acids are quickly released from muscle tissues and converted to glucose in the liver.
- Free fatty acids are also released from fat depots.

The net catabolic result of these hormonal responses is an increasing urinary nitrogen, muscle loss, and weight loss, as the body attempts to meet its energy requirements.

(*Note:* Body weights taken during this critical phase do not reflect the true lean body mass, for areas of depletion are replaced by water and sodium.)

As injury and trauma resolve, there is a *reversal* of the above responses:

Diminution of catecholamine secretion

Return to a normal insulin glucagon ratio in the blood

Decrease in renin secretion

Decrease in aldosterone secretion and restoration of free water diuresis

Wound Healing

Moore and Brennan describe postoperative wound healing as a phase of "convalescent anabolism," a period lasting 5 to 15 days during which time the wound is given high biological priority for energy, amino acids, and nutrients.[3]

In the initial phase of wound healing, amino acids, energy, and vitamin C are essential. Sources of amino acids and energy are derived from gluconeogenesis. Vitamin C may be administered parenterally or orally (e.g., 500 mg/orally). The vitamin and amino acids are necessary for collagen synthesis, especially the initial step in wound healing, the formation of collagen fibrils and reticulum. Vitamin C is required for the pathway in which proline is hydroxylated to hydroxyproline to form collagen.[4]

It is ironic that the primary stage of healing occurs during negative oral intake, again illustrating the need for sound nutritional status prior to surgery.

In addition, trace minerals, especially zinc may, aid in wound healing.[5] It is suggested that zinc is an essential cofactor in many enzyme systems, e.g., pancreatic carboxypeptidase and glutamic dehydrogenase (both are important in protein metabolism). Its exact role in wound healing is still being researched.

Results of a study on vitamin E and wound healing in rats suggest that the vitamin produces an adverse effect. In exerting an anti-inflammatory effect on the wound, vitamin E suppresses early collagen synthesis and causes weakening of young wounds. Present research indicates no role for vitamin E in wound healing.[6]

The wound achieves tensile integrity, the point at which the wound is strong enough for suture removal, approximately 7 days after surgery.[7] Prior to this time, there are clinical signs of improvement as the stress factors are reduced. Pain is lessened; appetite is increased; peristalsis returns; the insulin/glucagon ratio is restored (blood insulin levels are again greater than levels of glucagon)—all signal the start of the anabolic phase of healing. The priority at this time is to provide and assure an adequate oral intake of protein and energy for continued protein synthesis and repletion. When there are postoperative complications or extensive surgical procedures, nutritional support by means of nasogastric tube feedings, intravenous therapy, or total parenteral nutrition may be necessary.

As a consequence of inadequate nutrition,

oral or parenteral, wound healing deteriorates. The wound itself becomes a nitrogen donor to the general metabolic pool and competes for nutrients with other tissues. This state, described as "late post-traumatic starvation or nutritional failure," results in persistent infection and failure of wounds to close and heal.[8]

Immune Response

The relationship of nutritional status to the immune response is well documented in the literature (see Chap. 16). The increased susceptibility to infection in cases of kwashiorkor or severe protein-calorie malnutrition in children has been fully cited. An increased incidence of surgical infections is also felt to be strongly related to the poor nutritional status of hospital patients.

The immune response system is the body's natural defense system. It is the reactive response of humoral (circulating antibody) and cell-mediated (lymphocytic response) mechanisms to disease and infection. Its integrity, as measured by neutrophil action, serum albumin, antibody-antigen interaction, immunoglobulin concentration, lymphocytic responses, etc., is felt to be greatly influenced by nutrition.[9-11]

Current research suggests that dietary protein, vitamin B_6, and pantothenic acid are essential in maintaining and preserving the effectiveness of the system. Vitamins A and B_{12} are also considered significant. Worthington suggests that a deficiency of these nutrients (all are vital for DNA-protein synthesis and for release of circulatory antibodies) results in an impairment of antibody synthesis.[12] Investigators support the theory that in conditions in which circulating antibody cells are reduced, the organism becomes more susceptible to disease and is hindered in its recovery from infection.

Lack of adequate protein and B_6 intake may also lead to thymus gland atrophy. Consequently, synthesis and action of lymphoid cells is greatly reduced. This is demonstrated in malnourished populations by graft rejections and delayed hypersensitivity reactions.

More important, when the nutritional status of children and malnourished hospital patients is improved by proper nutrition therapy, there are increased lymphocytic counts and a rise in serum immunoglobulins, both of which suggest the role of sound nutrition in preserving effective immune system responses.[13]

The immune response, along with the body's catabolic response to stress, and the need for specific nutrients for wound healing reinforce the need for a period of preoperative nutrition.

Evaluation of Nutrient Needs of the Surgical Patient

Nutrient needs during stress are not known, but the recommended dietary allowances (RDA) (see App. Table A-1) can serve as a realistic base in planning diets for routine nonextensive surgery in well-nourished patients.

Trauma may increase these nutrient requirements well above the recommended levels of intake. An example would be the escalation of vitamin C requirements during stress as compared to nonstress periods (see Table 24-1. It is estimated that in some instances of stress, such as is encountered in the burn patient, 100 times the RDA may be required.

Careful clinical and dietary monitoring aids in assuring that adequate nutrient therapy is provided. Monitoring of trays at meal service by nursing and dietary personnel will provide an estimate of nutrient intake.

For the most part, individuals who require surgery are in relatively good nutritional status (exceptions may be the poor, the elderly, or patients suffering from other disease states). For this group, surgical needs are supportive. Human and technical measures can be planned without complications.

On the other hand, supervising those who are in a debilitated preoperative state requires the efforts of the patient care team, as management prior to and after surgery is complex.

Butterworth and Blackburn forcefully describe the need to identify surgical and medical patients in hospitals who may be classified as high-risk due to the inherent malnutrition of disease, inadequate and improper diets, or hospital-induced malnutrition (known as iatrogentic malnutrition).[14] This state results when the assessment of nutritional status and appropriate nutritional management have not been planned for and implemented.[15]

These high-risk patients require aggressive, ongoing nutritional support in order for the outcome of surgery and rehabilitation to succeed. Toward this end, they advocate the need for nutritional assessment as an integral aspect of patient management, including evaluation of nutritional status by anthropometric measurements (if possible), clinical indices, interviews with the patient, etc. (See Chap. 15.) All of these indicators of nutritional assessment should be reviewed at patient care conferences where individualized therapeutic diets and an effective dietary plan can be formulated and thereby integrated into the patient's medical and surgical treatment.

PREOPERATIVE NUTRITION

The goal of preoperative nutrition therapy is directed toward physiological and nutritional repletion so as to better enable an adult or child to meet the catabolic stress of surgery. Furthermore, a well-nourished state optimizes wound healing, increases resistance to infection, and hastens convalescence and recovery.

Goals of Preoperative Nutrition

1 *Restoration of nitrogen balance* In the preoperative and postoperative management of the "surgical risk" patient (one who is protein-depleted), as well as in any instance of severe trauma, especially severe burns, strong efforts at reversing the marked nitrogen loss must be made for several reasons.

- There is increased nitrogen loss during the postoperative period. The lengthy postoperative period is one of semistarvation, during which time a patient is supported nutritionally by intravenous fluids and a minimal oral intake. This further increases nitrogen losses, depletes nitrogen stores, and prolongs convalescence.

2 *Wound healing* Sources of nitrogen in the form of amino acids (protein) are necessary for wounds to heal properly and for tissue repair to occur. (Protein is essential for amino acid synthesis, as well as for antibody, enzyme, and hormone synthesis.)

3 *Maintenance of serum protein levels* Normal serum protein levels must be maintained, with serum albumin levels monitored closely to assure normal blood volume and concentration and to prevent edema and threat of sepsis. Weight loss and hypoproteinemia (serum albumin less than 3.5 mg/100 ml) are indicators of diminished protein reserve. Table 24-2 shows the protein reserve status as reflected by serum albumin levels.

4 *Carbohydrate stores* Adequate carbohydrate intake is essential to maintain a liver replete with glycogen, a necessary defense against the burden of anesthesia and stress.

TABLE 24-1 VITAMIN C REQUIREMENTS* DURING NON-STRESS AND STRESS

	Nonstress	Stress (e.g., burns)
Adult	45 mg	500–1500 mg
Child	35 mg	Same as above

* 100 times the recommended dietary allowance (see Appendix, Table A-1) may be required.

TABLE 24-2 PROTEIN RESERVE AS REFLECTED IN SERUM ALBUMIN LEVELS

Serum albumin	Interpretion
3.5 mg/100 ml	Normal
3.0 mg/100 ml	Beginning protein depletion
2.7 mg/100 ml	Moderate protein depletion
2.4 mg/100 ml	Severe protein depletion Acute period of stress and trauma

These preoperative goals may be met by any of the following methods used singly or in combination with one another.

Oral intake

Intravenous therapy

Tube feedings

Total parenteral nutrition

Preoperative Diets

An adequate energy intake with a good source of protein of high biological value (HBV) must be planned for and the intake monitored.

The body must meet its crucial energy requirements with a food intake (preferably oral) of sufficient kilocalories (kilojoules); if this is not met, the body will catabolize its protein reserves. It is ironic that high-protein regiments, in which the protein intake is intended for anabolism and synthesis, are self-defeating when planned without an adequate energy intake. In addition, such regimens may further compromise an already stressed kidney by the increase of urinary nitrogenous wastes. There is much danger of osmotic diuresis and dehydration if increased water requirements are not met to aid in the excretion of these wastes.

Also, the antiketogenic effect of carbohydrate and its protein-sparing action are universally recognized. For practical purposes, 0.8 to 1.5 g of HBV protein/kg of body weight per day and 25 to 50 kcal/kg (105–210 kJ/kg) per day are recommended for adults as a sound plan that will meet energy requirements and allow for nitrogen repletion, balance, and protein synthesis. Table 24-3 suggests daily fluid, protein, and energy requirements for neonates and infants.

For those patients who require immediate surgery, and for whom there is no time for providing the benefits from a period of preoperative nutrition, giving whole blood or plasma raises the hemoglobin and hematocrit levels. Table 24-4 shows recommended blood values for adults and children. Promptly, the patient feels "stronger," and is psychologically better prepared.

Concern for adequate levels of vitamins C and K is real. Vitamin C is necessary for wound healing and closure. This is crucial, for an open, exposed wound is an invitation to infection. Adequate vitamin K and a normal prothrombin time are insurance for proper clotting, thus lessening the danger of hemorrhage.

High-energy Moderate-Protein Diet

A high-energy, moderate-protein diet is recommended preoperatively. It is given in small

TABLE 24-3 RECOMMENDED DAILY REQUIREMENTS FOR NEONATES AND INFANTS

Age	Energy		Protein, g/kg	Fluids, ml/kg
	kcal/kg	kJ/kg		
Newborn (0–6 months)	120	504	2–4	100–150
Infants (6 months–1 yr)	50–100	210–420	1.5–2	50

TABLE 24-4 RECOMMENDED BLOOD VALUES FOR CHILDREN AND ADULTS

Total Protein (TP)	5 g/100 ml
Albumin	4.5–5.5 g/100 ml
Hematocrit	40–45%
Hemoglobin	12–14 g/100 ml

frequent meals and achieved by the use of supplemental high-energy, high-protein drinks. (See Table 24-5.)

Care and restraint must be exercised. Large amounts of food may defeat patients who know that they must eat and force themselves to do so. Consuming a small meal in its entirety is a victory and reinforcing; too large a meal may further depress or discourage an appetite strained by bouts of nausea, vomiting, and anxiety.

Mealtimes should be quiet and as pleasant

TABLE 24-5 HIGH-ENERGY HIGH PROTEIN DIET

Approximate Composition:

2500 kcal (10.5 MJ)

345 carbohydrate

110 g protein

120 g fat

Protein is increased by addition of high-caloric, high-protein supplements; e.g., Sustacal

Nutrients for a 50-kg female, 23 years of age, 2 weeks postoperative:

50 kcal (210 kJ)/kg body weight

(approx) 2 g protein/kg body weight

(approx) 25 nonprotein calories/g of protein

Sample menu	
Breakfast	*Lunch*
½ cup Orange juice	½ cup Cream of asparagus soup
1 slice White toast with butter and jelly	½ cup Salmon with mayonnaise
1 Soft boiled egg	2 Saltines, butter
Tea, 2 tsp sugar	Coffee ice cream
	Vanilla Wafers
	Tea, ½ cup milk, 2 tsp sugar
10:00 A.M. snack:	*2:00 P.M. snack:*
250 ml Sustacal*	250 ml Sustacal
2 Uneeda biscuits, jelly	4 Arrowroot biscuits
Supper	*Bedtime snack*
2 oz Baked meatloaf with plain gravy	Cornflakes with 1 cup milk, sliced
Mashed potato	peaches, and 2 tsp sugar
Baked hubbard squash with butter and brown sugar	
Cottage cheese with french dressing	
Fruited Jello with cream	
Sanka, cream, 2 tsp sugar	

* Reduced lactose—6 g/12 fl oz

as possible, and not associated with blood tests, examinations, etc. This is hard to achieve in a hospital environment, but is an important goal to meet for a patient to eat well and be rested.

Patients accept liquids well. Some prefer them less sweet; dilution of these drinks with skim milk, albeit this reduces the calories (joules), nevertheless is more acceptable.

Timing is also important. Supplemental feedings scheduled close to mealtimes interfere with intake.

Elemental Diet

An elemental diet of low-residue food is a chemically defined, synthetic mixture of carbohydrates, amino acids, and essential fatty acids with added vitamins and minerals. The diet is bulk-free, easily absorbed and assimilated, and is designed as a sole source of nutrition. Products such as Vivonex and Precision typify elemental diets. *Oral alimentation,* or use of the elemental diet, has been advocated as a component of preoperative as well as postoperative management in attempts to achieve a more satisfactory nutritional state. Its use has replaced, to a large degree, the traditional clear liquid diets that have concerned individuals awaiting colonic surgery. Nutritional comparisons are shown in Table 24-6.

In conditions when it is necessary to have a "clean empty" bowel, clear liquids and Vivonex or Precision are ordered 2 or 3 days preoperatively so as to ensure this goal. More importantly, their use allows a patient to meet surgical stress in a well-nourished state of positive nitrogen balance, rather than in the semi-starved state of the clear liquid diet.

A fuller discussion of the composition of elemental diets is given under "Tubal Alimentation," below (see p. 526).

NPO

The surgeon may order that the patient be given nothing by mouth (NPO = nothing per os). Patients may be unable to take food orally (the preferred route) because of intractable vomiting, obstruction, etc. Preoperative repletion may be supported by the following measures:

Parenterally—i.e., with 5 percent dextrose in water (D_5W) and isotonic amino acids

With peripheral infusions of fat emulsions

By total parenteral nutrition

By tubal alimentation with elemental diets, administered slowly (drip method) or given by mouth very slowly.

These may provide a degree of support in patients with partial obstruction and who now await surgical intervention.

TABLE 24-6 COMPARISON OF CLEAR LIQUID AND ELEMENTAL DIET

Type	Volume	Carbo-hydrate, g	Protein, g	Fat, g	kcal	kJ
Clear liquid (tea, sugar, broth, Jello)	1800 ml	110	10	—	480	2016
Vivonex Standard*	1800 ml	407	31	1	1800	7560

* Mixing directions: 6 pkg Vivonex Standard (unflavored), 6 pkg flavoring of choice, 1530 ml water.

1 Blend all of above in mixer.

2 Allow to stand and settle for 5 min.

3 Bring to 1800 ml volume with additional water.

POSTOPERATIVE
DIETARY MANAGEMENT

Postoperatively, adults and children in a well-nourished state have reserves of nutrients. This enables them to endure the short period (3 or 4 days) of semistarvation without severe physiological insult to their system. Intravenous therapy provides fluid, electrolyte, and nutritional support. Management during this time is directed at maintaining the body's fluid and electrolyte balance, preventing dehydration, and providing some calories (joules) for energy needs until the gastrointestinal tract resumes normal functioning and the patient is able to take liquids and nourishment by mouth.

The postoperative course is a time of semistarvation. It is characterized by the catabolic response to stress that was described earlier, with the net outcome of hormone release being:

Increased gluconeogenesis with mobilization of amino acids from muscle

Increased release of free fatty acids

Increased urinary nitrogen and potassium

In addition to these responses, losses of water, blood, and nitrogen must also be considered.

Water losses   There is loss of water and other body fluids and electrolytes (sodium, potassium) due to wound drainage, nasogastric suctioning, vomiting, and fever. Immediate replacement is essential in order to prevent dehydration, especially in infants and children who have a high body water content.

Blood losses   Plasma protein, especially in children, requires immediate replacement so that adequate blood volume and flow are maintained. Use of plasma or albumin, or isotonic saline, is necessary in infants in order to expand or restore blood volume. Loss of plasma poses a serious threat to infants, who have a rapid basal metabolic rate (BMR) and a large body surface area. (Adequate albumin concentration is required to ensure colloidal osmotic pressure.) Total serum protein in infants, children, and adults should be maintained at 5 g/100 ml or higher. Common parenteral solutions are presented in Table 24-7.

Nitrogen losses   Nitrogen losses can be ameliorated by an exogenous source of glucose, which also serves to provide energy to the brain and other vital organs. This also prevents the development of ketosis (100 to 150 g of glucose is required daily to prevent ketosis).

At the point of anabolism, when the patient is ready to eat, and peristalsis has returned, it is essential to plan for proper energy levels and protein in the diet. It is also important to monitor the intake at meals, especially in the at-risk patient. Proprietary and commercial supplements are nutritionally designed toward meeting this goal (see "Supplementary Feedings," p. 528). In addition, they have added vitamins and minerals, especially those (vitamins C and B_6, zinc) which are involved in protein synthesis and wound healing.

Initial Postoperative Diet

During the uncomplicated initial postoperative period intravenous therapy is employed for short-term support. It is used to restore obligatory basal fluid and electrolyte losses and to maintain homeostatic balance. A sample plan for replacement needs for adults is shown in Table 24-8.

Adequacy of intravenous fluid and electrolyte therapy can be assured by monitoring *urinary output* and *serum sodium and potassium levels;* when all values fall within normal range, fluid and electrolyte needs are met. Careful attention to accurate "intake and output" ("I and O") recording by the nursing staff following surgery is essential. In addition, the degree of dehydration may also be estimated by body weight losses; e.g., a 6, 8, or 10 percent weight loss reflects a comparable severity of dehydration. Daily weight records are therefore recommended.

TABLE 24-7 COMMON PARENTERAL SOLUTIONS

Component	Solution	Use	Comments
Glucose	D₅W (5% dextrose in water)	*Isotonic* 1 l = 50 g glucose 190 kcal (798 kJ) 1 g = 3.8 kcal (16.1 kJ) (anhydrous glucose used)	Basal caloric requirements are 1500–2300 kcal (6300–9660 kJ) daily. Traditional IV therapy cannot meet this requirement without overloading the body with water—2000–2500 ml/24 h = maximum allowance for fluid 100–150 g glucose per day will exert a protein-sparing effect, prevent starvation ketosis, and provide energy for the brain
	D₁₀W (10% dextrose in water)	*Hypertonic* 1 l = 100 g glucose 380 kcal (1596 kJ)	Use must be carefully monitored for danger of venous thrombosis or signs of diarrhea
SPA (salt-poor albumin) Plasma Dextran 40 Dextran 70 Plasmanate	Same as components	Blood volume expanders	These solutions are used to maintain adequate blood flow. Albumin is especially needed to maintain colloidal osmotic pressure
Saline	0.9%	Isotonic (154 meq)	Replacement needs—to maintain serum Na⁺ levels at 136–145 meq/l
Amino acids	Amigen (Casein hydrolysate) Aminosol (Fibrin hydrolysate) Freamine (Synthetic amino acids)	Source of amino acids	Abate muscle catabolism (5% solutions are isotonic)
Lipids	Intralipid* 10% or 20% soybean emulsions Lipofundin 10% or 20% soybean emulsions	Concentrated source of kcals (1.1 kcal/ml) 110 kcal/100 ml (4.62 kJ/100 ml) Isotonic 280 mosmol	Administered by peripheral vein No "fat overloading syndrome"
Whole blood Packed cells	Same as components	Restoration and maintenance of adequate blood volume and flow—crucial to survival	All tissues require adequate perfusion of blood as oxygenation and nourishment are necessary for their integrity
Parenteral vitamins	C, K, B complex	Wound healing; blood clotting; carbohydrate metabolism	Multivitamin preparations may be given by mouth when a patient is able to take them

* Contents: 10% soybean oil, 1.2% egg yolk, phospholipids, 2.5% glycerol

TABLE 24-8 24-H INTRAVENOUS THERAPY FOR ADULT REPLACEMENT NEEDS FOLLOWING ROUTINE NONEXTENSIVE SURGERY

	Solution	Volume	Glucose, g	Water, ml	Sodium, meq	Potassium, meq		Comments
1	0.45% Saline with D₅W	500 ml	25	500	38.5	—	1	Source of sodium for routine replacement
2	D₅W with KCl	1000 ml + 20 meq K	50	1000	—	—	2, 3	125 g glucose for sparing protein and preventing ketosis. Potassium given to prevent deficit (especially if there has been GI suctioning)
						20		
3	D₅W with KCl	1000 ml + 20 meq K	50	1000	—	—	4	Fluid (as water) needs: urine losses 800–1000 ml insensible losses (lungs and skin) 700 sweat 600 GI losses 300
						20		
	Input	2500 ml-water + 40 meq KCl	125 g*	2500	38.5	40		Output 2400 ml

D₅W = 5% dextrose in water; KCl = potassium chloride; GI = gastrointestinal.
* 125 g glucose equals 475 kcal (1995 kJ)

Fluid therapy in *infants and children* (see Table 24-9) is required in order to provide energy support and to prevent dehydration. The energy reserve of the newborn is very small, and the BMR is high; therefore, energy deprivation and acidosis can be a very sudden and life-threatening situation. Preoperatively, 50 ml of intravenous maintenance fluid/kg of body weight is administered daily. Postoperatively, the nurse must carefully and closely monitor infants and young children receiving intravenous therapy, to ensure adequate urine output so as to avoid water overloading and intoxication.

Following uncomplicated procedures, there is rapid progression to oral fluids so as to establish full energy and protein intake as soon as possible.

The first oral fluid may be glucose and water.

This is followed by dilute commercial formula (later, the child is given the formula in full strength) appropriately planned for age and weight.

Postoperative Diets: A Progression From Liquid to House Diet

In routine nonextensive surgery in a well-nourished patient, an established pattern of management is followed. Intravenous fluids are supportive until a patient is able to take sufficient fluids and some nutrients by mouth; thereafter, when bowel sounds return the patient progresses rapidly to solids.

After minor surgical procedures, once the patient is fully reactive and recovered from anesthesia, often *diet as tolerated* is ordered. Consultation with the patient by dietary personnel is strongly recommended. A simple meal of tea, toast, and custard may be preferred over a large meal planned without such an interview. This again illustrates the need for the dietitian, nurse, or other appropriate personnel to continuously interact with patients in order to determine their needs. In addition, the dietitian and nurse can observe limitations,

evaluate status, and recommend or advise. Such contact is an important exchange postoperatively as well as preoperatively.

After more complicated surgery, the patient is kept NPO, and maintained on intravenous therapy for fluid and energy support. This regimen is maintained until ambulation and peristalsis are resumed, and satisfactory fluid intake and urinary output are achieved. The objective in resuming oral intake as soon as possible is to prevent severe energy and protein losses. The patient at this stage is started on sips of water, or clear liquids (tea, broth, or Jello), 30 ml, 60 ml, or 90 ml given hourly; progression is planned according to the patient's increased tolerance, signs of hunger, absence of vomiting, passage of flatus, and presence of active bowel sounds. Rapid progress is made to unrestricted intake of clear liquids (1000 to 1500 ml daily), and to full liquids—avoiding coffee and spicy broths. With children, knowledge of their favorite juices and (if not weaned) provision of their own bottle are important.

When diet must be related to a surgical procedure it is planned according to the physician's request or dietitian's recommendation.

Table 24-10 summarizes common surgical procedures and postoperative dietary management.

In monitoring nutrient and fluid intake, careful "I and O" (intake-output) records must be maintained. It is most important to be cognizant of all potential sources of nutrients in determining nutrient intake. These include:

Foods: Solids, liquids
Intravenous fluids: D_5W
Tube feedings

PARENTERAL AND OTHER NUTRITIONAL SUPPORT SYSTEMS

Parenteral and other support systems become the choice of management for those patients whose energy and protein needs are great and

TABLE 24-9 24-H MAINTENANCE INTRAVENOUS FLUID THERAPY FOR PREMATURE, NEWBORN, AND OLDER CHILDREN

Condition and weight	Water, ml/kg	Calories, cal/kg	Kilojoules, kJ/kg	Sodium, meq/kg	Potassium, meq/kg	Chloride, meq/kg	Expected urine output, ml/kg
Premature	40	50	210	0.5	0.5	0.5	30 ml total in first 24 h
Newborn First week	50–60	60	252	0.5	0.5	0.5	30–110
After first week	100–110	100–110	420–462	1.5–2	1–1.5	1.5	30–110
Older Infants 1–10 kg	100	100	420	1.5–2	1–1.5	1.5	30–110
11–20 kg	1000 ml + 50 ml/kg for wt over 10 kg	1000 kcal + 50 kcal/kg for wt over 10 kg	4200 kJ + 210 kJ/kg for wt over 10 kg	—	—	—	—
20 kg and over	1500 ml + 20 ml/kg for wt over 20 kg	1500 kcal + 20 kcal/kg for wt over 20 kg	6300 kJ + 84 kJ/kg for wt over 20 kg	—	—	—	—

Source: A. S. Besser and H. Firor, "Pediatric Surgery," in R. E. Condon and L. M. Nyhus (eds.), *Manual of Surgical Therapeutics*, 3d ed., Little, Brown and Company, Boston, 1975, p. 336 (used with permission).

cannot be met solely by oral intake. These systems have been designed to ensure maximization of protein intake for synthesis and positive nitrogen balance, with resultant healing and repair. They are also used in children to prevent dehydration, provide calories (joules), and maintain adequate blood volume. Such nutritional support systems are classified as:

1　Intravenous or parenteral alimentation
2　Total parenteral nutrition (TPN or Hyperalimentation)
3　Tubal alimentation

Intravenous (Parenteral) Alimentation

Intravenous therapy used as a short-term support system is continued when a patient has not resumed eating within 4 days postoperatively. Sources of nutrients are delivered by peripheral vein; however, adequate absorption of calories (joules) and protein is limited because of the danger of fluid overload and subsequent compromising of the circulatory system—this is especially hazardous in the young child and the elderly. For long-term support, intravenous fat and glucose, or TPN solutions are used. Glucose-free amino acid solutions are advocated by certain investigators.

(Note: The appropriateness of parenteral support systems is reflected in clinical signs of improvement. Early indications of progress—often seen before true weight gain—are weight stabilization, alertness and awareness of the environment, and absence of diarrhea.)

Glucose-Free Amino Acid Solutions

Blackburn supports the concept of effective intravenous alimentation by use of glucose-free amino acid solutions.[16] This is based on the fact that the glucose-free solution serves to decrease the stimulation and release of insulin, which has an antilipolytic activity. As a result, there is an increased mobilization of fat stores, and increased release of free fatty acids for energy needs, so that gluconeogenesis and muscle catabolism are no longer necessary for

meeting energy requirements. The intravenous amino acids provide a source of nitrogen for tissue repletion and synthesis.

The concept is physiologically sound; however, the theory presupposes that the patient has adequate fat reserves. The use of glucose-free amino acid solutions is not widespread or generally accepted as a standard mode of support.

Total Parenteral Nutrition (TPN; Hyperalimentation)

As a lifesaving alternative to conventional therapy, which cannot satisfy the great nutritional demands of severe trauma, sepsis, and burns, Dudrick and colleagues in recent years have pioneered the design and application of total parenteral nutrition (TPN). This is a nutritional support system for patients whose nutritional requirements for energy and protein are large and for whom intravenous, oral, or tubal alimentation is inadequate or contraindicated.[17-21]

The infusions are designed to provide sufficient energy as hypertonic glucose (25 to 50 percent); L-amino acids (3, 5, or 8 percent); and maintenance requirements for sodium, potassium, phosphorus, and vitamins A, D, E, and C in a ratio that is favorable to nitrogen repletion and wound healing. Optional additions are vitamins K and B_{12}, folic acid, and iron.

It has been reported that TPN is successful in providing effective nutritional support for:

Short bowel syndrome
Advanced inflammatory bowel disease
Intestinal fistulas
Gastrointestinal anomalies (omphalocele and Gastroschisis) of the newborn, which can be repaired while the infant is being adequately nourished

TPN promotes wound healing and weight gain in postoperative patients, burn victims, etc., and supports normal growth and development in newborns and infants. Table 24-11

TABLE 24-10 POSTOPERATIVE DIETARY MANAGEMENT

Focus	Disorder	Surgical procedure	Feeding method	Dietary modification	Comments
Head	Head injury	Burr holes	Nasogastric tube feeding	Standard tube feeding	Patient unconscious
Cranium, ear, nose, throat, eye	Tonsillitis	Tonsillectomy	By mouth	Liquids to soft foods	Not by straw
Mouth	Cataract	Removal	By mouth	As tolerated	
	Cancer	Cryosurgery	Nasogastric tube feeding or gastrostomy	Standard tube feeding	High-energy, high-protein
Jaw	Caries	Full mouth extraction	By mouth	Liquids to soft foods	Cool liquids to room temperature
	Cancer	Radical excision	Nasogastric tube feeding or gastrostomy	High-energy, high-protein	
Cheek	Fracture	Wiring and repair	By mouth	High-energy, high-protein liquids	By straw
	Tumor	Cryosurgery	Nasogastric tube feeding or gastrostomy	High-energy, high-protein	
Esophagus Larynx	Cancer Cancer	Surgical repair Removal	Nasogastric tube feeding or gastrostomy	High-energy, high-protein Elemental diets Baby foods, liquids	
Stomach	Hiatus hernia	Repair	By mouth	Liberal bland to house diet	Liquids after meals
	Cancer; Zollinger-Ellison syndrome	Subtotal to total gastrectomy	By mouth	Blenderized diet ↑ protein, ↑ fat, moderate carbohydrate	Small frequent feedings. Hypoglycemia, loss of intrinsic factor may occur
	Peptic ulcer	Pyloroplasty, subtotal Billroth gastrectomy I or II	By mouth	Anti-dumping diet ↑ protein, ↑ fat, moderate carbohydrate	
Small intestine Duodenum	Ulcer Cancer	Resection	By mouth	As tolerated	
Jejunum	Crohn's disease (regional ileitis)	Resection	By mouth	Diet for "short bowel" dilute elemental diets +	
Ileum		Resection	By mouth	MCT Oil	Loss of vitamin B_{12}, water, electrolytes; ↑ lactose intolerance, fat intolerance; ↑ diarrhea, steatorrhea

Organ	Condition	Surgery/Procedure	Route	Diet	Comments
Colon	Cancer	Colectomy (subtotal or total); colostomy	By mouth	Low roughage, increased as tolerated	
	Ulcerative colitis		By mouth		
	Diverticulitis		By mouth	May have increased bulk, increased roughage (With physician's approval)	Bran (2 tbsp tid) may be added to diet
Rectum	Fissure	Fissurectomy			
	Hemorrhoids	Hemorrhoidectomy	By mouth		
Heart	Stroke	Embolectomy	Nasogastric tube feeding	Standard—baby foods if tolerated	Saturated fat decreased; polyunsaturates increased
	Acute sclerotic heart disease—coronary arteries	CABG (coronary artery bypass graft)	By mouth	No added salt (2–4 g sodium)	
Gallbladder	Cholecystitis	Cholecystectomy		Low fat	Gas-forming vegetables may not be tolerated
	Cholelithiasis	Cholecystectomy	By mouth	House diet as tolerated	
Genitourinary	Nephrolithiasis	Nephrectomy	By mouth	Forced fluids	Calcium or uric acid may be restricted
Kidney	Cancer		By mouth		
	Fibrocystic disease	Transplantation	By mouth	Individualized according to bio-chemical profile	

TABLE 24-11 RECOMMENDED DESIGN FOR 24-HR TOTAL PARENTERAL NUTRITION (FOR SUPPLYING ENERGY AND PROTEIN)

	Kcal/kg body weight	kJ/kg body weight	Nitrogen, g/kg weight
Adults	30–50	126–210	0.2
Infants	125–130	525–546	0.6–0.74

gives a recommended basis for planning TPN solutions.

Problems of TPN Solutions

There are certain problems encountered in attempting to provide nutritional adequacy by means of parenteral solutions. They are as follows:

1 In meeting the great need to deliver sufficient energy for anabolism, the traditionally used hypertonic glucose presents many dangers. Two important ones are
   - Thrombosis
   - Hazards of septicemia (glucose is an excellent growth medium for bacteria and fungi)

2 The source of protein (i.e., of amino acids for nitrogen metabolism) that is used to favor repletion, growth, and development may vary.
   - It is suggested that synthetic amino acids be used to provide the protein source in TPN solutions. This will allow individualized planning to meet amino acid requirements and will help to avoid the danger of hyperchloremia in infants. (The use of 3 percent Freamine is advocated.)
   - Solutions of casein hydrolysate (Amigen) yield peptides as well as free amino acids (by the enzymatic hydrolysis of casein) (Aminosol is a fibrin hyroly-

TABLE 24-12 TOTAL PARENTERAL SOLUTIONS FOR ADULTS

	Volume	Concentration of nutrients per liter	Calories (joules)	Nutrient per liter
Freamine II Crystalline amino acids*	500 ml	8.5% (Protein)	153 kcal (643 kJ)	42.5 g
Dextrose	500 ml	50% (Carbohydrate)	850 kcal (3570 kJ)	250 g
Sodium				5 meq
Phosphate				10 meq
Osmolarity				1700–1750 mosmol
pH				6.5
The following may be added				
KCl (Potassium chloride)				80 meq/l
Magnesium sulfate				8.2 meq/l
Calcium				4.5 meq/l
MVI (Multivitamins for injection) or				
Berocca-C (Vitamins B & C)				
Solu-B-Forte (Water-soluble vitamins)				
Vitamin K is given intramuscularly				

* Isolated and purified from edible soy bean hydrolysate or synthesized.
Source: Reprinted with permission of Beth Israel Hospital, Boston, Mass.

TABLE 24-13 TOTAL PARENTERAL SOLUTIONS FOR CHILDREN

Source of nutrients	Calories (joules)	Concentration of nutrient per liter*
Protein hydrolysate	108 kcal (454 kJ)	30.0 g
Dextrose (hydrous)	668 kcal (2806 kJ)	196.6 g
Potassium		12.0 meq
Sodium		15.0 meq
Calcium		540 mg
Phosphorus		155.0 mg
Magnesium		7.6 meq
Chloride		10.8 meq
Folic acid		0.5 mg
Multivitamins		5.0 ml
Vitamin K_1		0.2 mg
Vitamin B_{12}		6.6 μcg
Trace elements (zinc, copper, iodine, fluoride, manganese) solution		2.0 m

* Each liter contains approximately 41 g nitrogen and 800 kcal (3360 kJ). 135 ml/kg body weight per day provides 108 kcal (454 kJ)/kg of body weight day. Use for infants and children; additional fluid losses replaced by peripheral intravenous therapy; if rate of infusion is exceeded, hyperglycemia may result.
Source: Reprinted with permission of the Children's Hospital Medical Center, Boston, Mass.

sate; Freamine is a crystalline L-amino acid solution.) However, a large percentage of peptides are lost in the urine and not utilized; e.g., 36 to 53 percent of Amigen infusion is excreted as compared to a 2.4 to 6 percent loss of free amino acids.

3 Overaddition of multivitamin preparations, especially vitamins A and D, to TPN solutions may carry the danger of hypervitaminosis in infants and children.

4 Inadequate monitoring of serum trace elements may lead to potential difficulties; e.g., prolonged TPN use without appropriate supplementation may result in depressed copper and zinc levels; these elements are considered necessary micronutrients in wound healing.[22]

Tables 24-12 and 24-13 give sample solutions for TPN in adults and children, respectively. Figure 24-2 compares the energy densities of several parenteral solutions.

(Note: The cost of TPN warrants thorough investigation of other alternatives before a final decision for its use is made. TPN is indicated in long-term use in specific patients who *cannot* be managed by traditional methods. The expense of TPN therapy is 7 times the expense of a hospital meal.)

Fat Emulsions

The use of fat emulsions as an aspect of TPN is gaining in application in the United States.[23] Intralipid, a soybean oil derivative, is most commonly used. It is isotonic when delivered by peripheral vein and provides 1.1 kcal (4.62 kJ)/g. The use of fat emulsions is also instrumental in preventing the essential fatty acid deficiency that may result from long-term TPN. It is recommended that fat emulsions should not constitute more than 60 percent of the total calories.[24] (It may still be necessary to provide sufficient glucose calories by the subclavian vein.) Adults can easily be given 1000 kcal (4.2 MJ) daily. Tables 24-14 and 24-15

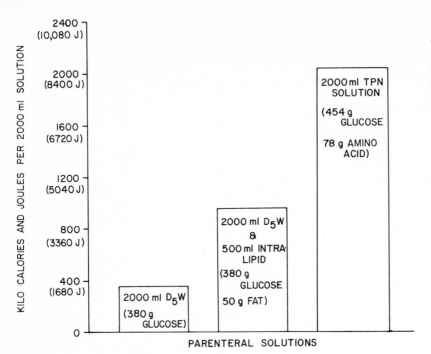

Figure 24-2

A comparison of parenteral solutions. Equal volumes of three different parenteral solutions vary markedly in energy potential.

TABLE 24-14 RECOMMENDED INFUSION RATE FOR INTRALIPID*

Adults: 0.5 ml/min initially, progressing to a maximum of 5 ml/min. Maximum single infusion, 500 ml; maximum total infusion, 7 l over a 14-day period

Children: 30 ml/kg body weight delivered over a 6 h period, every other day

---

* Cutter Laboratories, Inc. Intralipid may be infused simultaneously with 5% dextrose or 5% amino acid solutions. Adverse effects (fever and nausea) may be decreased with decreased dosage. Overloading syndrome (anorexia, fever, headache, sore throat, and pain) is not observed with prolonged use of Intralipid.

TABLE 24-15 RECOMMENDED DAILY DOSAGE FOR INTRALIPID

	g/kg body wt	Comments
Infants	2	May increase to maximum of 4 g/kg over several days
Adults	1.5–2	

show recommended infusion rates and dosages, respectively. Intralipid, like TPN solutions, is also very expensive.

Routes of Administration

TPN solutions, which are very concentrated mixtures, are delivered by insertion of a sterile catheter into a large central vein. The subclavian vein is commonly used, for at this point there is rapid blood flow into the superior vena cava. (In infants, the central vein is the route of administration.) This permits a rapid flushing and dilution of the hypertonic solution, thereby reducing the danger of thrombosis. In addition, it is important to remember that this is achieved in a volume of water that does not exceed the individual's daily fluid requirement (Figure 24-3).

The rate of flow of the infusion must be regulated so that a constant, uninterrupted flow is administered in order to avoid marked fluctuations in blood glucose.

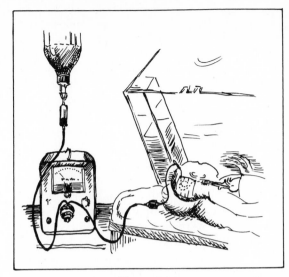

Figure 24-3

The "lifeline." The "lifeline" consists of (1) the nutrient solution, (2) calibrated burette, (3) infusion pump, (4) disposable tubing, (5) bacterial filter, (6) T connector, and (7) tubing held in place at the head by a sterile dressing. The tube is inserted through one of the jugular veins of the neck into the vena cava. After verification by x-ray the tube is further inserted under the skin to a point of exit on the head. It is difficult to otherwise keep the lifeline clean and secured at the neck.

Table 24-16 gives recommendations for clinical and biochemical signs to monitor.*

Risk Factors

1 *Insulin reaction* In response to the hypertonic glucose of TPN solutions, there is an increased secretion of insulin (as well as added parenteral insulin administration). Rebound insulin shock, or hypoglycemia, may occur if solutions are abruptly stopped. When oral feedings are to be resumed, it is also recommended that TPN solutions be tapered off over a 48-h period.

* Parents and staff involved in the care of young children receiving TPN are encouraged to hold and interact with the children in attempts to normalize and foster their psychosocial development.)

TABLE 24-16 CLINICAL AND BIOCHEMICAL MONITORING IN TOTAL PARENTERAL NUTRITION*

Factor	Frequency
Electrolytes (Na^+, K^+, Ca^{2+}, Cl^-, P)	Daily, then 2 or 3 times/week
Weight (Fluid intake and output)	Daily
Vital signs	Daily
Blood urea nitrogen	Daily
Serum glucose	Daily
Urinalysis (glucose)	Daily (Cover with sliding scale insulin)
Complete blood count	Weekly
Creatinine	Weekly
Fibrinogen	Weekly
Magnesium	Weekly
Copper†	Weekly
Zinc†	Weekly

* Urinary and fecal nitrogen determinations will determine if positive nitrogen balance is achieved and maintained.

† Recent research indicates the need to monitor copper and zinc levels. (See C. R. Fleming et al., "Prospective Study of Serum Copper and Zinc Levels in Patients Receiving Total Parenteral Nutrition," *American Journal of Clinical Nutrition,* **29:**70, 1976.

2 *Contamination* Strict control in defined pharmacy areas must be assured in order to prevent bacterial contamination.

3 *Infection* Catheter contamination at the entry site or contaminated solutions may lead to septicemia. The patient may already be predisposed to monilial infection because of his poor nutritional state as well as the use of broad-spectrum antibiotics.

4 *Metabolic complications* Some are:
- Too rapid infusion and prolonged use of hypertonic solutions can lead to hyperosmolar reactions and coma.
- Vitamin toxicity may result in hypercalciuria and renal stone formation.
- Essential fatty acid deficiency may result if fat is not supplied; therefore, addition of fat emulsion to the regimen is recommended.

Tubal Alimentation (Enteral Nutrition)

When an individual is unable to take food orally, an artificial route may be created as a nutritional support system. Causes include fractures of the jaw, cancer of the mouth or esophagus, esophageal fistula of the newborn, and anorexia of long-term illness.[25] The type of feeding and the route of administration are determined by the nature of the case and the philosophy of the physician.

Table 24-17 lists some common tube feeding formulas. Beyond 1 kcal/ml (4.2 kJ/ml), mixtures are hypertonic or viscous as a result of the increased addition of carbohydrate sources or protein hydrolysates. As a result, the formulas must be diluted, thereby decreasing nutrient intake.

In the debilitated, the elderly, the very young, or the postoperative patient, it is judicious to proceed cautiously when planning tube feeding methods.[26] Food intake over a period of time has been limited or decreased. Too rapid or forced feedings of large volumes of concentrated mixtures may result in vomiting and diarrhea. Mixtures containing large solute concentrations and increased levels of protein, when administered without sufficient water, may result in osmotic diuresis and the danger of dehydration. These are serious setbacks to recovery that most patients can ill afford.

Monitoring for symptoms of thirst, cramping, diarrhea, and urinary output is necessary.

The initial goal should be to give 1000 kcal (4.2 mJ), as a solution containing 0.5 kcal/ml (2.1 kJ/ml), over a 24-h period without causing signs of cramping or diarrhea. Such tolerance, indicative of absorption and assimilation when achieved, will allow for gradual addition of calories (joules) and an increase in concentration.

It is ironic that a conscious patient for whom a nasogastric tube feeding has been planned may request a change in flavor. It is not uncommon for such patients to claim that they can taste the feeding.

In addition to the formula composition (i.e., increased lactose levels, and hypertonicity) there are other causes for diarrhea: contamination, bacterial infections, use of antibiotics are all factors to be considered. Poor sanitation and handling as possible causes re-

TABLE 24-17   CLASSIFICATION OF COMMON TUBE FEEDINGS

	Type	Characteristics	Observations
1	Blenderized (Meat base)	Mixtures of natural foods, blenderized in high speed blenders. Simulates diet to which the adult gastrointestinal tract is accustomed	Well tolerated
2	Milk base	Egg-milk-sugar mixtures with skim milk powder and casein hydrolysates added. This is *not* a mixture which the gastrointestinal tract readily tolerates	High in lactose and simple sugars. May result in diarrhea (lactose is acted on by bacteria to form lactic acid; this causes increased gastrointestinal motility)
3	Proprietary		
a	Elemental diets Vivonex Precision	Glucose, L-amino acids, linoleate, added vitamins and minerals. Hyperosomolar; sole source of nutrition	Standardized; sanitary; labor-saving, expensive. Easy passage through feeding tubes
b	Ensure	Soybean derivative	Lactose-free (see Table 24–20)
c	Isocal	Medium-chain triglycerides, peptides	350 mosmol/l
d	Sustagen	Milk-base, added simple sugars. Dehydrated; relatively easily prepared and well tolerated	See Table 24–20
e	Gerber's Meat Base Formula	Milk replacement: beef hearts are the source of protein. Isotonic	1 liter = 822 kcal (3452.4 kJ); carbohydrate 59.5, protein 40.8, fat 46.8, solute 270 mosm; lactose-free

TABLE 24-18 METHODS OF TUBE FEEDING ADMINISTRATION

Route	Recommendations	Observations
Nasogastric *(Intragastric)*	1 Use in all types of feeding 2 Use polyvinyl tubes; these are soft and comfortable but the narrow lumen precludes use of tube feedings that are viscous	Long-term extended use may result in nasal erosions or esophageal strictures
Gastrostomy *(An opening is made in the abdominal wall; a tube is inserted and is sutured in the opening of the stomach)*	Use in long-term management of: 1 Inoperable cancer of the mouth, esophagus, or larynx 2 Esophageal atresia of the newborn	Hold feedings for 2–3 days, until full peristalsis is resumed and wound closure is assured.
Jejunostomy *(An opening in the vicinity of the jejunum)*	Used in inoperable cancer with obstruction 1 Dilute elemental diets 2 Mixtures of simple sugars and peptides or amino acids (simulate jejunal contents)	Limited success

quire close investigation when cases of diarrhea occur. Feedings should be refrigerated; only a 24-h supply should be prepared and on hand, and only the amount required for the feeding should be removed and allowed to come to room temperature prior to administration.

Administration

Table 24-18 summarizes methods of tube feeding administration, and Fig. 24-4 illustrates tube feeding sites.

Quantity and frequency of tube feedings 180 to 200 ml of formula followed by 50 to 100 ml of water, if tolerated, is recommended in those patients who are not severely debilitated. Otherwise, 120 ml of the tube feeding is recommended until tolerance is reached. In young adult patients with large nutrient requirements, 250 to 300 ml every 3 to 4 hours is the ultimate goal, if tolerated. Feedings may be given every 3 h with reasonable safety and success. Sufficient water must be given to ensure adequate urinary output.

For loose stools or simple diarrhea, tincture of opium, codeine, or Kaopectate may be given to control it.

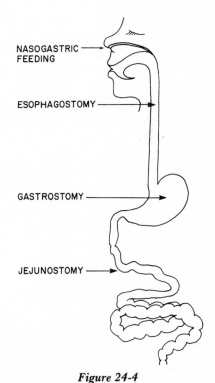

NASOGASTRIC FEEDING

ESOPHAGOSTOMY

GASTROSTOMY

JEJUNOSTOMY

Figure 24-4

The nature of the pathological condition determines the anatomical site for enteral feeding.

TABLE 24-19   TUBE FEEDING DELIVERY SYSTEMS

Delivery system	Method (head of patient or bed must be raised)
Asepto syringe	Quantity of feeding is measured into syringe and released slowly into feeding tube. Strict nursing supervision is required
Gravity drip	Feeding bag or commercial tube feeding set is used. Predetermined quantity is placed in bag; flow is regulated by stopcock. Flow is increased from 30 drops/min to 60 if tolerated
IVAC infusion pump (for TPN solutions)	Electronic regulation of flow into tube over 24-h period; used primarily in TPN delivery system
Food pump	Mechanical pump regulates predetermined flow over a 24-h period

Procedure for determining gastric residua   Gastrointestinal tonus is sluggish, especially in immobilized patients. Therefore it is essential to determine the gastric contents before giving a tube feeding. The stomach is aspirated by means of a large syringe. If the gastric residuum (undigested tube feeding material) exceeds one-half of the planned feeding, the feeding is postponed. Failure to do this may result in overfeeding and regurgitation of gastric contents with potential aspiration pneumonia or choking as the consequences. Delivery systems are summarized in Table 24-19.

Supplementary Feedings

These preparations (see Table 24-20) may be taken by mouth or given by tube. They are frequently milk-derived, with added carbohydrate, protein hydrolysates, fat, minerals, and vitamins; many are designed for use as the sole source of nutritional support. They provide a sound balance of energy and protein, and are easily digested and assimilated. They are easily obtained from local pharmacies after hospital discharge; however, they are relatively expensive.

Tube Feeding for Infants and Children

Unconscious infants and low-birth-weight neonates (1.2 to 2.5 kg) who are unable to take adequate nourishment orally because of immaturity (i.e., inability to suck) are supported by:

Gavage or nasogastric tube feedings
Gastrostomy feedings

In addition, supplemental intravenous glucose may be necessary for low-birth-weight infants (less than 1.2 kg)—administered within the first 3 to 6 h of life—in order to prevent acidosis and hypoglycemia

Plans for enteral feedings are individualized according to:

Gestational age
Extrauterine adjustment
Clinical status

The quantity and frequency of feeding, as well as the concentration of formulas, must be based on individual requirements. Commercial infant formulas may be used. Small quantities—3.5 or 7 ml—are given every 1 to 3 h, and are increased in volume, concentration, and frequency as tolerance increases. (See "Low-Birth-Weight Infants" in Chap. 26.)

Tube Feeding for Older Infants and Young Children

Commercial infant formulas, individualized according to energy needs, may be used as tube feedings. Consideration must be given to protein, mineral, and vitamin levels, and to fluid needs, especially in those who are unable to express thirst.

The danger of solute overload (protein and electrolyte) becomes especially hazardous when the tube feeding is not followed by added water. This is mandatory in order to ensure adequate urine output (240 to 600 ml per

TABLE 24-20 PROPRIETARY SUPPLEMENTS

Brand (Major ingredients)	Carbohydrate, g/l	Protein, g/l	Fat, g/l	Kcal/l (kJ/l) estimate	Comments
Sustacal (liquid) (Sucrose, concentrated sweet skim milk, corn syrup, soy oil, sodium and calcium caseinate, soy protein plus vitamins and minerals)	138	60	23	1000 (4200)	6 g lactose/12 fld oz 14.4 meq Na/12 fld oz may be used as a tube feeding
Meritene (liquid) (concentrated sweet skim milk, corn syrup solids vegetable oil, sodium caseinate, sucrose), vitamins, minerals	115	60	33	1000 (4200)	May be used as a tube feeding formula
Eggnog (Egg, milk mixture)	129	52	30	994 (4175)	Delmark brand made with whole milk
Sustagen (powder) (Powdered whole milk solids, calcium caseinate, Dextrimaltose, dextrose, vitamins, and iron)	300	105	15	1750 (7350)	3 cups Sustagen powder + 3 cups water = 1 qt (1l) may be used as a tube feeding
Carnation Instant Breakfast (powder) (similar design to "Sustagen")	140	70	36	1200 (5040)	4 packages powder, plus 1 qt whole milk
Controlyte (powder) (Enzymatic hydrolysate of corn starch; polysaccharides, vegetable oil)	143	0.08	48	1008 (4234)	Concentrated source of kcal (kJ); essentially protein-free; low in electrolytes
Ensure Soy and casein isolate, corn oil, corn syrup solids, vitamins, minerals	145	37	37	1060 (4452)	460 mosmol may be given orally (variety of flavors orange, vanilla, cherry, strawberry, etc.) or as tube feeding; lactose-free

day in young children) and to prevent dehydration.

The nurse must be alert for symptoms of vomiting, diarrhea, high fever, and delirium.

Elemental Diets (Chemically Defined Low-Bulk, or Low-Residue Foods)

Chemically defined, nutritionally sound diets have gained prominence in recent "space age" years. These foods are water-soluble mixtures of glucose, glucose derivatives, dextrins, L-amino acids, and essential fatty acids (linoleate), with added vitamins and minerals, although it may be necessary to monitor for vitamin K levels and give this vitamin parenterally. They are lactose-free, essentially fat-free, and leave little residue in the lower bowel. They reduce stool size, volume, and frequency, and allow the lower bowel to rest.

Table 24-21 is a summary of some available elemental diets and low-residue foods. One popular preparation has egg albumin as the source of available nitrogen; another is a mixture of peptides derived from casein hydrolysate. Some preparations provide standard amounts of nitrogen (1 g/300 kcal or 1 g/1260 kJ) and others have a high nitrogen content (2 g/300 kcal or 2 g/1260 kJ).

These preparations are designed for use as the sole source of nutrition, and are essential components of managing many surgical and medical disease states: inflammatory bowel disease (regional enteritis, ulcerative colitis),

TABLE 24-21 COMMON ELEMENTAL DIETS AND LOW-RESIDUE FOODS

Estimated nutrient values/l

Name	Highlights	Estimated nutrient values			Approximate kcal (kJ)	mosmol/l*	Available flavors
		Carbohydrate, g	Protein, g	Fat, g			
Vivonex							
1 Standard	Glucose + glucose oligosaccharides, unflavored amino acids†	226	20.4	0,1	1000 (4200)	500	Cherry, strawberry, orange, beef broth, etc.
2 High nitrogen	Unflavored (give by tube)	210	41.7	0.4	1000 (4200)	844	
Flexical	Sucrose, malto-dextrin, hydrolyzed casein	155	21.8	34 soy oil MCT‡ Oil	1000 (4200)	805	Vanilla, orange
Precision LR							
1 Standard	Egg Albumin, Malto-dextrin, sucrose	226	22	0.7	1000 (4200)	600	Cherry, orange
2 High nitrogen		207	42	0.5	1000 (4200)	580	Citrus
3 Moderate nitrogen		150	33	31 vegetable oil	1000 (4200)	475	Orange, vanilla
4 Isotonic		150	30	31 vegetable oil	1000 (4200)	300	Vanilla

* Attempts have been made to design the solutions so that they simulate the osmolality of blood plasma (280–330 mosmol/l).

† Some diets are unflavored and offer a variety of flavor packets to help overcome monotony and off-taste.

‡ Medium-chain triglycerides.

TABLE 24-22 NORMALLY RECOMMENDED INTAKES OF ELEMENTAL DIETS[22]

	Wt/vol	kcal/ml	kJ/ml	Strength*
Adult	25%	1	4.2	Full strength
	12.5%	0.5	2.1	½ Strength
Children†	10%	0.4	1.7	Less than ½ strength
Newborn†	7.5%	0.3	1.3	

* Very dilute solutions are first introduced so that the gastrointestinal tract has time to adjust. Thereafter, concentration may be increased to tolerance. (See Table 24–23.)

† Infants and children are very sensitive to hypertonic solutions.

bowel fistulas, malabsorption, short-bowel syndrome, pancreatic disease, etc.[27] Other indications for use have already been mentioned: preoperatively for bowel preparation and nutritional support; they are also useful in preparation for colonic x-rays.

The preparations may also be used as adjuncts to oral intake; however, this is not advocated because elemental diets are expensive, and can become monotonous and nauseating because of their characteristic smell and taste of amino acids. Moreover, there are other supplements that are as well utilized and better accepted (e.g., Sustacal).

Absorption The elemental diets require a minimum of digestion by pancreatic and biliary secretions. They are absorbed in the upper part of the small intestine (jejunum), and as a consequence should not be mixed with solid foods which are digested and absorbed further along in the gastrointestinal tract.

Administration In addition to supervising intake (some patients have been known to dispose of feedings in sinks) and advising patients of the need for the diet, one must monitor patients for symptoms that indicate hyperosmolar sensitivity and intolerance.

Some individuals with normal gastrointestinal tracts, and in well-nourished states, may still exhibit signs of excessive thirst, cramps, or diarrhea. The solutions which have high solute concentrations and simple sugar levels, and are very concentrated (1 kcal/ml or 4.2 kJ/ml) must be planned carefully, for the danger of solute overload and osmotic dehydration is very real.

Normally recommended intakes are shown in Table 24-22, and Table 24-23 represents a sample plan of feeding.

Adult patients must be advised to sip the mixture very slowly over a period of time. Giving these mixtures over ice or as slush increases their acceptance. At the first signs of intolerance (cramping is common) the feedings should be stopped for 24-h. Refeeding is commenced at one-quarter strength (this, rather than full-strength, is recommended as the strength of choice for severely debilitated patients), and the concentration is increased daily to individual tolerance. In adults who require tube feedings, one-half strength (0.5 kcal/ml, or 2.1 kJ/ml) of an elemental diet, given at the rate of 40 to 60 ml/h, is recommended as an initial concentration.

TABLE 24-23 RECOMMENDED ADMINISTRATION OF ELEMENTAL DIET TO AVOID OSMOTIC DEHYDRATION

Day	Strength	Volume of water	kcal/ml	kJ/ml
1	¼	1800 ml	0.25	1.05
2	½	1800 ml	0.5	2.1
3	¾	1800 ml	0.75	3.15
4	Full	1800 ml	1	4.2

However, those patients in a severely debilitated state require one-quarter strength initially.

Careful addition of water to regimens featuring elemental diets is vital. Patients must be instructed to drink sufficient water in addition to the planned diet. This will help in avoiding the intolerance that may occur. In addition, periodic clinical monitoring of blood and urine for glucose and of blood for electrolyte levels is essential.

Elemental Diets for Infants and Children

Children are very sensitive to concentrated solutions containing high solute loads. In infants, one-third strength solutions (0.33 kcal/ml, or 1.4 kJ/ml) are recommended by Randall as an initial course.[28] This is gradually increased over several days, according to tolerance and absence of danger signs. One-half strength is considered the limit of tolerance. Older children may be able to tolerate full-strength mixtures (1 kcal/ml, or 4.2 kJ/ml); however, one-half strength (0.5 kcal/ml, or 2.1 kJ/ml) is recommended as the starting level, gradually increased to the level of tolerance as the gastrointestinal tract adjusts.

Infants and young children can be given the elemental diets from nursing bottles; its taste—similar to the taste of Kool-Aid—is better accepted by children than by adults.

BURNS

CLASSIFICATION OF BURNS (SEVERITY AND DEPTH)

Degree of Severity

Burns may be classified according to severity in the following manner:

Small burns   Less than 15 to 20 percent of the total body surface area (BSA) is affected.

Intermediate burns   20 to 40 percent of BSA is affected.

Large or *severe burns*   More than 40 to 50 percent of BSA is affected.

Depth of Injury

Depth of injury is classified in the following manner:

Full-thickness burn   all epithelial remnants are destroyed; autografting is required.

Partial-thickness burn   remaining epithelium is present which will spontaneously re-epithelialize the area.

We will focus on the intermediate-burn patient, bearing in mind that increased nutritional demands and requirements must be met for all cases of burn injury.

Metabolic Sequelae of Burns

The burn patient, in previously good health and sound nutritional status, now develops metabolic sequelae, which are summarized as follows:

1   There is marked hormonal response to the severe trauma of thermal injury.
    a   Increased catecholamine secretion results in increased glucagon secretion and increased heat production (elevated basal metabolic rate) that usually lasts 6 to 8 weeks after injury.
    b   Action of insulin is depressed and glucose intolerance, simulating diabetes, is common.
2   The loss of skin surface represents the loss of an effective defense against infections. This loss of protection results in huge water losses; in addition, much energy is expended in the process of evaporation, so that energy requirements are well above basal needs. This emphasizes the need to close the wounds (by grafting if necessary) as soon as possible.
3   There is marked protein catabolism.
    a   Increased glucocorticoid activity results in mobilization of tissue amino acids as

the need for energy becomes urgent. This is reflected in increased urinary nitrogen and potassium.

b There is increased loss of albumin and other plasma proteins from the oozing exudates of the open wound.

Goals of Management

The goals of management are to support the patient's (adult's or child's) respiratory and circulatory system, and to sustain him or her until skin cover is achieved and basal metabolic rate is normalized.[29–31]

Fluid and Electrolyte Replacement

Initial care is directed toward the restoration of fluid and electrolyte balance and of blood volume, in order to prevent dehydration, shock, and metabolic acidosis. This is accomplished with the following techniques:

Intravenous support with glucose, electrolyte, colloid, and water is crucial.

Blood transfusions may be necessary within 24 to 36 h. The blood replacement is required because there is increased blood loss from the wound as well as depressed erythrocyte formation by the bone marrow.

Plasma or albumin may be required to support blood volume. *Glucose* is given to prevent acidosis.

The formulas in Table 24-24 provide a guide for immediately determining the water, colloid, and electrolyte needs.

Burns in infants and children require special attention since shock and acidosis within 18 to 24 h of injury are the usual consequence. As a precaution, children are given intravenous therapy regardless of the extent of the burn injury.

Urine output is monitored hourly so as to assure adequate fluid therapy (see Table 24-25). Oliguira may be present, but it is usually resolved within 48 h.

Children are kept NPO (given nothing by mouth) for the first 48 h. After this time, the danger of vomiting has lessened and small amounts of fluid (30 to 60 ml) may be given. The child is rapidly advanced to high-energy, high-protein liquids and then to an appropriate individualized high-energy, high-protein diet.

Prevention of Infection

The loss of skin cover represents the loss of an effective barrier against infection. The burn wound itself is often a source of bacterial contamination. In addition, there is an early lack of resistance as the individual's defense system is lowered. Lymphadenopathy, decreased antibody response, and gamma globulin destruction often result as a consequence of burn injury. All patients with full-thickness burns are given tetanus immunizations or boosters; infants and young children are given gamma globulin. Antibiotics, intravenous and topical (e.g., penicillin), are also administered.

Burn unit To help control the spread of infection, assure aseptic technique, and control evaporative water losses (in a 20 to 40 percent BSA burn, 1 to 2 l of water are lost through evaporation daily), special environmentally controlled burn units are used. These "plastic tents" have controlled humidity (20 percent) and temperature (30°C), as well as a flow of sterile air. They provide a bacteria-controlled, psychologically acceptable environment (the patient is able to see his surroundings, from within the transparent tent) that fosters survival.

Gastrointestinal Atony

Gastrointestinal atony or ileus may occur over a period of 24 to 36 h.[32] It is managed by nasogastric tube insertion and suction. When peristalsis is resumed, the objective is to provide sufficient food to meet the great, critical energy and protein requirements. Nutritional assessment and an individualized plan of action are imperative.

The patient with a normal gastrointestinal

TABLE 24-24   FORMULAS FOR CALCULATING FLUID REQUIREMENTS

Evans formula

Day 1   % BAS* burned × body weight (kg × 1 = ml colloid
        % BSA burned × body weight (kg) × 1 = ml 5% dextrose in normal saline } one-half given in first 8 h
        Plus maintenance fluids: 2000 ml 5% dextrose in water per day

Day 2   % BSA burned × body weight (kg) × 0.5 = ml colloid
        % BSA burned × body weight (kg) × 0.5 = ml 5% dextrose in normal saline
        Plus maintenance fluids: 2000 ml 5% dextrose in water per day

Day 3   and thereafter—intravenous fluids as indicated (burns over 50% BSA calculated as 50% burn)

Brooke Army Formula

Day 1   % BSA burned × body weight (kg) × 1.5 = ml 5% dextrose in normal saline } one-half given in first 8 h
        % BSA burned × body weight (kg) × 0.5 = ml colloid†
        Plus maintenance fluids: 2000 ml 5% dextrose in water per day

Day 2   % BSA burned × body weight (kg) × 0.75 = ml 5% dextrose in normal saline
        % BSA burned × body weight (kg) × 0.25 = ml colloid
        Plus maintenance fluids: 2000 ml 5% dextrose in water per day

Children's Hospital of Michigan formula

Day 1   % BSA burned × body weight (kg) × 2 = ml 5% dextrose in lactated Ringer's solution two-thirds in first 8 h
        Plus maintenance fluids: 1500 ml 5% dextrose in lactated Ringer's solution per square meter BSA per day
        For burns of 40–60% BSA, add 50 meq sodium bicarbonate to each liter of fluid and reduce rate by 10%
        For burns over 60% BSA, add { 40 meq sodium bicarbonate to each liter of fluid
        50 meq sodium chloride (12.5 ml of 15% saline) to each liter of fluid; slow rate by 20%

Day 2   Same fluids, but for burns over 40% with hyperosmolar solutions in use, monitor electrolytes at 18, 24, 30 and 36 h and q4 h thereafter. Stop hyperosmolar solution when serum sodium rises to or above 150 meq or serum osmolarity exceeds 350 millimoles. Resume 5% dextrose in lactated Ringer's at original rate

Day 3   and thereafter—5% dextrose in lactated Ringer's solution at a rate sufficient to maintain urinary output of 40 ml/m² BSA per hour

---

* BSA = body surface area.

† Because colloid is now considered ineffective during the first 24 h after a burn, some authors advocate eliminating colloid from the Brooke formula.

tract and no sepsis may be started on clear liquids and should rapidly progress to full liquids within 24 h after injury. Patients with large burns are usually not fed for 3 days.

Nutritional Support

The body's demand for energy and protein, and the need to control weight loss, are paramount. Sufficient calories (joules) for energy needs and protein synthesis must be consumed or delivered by a nutritional support system—protein utilization for wound healing and prevention of hypoproteinemia are of primary importance. The burn patient with adequate nutrient intake has greater success with the

TABLE 24-25   GUIDE TO MONITORING HOURLY URINES IN PATIENTS WITH BURNS

Patient	Age, yr	ml/h
Infants	Under 1	5–10
Children	1–10	10–20
	over 10	15–30
Adults		30–50

grafting procedure, has better healing at graft sites, and is less threatened by infection. Table 24-26 represents a plan for nutrient requirements.

Multivitamin preparations, especially vi-

TABLE 24-26 RECOMMENDED NUTRITIONAL DESIGNS FOR BURN PATIENTS

	Protein			*Energy*		
	g/kg body weight + g/each 1% BSA burned			*kcal/kg (kJ/kg) body weight + kcal/1% (kJ/1%) BSA burned*		
Children (up to 12 years of age)	3	+	1	60 (252)	+	35 (147)
Adults	1	+	3	20 (84)	+	70 (294)

BSA = body surface area.

tamins C and B complex, are given. (The recommended dose of vitamin D is 500 mg to 1.5 g daily.) Iron may be required for patients who become anemic. Serum zinc levels were found to be low in burned patients. Zinc supplementation, however, was not felt to be necessary since adequate oral intake soon results in normalization of zinc levels.[33]

Dietary regimens As a daily dietary program for burn patients, 3000 to 5000 kcal (12.6 to 21 MJ) and 150 to 200 g of protein is not uncommon. All routes—oral, artificial, and in some cases TPN—are utilized so as to achieve this critical goal. All possible methods must be employed, because the patient realistically cannot take this amount of food solely by mouth because of pain, shock, depression, etc.).

1 *Oral route* High-energy, high-protein liquids, milk shakes, and cream soups are given frequently, and are well accepted.
2 *Tube feedings* High-nitrogen elemental diets have successful application.[34] They are first given at one-quarter strength and increased to full strength as tolerance increases.
3 *TPN* This route requires careful supervision, but it is finding greater application. The danger of contamination and possible monilial sepsis is always present.
4 *Fat emulsions* Use of intravenous fat has great potential in meeting energy requirements, as well as exerting a protein-sparing effect.

Monitoring of nutrient needs by checking the patient's tray and careful documentation of intake and output records further serve to intensify the role of the dietitian and nurse, who must set rehabilitative goals and direct the efforts made toward meeting them.

In the attempt to reach this great nutritional goal, overstimulation of the gastrointestinal tract by the large volume of nutrient-rich material may occur and hemorrhage may result; therefore, aggressive concern must be tempered with caution.

Emotional Support

In addition to technical and nutritional support, emotional support must be given. There may be psychological scars as well as physical ones. Hospitalizations are long; wound debridement is painful and discouraging. Regrafting due to failure of a graft to "take" is common. The road back to health and normalcy is rugged, and the patient requires the constant support and encouragement of all.

Severely burned children must now endure and overcome an abrupt psychological as well as physical insult to their normal development. Children may experience grief and anger over body disfigurement; skin grafting and release of disabling, painful contractures are essential.

As children learn new methods of coping,

they may become manipulative, uncooperative, rebellious, or depressed.[35] Campbell, and Holli and Oakes, make several sound observations and give practical suggestions in managing and feeding burned children.[36,37] They suggest that there is complete loss of autonomy in many burn cases; since the patients are now totally dependent on others for their survival, they may resort to behavior that will give them some degree of self-control.

There is, therefore, great need to encourage verbalization of feelings as well as to provide opportunities for choosing or for simple decision-making on the patient's part. As best as possible and with guidance, the patient should be allowed to help plan and select a menu. Individualized diets should include popular and familiar foods, such as hot dogs, hamburgers, high-energy, high-protein milk shakes, and pizza. Trays should be placed where patients can see them, and should be attractive and colorful. All attempts at continuing interaction with burn patients and normalization of activities should be encouraged.

INTERDISCIPLINARY TEAM

Nutrition is paramount to the recovery of the surgically stressed or burned patient and requires the team approach. For example, in managing the burn patient, the combined efforts of the burn team—the doctor, nurse, nutritionist, respiratory therapist, social worker, etc.—must be executed judiciously, efficiently, and without delay. The toll of surgery or severe burns is great, often devastating; and rehabilitation is long and marred by many painful episodes and setbacks.

In the team approach, the special roles of the nurse and dietitian are prominent. The dietitian is specially trained to help in establishing the patient's nutritional needs and in providing the appropriate dietary intervention. The dietitian's role is one of a translator; that is, to take those nutritional needs that are determined by assessment techniques and translate them into food.

The nurse with continuing patient contact can closely determine the effectiveness of the diet: monitoring the clinical signs (weight, fluid intake and output), appraising moods, helping with menu selection, and verbalizing the patient's requests. Together with the patient, the nurse and dietitian can plan a diet that is psychologically responsive to the human need. It should be remembered that despite all good intentions and impressive plans, if a patient will not eat, all skill and knowledge are wasted.

This chapter serves to reaffirm the need to provide human as well as technical support for those who must overcome and survive surgery, stress, or burns.

STUDY QUESTIONS

1 Describe the body's catabolic hormonal response to stress, surgery, and burns.
2 What are the goals of postoperative nutritional management?
3 Is it possible to maintain a patient on 5% dextrose in water postoperatively for an extended period of time?
4 What clinical and laboratory signs should be closely monitored in patients receiving TPN?
5 What are signs of intolerance in patients receiving tube feedings?

CASE STUDY 24-1

A 23-year-old female was admitted to the hospital because of progressive cachexia, cramping, and diarrhea.

The diagnosis of Crohn's disease was made at age 16. Past hospitalizations included fistula repair at age 16 and excision of a perirectal abscess and fistula at age 21. Her present medical management includes 25 mg prednisone, Lomotil, and no dietary restrictions. In the past 6 months she has lost 10 lb.

On physical examination the patient was found to be a lethargic woman 5 ft 4 in tall and weighing 110 lb. Laboratory data revealed total plasma protein 7.1 g/100 ml, albumin 2.99 g/100 ml, hemoglobin 10.7 g/100 ml, and hematocrit 32.2 percent. Barium enema x-ray studies established the diagnosis of perirectal abscess secondary to Crohn's disease. The following care plan was established:

1 Surgical incision and drainage of the abscess

2 Steroids and ampicillin

3 Nutritional support—preoperative and postoperative use of Vivonex

Case Study Questions

1 Apply the concept of the body's catabolic response to stress to the case, considering the significance of the low serum albumin, low hematocrit, and hemoglobin level.

2 Why are elemental diets advocated as primary support in inflammatory bowel disease?

3 What might future medical and dietary management offer?

REFERENCES

1 W. Stahl, *Supportive Care of the Surgical Patient,* Grune and Stratton, Inc., New York, 1972.

2 H. A. Zintel, "Nutrition in the Care of the Surgical Patient," in M. G. Wohl and R. S. Goodhart (eds.), *Modern Nutrition in Health and Disease,* 4th ed., Lea and Febiger, Philadelphia, 1973.

3 F. D. Moore and M. F. Brennan, "Surgical Injury," in W. F. Ballinger et al. (eds.), *Manual of Surgical Nutrition,* W. B. Saunders Company, Philadelphia, 1975.

4 E. Peacock and W. Van Winkle, "Biochemistry and Environment of Wounds," in E. Peacock and W. Van Winkle, *Surgery and Biology fo Wound Repair,* Saunders Company, Philadelphia, 1970.

5 D. O'Berleas et al., "Effect of Zinc Deficiency on Wound Healing in Rats, *American Journal of Surgery* 121:556, 1971.

6 I. K. Hunt, "Inhibitory Effects of Vitamin E on Collagen Synthesis and Wound Repair," *Annals of Surgery,* 175:235, 1972.

7 F. D. Moore and M. F. Brennan, op. cit.

8 Ibid.

9 "Cellular Immunity and Malnutrition," *Nutrition Reviews,* 30:523, 1972.

10 D. G. Jose, "Cancer Connection with Immunity and Nutrition," *Nutrition Today,* March-April 1973, p. 4.

11 A. E. Axelrod, "Nutrition and Acquired Immunity," *Food and Nutrition News,* October-November 1974.

12 B. Worthington, "Effect of Nutritional Status on Immune Phenomena," *Journal of The American Dietetic Association,* 65:123, 1974.

13 D. K. Law, S. J. Dudrick, and N. I. Abdou, "Effects of Protein-Calorie Malnutrition on Immune Competence of the Surgical Patient," *Surgery Gynecology and Obstetrics,* **139:**257, 1974.

14 C. E. Butterworth, Jr., and G. L. Blackburn, "Hospital Malnutrition and How To Assess the Nutritional Status of a Patient," *Nutrition Today,* March-April 1975.

15 Ibid.

16 G. L. Blackburn, *Adaptation to Starvation,* Intake: Perspectives in Clinical Nutrition, Eaton Laboratories, Norwich, New York, 1973.

17 M. Asch and E. Fonkalsrud, "Special Pediatric Considerations," in W. F. Ballinger et al., op. cit.

18 D. O'Brien and H. P. Chase "Parenteral Nutrition in Infancy," in S. S. Gellis and B. M. Kagan (eds.), *Current Pediatric Therapy,* W. B. Saunders Company, Philadelphia, 1974.

19 M. E. Shils, "Total Parenteral Nutrition," in R. S. Goodhart and M. E. Shils (eds.), *Modern Nutrition in Health and Disease,* 5th ed., Lea and Febiger, Philadelphia, 1973.

20 C. R. Fleming et al., "Total Parenteral Nutrition," *Mayo Clinic Proceedings,* 51:187, 1976.

21 M. Shils, "Guidelines for Total Parenteral Nutrition," *Journal of The American Medical Association,* **22:**1514, 1972.

22 C. R. Fleming et al., "Prospective Study of Serum Copper and Zinc Levels in Patients Receiving Total Parenteral Nutrition," *American Journal of Clinical Nutrition,* 29:70, 1976.

23 M. Asch and Fonkalsrude op. cit.

24 C. R. Fleming, op. cit.

25 A. Gormican, "Tube Feeding," *Dietetic Currents,* April-May-June 1975.

26 J. C. Dougherty, "Influence of High Protein Diets on Renal Function," *Journal of The American Dietetic Association,* **63:**392, 1973.

27 H. T. Randall, "Diet and Nutrition in the Care of the Surgical Patient," in R. S. Goodhart and M. E. Shils, op. cit.

28 H. T. Randall, op. cit.

29 B. A. Pruitt, "Postburn Hypermetabolism and Nutrition of the Burn Patient," in: W. F. Ballinger et al., op. cit.

30 J. Long and B. A. Pruitt, "Nutritional Care of the Burn Patient," *Dietetic Currents,* January 1974.

31 C. Crenshaw, *Nutritional Support for Burn Patients,* Intake: Perspectives in Clinical Nutrition, Eaton Laboratories, Norwich, New York, 1973.

32 B. Harpole et al., *Nutritional Management of Problem Patients,* Intake: Perspectives in Clinical Nutrition, Eaton Laboratories, Norwich, New York, 1975.

33 I. Cohen et al., "Hypogeusia, Anorexia and Altered Zinc Metabolism Following Thermal Burn," *Journal of The American Medical Association,* **223:**914, 1973.

34 B. Harpole, et al. op. cit.

35 L. Campbell, "Special Behavioral Problems of the Burned Child," *American Journal of Nursing,* **76:**220, 1976.

36 L. Campbell, op. cit.

37 B. Holli and J. Oakes, "Feeding the Burned Child," *Journal of The American Dietetic Association,* **67:**240, 1975.

CHAPTER 25

FOOD ALLERGY

Mary Alice Marino

KEY WORDS
Antigen
Antibody
Allergen

INTRODUCTION

A problem specific to childhood but occurring at all ages through the life cycle is that of *food allergy*. Because of the possible effect of food allergy on nutrient utilization and the stress on the body imposed by the allergy, individuals are placed at nutritional risk, with the growth and development of children particularly threatened. Good management is imperative and includes strict avoidance of the offending foods, and awareness of the age-specific nutritional needs.

An *allergy* is the abnormal reaction or hypersensitivity to a substance which produces symptoms in the allergic individual. Although the allergy can appear at any age, it is far more common in infants and children. It has been estimated that approximately half of adult allergies begin in childhood.[1] The sensitivity to a particular food may seem to disappear with increasing age, but the tendency is never completely outgrown.

IMMUNOLOGICAL BASIS OF ALLERGY

To understand food allergy, it is necessary to consider the allergic reaction as a response of the body's immune defense system, whereby the body guards against the intrusion of a foreign substance, the *antigen*. (See Chap. 16.) In the case of food allergy, the antigens are natural products, usually protein, that are ingested in food. Since the body regards these as intruding substances, it produces an *antibody* which binds the antigen. Antibodies, also known as *immunoglobulins,* are found in the blood or tissues of all healthy persons. However, the allergic individual produces a greater quantity than normal of a particular immunoglobulin, IgE, which creates an overreaction of this protective mechanism. IgE is present in high concentration in the mucosa of the gastrointestinal tract, bronchial tubes, and nose. These are referred to as the allergy "shock organs" and are very frequently the sites for the antigen-antibody reactions of food allergy.

During the process of digestion, most food antigens are destroyed by the gastrointestinal tract. Because the protein molecules are very large, they rarely enter the bloodstream. The higher incidence of food allergy in infants and young children is thought to be related to the lower efficiency of their immature gastrointestinal systems. This allows more incompletely digested food and consequently more antigens or food *allergens* to be absorbed into the blood stream for reaction with antibodies.

SYMPTOMS

Because there are no specific criteria by which a diagnosis of food allergy can be made, and because the symptoms are so varied, the topic of food allergy is a subject of much confusion and debate. There are no immunological methods for accurately confirming or predicting the allergic symptoms that may follow ingestion of any food.[2] The reactions may occur in almost any body system—gastrointestinal, respiratory, cutaneous, urinary, or nervous system, mucous glands, and mucous membranes.

Table 25-1 shows the diversity of the symptoms which have been attributed to food allergy. Although the allergy may be as localized in manifestation as the appearance of eczema of the hands, it often occurs as a generalized and diffuse reaction with such symptoms as headache, vomiting, and urticaria (hives), involving many body systems. One particular food may be responsible for a variety of symptoms in the same individual. The diagnosis of food allergy is further complicated because the symptoms often duplicate those of other disorders.

FOOD ALLERGENS

Although almost any food could be the cause of an allergic reaction, certain foods are known to be particularly potent allergens. Some of the most common offenders are milk, egg, wheat, chocolate, nuts, fish and shellfish, citrus fruit, tomatoes, legumes, and corn. It is the protein component of the foods which is considered to be the cause of the allergy.

Milk Allergy

Milk allergy is usually thought to be the most common allergy in infants and young children.[3] The estimated frequency of occurrence in children ranges from 0.3 to 7 percent, with the onset most commonly prior to 1 month of age.[4] Part of the reason that milk is such a frequent offender is its high level of consumption, particularly in infancy. The sensitivity may be due to one of three proteins found in milk: lactalbumin, lactoglobulin, and casein. Lactalbumin plays the primary role in allergic reactions. Symptoms often related to milk allergy are eczema, colic, mucous and bloody diarrhea, and asthma.

Iron-deficiency anemia and intestinal loss of blood and protein have been noted to result from high intakes of pasteurized cow's milk. These conditions occur primarily in babies under 1 year of age whose milk intake is over 1 liter per day. Heat treatment of commercially prepared formulas seems to alleviate this problem, thus making heat-labile milk protein the suspected cause of the infant's difficulty.

TABLE 25-1 COMMON ALLERGIC SYMPTOMS

System	Symptoms
Gastrointestinal	Canker sores, cheilitis, colic, colitis, diarrhea, malabsorption, enteropathy, vomiting
Respiratory	Rhinitis, cough, asthma, bronchitis
Cutaneous	Angioedema, eczema, pruritus, purpura, urticaria
Central nervous system	Headache, neuralgias, irritability, personality change
Miscellaneous	Pallor, enuresis, retarded growth, menstrual irregularity

Wheat Allergy

There are many proteins in wheat that may act as antigens. These allergens are responsible for celiac disease, the intestinal malabsorption condition that occurs in children. Antibodies are produced in the intestinal mucosa and form an immune reaction following ingestion of wheat. The antigen-antibody complex injures the mucosa, resulting in loss of protein from the gut. Wheat allergy is the most common cereal allergy, but many children are also sensitive to corn. Rice is the grain that is least likely to produce an allergic manifestation.

Egg Allergy

Egg is an important allergen, frequently causing violent and almost instantaneous reactions. Egg allergy, often manifesting as eczema or urticaria, is most common in infancy and early childhood. The sensitivity is in response to the *albumin,* the protein in the egg white, and may even be induced by inhaling the odor of cooking eggs. Although not as commonly a problem as the albumin of the egg white, the egg yolk can also cause symptoms. Because many vaccines are often grown on egg or chick embryo, the egg-sensitive child must be guarded against such inoculations, which may have dangerous effects.

Other Allergies

The fruits most commonly producing an allergy in children are citrus fruits, strawberries, and melons. Group allergies may occur among fruits. For example, a child who is allergic to oranges may often be sensitive to other citrus fruits—lemon, grapefruit, and lime. Urticaria seems to be a symptom often associated with fruit allergies. Of the vegetables, tomatoes and the legumes, (including peanuts) are the most common offenders.

Fish and seafood are also potent allergens. Some children are sensitive to fish but can tolerate shellfish, whereas others have a generalized allergy to all types of seafood. Symptoms often reported from fish allergy include urticaria, gastrointestinal problems, and migraine headaches. Beef, pork, and poultry may cause cutaneous and respiratory problems. Of all the meats, lamb is the least common offender.

Nuts, chocolate and cocoa, mustard, black pepper, cloves, and food additives are other reported sources of food allergy. Food additives have been implicated as a causative factor in hyperactivity, although there is no definitive evidence for this (see "Food Additives and Hyperactivity" in Chap. 22).

DIAGNOSIS

Since there are no clear-cut immunological diagnostic tests, the diagnosis of food allergy is a particularly challenging problem. Although skin tests will not determine which foods are causing the allergy, skin tests of a few suspected foods are useful in establishing an allergic tendency. The actual diagnosis is the result of a complete clinical study, followed by an elimination trial and challenge of the suspected foods.

Clinical Study

The clinical study, which includes a family history and diet history, a physical examination, and laboratory studies, is important. There are hereditary factors present in food allergies in terms of both the offending foods and the symptoms that occur. It has been noted that a child has nearly a 75 percent chance of having a food allergy if both parents have allergies, and a 50 percent chance if one parent is affected.[5] A food diary, including a detailed record of all foods and beverages consumed in a 24-h period, is an important diagnostic tool. Not only are the foods recorded, but also the symptoms are noted. If the symptoms are immediate, the offending food is easily detected. Another possible use of the food diary is to determine which foods the child obviously avoids, since children may instinctively avoid the troublesome foods. If the 24-h history is not conclusive, the parents are asked to keep a 14-day diet record. Laboratory studies and procedures are sometimes necessary in order to rule out other disorders with similar symptoms, such as cystic fibrosis, infections, enzyme defects, and gastrointestinal malformation.

Elimination Diets

The elimination diet may be one of two types. A single suspected food item may be avoided, or all foods known to be highly allergenic may be avoided. In the latter type, only hypoallergenic foods would be allowed: tea (with sugar), olive oil, lamb, beets, spinach, sweet potatoes, apricots, cherries, peaches, and plums. Either of these trials must be conducted for at least a week, and the effects observed. Optimal nutrition is not a vital issue during these short-term trials, although it is of much concern after therapeutic restrictions are initiated.

In the challenge period one particular food is given in gradually increasing amounts. The food is one that is suspected of producing the allergy and its effects must be observed for at least one week before another food is added.

TREATMENT

Once the source of the allergy is determined, treatment is that of strict avoidance. The second, and also important, aspect of management involves a careful assessment of the nutritional adequacy of the diet. Comparable foods must be substituted for the foods eliminated, particularly when they represent important sources of energy, protein, vitamins, and minerals. The three allergens which require the most aggressive management in relation to both ensuring optimal nutrition and maintaining consistent avoidance are milk, wheat, and egg.

Milk-Free Diet

Since milk is the primary source of nutrients in infancy and continues to function as a valuable contributor of protein, energy, calcium, and riboflavin during childhood and into adult life, the child with milk allergy requires special consideration. The milk-sensitive infant may be given one of the soybean or hypoallergenic milk substitutes. (See Table 25-2.) Also available on the market is Gerber's Meat Base Formula, a combination of strained beef hearts, sucrose, sesame oil, tapioca, calcium ascorbate, and vitamins A and D. This is perhaps useful for infants who are allergic to both cow's milk and soybean milk. Some children who are sensitive to the lactalbumin in milk may be able to tolerate goat's milk as a substitute because the whey portion, which is the lactalbumin portion, is different in goat's milk and cow's milk. It is important to note, however, that a macrocytic anemia due to a deficiency of vitamin B_{12} in goat's milk sometimes occurs in the children receiving this substitute.

In order children, adherence to a milk-free diet is more difficult, since milk is such a common ingredient in foods. Some children are able to tolerate milk after it is heated, and therefore are allowed custards, puddings, cakes, breads, and soups made with milk. For other children, however, heat treatment has no effect on the allergic response to milk. Table 25-3 presents a milk-free diet, which would be necessary for the management of this allergy.

Wheat-Free Diet

Since most baked and commercial products use wheat flour as an important ingredient, strict adherence to a wheat-free diet is a particular challenge. Obtaining an adequate energy intake is often difficult on this regimen. (See Table 25-4.) The avoidance of enriched wheat flour removes a good source of iron, thiamin, niacin, and riboflavin from the child, and care must be taken to ensure that these nutrients

TABLE 25-2 SOY AND HYPOALLERGENIC FORMULAS

Formula	Company	Protein Source
Isomil	Ross Laboratories	Soy protein isolate
Meat Base Formula	Gerber Products Co.	Beef hearts
Mull-Soy	Borden Inc.	Soy protein isolate
Neo-Mull-Soy	Borden Inc.	Soy protein isolate
Nutramigen	Mead Johnson & Co.	Hydrolyzed casein
ProSobee	Mead Johnson & Co.	Soy protein isolate
Sobee	Mead Johnson & Co.	Soy protein isolate
Soyalac	Loma Linda Food Co.	Soy protein isolate

TABLE 25-3 MILK-FREE DIET

Type of food	Foods allowed	Foods avoided
Beverages	Carbonated drinks, Kool-Aid, fruit juices, cocoa made with water, lemonade, tea. Special formulas: See Table 25–2	Fresh, dried, or evaporated milk, malted milk, cocoa made with milk solids
Bread and crackers	French bread, rye bread, ryKrisp, homemade bread made without milk, pretzels, Ritz crackers, Triscuit, graham crackers, saltines, soda, Premium, Uneeda	Bread unless made without milk; hot breads (pancakes, waffles, griddle cakes, muffins, biscuits)
Cereals	Any cereal served with fruit juice or milk substitute	Cereals if served with milk or cream
Meat, fish, and poultry	All, if prepared without sauces made with milk or cream	Wieners and bologna if milk solids added in processing (check labels)
Eggs	In any form, if milk is not added	None, if milk is not added
Cheese	None	In all forms
Desserts	Fruit, Popsicles, fruited Jello, homemade puddings made without milk (tapioca, junket, cornstarch pudding), fruit ice, water ice, homemade pies, cakes, cookies made without milk	Ice cream, sherbet, all puddings, custards, cakes, pies, and cookies made with milk, yogurt
Fats	Vegetable oils, lard, margarines without added milk solids (kosher margarine)	Butter, cream, sour cream, margarine with added milk solids, salad dressings with milk added
Potato and substitutes	Potato, rice, pastas (spaghetti, macaroni, noodles) if milk or cheese is not added	None, if milk, cream, butter, or cheese is not added
Soups	Broth, clear consomme, bouillon, broth-based	Creamed soups
Vegetables	All	None, if milk, cream, butter, or cheese is not added
Fruits	All	None
Miscellaneous	Moderate amounts of sugar, jams, jellies, lollipops, hard candies, peanut butter, nuts, corn chips, potato chips, popcorn (without butter added), pickles, olives, meat juice gravy	Candy made with milk (caramels, milk chocolate, fondant, nougat), hollandaise sauce

TABLE 25-4 WHEAT-FREE DIET

Type of food	Foods allowed	Foods avoided
Beverages	Milk, carbonated drinks, Kool-aid, fruit juices, lemonade, hot chocolate	Postum, Ovaltine
Breads and crackers	Rye bread if 100% rye, RyKrisp, corn bread or muffins, rice flour bread or muffins if made at home without wheat flour added	All other breads, rolls, crackers
Cereals	Any corn, oat, or rice cereal	Wheat cereals—farina, bran, puffed wheat, shredded wheat
Meat, fish, and poultry	Plain meats, fish, and poultry prepared without breading and without gravy made with flour	Breaded meats, processed meats (wieners, hot dogs) if bread fillers added, meat loaf, croquettes, meatballs if bread added
Eggs	Fried, poached, boiled, scrambled, baked	None
Cheese	Cheddar, American, Swiss, cottage, farmer	None, unless flour is added to processed cheese foods
Desserts	Fruits, Jello, fruit ice, sherbet, ice cream, custard, Junket, puddings made from rice or cornstarch	Cakes, pies, cookies, doughnuts (except if made with rice flour)
Fats	Vegetable oils, butter, margarine, lard	Salad dressings, gravy, if thickened with flour
Potato and substitutes	Potato, rice	Spaghetti, noodles, macaroni, stuffing unless made with rice, dumplings
Soups	Homemade soups, consomme, made without flour	All canned soups
Vegetables	All	Only if sauce made with flour is added
Fruits	All	None
Miscellaneous	Moderate amounts of sugar, jams, jellies, peanut butter, nuts, potato chips pickles, olives, meat juice gravy	Beer, pretzels

are provided from other sources. Rice flour may be substituted in most recipes, in the proportion of ¾ cup of rice flour for 1 cup of regular wheat flour.

Egg-Free Diet

Egg has many uses in cooking, and therefore its presence in foods is extremely common. Other foods rich in protein and iron, such as meat, fish, and poultry, can be substituted for egg. The primary nutritional concern in the growing child who is egg-sensitive therefore relates to ensuring adequate calories, since a great majority of baked goods contain egg and need to be avoided. Egg is used as a binder and to add volume to cakes, as a thickening agent in creamed dishes and sauces, to help pies and cookies brown, and as a glaze for breads. To replace egg as the binding substance in cakes, an equal amount of mashed banana may be substituted. An extra ½ teaspoon of baking powder can also be added to the egg-free cake recipe to make up for the loss of volume. In creamed dishes and sauces, extra flour or cornstarch can be added to replace the thickening action of the egg. Table 25-5 lists the allowable foods and those which must be avoided by the egg-sensitive child.

TABLE 25-5 EGG-FREE DIET

Types of food	Foods allowed	Foods avoided
Beverages	All except those which have egg added	Eggnog
Breads and crackers	Saltine crackers, soda crackers, graham crackers, white, wheat, rye, French, pumpernickel breads	Hot breads or any breads and crackers made with egg, French toast
Cereals	Any	None
Meat, fish, and poultry	All except those with egg added	Any prepared or coated with egg; sausage, croquettes, meat loaf
Eggs	None	All
Cheese	All	None
Desserts	Fruits, Jello, fruit ice, sherbet, ice cream, puddings if made without egg, pies if made without egg	Cakes, cookies, frostings, French ice cream made with eggs, meringue, custards, Bavarian creams
Fats	Vegetable oils, butter, margarine, lard	Salad dressing if egg added
Potato and substitutes	Potato, rice, noodles except those with added egg, macaroni, spaghetti	Egg noodles
Soups	All except those with egg or egg noodles added	Soups with egg or egg noodles
Vegetables	All	None
Fruits	All	None
Miscellaneous	Moderate amounts of sugar, jams, jellies, lollipops, hard candy, candies made without egg, peanut butter, nuts, potato chips, corn chips, pretzels, pickles, olives	Hollandaise sauce, candies made with egg

LABEL READING

An important habit to foster in proper management of food allergy is reading the labels of all prepared and processed foods. The offending allergen may be present in unexpected sources and may be listed in unfamiliar terms. The following ingredients indicate that milk or a milk derivative has been added: *lactose, caseinate, sodium caseinate, casein, lactalbumin, curds,* and *whey.* Eggs may be added to foods in the following forms: *albumin, vitellin, livetin, yolk, powdered* or *dried egg, globulin, ovomucoid,* and *ovomucin.*

DIET COUNSELING

Although food allergy presents a confusing array of symptoms and is difficult to diagnose, it *is* a manageable problem. Successful treatment depends on good counseling based on the following considerations:

1 A thorough diet history must serve as the basis for counseling.

2 When an important nutrient source or an entire food group must be eliminated because of the allergy, alternate food sources must be included.

3 Special help with food selection must be given. Prepared, processed, and mixed dishes often are a particular hazard. Shopping for foods must be done with a careful eye on labels. Also, guidelines for restaurant choices and other meals eaten away from home are important for proper treatment.

4 Another area of concern is advice regarding recipes appropriate for milk-free, wheat-free, and egg-free diets. (See Table 25-6.)

TABLE 25-6 SOURCES OF RECIPES FOR ALLERGY DIETS*

Allergy Recipes
    The American Dietetic Association
    430 North Michigan Avenue
    Chicago, IL 60611

Baking for People with Food Allergy
    Superintendent of Documents
    U.S. Government Printing Office
    Washington, DC 20402

Carnival Recipes (Party food ideas for egg-free, wheat-free, and milk-free diets)
    General Foods
    Box 130
    Coubourg, Ont., Canada

125 Recipes for Allergy Diet
    Good Housekeeping
    959 Eighth Avenue
    New York, NY 10019

Wheat, Milk, and Eggfree Recipes from Mary Alden
    Quaker Oats Co.
    Merchandise Mart Plaza
    Chicago, IL 60654

* Although many recipes are free, some do require a fee. It is best to contact the individual company for a current cost policy.

5 In certain instances it may be necessary to supplement the diet with vitamin or mineral preparations (e.g., calcium), or both, if alternative food sources cannot be successfully added.

Strict avoidance of the food allergen and relief of the troublesome symptoms are vital concerns in the management of food allergy, but also necessary is a sensitivity to the nutritional and emotional needs of the child. Nutritional adequacy, interest, and variety are important goals in the food allergy diet.

STUDY QUESTIONS

1 What is an allergic reaction?

2 What are some of the common allergic symptoms related to food allergy?

3 What diagnostic tools are used in establishing the diagnosis of food allergy?

4 What are the nutritional concerns for a child with milk allergy? Wheat allergy? Egg allergy?

5 List the five important considerations when counseling the allergy patient.

CASE STUDY 25-1

Julie, a 7-month-old baby girl, was admitted to the hospital with a 3-week history of diarrhea, vomiting, and irritability. Her weight had dropped from 7.3 kg at age 6 months to a present weight of 6.5 kg. Whereas she had originally been growing in the 50th percentile for weight,

her growth rate at the time of admission was between the 3d and 10th percentiles. Julie's length at age 6 months was 67 cm (75th percentile), and on admission it was measured as 68 cm (50th to 75th percentile)

Julie's early history was unremarkable, the

baby having had no significant problems before the current onset of symptoms. She had been breast-fed from birth and had always been a good feeder. At 3 months her mother had introduced cereals; at 3½ months, strained fruits. Both had been well accepted. When Julie was 6 months old, 4 weeks prior to admission, her mother began weaning her from the breast, introducing 2 bottles of cow's milk each day. A week later, her symptoms began.

Case Study Questions

1 *What are the possible diagnoses that might be suggested by this presentation of symptoms?*

2 *What would be the appropriate dietary intervention, considering the suspected food allergy?*

3 *What must be considered in planning the diet for this child with this food allergy?*

REFERENCES

1 C. A. Frazier, *Coping with Food Allergy,* Quadrangle/The New York Times Co., New York, 1974, p. 6.

2 S. J. Fomon, *Infant Nutrition,* 2d ed., W. B. Saunders Company, Philadelphia, 1974, p. 414.

3 Frazier, op. cit., p. 9.

4 Fomon, op. cit., p. 436.

5 Frazier, op. cit., p. 4.

CHAPTER 26
SPECIAL
NUTRITIONAL
CONCERNS

Nancie H. Herbold
Carol Hum
Edith L. Getchell

INTRODUCTION

This final chapter addresses three growing areas of nutritional concern; cancer, inborn errors of metabolism, and nutritional needs of the low-birth-weight infant. The poor nutritional status of cancer patients has long been ignored and accepted as the sequela of the disease state; and until recently the possible carcinogenic properties of food were not even considered. Research has led diet to the forefront in the prevention of the mental retardation that occurs with some inborn errors of metabolism, and in the treatment of the low-birth-weight infant with its highly individualized nutritional needs. We feel that each of these areas needs a special focus.

FOOD, NUTRITION, AND CANCER

Nancie H. Herbold

INTRODUCTION

Cancer is one of the major health problems in the United States today. Approximately one out of every four individuals in the United States will develop cancer in their lifetime.[1] In children under the age of 15, cancer is second only to accidents as the leading cause of death.[2] The interrelationship between food, nutrition, and cancer is unclear. For example, in Japan, where there is a low incidence of cancer of the colon, the diet is low in unsaturated fat. However, among Japanese people who immigrate to the United States, the incidence of cancer of the colon increases, as does the intake of saturated fat.[3] Also, cancer of the colon has been associated with diets low in fiber and high in refined foods. In primitive societies the fiber intake is high and there is little cancer of the colon, whereas in more industrialized societies the fiber intake is low and the incidence of cancer is high. Cancer of the breast is more frequently seen in women who are overweight and have a high fat intake, whereas cancer of the esophagus has been associated with smoking and alcohol. Malnutrition is known to decrease most resistance; therefore, malnourished tissues may be more susceptible to cancer invasion.

More investigation needs to be conducted before we have definite answers, but in the meantime adoption of a "prudent diet," low in fat, high in fiber, and with representatives from the basic food groups, is recommended. In this section we will focus on:

1 The possible carcinogens in our food supply
2 Nutritional therapy for the cancer patient

Food itself may be considered a possible carcinogen or it may be considered a precursor of a carcinogen. The food may take on carcinogenic properties by virtue of its own natural organic properties which stimulate the formation of harmful compounds, or the carcinogenicity may be due to effects of processing.

CARCINOGENS

Polycyclic Aromatic Hydrocarbons

Polycyclic aromatic hydrocarbons are found in cigarette smoke, barbecued food, smoked fish, ham, cooking oils, and coffee. Epidemiologic evidence shows that populations who consume a large amount of smoked fish are at high risk of developing stomach cancer.[4] Yet smokers swallow some polycyclics and there does not seem to be a strong link between smoking and cancer of the stomach. In the United States air pollution, smoking, and industrial exposure to polycyclics seem to pose more of a problem than does food in cancer development.

Nitrosamines

Nitrosamines are formed by the combining of nitrites, which are added to food as a preservative, with amines, found in the stomach as well as in some foods, or by bacterial reduction of nitrate to nitrite. Nitrosamines, which are known carcinogens in animals, can form in the soil, during food storage or preparation, and after ingestion into the body.

Nitrites and nitrates are found naturally in small amounts in food such as carrots, spinach, beets, and water. Nitrates are used as preservatives to prevent botulism and to fix color in such foods as: bacon, sausage, frankfurters, ham, and various luncheon meats. Ascorbic acid seems to have an inhibitory effect on nitrosamine formation. Therefore, drinking orange juice before consuming any of the previously mentioned foods may produce a protective benefit.[5] Many consumer advocates are attempting to prevent the use of or decrease the amount of nitrates being added to foods. Though nitrosamines are known to be carcinogenic in rats, there has not yet been conclusive evidence that they are directly associated with cancer in humans.

Saccharin

Saccharin produced cancer in rats when large amounts were implanted in their bladders. Tumors were also produced when rats were fed diets high in saccharin. It was this evidence which was recently released by the Canadian government that prompted the U.S. Food and Drug Administration to enact a ban on saccharin. The proposed regulations of this ban include:

1 Treatment of saccharin as a nonprescription drug.
2 Labeling that must include the warning that, "saccharin may cause an increased risk of cancer and should be used only as medically indicated," i.e., by persons such as diabetics who must restrict their intake of sugar.
3 Saccharin will no longer be permitted as an ingredient in food and beverages.

It has been recommended that human consumption not exceed 1 g/day for an adult.[6] It has also been recommended that individuals consuming saccharin on a regular basis (e.g., diabetics) eliminate it from their diet periodically for 2 or 3 days so that any buildup can be metabolized and eliminated.

Aflatoxins

Aflatoxins are natural carcinogens produced by strains of *Aspergillus flavus*. This mold can be found growing on peanuts and other grains when storage humidity is high. Aflatoxins can produce liver cancer in rats. In parts of the world where environmental conditions are conducive to aspergillus growth there is an increased incidence of liver cancer. Aflatoxins are not a problem in the United States because storage conditions are controlled. Imported products are more likely to be a source of *Aspergillus flavus*. These products are monitored by the U.S. Department of Agriculture and the U.S. Food and Drug Administration (FDA) to check for contamination.

DES (Diethylstilbestrol)

DES is a hormone used in animals to increase their weight, thereby improving the net meat yield. In the 1940s DES pellets were implanted in poultry to produce tender chickens. However, evidence became available proving that DES was carcinogenic in the mouse when given in large quantities. Since small amounts of DES could be detected in the chicken fat of implanted birds, the FDA banned its use. However, the FDA permits the addition of DES to cattle feed, with the stipulation that it be removed from the feed 48 h prior to the slaughter of the animal.

These are some of the current food-related concerns pertaining to diet and cancer. They have been discussed so that you, as a nutrition educator, will be able to dispel some of the misinformation that commonly surrounds food and cancer.

NUTRITION AS A COMPONENT OF TREATMENT FOR THE CANCER PATIENT

Before we can discuss the treatment of cancer patients it is necessary for the student to understand some of the terminology associated with cancer. *Cancer* itself is defined as "a cellular tumor, the natural course of which is fatal and usually associated with the formation of secondary tumors."[7] *Neoplasm* is commonly used interchangeably with cancer or malignant tumor. The Committee on Professional Education of the International Union Against Cancer defines a neoplasm as follows:

A neoplasm or tumor is a distribution of growth characterized primarily by an excessive proliferation of cells without apparent relation to the physiological demands of the organ involved.[8]

Tumors can be classified into two broad categories:

1 Benign
2 Malignant

Benign tumors are nonspreading localized tumors which usually do not produce serious illness. *Malignant tumors* grow rapidly and spread (*metastasize*) to other areas of the body and if not treated early can cause serious illness.

Weight loss and a lack of appetite may be one of the first symptoms associated with cancer. The anorexia of cancer is defined as follows:

Food intake is inadequate to meet the combined needs of the host and tumor even if food intake remained constant this could result in a loss of carcass weight in a tumor bearing host.[9]

The *cachexia* (loss of carcass weight) associated with malignancy is due to the effects of anorexia, a decrease in calories (kilojoules) consumed, and an increase in energy expenditure. Patients are frequently in an energy deficient state and have increased basal metabolic rates. Generally patients are in a state of negative nitrogen balance; however, some patients have been seen who are energy deficient but are in positive nitrogen balance. The explanation for this positive nitrogen balance may be attributed to the capacity of the tumor to retain nitrogen from both dietary nitrogen and nitrogen released from tissue.

Patients may develop side effects (nausea, vomiting, diarrhea) from the various modalities of treatment, which will need monitoring by the medical team. In the following section three types of treatment will be discussed—radiation, surgery, and chemotherapy—and the nutritional problems and methods of nutritional treatment associated with each type.

Radiation

Patients may receive radiation as a form of treatment by itself or in conjunction with chemotherapy and surgery. Radiation acts to selectively destroy abnormal cells within the body. Generally, patients are irradiated 5 days per week for approximately 4 to 6 weeks. Depending upon the site of radiation a variety of nutritional problems may arise.

Head and Neck Region

Patients receiving radiation therapy to the head and neck area, particularly radiation to the tonsillar region, palate, tongue, and nasopharynx, present numerous nutritional problems. Patients undergoing radiation to these areas frequently complain of: altered or unpleasant sense of taste, a loss of or a reduction of taste acuity, pain upon swallowing, burning sensations, dryness of the mouth, and a general lack of appetite. Taste may be altered by damage from radiation to the taste buds. Patients whose radiation field includes the salivary glands will notice a decrease in salivation and a change in the saliva composition. Saliva that is present becomes thick and viscous, making it difficult for the patient to swallow.

Alcoholics, heavy smokers, patients with poor oral hygiene, and patients with chronic poor nutrition are at risk of developing mandible necrosis.

Dietary treatment Diet therapy includes modifying the texture of the food to prevent pain on swallowing. Acid foods such as orange juice may need to be diluted or eliminated from the diet. Spices may be an irritant to the oral mucosa, as may very hot or very cold foods. For the patient with reduced salivation, moist foods, foods mixed with sauces or broths, soups, custards, and puddings may aid in swallowing and thus help to keep energy intake adequate (see Table 26-1).

Patients with reduced salivation are more susceptible to dental caries (see Chap. 23). In the past, these patients would have their teeth extracted to prevent osteoradionecrosis. Today all efforts are made to preserve the patient's teeth. The nutrition educator must work with patients to decrease the sucrose content of their diet while maintaining adequate energy. Patients are also given, as a prophylactic measure, a 1 percent sodium fluoride gel contained in a dental tray (mouth guard) which is inserted into the mouth for 5 min/day.

If the patient is experiencing severe swallowing problems, a liquid dietary supplement or blenderized diet (see Chap. 24) may be needed, along with vitamin and mineral supplementation. High-protein milk (whole milk

TABLE 26-1 DIETARY SUGGESTIONS FOR PATIENTS RECEIVING RADIATION THERAPY TO THE HEAD AND NECK AREA

1 Swallowing can be made easier when liquids are taken by straw.
2 Tilting the head back when eating may make swallowing easier.
3 Avoid foods that may irritate the oral mucosa or throat, such as highly seasoned, abrasive foods and very hot or cold foods.
4 Use noncariogenic foods such as sugarless gum and sugarless mints to stimulate saliva production.

with added dry powdered skim milk) should be encouraged for use in eggnogs, frappes, soups, puddings, and custards. The commercially prepared supplement often proves to have an advantage over home-prepared foods, as the patient associates it with medicine and gives better compliance, resulting in a higher energy intake. Small frequent feedings are advised for the patient who has a lack of appetite or is experiencing pain. Xylocaine, a local anesthetic, may be useful for the patient who is unable to swallow because of pain. If a patient is unable or unwilling to take anything by mouth, artificial tube feeding may be necessary (See Chap. 24.) When the tumor is located at a site that would interfere with the use of a nasogastric tube, a gastrostomy may be the alternative feeding method.

Hyperalimentation has recently gained use in the treatment of the patient who is undergoing head and neck radiation. It has been used with patients who were 10 lb below their ideal or usual body weight and whose serum albumin was less than 3.6 g/100 ml.[10] When elemental diets produced diarrhea or abdominal cramps patients were given intravenous hyperalimentation of 2500 to 3000 kcal/day (10.5 to 12.6 MJ/day) until they were able to consume enough food enterally to maintain adequate nutrition.

Keeping the patient in positive nitrogen balance and a positive nutritional state is most important since the rate of wound healing and tissue tolerance for radiotherapy are related to the nutritional status of the patient.[11]

Steiger et al. reported that in experiments with rats, well-nourished rats seemed to support tumor growth while malnourished rats did not.[12] This same investigator reported that in patients a positive nitrogen balance did not favorably alter their clinical course and that tumor growth may be exacerbated by hyperalimentation. This information must be weighed against the evidence which shows that patients who are well nourished will tolerate radiation therapy better and will react more favorably to chemotherapeutic agents.

It must be emphasized that nutritional treatment is always individualized to meet each patient's particular need.

Gastrointestinal and Genitourinary Tracts

One of the most frequently reported side effects of radiation to the gastrointestinal or genitourinary tract is diarrhea. Many patients will develop diarrhea after approximately 2 weeks of treatments.

Dietary treatment   A low-roughage or a low-residue diet may be efficacious for some patients, while eliminating lactose, or a combination of these procedures, may prove beneficial for others. Adequate fluid intake is important to prevent dehydration. If diarrhea persists, the implementation of an elemental diet (see Chap. 24) would be the treatment of choice.

Surgery

It is important that patients come to surgery well nourished and in positive nitrogen balance. The nutritional guidelines for cancer-surgery patients are generally the same as those for any surgical patient (see Chap. 24).

Chemotherapy

Drugs used in cancer treatment (antineoplastic agents) are cytotoxic not only to the neoplastic cells but to the normal cells as well and must be administered with great caution. Antineoplastic agents can be classified in five categories, depending upon their mode of action: alkylating agents, antimetabolites, antibiotics, alkaloids, and miscellaneous (see Table 26-2).

Patients receiving chemotherapy are susceptible to many side effects which may alter their ability to eat. Some of the more common side effects include nausea, vomiting, mucositis (inflammation of the mucosa), ulcerations of the mouth, anorexia, and diarrhea (see Table 26-2). The astute nurse and dietitian will be familiar with these symptoms and will adjust the patient's diet accordingly. In general, soft,

TABLE 26-2 SIDE EFFECTS OF COMMONLY USED ANTINEOPLASTIC AGENTS

Drug	Side effects
Antibiotics	
Dactinomycin (actinomycin D) (Cosmegen)	Stomatitis, anorexia, nausea, vomiting, diarrhea, oral ulceration
Bleomycin (Blenoxane)	Stomatitis, anorexia, nausea, vomiting, fever, oral ulceration
Alkylating agents	
Cyclophosphamide (Cytoxan)	Anorexia, vomiting, nausea, hemorrhagic cystitis, hemorrhagic colitis, mucosal ulceration
Nitrogen mustard (Mustargen)	Anorexia, vomiting, nausea, diarrhea, metallic taste
Antimetabolites	
Cytarabine (Cytosar)	Anorexia, nausea, vomiting, diarrhea, megaloblastic anemia; antagonist to pyrimidine
5-Fluorouracil	Stomatitis, anorexia, nausea, vomiting, diarrhea, gastrointestinal ulceration, and bleeding
6-Mercaptopurine	Stomatitis, nausea, vomiting, diarrhea, fever; antagonist to purine and pantothenic acid
Methotrexate	Stomatitis, anorexia, nausea, vomiting, diarrhea, gastrointestinal ulcerations, abnormal liver function
Miscellaneous	
Quinacrine (Atabrine)	Fever, nausea, vomiting

Sources: (1) D. C. March, *Handbook: Interactions of Selected Drugs with Nutritional Status in Man,* American Dietetic Association, October 1976, pp. 25–28; (2) M. J. and D. W. Smith, *Pharmacology and Drug Therapy in Nursing,* J. B. Lippincott Company, Philadelphia, 1968, pp. 617–622.

low-roughage, or elemental diets, as determined by individual need, may be used for the patient who is experiencing side effects from a chemotherapeutic agent. When mucositis and stomatitis are present, acid foods should be avoided. Small frequent feedings may be helpful in treating the patient who is experiencing nausea or anorexia. When fever, diarrhea, and vomiting are present an increased fluid intake must be encouraged. Patients receiving the drug Cytoxan should have a fluid intake of 2 to 3 l/day to prevent hemorrhagic cystitis.[13] Patients respond best to chemotherapy when they are in a positive nutritional state.

INBORN ERRORS OF METABOLISM

Carol Hum

INTRODUCTION

In the past 20 years, the discovery of new inborn errors of metabolism has increased dramatically in rate. This has been the result of the development of new techniques for the quantitative determination of metabolites in blood and urine, and the recent increase of interest in the biochemical causes of disease and mental retardation. For the most part, metabolic diseases are rare; however, recognition of and interest in them has spread, because the dietary management of several of the inborn errors offers one of the few instances of effective prevention of mental retardation.

BIOCHEMICAL DEFECT

The inborn errors of metabolism are inherited biochemical disorders which result from a defect in enzyme activity. These diseases originate in mutations of single genes which are responsible for the synthesis of specific enzymes. The gene mutation either results in the production of a structurally altered enzyme that is incapable of normal catalytic activity, or causes an inhibition of enzyme synthesis.[14] In both cases, the nonfunctioning enzyme produces a block in the metabolic pathway at a specific point and leads to an abnormal accumulation of large amounts of substrate before the block (see Fig. 26-1). Substrate, or metabolites of the substrate formed by subsidiary pathways, can be found in increased levels in the blood, urine, and tissues.

CLINICAL MANIFESTATIONS

The pathological consequences of enzyme deficiency diseases are attributed to the disordered pattern of metabolism and resulting biochemical imbalance. Clinical symptoms vary widely (see Table 26-3). There are some defects that have no clinical effect on the individual, while others (e.g., homocystinuria) may cause mental retardation and serious disease affecting several organ systems. In some (e.g., phenylketonuria) neurological damage is slowly progressive, and is often without no-

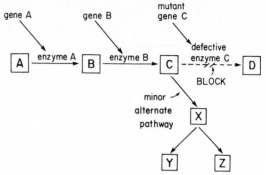

Figure 26-1

Schematic representation of an altered metabolic sequence. A genetic defect in enzyme C produces a block in the reaction that leads to accumulation of substrate C and an increased utilization of the minor alternate pathway, which produces metabolites X, Y, and Z.

ticeable signs in the first months of life. Still others (e.g., maple syrup urine disease and galactosemia) are associated with a rapidly deteriorating neonatal course leading to early death unless immediate treatment is instituted. Although the primary enzymatic defect has been identified in many of the diseases, the exact processes which produce the clinical manifestations often remain unclear.[15]

INHERITANCE

In spite of the wide range of clinical abnormalities, the majority of metabolic inborn errors share an autosomal recessive mode of transmission[16] (see Fig. 26-2). Persons carrying the mutant recessive gene do not show any clinical manifestations of the disease, but when both parents are carriers, each pregnancy carries a 1 in 4 chance of transmitting the disease to the offspring.

DIAGNOSIS

It is important to note that the majority of enzymatic defects do not have specific, clear-cut clinical features which would immediately

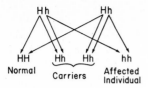

H - dominant gene

h - recessive gene

Figure 26-2

Inheritance pattern for an inborn error. Homozygotes (hh) with the inborn metabolic error must inherit the disease from both parents who are heterozygotes (Hh), or carriers of the disease.

draw attention to the presence of an inborn error of metabolism. The high morbidity and mortality in unrecognized and untreated cases of inborn errors such as galactosemia and maple syrup urine disease make their early diagnosis essential if clinical complications and even death are to be prevented. Thus, when unexpected symptoms or crisis occur in early infancy, such as failure to eat, vomiting, irritability, lethargy, coma, acidosis, enlarged liver, or jaundice, which persist or do not respond to conventional treatment, the possibility of an inborn error of metabolism should be considered.[17] Appropriate screening tests or quantitative analysis of plasma or urine can then be made to detect any signs of biochemical abnormality. The early detection of phenylketonuria well in advance of the onset of clinical symptoms is now possible through mass screening of newborns.

When the enzyme deficiency or the presence of abnormal levels of metabolites is detectable in amniotic fluid cells, prenatal diagnosis of an inborn error is possible by amniocentesis (a special process whereby the amniotic fluid surrounding the fetus is withdrawn and analyzed).[18] Amniocentesis is offered to families in which a high risk for a specific inborn error has been established by the diagnosis of the disorder in an affected child.

TREATMENT

Early treatment is essential, if mental retardation and other serious sequelae associated with many of the inborn errors are to be prevented. The rapidly developing central nervous system of the infant is particularly vulnerable to the defects in metabolism which can interfere with its growth.

For several inborn errors treatment is possible by restriction or elimination of the substrate (a carbohydrate or a protein) from the diet. Dietary treatment has been applied to a number of hereditary metabolic diseases with varying degrees of success. The control of substrate accumulation is possible when the substrate is a nutrient which the body cannot synthesize (e.g., phenylalanine in phenylketonuria) or if it is derived primarily from the diet (e.g., galactose in galactosemia).

A number of semisynthetic dietary products are available for use in the treatment of specific disorders of amino acid metabolism in which it is necessary to restrict one or more amino acids to the level of the minimum requirement.[19] The products are based either on specially treated protein hydrolysates or on mixtures of pure amino acids so that the resulting diet can be extremely low in or devoid of the implicated amino acid. Generally, the product will also contain additional formulations of carbohydrate, fat, vitamins, and minerals to meet the body's requirements for these nutrients. Natural foods containing known amounts of the restricted amino acid are then incorporated into the diet to supply just the amount required for normal metabolism.

Specific inborn errors of carbohydrate metabolism may be treated by the total elimination of the implicated carbohydrate from the diet. Dietary management is relatively less difficult for carbohydrate disorders than for amino acid disorders since specific disaccharides and monosaccharides are not essential nutrients and may be synthesized within the body as they are needed. Care must be taken to ensure that a balanced selection of

TABLE 26-3 EXAMPLES OF CLINICALLY SIGNIFICANT INBORN ERRORS OF AMINO ACID AND CARBOHYDRATE METABOLISM TREATABLE BY DIET

Disorder	Incidence	Biochemical defect	Biochemical analysis	
			Blood	Urine
Phenylketonuria	1:10,000	Defective phenylalanine hydroxylase (Phenylalanine, an essential amino acid, is not converted to tyrosine, a nonessential amino acid)	Increased phenylalanine	Increased phenylacids: phenylpyruvic acid, phenylacetic acid, orthohydroxyphenylacetic acid
Galactosemia	1:100,000	Defective galactose-1-phosphate uridyl transferase (Galactose, a monosaccharide, is not converted to glucose)	Increased galactose-1-phosphate	Increased galactose; generalized aminoaciduria
Homocystinuria	1:180,000	Defective cystathionine synthetase (Homocysteine, an intermediate product of the essential amino acid, methionine, does not react with serine to yield cystathionine)	Increased methionine and homocysteine	Increased homocysteine
Maple syrup urine disease (MSUD)	1:200,000	Defective oxidative decarboxylase (Keto acids of the branched-chain amino acids—leucine, valine, isoleucine—are not converted to simple acids)	Increased leucine, valine, isoleucine, and their keto acids	Increased leucine, valine, isoleucine, and their keto acids
Tyrosinemia	Not determined	Defect in parahydroxyphenylpyruvic acid (Tyrosine, a nonessential amino acid, is not converted to homogentistic acid)	Increased tyrosine	Increased parahydroxyphenylpyruvic acid; generalized aminoaciduria
Fructosemia	Over 40 reported cases	Defect in fructose-1-phosphate aldolase (Fructose, a monosaccharide, is not converted to glucose)	Increased fructose	Increased fructose

(continued)

TABLE 26-3 *(continued)*

Clinical Symptoms	Treatment	Comment
Normal at birth followed by hyperactivity, irritability, persistent musty odor, severe mental retardation, decreased pigmentation, eczema, if untreated	Phenylalanine-restricted diet: No milk, milk products, meat, fish, poultry Breads, cereals, fruit, vegetables in controlled amounts Special formula low in phenylalanine Special low-protein flour	Phenylalanine must be provided in amounts sufficient to support growth As the child progresses from bottle to cup, from strained to junior and table foods and self-feeding, phenylalanine intake may vary considerably
Normal at birth with symptoms developing after feedings containing lactose; anorexia, vomiting, occasional diarrhea, lethargy, jaundice, hepatomegaly, increased susceptibility to infection. Later: cataracts, physical and mental retardation	Rigid exclusion of lactose and galactose from the diet (hydrolysis of lactose yields glucose and galactose) Milk-free, galactose-free diet: No milk, milk products Use of special formula, "CHO-Free" (Syntex)	Prenatal diagnosis by amniocentesis is possible Children may not accept "CHO-Free" formula because of its taste. Therefore, diet will need nutrient supplementation
Possible mental retardation; lens dislocation, limb overgrowth, connective-tissue defect leading to scoliosis, osteoporosis, vascular thrombosis, fair hair and skin	Methionine-restricted diet supplemented by cysteine (cysteine, a product of methionine, becomes an essential amino acid when methionine is limited)	Some patients are responsive to high doses of pyridoxine (vitamin B_6), a coenzyme of cystathionine synthetase Prenatal diagnosis by amniocentesis
Normal at birth with symptoms showing in the first few days: difficulty with sucking and swallowing, irregular respiration, intermittent rigidity and flaccidity, possible grand mal seizures; urine has the odor of maple syrup. If infant survives, mental retardation is severe	Diet restricted in leucine, valine, and isoleucine Special formula is prepared	Prenatal diagnosis by amniocentesis For the child with transient MSUD maintained only on a low-protein diet, vitamin supplementation is necessary
Enlargement of liver and spleen noted early in infancy; abdominal distention, liver and renal damage, vitamin D–resistant rickets	Diet restricted in tyrosine and phenylalanine (the essential amino acid, phenylalanine, is a precursor of tyrosine)	Ultimate success of diet treatment in preventing the disease process has not been determined
Infants: anorexia, vomiting, failure to thrive, hypoglycemic convulsions, dysfunction of liver and kidney Older children: spontaneous hypoglycemia, nausea and vomiting on ingestion of fructose	Elimination of fructose and sucrose from the diet (hydrolysis of sucrose yields glucose and fructose)	Differentiate from transient neonatal tyrosinemia

appropriate foods is provided, and that the foods are free of the implicated carbohydrate as a sweetener or ingredient.

Although the dietary management of inborn errors may appear simple in theory, the complexities of practical application must not be overlooked. In order to illustrate the broader dimensions of disease detection, therapy, and prognosis, the remainder of this section will be devoted to a discussion of phenylketonuria, the inborn error of metabolism for which dietary treatment is longest established.

PHENYLKETONURIA

Primary Defect

In phenylketonuria (PKU) there is a defect in the enzyme *phenylalanine hydroxylase,* which is necessary for the conversion of the essential amino acid, phenylalanine, to tyrosine. As a consequence, phenylalanine and its metabolites accumulate in large amounts in the blood, and phenylacids produced by compensatory pathways are excreted in the urine (see Fig. 26-3).

Figure 26-3

The primary defect in phenylketonuria. A defect in the enzyme phenylalanine hydroxylase leads to an accumulation of the substrate phenylalanine in the blood and the excretion of its degradation products in the urine.

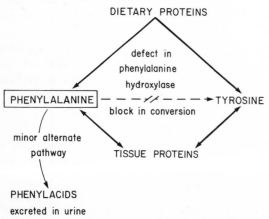

DIETARY PROTEINS

defect in
phenylalanine
hydroxylase

PHENYLALANINE ─ ─ ─ ─/ /─ ─ ─ → TYROSINE
block in conversion

minor alternate
pathway

TISSUE PROTEINS

PHENYLACIDS
excreted in urine

If abnormally elevated levels of phenylalanine and its metabolites persist, they produce deleterious effects on brain metabolism and lead to profound impairment of mental development. In addition, untreated individuals may exhibit aggressive behavior, hyperactivity, neuromuscular instability, seizures, and eczema. Blonde hair, fair complexion, and blue eyes, due to decreased pigmentation, are also common findings.

PKU Screening

The development of a simple screening test in the early 1960s has made the widespread screening of newborns for PKU possible.[20] The Guthrie test is an assay for phenylalanine which can be performed on blood specimens taken from the baby's heel. Normally, the blood contains a small amount of phenylalanine, approximately 1 to 2 mg/100 ml of plasma. However, when the infant with PKU begins formula or breast-milk feedings, the phenylalanine derived from the milk protein causes a significant rise in blood phenylalanine levels which may reach 15 to 30 mg/100 ml or higher, in the first week of life.

The Guthrie test, when performed in early infancy, detects the elevated levels of phenylalanine and allows for diagnosis in the symptom-free interval before irreversible neurological damage has taken place. However, since there are also transient states of hyperphenylalaninemia and variants of PKU that do not require dietary treatment, the results of a positive PKU Guthrie screening test must be followed by additional tests to confirm the diagnosis of PKU before diet therapy is initiated.

At present, 43 states have laws mandating PKU screening of all newborns, while the remaining states provide voluntary screening.[21] Current practice involves performing the test within the first week following birth, generally just before discharge from the nursery. A second determination of blood phenylalanine is recommended for all infants at or before 1 month of age to detect infants with PKU who had low concentrations of phenylalanine in the first few days.[22,23]

Treatment

A significant factor in determining the success of therapy in terms of intellectual development is the age at the time of diagnosis and initiation of therapy. The earlier treatment is begun, the better the prognosis. When PKU is detected in early infancy and a low phenylalanine diet is instituted and properly maintained, mental retardation and other symptoms associated with the disease can be prevented.

Normal physical and mental development have been shown to occur when the diet was started within the first 2 months of life, and particularly during the first month.[24,25] As treatment is delayed, the likelihood of satisfactory mental development decreases. While the late treatment of infants and young children may reestablish mental development and improve behavior, it will not be effective in reversing early retardation that has taken place.

Phenylalanine-Restricted Diet

The basis of treatment is to provide a diet low enough in phenylalanine to maintain blood levels between 3 and 10 mg/100 ml, while supplying enough of the amino acid to support needs for normal physical growth and health.[26] Phenylalanine requirements range from 65 to 90 mg/kg of body weight during the newborn period to 20 to 25 mg/kg at 2 years.[27]

Phenylalanine is an essential amino acid which must be obtained from food protein since it cannot be synthesized in the body. It is required by all persons, including individuals with PKU. Phenylalanine occurs in all natural protein, making up approximately 5 percent of the total protein. The amount obtained in a normal diet is far in excess of the required amount. In order to control elevations of blood phenylalanine in the child with PKU, artificial replacement of natural protein is required. This is achieved by the use of one of several low or phenylalanine-free protein sources that have been developed.

Lofenalac, a widely used product, is a casein hydrolysate from which 95 percent of the phenylalanine has been removed. It is a formula fortified with vitamins and minerals, and is nutritionally complete except for phenylalanine. It is the major source of nourishment in the low-phenylalanine diet. However, since the phenylalanine content of Lofenalac is less than 1 percent, used alone it will not supply adequate amounts of the amino acid to support growth and the maintenance of tissues. Measured amounts of natural foods that are low in protein are included in the diet to provide the amount of phenylalanine required.

In early infancy, a small amount (2 to 6 oz) of cow's milk is usually added to the Lofenalac formula to meet the need for phenylalanine. As the infant grows, restricted amounts of solids are calculated into the diet with the aid of phenylalanine exchange food lists which include cereals, vegetables, and fruits. Each food listed contains approximately 15 mg of phenylalanine and may be exchanged for any other serving of food. For example:

2 tablespoons rice cereal = 1 equivalent
½ cup peaches = 1 equivalent
7 tablespoons carrots = 1 equivalent

Since meat, fish, poultry, and dairy products are so high in phenylalanine, they are totally excluded from the diet. Special low-protein flour products ("apoprotein" products) are also available.

The diet is planned so that the young child is introduced to increments in food texture and self-feeding practices at the same times as other children. (See Table 26-4.)

Monitoring Treatment

Since considerable variation exists among PKU individuals in regard to phenylalanine requirements and tolerance, regular monitoring of blood phenylalanine is essential. The phenylalanine level reflects the biochemical response

TABLE 26-4 DIETARY PROGRESSION OF AN INFANT WITH PKU

1-Month-old girl

Diet: Formula: ½ cup Lofenalac + 4 oz whole milk + 1 tbsp corn oil to a volume of 28 oz

Weight: 4.18 kg (10th percentile)

Height: 5.2 cm (10th percentile)

Sample feeding schedule: 3.5 oz in 6 feedings per day

	Phenylalanine, mg	Protein, g	Energy kcal	kJ
Mean intake per day	268	15.6	476	1989
Intake/kg body weight per day	63.8	3.7	114	479

4-Month-old girl

Diet: Formula: ¾ cup Lofenalac + 2½ oz whole milk to a volume of 30 oz

      Food: 4 Equivalents

Weight: 6.04 kg (25th percentile)

Height: 61 cm (25–50th percentile)

Sample feeding schedule:

AM 8:00	Lofenalac	6 oz	
PM 12:00	Lofenalac	6 oz	
	Mixed cereal	2 tbsp	(2 equivalents)
	Strained applesauce	2 tbsp	(0 equivalents)
3:30	Lofenalac	5½ oz	
	Strained green peas	1½ tbsp	(1½ equivalents)
	Strained peaches	4 tbsp	(½ equivalent)
7:00	Lofenalac	6 oz	
11:30	Lofenalac	6 oz	

	Phenylalanine, mg	Protein, g	Energy kcal	kJ
Mean intake per day	275	22	609	2558
Intake/kg body weight per day	46	4	102	428

(continued)

to dietary manipulations and the degree of dietary control. A suitable schedule for blood phenylalanine determinations is:

1 Twice weekly during the initial diet stabilization

2 Weekly in infants

3 At 2- to 3-week intervals in toddlers

4 Monthly thereafter for the duration of the diet.[28]

The blood phenylalanine level and the rates of weight gain and growth determine when additional phenylalanine is needed in the diet. The diet is monitored for phenylalanine, protein, and calories (Lofenalac is supplemented with vitamins and minerals). Inadequate intake of phenylalanine can lead to anorexia, rash, listlessness, and failure to grow. If not recognized and treated, the deficiency can impair intellectual function, lead to severe illness, and eventually be fatal.

During periods of illness and fever, phenylalanine blood levels increase; however, the child is managed as is any other pediatric patient, with treatment appropriate to the condition and not to the dietary control.

TABLE 26-4 (*continued*)

8-Month-old girl

Diet: Formula: 1 cup Lofenalac + 2 oz whole milk to a volume of 20 oz

Food: 6 Equivalents

Weight: 8.79 (75th percentile)

Height: 70 cm (75th percentile)

Sample feeding schedule:

AM	7:00	Lofenalac	5 oz	
	11:00	Lofenalac	4 oz	
		Mixed cereal	2 tbsp	(2 equivalents)
		Table applesauce	3 tbsp	(0 equivalents)
PM	1:00	Table applesauce	3½ tbsp	(0 equivalents)
	3:00	Lofenalac	5 oz	
		Saltine cracker	1	(1 equivalent)
		Junior blueberries	2½ tbsp	(½ equivalent)
	7:00	Lofenalac	4 oz	
		Junior corn	2½ tbsp	(2½ equivalents)
		Table applesauce	2 tbsp	(0 equivalents)
	8:30	Lofenalac	1 oz	

| | | | | Energy | |
	Phenylalanine, mg	*Protein, g*	*kcal*		*kJ*
Mean intake per day	314	26.6	895		3759
Intake/kg body weight per day	35.7	3.0	102		428

Diet Discontinuation

The length of time that diet therapy should be continued is still in doubt. Some centers terminate the diet at school age on the grounds that near-maximum growth of the brain has been achieved by this time. (See Table 26-5.) Others, on the basis of uncertainty as to the consequences of a return to high blood levels of phenylalanine, maintain the diet indefinitely. As experience and information in this area continue to increase a more definitive answer should be forthcoming.

As diet discontinuation commences, both child and family may undergo a stressful period of transition. New foods that were once restricted are now allowed. Both parent and child must adapt to this new food experience as the parent is now in the position of encouraging formerly forbidden foods and the child is exposed to the new taste of milk and meat. Vitamin and mineral supplementation of the diet is recommended while the child broadens his or her pattern of food acceptances.

Maternal PKU

The problem of maternal PKU arises with the pregnancy of the female with PKU. Increased concentrations of phenylalanine in the mother appear to have a toxic influence on the fetus, and result in the birth of an infant who manifests intrauterine growth retardation, profound retardation in mental development, and congenital anomalies. In order to avoid the teratogenic effect of phenylalanine in women with PKU who wish to bear children, a carefully controlled phenylalanine-restricted diet during pregnancy is recommended;[29] the outcome of such a pregnancy is unknown.

THE LOW-BIRTH-WEIGHT INFANT

Edith L. Getchell

Birth precipitates a series of physical and biochemical adjustments. A newborn infant,

TABLE 26-5 DIET DISCONTINUATION AT AGE FIVE

Children's Hospital Medical Center, Boston, Mass., with 8 years of experience in treating children with phenylketonuria, has provided evidence which strongly supports the following in regard to diet discontinuation at 5 years of age:

1 Following diet discontinuation, the child with PKU will indeed show a notable rise in blood phenylalanine levels. However, since brain development and growth are largely complete by age 5 years, such rises have no known liability.

2 There are no significant changes in intelligence or behavior when the special diet is discontinued at 5 years of age.

3 Physical growth continued normally following diet discontinuation.

4 Diet discontinuation allows easier mealtime management and more comfortable peer-related food experiences. There can be a decrease in family tension.

5 Diet discontinuation does require a period of adjustment for the child and the family.

A national collaborative study currently being conducted on PKU also reports no significant differences in behavior, intelligence, or growth of children following diet discontinuation.

Diet discontinuation procedures on the fifth birthday are the same for all children—males and females. The one important exception to diet liberalization is the pregnant woman with PKU. During pregnancy she must return to her phenylalanine-restricted diet and special formula, to help prevent damage to her unborn child.

---

abruptly severed from a continuous supply line, must adapt to an extrauterine environment where nourishment is provided sporadically and requires complex processing prior to utilization. As a fetus, oral intake begins perhaps as early as 16 to 17 weeks gestation, with the swallowing of small amounts of amniotic fluid (2–7 ml/24 h). By term, swallowing increases intake to 450 ml daily.[32] Apparently fetal swallowing contributes to the regulation of amniotic fluid volume; however, it may likewise be of some nutritional import. Energy contributions are minimal, as glucose concentrations never exceed maternal plasma and decrease during gestation, providing only 15 mg/100 ml at term. Protein, however, is present in a range of 0.3 to 0.6 g/100 ml, the peak occurring between 25 and 28 weeks gestation. If the protein present in amniotic fluid at term can be fully utilized, 14 percent of the RDA for a 3-kg newborn is provided. While oral intake of amniotic fluid may have contributed to some degree during gestation, nuriture was primarily delivered preprocessed directly into circulation.

The well-nourished 40-week full-term infant, with a well-developed gastrointestinal tract, requires a considerable period of adjustment and further refinement before he or she ingests, digests, and absorbs food efficiently. The following discussion will consider the premature end products of undernourished gestations, whose adjustment to extrauterine existence is more dramatic and difficult, and who require precise and finely tuned nutritional management. Neonatal capacities for adaptation, postnatal ontogeny, and environmental adjustments which minimize stress and compensate limitations will be reviewed.

CLARIFICATION OF TERMS

Infants born before the 37th week of gestation are commonly considered *premature*. Birth weight in relation to fetal age is an indicator of the quality of fetal development, and, using intrauterine growth rates,[33] infants are classified as *appropriate for gestational age* (AGA), or *small for gestational age* (SGA), or *small for date* (SFD). SGAs and SFDs include newborns whose birth weights are below the third percentile of expected weight for gestational age. SGAs and SFDs then include full-term infants, as well as prematures, who were victims of fetal malnutrition. Intrauterine growth retardation is most often the consequence of placental insufficiency, although severe maternal malnutrition can also be the cause. The term *low birth weight* (LBW) is applied to weights of 2500 g or less, and while LBWs account for only 7 to 10 percent of live births, they make up two-thirds or more of neonatal deaths.[34] Extremes of underweight are designated by the term *very low birth weight* (VLBW), which is used by some authors to describe birth weights of less than 1500 grams.

Until recent years, some 70 percent of LBW infants who managed to survive the precarious neonatal period have been left with neurological impairment, including motor and sensory disorders and mental retardation. Advances in neonatal care have improved the prognosis. Management of metabolic problems has become more efficient, and infants at risk receive more immediate care at regional intensive neonatal care units. Improved nutritional treatment during the first week of life has also been identified as a major contributing factor. Lubchenco reported over 70 percent of infants weighing less than 1000 g, and later found to have IQ scores below 90, had an average caloric intake of only 25 kcal (105 kJ)/kg of body weight per day during their first week of life.[35] Grassy, in follow-up studies of 28 survivors receiving intensive neonatal care, reported higher average caloric intakes of 60 kcal (252 kJ)/kg of body weight per day during the first week of life. Of the eight infants with neurological impairment at 12 to 51 months, six had received less than 50 kcal (210 kJ)/kg of body weight per day. In contrast, only 3 of the 10 without such impairment had received less than 50 kcal (210 kJ)/kg of body weight per day.[36] Clearly, early adequate alimentation is essential.

Currently accepted is the belief that nutritional deprivation which alters cell division may have permanent consequence, whereas that which occurs when cells are increasing in size is largely reversible with the restoration of adequate nutrition. Validity of this concept imposes responsibility for early establishment of optimal nutrition, particularly in relation to neuronal division which may last well into the neonatal period.[37]

For all attempts at sophistication of feeding regimens for the premature infant, nothing has yet been designed—or is ever likely to be—which provides the benefits of intrauterine nutriture. However, in absence of the perfect environment, nutritional management nonetheless attempts to support normal intrauterine growth rates by customizing composition of the food as well as mode and rate of delivery.

The full-term SGA infant is not as compromised developmentally as the premature infant. SGA neonatal mortality, while 10 times that of the full-size term infant, is less than one-half that of their preterm weight peers.[38] Custom blending of ingredients becomes less of a factor in his management than determining appropriate amounts. Potential for "catch-up growth" must be encouraged.

NUTRITIONAL HAZARDS OF PREMATURITY

The cyclical contributing factors which precipitate and perpetuate nutritional deficits in the premature are summarized in Fig. 26-4.

Marginal Birth Stores

The SGA and premature infant have increased risk for hypoglycemia (blood glucose <20 mg/100 ml) as a consequence of their inadequate glycogen stores. This characteristic risk is associated with long-term prognosis of impaired CNS function. Glycogen is at best a short-term fuel, which is depleted within 24 h in the normal full-term newborn. At birth, with sudden departure from a fetal carbohydrate diet, and as a consequence of delayed feedings, fatty acids mobilized from adipose tissue become the major energy source. Increasing deposition of white adipose tissue from the 34th week of gestation provides the full-term infant with a fat storage supply that is 13 percent of his body mass. The newborn premature may have less than 3 percent.[39] This fat supply metabolized in a carbohydrate-poor environment yields ketones which can be utilized by the newborn brain. Enzymes for metabolism of ketones in the brain have been seen as early as 8 to 10 weeks gestation.[40]

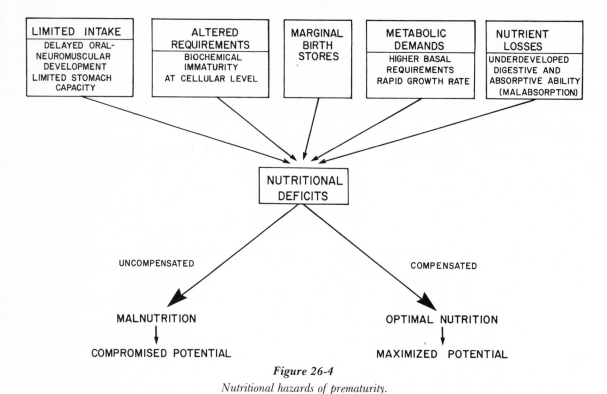

Figure 26-4

Nutritional hazards of prematurity.

Altered Fluid and Nutrient Needs

Established requirements and recommended allowances for the full-term infant do not apply to the premature. Lack of knowledge on vitamin requirements during fetal development leads to the reasonable practice of providing most vitamins at levels recommended for full-term infants. Analysis of body composition changes occurring during gestation provides the basis for recommending advisable protein and mineral intakes. The caloric cost of growth for LBW and SGA infants per unit of body weight greatly exceeds that of the term newborn. The energy required for deposition of body protein and fat can be estimated by relating body composition changes occurring during fetal development to the energy requirements observed in animal growth studies (7.5 kcal (31.50 kJ)/g of protein and 11.6 kcal (48.72 kJ)/g of fat).[41]

Fluid requirements will vary with maturity

of renal function and homeostatic mechanisms. Close monitoring and frequent tailoring of water intake and electrolyte balance is required. In utero, enormous volumes of water exchange between mother, fetus, and amniotic fluid. The hourly exchange between mother and fetus is estimated at 3500 ml.[42] At birth, the infant begins adapting to major changes in both magnitude and routes. The transition is accompanied as well by the establishment of a new route—that of water *loss* from skin and lungs. Term and premature infants experience weight loss over their first few days of life which is largely accounted for by water loss.[43]

Nephrogenesis is complete by the 35th week of gestation, and a full complement of nephrons is present at term. Glomerular filtration rate is low at birth, and increases with postnatal age. Infants normally demonstrate slow diuretic response to water loads during the first 3 postnatal days. Although maximum dilution is achieved after about 5 days, the rate of excreting a water load is much slower than that of the adult. This lag is more accentuated in the premature.[44] The premature newborn kidney also has a relatively low concentrating ability, resulting from the lack of osmotically active substances as well as the state of renal immaturity. Renal solute load is composed primarily of electrolytes and end products of protein metabolism. If no growth occurs, the "potential" renal solute load—i.e., the total provided by intake (approximately 4 mosmol/g protein and 1 mosmol/meq of Na, K, and Cl) will be presented to the kidney for excretion. Zeigler has suggested that the percentage of "potential" renal solute which is diverted into new tissue is greater for the growing premature than the growing full-size infant.[45] He estimates retention to be 1.27 mosmol/g of weight gain. In other words, appropriate levels of fluid intake and electrolyte concentration are determined by rate of growth as well as by consideration of renal function. With desired levels of growth and with commonly used formulations, water balance in the LBW is a concern primarily when intake is small and extrarenal losses increase. The premature kidney, even with lessened capacity is still able to achieve sufficient urine concentration. In the absence of growth, renal solute may become a larger factor in management. A urine osmolality of 75 to 300 mosmol/kg indicates that renal concentrating or diluting mechanisms are not unduly stressed. Although some research indicates ADH (antidiuretic hormone) in prematures is limited, and that renal tubules may not be responsive, the deficiencies are not of a magnitude to significantly affect renal concentrating requirements.[46]

Maturational lags in the synthesis of specific amino acid metabolizing enzyme systems affects amino acid essentiality, and in some instances can affect advisable intakes of other nutrients. To illustrate, the enzyme cystathionase, deficient in human fetal liver, is necessary to convert methionine, an essential amino acid, to cystine, not normally considered essential.[47] Tyrosine, synthesized from phenyl-

alanine, has also been suggested as essential for the premature and perhaps some full-term infants in the early months of life.[48] While tyrosine is essential, it can also accumulate to undesirable levels in the premature (transient tyrosinemia), due to an inability to catabolize the amino acid. Insufficient ascorbic acid inhibits the enzyme involved. With daily protein intakes of 2 to 3 g/kg, 50 to 100 mg ascorbic acid daily eliminates tyrosinemia in most infants.[49]

Altered Metabolic Demands

Basal metabolic rates, determined by the measurement of O_2 uptake and CO_2 excretion at rest, are expressed in relation to body surface. LBW and SGA infants, by virtue of smaller body size, have more surface area than do full-sized term infants, and therefore basal needs per unit body weight are higher. Sinclair estimated daily resting energy expenditure (exclusive of activity or cold stress) to be 34 to 50 kcal(142 to 210 kJ)/kg.[50] Heat production (i.e., O_2 consumption) depends on activity, food, and temperature. While the effects of activity and food on metabolic rates have been appreciated for some time, the crucial importance of temperature in determining metabolic rates of newborns has not. It is now realized that all newborns, including premature infants, respond to cold stress with increases in heat production that can be greater than that due to activity or food.[51] The premature's lack of adequate adipose insulation accelerates heat loss, straining homeothermic capacity.

For both LBW and full-size infants, a rise in O_2 consumption occurs early postnatally. However, in the first 10 days of life, O_2 consumption per unit of body weight is slightly lower for LBW than for full-size infants, and lower for VLBW infants. After 2 weeks, O_2 consumption per unit weight rises. The apparent contradiction of recent studies—that LBW infants have lower rates of heat production rather than higher rates as compared to full-term newborns—may be the result of the inclusion of cold-induced metabolic increases in the earlier estimates.[52]

SGA infants show a marked rise in metabolic rate postnatally. Their O_2 consumption exceeds that of similar weight, less gestationally mature infants. This distinctive hypermetabolism, suggestive during the first 12 h of life, becomes more pronounced after 2 to 3 days of age, and continues after 10 days. This postnatal response is similar to that observed in the early recovery stages of infant malnutrition, indicating capacity for cellular metabolism was limited by the poor energy-nutrient delivery in the uterine environment.[53]

Increases in metabolism to accommodate cold stress may seriously restrict calories available for growth. Capacity for response to heat loss is present shortly after birth, less on the first day than thereafter. LBW infants' response is quantitively smaller than full-size babies on the first day of life, but improves with increasing postnatal age. It is important to remember that response can be modified by illness and thermal environment.[54]

Increased muscular activity (with or without shivering) contributes to increased heat production; however, infants usually rely on nonshivering thermogenesis, and O_2 consumption increases in the absence of observable muscular response. Cold may stimulate production of catecholamines, which initiates metabolism of brown adipose tissue.[55] Brown adipose tissue has been found in five sites in the newborn: between scapulae, around muscles and blood vessels of the neck, in axillae, in the mediastinum between esophagus and trachea, and around kidney and adrenals. Brown adipose tissue, differentiating from reticular cells at 26 to 30 weeks gestation, is not completely formed at term, but continues to develop after birth. Indirect evidence supports the role of brown fat in thermohomeostasis. Capacity for nonshivering thermogenesis continues to develop after birth, particularly in premature infants. Term SGA infants, while they share with the premature a limited ability to conserve body heat, have better resistance to cold as a result of their better flexor tone and higher rates of resting heat production. Capacity to increase heat production is well developed, and accomplished by increasing muscle activity and by heat production in brown adipose tissue.[56]

Limited Intake

As Ghadimi has pointed out, because of the premature's "feeble ability to accept and retain food, nutritional deprivation under conditions of oral feeding is almost inevitable."[57] Even in the absence of anatomic defects, physical and oral neuromuscular limitations, varying in degree with maturation, seriously limit possibilities for oral nutrition.

Coordination between sucking and swallowing is poorly developed, especially in infants less than 34 weeks gestation. With failure of the epiglottis to close and thereby inhibiting respiration, the LBW infant aspirates. Various motor abnormalities, as pharyngoesophageal incoordination or gastroesophageal sphincter incompetance, may produce vomiting and regurgitation. Premature infants over 2000 grams and normal newborns less than 12 h of age have poorly coordinated responses to swallowing, including rapid peristalsis, biphasic waves, and often nonperistaltic simultaneous contractions along the entire length of the esophagus. Peristalsis becomes more coordinated, rate slows, and simultaneous contractions decreases in frequency as infant develops. Lower esophageal sphincter (LES) pressure levels have been shown to be lower in infants experiencing chalasia (regurgitation) than in adults. LES pressure approaches adult levels at 3 to 6 weeks of age.[58] Aspiration and regurgitation is further complicated by weak respiratory muscles and the absence of a cough reflex in the very LBW infant.

Stomach capacity is limited, varying from 3 to 40 cc in the 800- to 4000-g neonate. Delayed stomach emptying limits frequency and total volume of feedings. At 32 weeks gestation, as much as 9 h is required for progression of contrast material to the colon. Gastrointestinal motility advances with fetal age, and by term, transit time is reduced to 4½ to 7 h.[59]

Term SGA infants are more neurologically mature, able to suck better, and capable of accepting higher caloric intakes.

Nutrient Losses

Nutrient deficits, the consequence of limited intake, become more pronounced as oral intake is processed by immature digestive and absorptive systems. The premature is characterized by poor fat absorption, transitory lactose intolerance, and apparent delay in intestinal rejuvination following trauma.

All neonates are characterized by a temporary inability to absorb fat. The normal full term breast-fed infant will exhibit a physiological steatorrhea accounting for 10 percent of his fat intake. The premature's absorption of dietary lipid is less efficient, 60 to 85 percent of intake, depending on the type and the amount. As monoglycerides and unhydrolyzed triglycerides are found in newborns' feces, the intraluminal phase of fat absorption would seem incomplete. Pancreatic lipase activity is present by 34 to 36 weeks gestation. Prematures born at this age exhibit a fivefold increase in lipase activity during their first week of life.[60] After 1 week of life, when pancreatic lipase levels become adequate for lipolysis, intestinal bile-salt concentrations continue to remain too low to form the necessary micellar complexes required to ferry lipid into the intestinal epithelial cell. Intestinal reabsorption of bile salts may be incomplete. Unlike adults, variations in bile-salt pool size are not compensated for by increased recycling frequency or by increased secretion rates.[61] Improvement of lipid absorption over the first 4 to 6 weeks of life is closely correlated to increased intraluminal bile-salt concentrations, a function of both liver and gastrointestinal maturation. Interest has been given recently to possible advantages in the use of MCT (medium-chain triglycerides) in formulation for the premature.[62]

Carbohydrate absorption likewise has maturational implications. While sucrase, maltase, and lactase are present in small-intestinal mucosa very early in gestation, lactase attains maximal activity only close to term. Seven- to eight-month prematures may have enzyme deficiencies capable of causing diarrhea and energy loss when given sufficient lactose load.[63] While the potential exists, occurrence of lactose intolerance is quite uncommon.[64] After birth, lactase activity in LBW infants rapidly reaches values of the term baby. As the presence of lactose provides bacteriostatic benefit, its elimination in the absence of intolerance should be avoided. Lactose lends to the development of a fermentive bacterial flora, *Lactobacillus,* which may provide protection against gram-negative sepsis.[65]

Observed differences in small-intestinal cellular proliferation and migration may be of importance to the sick full-term and LBW infants in management of diarrhea and intestinal disease. In the mature human intestine, cells require only 2 to 3 days to migrate from the crypt. While cell turnover and migration have been studied in only one anencephalic newborn, the rate was found to be one-third to one-half that of an adult. Suckling rats have also been found to have a slower migration rate than mature animals. Although this has not been true in the pig or guinea pig, possibilities that the infant intestine may require more time to recover from intestinal trauma is of interest.

NUTRITIONAL GOALS AND PARAMETERS

Using birthweight data on 5635 live-born Caucasian infants of 24 to 42 weeks gestational age, Lubchenco has presented weight curves in the form of percentiles.[66] These curves can be used as standards for the adequacy of an individual infant's weight before and after birth. Determination of a newborn infant's position on the intrauterine growth chart indicates the appropriateness of weight in relation to gestational age. Extremes can be evaluated, and possible cause investigated. Unusually large infants might identify incorrect estimates of gestational age, or, with parents of average size, may indicate a diabetic or prediabetic mother. After birth, comparing postnatal growth to intrauterine growth standards assists in identifying when an infant has "caught up" to his or her birth percentile (weight loss following birth results in a downward curve deviation), or in identifying when the weight deviates substantially from expected prenatal growth. Adequacy of nutrition can be evaluated. More importantly, an estimate of growth that can reasonably be expected provides the basis for establishing levels of advisable nutrient intake. Weights at the 10th, 50th, and 90th percentiles as documented by Lubchenco are presented in Table 26-6.

Growth Standards

If the attainment of normal intrauterine growth is the established goal in the nutritional management of LBW infants, an average weight gain of approximately 20 to 30 g/day would be desired. Lubchenco's data indicates an 18-g increase per day between 28 and 32 weeks gestation, with approximately 36 g/day added between 32 and 36 weeks. Weight gain is not as rapid after the 36th week, as placental transport does not continue to support as accelerated a gain. The term newborn, after an extrauterine adjustment of about 1 week, demonstrates a growth spurt which surpasses his gestational rate. Daily he increases his weight by 38 g (male at the 50th percentile). Foman speculates that this represents "catch-up" growth, and that it is reasonable to assume that growth potential of the premature is of a magnitude to achieve fetal rates of growth. LBW infants who are SGA may exhibit a more rapid postnatal catch-up growth and gain than their AGA peers.[67] Heird, on the other hand, questions the appropriateness of establishing intrauterine growth as the standard, and

suggests that feeding methods that prevent weight loss might be as acceptable.[68] Presently, however, most investigators accept a goal of paralleling uterine growth rates.

Postnatal weight loss in the LBW infant is more hazardous than that of the term infant of normal weight. Rapid brain growth, by cell division, occurs in the last trimester and continues for the first half year of life. Concern for the long-term consequences of undernutrition has prompted Rickard and Gresham to define acceptable losses and desirable gains. They believe low weight should be reached between 2 and 8 days of age and should not exceed 5 to 10 percent of birth weight. For the VLBW infant, a loss not exceeding 5 percent is preferred. Their goal for regain of birth weight is between 1 and 2 weeks. For the 1- to 2-kg infant, a 20 g/day weight gain, and a 1 cm/week increase in length is desired.[69] Because Sinclair does not accept the premise that body water stores at birth meet early postnatal water requirements, he suggests that fluid losses account for a substantial portion of the weight loss, and that greater losses should be expected in the VLBW infants by virtue of their body water content. He therefore accepts a larger weight loss tolerance—10 percent for infants more than 1500 g at birth, with a loss not to exceed 15 percent in infants less than 1500 g.[70]

Energy and Protein Recommendations

The LBW infant has extraordinary needs for both energy and protein during the early weeks of life. Enzyme systems must mature rapidly and anabolic processes function at maximum rates. An energy intake of approximately 120 kcal (504 kJ)/kg is generally recommended.[71,72,73,74] As mentioned previously, initial metabolic rates are low, but increase over the first 2 weeks of life as extrauterine adaptations are achieved, and rapid growth begins. To support the intrauterine growth range of 18 to 36 g/day, intakes between 110 and 140 kcal (462 and 588 kJ)/kg of body weight per

TABLE 26-6   WEIGHTS OF LIVE-BORN CAUCASIAN INFANTS OF VARYING GESTATIONAL AGE, MALES AND FEMALES

Gestational age, weeks	Weight, g		
	10th percentile	50th percentile	90th percentile
24	530	840	1260
25	605	880	1305
26	685	955	1360
27	770	1045	1435
28	860	1150	1550
29	960	1270	1690
30	1060	1395	1840
31	1170	1540	2030
32	1290	1715	2280
33	1440	1920	2600
34	1600	2200	2940
35	1800	2485	3200
36	2050	2710	3390
37	2260	2900	3520
38	2430	3030	3640
39	2550	3140	3735
40	2630	3230	3815
41	2690	3290	3870
42	2720	3300	3890

Source: Adapted from L. A. Lubchenco et al., "Intrauterine Growth as Estimated from Liveborn Birth-Weight Data at 24–42 Weeks of Gestation," *Pediatrics,* **32**(5):793, 1963.

day would be required. Intakes above 120 kcal (504 kJ)/kg are difficult to achieve, and it can easily be seen how the stress imposed by illness, infection, or surgery will compromise desired growth rates. As Ghadimi has emphasized, providing for only basal energy needs during the first days of life addresses catabolic processes only, and is insufficient for premature survival.[75] Optimal growth supporting intakes need to be attained as rapidly as possible. Table 26-7 compartmentalizes energy requirements.

A protein intake over 2 g and less than 6 g/(kg · day) is generally regarded as sufficient to meet growth needs without contributing to complications of excessive intake (elevated BUN, acidosis, hyperpyrexia, lethargy, diarrhea, edema). Protein intakes of 6 g/kg have been associated with increased morbidity and mortality of LBW infants. Goldman reviewed the late effects of early dietary protein intake on LBW infants.[76] Over 300 infants with birth weights less than 2000 g were evaluated at 3 and at 5 to 7 years of age. The group of children who as young infants had been given 4 percent protein diets (6 to 7.2 g/kg) had a significantly increased incidence of low IQ scores when their birth weights were less than 1300 g. With birth weights below 1700 g, significantly increased incidence of strabismus was also noted on a 4 percent protein diet. Goldman concludes that advisable intake lies between 3

TABLE 26-7   ENERGY NEEDS OF THE PREMATURE

	Caloric requirements	
	kcal/kg/day	kJ/kg/day
Resting	50	210
Intermittent activity	15	63
Occasional cold stress	10	42
Specific dynamic action	8	34
Fecal calorie loss	12	50
Growth*	25	105
Total	120	504

* Energy requirements for growth may be decreased 10 to 25% when absorptive losses are eliminated by parenteral nutrition. Requirements are variable with rate of growth.

Source: Sinclair data: "Supportive Management of the Sick Neonate," *Pediatric Clinics of North America,* **17**:863, 1970.

and 6 g/(kg · day) when provided by cow's milk protein or human milk. When expected weight gains at various gestational ages are considered, protein recommendations can range from 2 to 5.1 g/(kg · day).[77] With a 20 g/day weight gain as the established goal, the youngest gestational age prematures (27 to 31 weeks) will require 3.8 g/kg, whereas that rate of growth will be supported by an intake of 2.4 g/kg in the 34- to 35-week LBW infant. Probably an intake of 3 to 4 g/(kg · day) is reasonable when nonhuman milk is the protein source. Intakes in excess of 4 g may not be advisable. Elevated BUN levels are commonly associated with high protein intakes. Raïhä suggests that intakes of 4.5 g/kg exceeds preterm infant synthesis needs, and questions the value of protein intakes greater than that provided by breast milk, particularly when protein source is casein-predominant rather than whey-predominant.[78] The role of breast milk in the management of LBW infants is presented on page 582. Appropriate protein intake must be individualized, and assumes adequate provision of calories. The smaller LBW infants are at greater risk of developing protein deficiency.

Because of the necessity for meeting energy needs in order to benefit from protein intake, advisable levels are often given as grams per 100 kcal (420 kJ). Foman has determined the daily protein needs for a 1250-g infant, gaining at the rate of 20 g/day, to be 4.4 g (3 g for growth, 1.2 g for nongrowth needs; 95 percent absorption assumed). Expressed in terms of body weight, the protein requirement is 3.5 g/(kg · day). If 155 kcal (651 kJ) are required daily to allow utilization of protein for other than energy purposes, the protein requirement, expressed in terms of energy requirement, would be given as 2.8 g/100 kcal (420 kJ).[79]

When protein is provided intravenously, requirements may be decreased. Snyderman places the protein requirement for the premature at 2.2 g/(kg · day),[80] and suspects the difference between oral and intravenous needs is not too great. However, infused amino acids bypass the liver where 20 percent or more of nitrogen is usually degraded to urea.[81] Concerns for elevated amino acid levels during total intravenous alimentation are discussed on page 576.

(Calorie and protein recommendations are summarized in Table 26-9.)

Fluid Requirements

Sinclair's recommended ranges of water intake required to replace insensible, urinary, and fecal water losses are presented in Table 26-8. Minimal activity, in a single-walled incubator, in a thermoneutral environment, with a relative humidity of 50 percent, is assumed. Increased metabolic rate caused by cold stress, activity, or illness increases water requirements substantially; necessary increments are noted in the table.

Vitamin and Mineral Concerns

Vitamins and minerals are often supplied according to the recommended dietary allowances for the full-term infant. Accelerated growth rates and immature homeostatic mech-

TABLE 26-8 WATER REQUIREMENTS FOR LBW INFANTS

Water losses	Water required, ml/(kg · 24 h)	
	1500 g body weight	*1500–2500 g body weight*
Insensible	30–60	15–35
Urine	50–100 ⟶	
Stool	5–10 ⟶	
Total	85–170	70–145
Increment for phototherapy	20	

Increased metabolic rate due to cold stress, activity, or illness increases water requirements. Totals may be increased to:

<1000 g	>200 ml/(kg · 24 h)
1000–1500 g	175–200 ml/(kg · 24 h)
1500–2500 g	150–180 ml/(kg · 24 h)

Source: R. Neil Roy and J. C. Sinclair, "Hydration of the Low Birth-Weight Infant," *Clinics in Perinatology,* **2**(2):400, 1975.

anisms alter advisable intakes. Supplements must be provided in relation to stores available at birth and levels of intake that can be achieved. Several nutrient concerns of current interest will be reviewed.

Calcium–Vitamin D

Eighty percent of the term skeleton is acquired during the final trimester. The fetal environment provides a net transplacental influx of 130 to 150 mg. calcium/(kg · 24 h).[82] Neither breast milk nor infant formulas can provide sufficient calcium to permit accretion at intrauterine rates. LBW infants are prone to become calcium deficient.

Maintenance of calcium homeostasis requires major physiologic adjustments after birth to accommodate the abrupt change in calcium flow. A transient functional hypoparathyroidism occurs normally in the neonate because fetal serum calcium levels exceed the threshold for parathyroid hormone release.[83] The parathyroid is stimulated to secrete PTH with low serum calcium levels. Response is understandably minimal the first day of life, increasing significantly after 50 h of age.

Transition from fetal to neonatal calcium balance is more difficult for premature infants. Early neonatal hypocalcemia (total serum calcium concentrations below 7 mg/100 ml, ionized calcium below 2.5 mg/100 ml) sometimes appearing within the first few hours, but usually within the first 3 days, occurs principally in products of complicated pregnancies and deliveries. LBW, SGA, asphyxiated infants, and infants of diabetic mothers are at high risk, with 30 to 50 percent of these births being affected. The degree and duration of hypocalcemia parallels the degree of immaturity, which is not too surprising, as serum concentrations of PTH increase during gestation.[84] Decreased PTH secretions also appear to be accompanied by peripheral unresponsiveness to PTH.

Neonatal hypocalcemia, the result of elevated dietary phosphate, usually occurs after the fifth day of life. If milk supplied has a high phosphate content, and an unfavorable calcium phosphorus ratio, the capacity of the neonatal kidney to remove excess phosphate may be exceeded, and hypocalcemia will be the natural consequence.

Brown examined the effects of oral calcium supplementation on premature and asphyxiated infants during their transitional period of establishing calcium homeostasis. In the study, 75 mg of elemental calcium/(kg · 24 h), in the form of calcium gluconate in syrup, was given just before, or within 1 h after feeding, for three days. Supplementation did not produce immediate effects on other homeostatic factors (as PTH, vitamin D, magnesium, or phosphorus), and maintained serum calcium at normal levels during supplementation and for more than 1 day after supplement was discontinued.[85] The only side effects noted were increased frequency of bowel movements, possibly related to sucrose medium for calcium; transient borderline hypercalcemia occurred in one patient. While increased serum calcium would seem beneficial to LBW infants at risk for hypocalcemia, marked increases are to be avoided, as the resultant hypercalcemia would repress the already insufficiently responsive parathyroid.

To supplement a deficient calcium intake, Chance provided calcium lactate, 800 mg/(kg · day), to LBW infants that were AGA and SGA, whose birth weights were less than 1300 g. Supplement was begun between 14 and 21 days of life and was accompanied by a vitamin supplement containing 500 IU vitamin D. Calcium retention equivalent to intrauterine accumulation was achieved with improved bone formation.[86] Calcium absorption was unexpectedly high compared to controls. Slight reduction in blood pH and absorption of fat and phosphorus were noted as side effects. Infants were followed until weights of 1800 g were achieved at a mean age of 54 days.

Vitamin D plays a role in calcium homeostasis. Provitamins, cholesterol-related compounds activated by ultraviolet light, are hydroxylated in the liver, forming 25-OHD. 25-OHD is later delivered to the kidney for further hydroxylation, which produces the physiologically active metabolite $1,25(OH)_2D_3$ (1,25-dihydroxycholecalciferol). Active D_3 increases calcium and phosphorus absorption in the intestine, stimulates resorption of calcium from the bone, and increases renal tubular permeability, which allows reabsorption of sodium, phosphate, and calcium. Maturity of the hydroxylation mechanisms in the liver and kidney of premature infants was investigated by Hillman and Haddad.[87] Maturational delays apparently prevent maintenance of normal 25-OHD levels before 36 to 38 weeks postconceptual age. Provision of 400 IU vitamin D supplements did not result in a rise in serum 25-OHD in the very premature. Suggestion is made that vitamin D in milk or as an oral or intravenous supplement is not effective before 38 weeks gestational age. Infants are routinely provided 400 IU vitamin D during their first year of life. Attempts to parallel intrauterine calcium accretion rates implies elevated D needs; however, potential for vitamin D tox-

icity must also be considered. Chance's use of 500 IU of vitamin D was accompanied by excellent calcium utilization and is suggestive of a reasonable level of intake.

Sodium

LBW infants, especially those with respiratory distress, are subject to hyponatremia (plasma sodium < 130 meq/l). Sodium losses exceed intake during the first weeks of life, as 2 to 6 weeks are required to develop sodium-conserving abilities. Even with low plasma sodium levels, large amounts of sodium can be excreted possibly as a result of decreased sodium reabsorption in the distal tubule, the probable site of aldosterone action. Hyponatremia of the VLBW infant can be prevented by small increases in dietary sodium [3 meq/(kg · day)]. Extreme prematurity may require very much higher intakes. The newborn preterm has lower limits of tolerance to sodium overload as well, and may respond to acute salt load by excreting too much. Sodium homeostasis apparently develops as a function of gestational rather than postnatal age.[88]

Iron, Vitamin E, and Folate

Closer examination in recent years of the interrelationships between iron and vitamin E have altered traditional recommendations for supplementation. Requirements for vitamin E are large in preterm infants; however, infants with birth weights less than 1500 g and 32 weeks gestation have impaired vitamin E absorption.[89] Absorptive capacity appears to be the limiting factor to the repair of the hemolytic anemia related to vitamin E deficiency. As an antioxidant, vitamin E protects cell membranes. It is also involved in the synthesis of heme. At birth, premature body stores of E are about $1/7$ those of the full-term infant: 3 mg as compared to 20.[90] LBW neonates provided alpha-tocopherol at levels 10 times that of the RDA have been unable to normalize their serum tocopherol levels. Only when weights approach gestational maturity is the absorption of E sufficient to maintain adequate plasma levels. Provision of iron in the presence of an E deficiency has been shown to further decrease the vitamin's absorption. The oxidant effect of iron on the fat-soluble vitamin at the intestinal level was considered responsible for decreasing the amounts of both tocopherol and iron available for absorption.

A recent study, using intramuscular vitamin E with and without intramuscular iron, demonstrates an E-iron interaction at the cellular level.[91] Iron dextran given alone produced a considerable oxidant effect in premature infants. The iron catalyzed the breakdown of red cell lipids resulting in blood cell hemolysis. However, when vitamin E was provided in a total dose of 125 mg/kg over the first week of life, E sufficiency was maintained during the first 6 weeks, even in the presence of intramuscular iron. Early attainment of E sufficiency by intramuscular medication may be a desirable goal in the care of the premature infant. As cell membranes other than RBCs are susceptible to oxidant induced injury, E deficiency together with oxygen administration—a common component of premature management—may have important implications.[92]

Iron status of the premature must be considered as a basis for determining appropriate supplementation. Dallman reviewed birth and postnatal iron status of the premature infant.[93] During fetal development approximately 75 mg iron/kg is accumulated, primarily in hemoglobin, but also in myoglobin, cytochromes, and other iron-containing proteins. At birth, the full-term infant has stores capable of sustaining health for months while on an iron-poor diet (about 15 mg/kg). The premature's stores are necessarily lower in relation to the degree of immaturity and consequently become depleted earlier.

Postnatal changes in the iron status of prematures occurs in three stages: (1) decreased erythropoiesis, starting at birth and continuing for 3 months; (2) resumption of a rapid rate of hematopoiesis, beginning between 1 and 3 months; and (3) exhaustion of iron stores, which occurs only when sufficient supple-

mental iron has not been provided. In utero, oxygen is received through the placenta, and the resulting relative tissue hypoxia increases erythropoietin production and subsequent red cell manufacture. At birth, with tissue oxygenation, hemoglobin synthesis decreases, and the iron which is released from dying cells is added to storage, further increasing the iron depot. Resumption of hematopoiesis occurs earlier in infants with lowest birth weights. Hemoglobin levels then rise as long as the iron supply lasts—usually for at least 1 month. It is important to note that the physiologic "anemia" of the first two stages is not the result of iron lack. Supplementation at this point will increase stores only, and cannot increase hemoglobin concentration.

There are then two avenues for prevention of iron deficiency: supplement early and build up marginal stores ensuring a safer iron supply for the resumption of red blood cell manufacture, or delay giving iron until the period when it is needed, i.e., when iron stores become depleted. The variable is timing, not dose, as 2 to 3 mg/kg is considered sufficient in either approach.[94] In view of iron-E interactions, providing iron prior to achievement of E sufficiency is not recommended. Vitamin E supplementation and serum tocopherol response will establish the timetable for initiating iron therapy. Supplements of E beyond the minimal amount provided by limited intakes of formula or breast milk are essential. Doses of 25 IU daily do not consistently raise serum tocopherol levels; however, higher doses are not recommended because of potential toxicity.[95] Water-soluble forms are better absorbed and demonstrate earlier maintenance of tocopherol sufficiency and a lesser decline in hemoglobin values.[96] Iron may be provided in the formula or given in medicinal form. Home administration of medicinal iron is inconvenient, unreliable, and not without the risk of acute poisoning with accidental ingestion by older family members. Speculation has been raised concerning possible disadvantages in providing iron in milk, particularly in the early months of life when concentrations of immunoglobins are low. Iron-binding proteins in milk, lactoferrin and transferrin, normally about one-third-saturated with iron, possess bacteriostatic properties. *Escherichia coli* are unable to proliferate without a good iron source. Lactoferrin, capable of binding iron, may be instrumental in limiting iron availability. Recently it has been suggested that when the iron-binding proteins become iron-saturated, they lose their antibacterial capacity. Theoretically, it is possible that amounts of iron added to formula would be sufficient to saturate iron-binding proteins.[97] Breast milk's low iron and high lactoferrin content suggests significance; however, the convenience and safety of fortifying formula with iron, along with the apparent effectiveness in doing so, outweighs theoretical disadvantages.

Need for folic acid is particularly high in rapidly growing premature infants. Folic acid, along with Vitamin B_{12}, is necessary for the synthesis of DNA, and hence for cellular growth. However, unlike B_{12}, whose stores may meet needs for the first year, folate stores are soon depleted and dietary supply may be insufficient. With intakes less than 20 μg/day, LBW infants will develop low serum folate after 2 weeks of age. As intakes of 50 μg/day maintain normal serum levels, supplements which augment intake to 50 μg are recommended for infants less than 2000 g who are otherwise well. The sick LBW infant will require 100 μg/day to maintain desired serum and erythrocyte folate levels.[98]

A summary of nutritional parameters as discussed above is provided in Table 26-9.

APPROACHES TO FEEDING THE LBW INFANT

The status of each LBW infant must provide the basis for the selection of his feeding regimen. Biochemical limitations and specialized needs, along with capacity for intake, will determine the best approach for obtaining acceptable levels of theoretically desirable goals. Maximizing potential will likely involve the combination of various approaches.

Total Intravenous Alimentation— Central Line

Use of total parenteral nutrition (TPN) in VLBW infants is considered an investigational procedure.[99] In light of limited knowledge regarding long-term developmental effects of TPN, it cannot be considered accepted routine care. It has been shown to produce satisfactory growth without undue risk when carefully monitored and controlled.[100-102]

Parenteral mixtures provide amino acids either as hydrolysates of fibrin or casein, or as a mixture of crystalline amino acids. Protein is generally given at levels between 2.5 and 4 g/(kg · day). Solutions are hypertonic, providing carbohydrate in a 20 percent concentration, usually in the form of glucose. A minimum of 25 to 30 g carbohydrate/day is required to meet energy requirements and ensure the utilization of amino acids. Electrolytes, minerals, and vitamins are furnished by additives to the infusate. Electrolytes are provided in relation to maintenance requirements. Parenteral requirements for vitamins and minerals are probably different from oral needs. However, in the absence of specific knowledge of these differences, oral requirements provide the guidelines. Essential fatty acids and trace mineral needs are not met by standard TPN solutions. Requirement for essential fatty acid (EFA) is small, only 1 to 4 percent of energy. Possibilities of providing it orally have been suggested. Absorption of EFA through the skin has been achieved by rubbing safflower oil into the skin. Copper is quite deficient in hyperalimentation solutions,[103] and many of the trace elements are present in small and varying quantities.

Because of the high osmolality (about 1740 mosmol/kg water), nearly 6 times isotonicity, a slow, continuous infusion into a large central vein is required, with constant infusion being

TABLE 26-9 NUTRITIONAL PARAMETERS FOR LBW INFANTS

Recommended energy[a] per kg/day	kcal	kJ	Minerals	Vitamins
Maintenance	50–60	210–252	Calcium:	Vitamin E (oral):
For 20 g/day gain	115–125	483–525	To prevent early neonatal	1U/day 25[e] To supplement
For 30 g/day gain	130–140	546–588	hypocalcemia in infants at risk.	poor intake and malabsorption.
			mg/(kg · 24 h) for 3 days 75[c]	Water-soluble form better
				absorbed.
Protein requirements[b]				
g/kg			To supplement marginal intake	Vitamin E (IM):
range	2.2–4.0		after establishment of Ca	mg/kg 125[g] Total dose, given in
VLBW	3.0–4.0		homeostasis. Total mg/day 800[d]	4 divided doses during 1st
LBW without				week of life.
exceptional stress	2.4–3.0			
g/100 kcal (9/420 kJ)			Iron:	Folic acid:
1250-g infant	2.8		mg/kg 2.5[e] mg/100 kcal/420 kJ	μ/day
2000-g infant	2.2		2.0 In formula or in medicinal	<2000 g
3000-g infant	1.6		form. Given shortly after birth	well premature 50[e]
			to augment stores, or initiated	<2000 g
			when iron stores depleted. Not	sick premature 100
			recommended in absence of	Vitamin D: IU/day 500[d]
			vitamin E deficiency	Ascorbic
				acid: mg/day 100[h]
			Sodium:	
			meq/(kg · day) 3[f]	
			To prevent hyponatremia	

[a] Higher figures related to smaller, more premature infants. Adapted from O'Donnell data as presented by Rickard and Gresham, *Journal of American Dietetic Association,* **66**(6):595, 1975; J. Sinclair et al., *Pediatric Clinics of North America,* **17**:863, 1970; S. J. Foman, E. E. Ziegler, and A. M. O'Donnell, *Infant Nutrition,* W. B. Saunders Company, Philadelphia, p. 498, 1974.

[b] S. J. Foman, E. E. Ziegler, and A. M. O'Donnell, *Infant Nutrition,* W. B. Saunders Company, Philadelphia, 1974.

[c] D. R. Brown, R. C. Tsang, and I. U. Chen, "Oral Calcium Supplementation in Premature and Asphyxiated Neonates," *Journal of Pediatrics,* **89**(6):976, 1976.

[d] G. M. Chance et al., "Growth and Mineral Metabolism in Very Low Birth Weight Infants, II Effects of Calcium Supplementation on Growth and Divalent Cations," *Pediatric Research,* **9**(7):568–575, 1975.

[e] P. R. Dallman, "Iron, Vitamin E, and Folate in the Preterm Infant," *Journal of Pediatrics,* **85**(6):742–752, 1974.

[f] R. N. Roy and J. C. Sinclair, "Hydration of the Low Birth-Weight Infant," *Clinics in Perinatology,* **2**(2):393, 1975.

[g] J. E. Graeber, M. L. Williams, and F. A. Oski, "The Use of Intramuscular Vitamin E in the Premature Infant," *Journal of Pediatrics,* **90**(2):282–284, 1977.

[h] C. L. Abitol et al., "Plasma Amino Acid Pattern During Supplemental Intravenous Nutrition of Low-Birth-Weight Infants," *Journal of Pediatrics,* **88**(2):178, 1976.

monitored by a pump (see Fig. 24-3). Glucose must be started at lower concentrations (8 to 10 percent) and gradually increased according to individual tolerance. Electrolytes and minerals are adjusted according to clinical and chemical feedback information. Achieving desired energy level without hyperglycemia usually requires 7 to 10 days. After 2 to 3 weeks of TPN, the clinical status of the patient should be assessed to determine the safety of beginning oral feedings. When oral route is established, the solution is proportionately decreased, and then discontinued when fluid and caloric requirements can be adequately met by enteral feedings alone. The time required to meet desired energy levels can be delayed by episodes of hyperglycemia, a common metabolic problem. Small doses of insulin (0.25 to 0.50 unit/(kg · day) minimize its occurrence and improve adaptation.

The investigational nature of TPN for LBW infants is easily understood when some of the complexities of management and solution formulation are considered. Metabolic complications such as hyper- or hyponatremia, kalemia, chloremia, calcemia, phosphatemia, and magnesemia are commonly iatrogenic. Constant monitoring and adjustment are required. Some complications are the result of protein source. Hyperchloremic metabolic acidosis occurs with the use of certain crystalline amino acids. Hyperammonemia is associated with protein hydrolysates which contain preformed NH_3. The more frequent and potentially hazardous complication of abormal aminograms likewise stems from currently available nitrogen sources.

Underdeveloped enzyme systems alter amino acid requirements for premature infants. Crystalline amino acid mixtures and protein hydrolysates have not been customized to these special requirements. Amino acids which bypass the liver are not subject to the usual liver control. With normal ingestion, digestion, and absorption, peripheral plasma will have maximal amino acid levels 2 h postprandially. Elevations are small in comparison with ingested food, and return to near fasting levels within 4 to 5 h. Parenteral amino acids, on the other hand, are delivered directly to the tissues, and in a different mixture. The premature infant may be at a disadvantage dealing with increased levels of some of the amino acids in light of his underdeveloped enzyme systems. Too rapid infusion rates may add to the difficulty of rearranging amino acid mixtures into the precise composition preferred by the tissue. Stegink, studying plasma amino acids of infants being alimented with casein and fibrin hydrolysates, noted that plasma patterns reflected compositional differences of the products and differed from normal fasting amino acid levels.[104] Current protein hydroly-

sates and crystalline amino acid mixtures are largely devoid of cystine and contain very low levels of tyrosine (both considered essential for the premature). Imbalances in the mixture of free amino acids normally found in cell sap may impede protein synthesis.

Abitol et al.[105] compared plasma aminograms of LBW infants with those of full-term infants and adults. Normal full-term infants had aminograms very similar to the adult. LBW patterns were significantly lower in some of the nonessential amino acids (glutamine, alanine, glycine, ornothine) and also low in the essential amino acid histidine. Weekly plasma amino acids of parenterally fed infants showed marked changes and identified the premature's increased "nonessential" needs. Although most amino acids did not exceed normal ranges in the parenterally fed, indicating efficient metabolism even in the face of high infusion concentrations, threonine, serine, and methionine accumulated to abnormal levels. Enzymatic deficiencies for metabolic pathways are suggested. The casein hydrolysate used as the nitrogen source in the Abitol study contained high concentrations of glutamic acid. However, the hypoglutaminemia characteristic of LBW infants was not improved. Deleterious effects of glutamate on the CNS have been demonstrated in animals, and low levels of glutamine may be associated with mental retardation. Conversion of glutamate to glutamine apparently is not managed well by the LBW infant. Nitrogen preparations which eliminate glutamic acid and provide glutamine instead would seem preferable. The hypermethioninemia also observed by Abitol indicates insufficient synthesis of cystine, and supports the essentiality of this amino acid for the LBW infant. All the LBW infants studied exhibited tyrosinemia. While infants were on intravenous alimentation, their plasma tyrosine returned to normal, but when the IV solution was discontinued, tyrosine levels almost doubled. Ascorbic acid, provided in the IV solution at the 100-mg level, acting as a reducing agent, substituted for the missing enzyme and enhanced tyrosine metabolism. Oral supplements given with the discontinuance of hyperalimentation provided only 60 mg of the vitamin, and did not sufficiently compensate for the enzyme lack.

The question of peptide utilization is another point of interest in the discussion of TPN management for LBW infants. Protein hydrolysates, unlike crystalline amino acids, have only 40 to 50 percent of their total N_2 as free amino acids; the remainder is in the form of peptides. Peptides are normally hydrolyzed at the brush border of the intestinal cell, with practically no peptides entering portal blood. However, when hydrolysates are used as the protein source in TPN, the peptides presented for utilization must be metabolized by the kidney or taken to the tissues intact. Little is known about utilization of these infused peptides. In addition, there is decreased availability of amino acids when hydrolysates are autoclaved with glucose during IV infusate preparation. Glucose reacts with certain amino acids to form sugar complexes, and reaction rates are accelerated by heat. The sugar–amino acid complexes formed during autoclaving cannot be utilized. When sterile glucose is introduced into hydrolysates just before infusing, utilization is increased substantially. Decreased formation of sugar complexes is also desirable as they have been found to chelate trace minerals, increasing urinary excretion of zinc, copper, and iron.[106]

Cautious exploration in the use of TPN in selected LBW infants is indicated, for with all its flaws, TPN has contributed to the survival of high-risk infants. Its use should be limited to those for whom there are no other reasonable alternatives. Risk of sepsis and possible deleterious consequences of amino acid imbalance are serious considerations. Long-term follow-up, with examination of risks and metabolic implications, applied to formulations and techniques of management, may justify expansion of its use. Winters summed it up well in his introduction to a conference on hyperalimentation:

What metabolic consequences result from providing a nutritionally complete intake of foods to an infant in whom the route of delivery bypasses the gastrointestinal tract and the liver? As someone has quipped, "to eat is human but to digest divine." . . . we want to know if our man-made attempts to replace the deity are good enough, or how they may be improved.[107]

Total Intravenous Alimentation— Peripheral

Providing total nutrition peripherally taxes fluid tolerance and the ability to maintain infusion sites. Reasonable volumes require highly osmolar solutions. The use of less concentrated mixtures often fails to meet nutritional requirements for growth due to volume limitations. Addition of a fat source, as Intralipid, increases calories without contributing to osmolality. The soybean oil mixture used provides 11 kcal (46.2 kJ)/10 ml. Because it is not miscible with amino acid solutions it must be infused separately, joining the carbohydrate–amino acid line just before entering the vein.

Nutrient mixtures are similar to those given by central line except that glucose solutions of only 8 to 10 percent are used. As potential metabolic complications are similar, chemical monitoring is likewise required. A major concern with the use of Intralipid is the rate of clearance of the lipid fraction by LBW infants. Serum lipemia should be measured daily, and with elevation, the fat mixture should be decreased or discontinued. Elimination curves in newborn LBWs were studied by Victorin.[108] Maximal removal capacity of both AGA and SGA infants of less than 2500 g birth weights were equal. However, the small-for-dates cleared fat more slowly. There is a similarity between the body's handling of natural chylomicrons and the Intralipid emulsion which delivers fat particles of similar size. Most of the IV fat is taken up by the liver to reappear as very low density lipoprotein or pre-beta-lipoproteins. Side effects from Intralipid have been minimal, and primarily febrile. Stability of the solution has been suggested as a possible factor, as particle size may increase if solutions are kept too warm.

Elevated serum triglycerides, observed with the use of Intralipid, can have varying affects. Glucose metabolism is inhibited by high concentrations of free fatty acids (FFAs), thereby decreasing glucose tolerance. Growth hormone is depressed by FFAs. Metabolic acidosis has been observed. Increased risk of kernicterus (deposits of bile pigments in basal ganglia) may also accompany elevated FFA levels, as fatty acids are believed to displace unconjugated bilirubin from albumin (the main carrier of FFA in the blood).

The possibility that fat particles might bind lipophilic free bilirubin, and thus be beneficial to the jaundiced infant, has been suggested. However, excess FFAs can competitively displace bilirubin from its primary binding site on albumin. Bilirubin will preferentially bind to albumin, plasma proteins, and red cells before adhering to Intralipid particles. To facilitate plasma transport, the FFAs metabolized from Intralipid bind to several sites on the albumin molecule, one of which is the primary binding site of bilirubin. Therefore, Intralipid is not recommended in the presence of jaundice.[109]

Elevated vitamin E needs should be considered, as Intralipid is a polyunsaturated fat.

Intralipid's caloric advantage must be weighed against its possible hazards. While increasing adequacy and efficiency of peripheral alimentation, this technique is not yet considered routine for LBW infants. Gaps in current knowledge must be filled to define clearly the acceptable tolerance for marginal intake—if indeed there is any. Suboptimal growth rates in the early neonatal period may contribute to nonrecoupable CNS deficits. The long-range consequences of providing too much too soon, in the presence of underdeveloped processing systems, likewise need to be known.

Intravenous Supplementation of Tolerated Oral Feedings

"Conventional" nutrition management of LBW infants presently supplements possible oral intake with 10 percent glucose by IV. Increasingly, supplemental IV includes amino acids and/or lipid. Infusion sites rarely last more than 24 h, and maintenance of infusion can become a serious limitation. Studies reviewed by Heird[110] indicate that the use of nitrogen-containing supplements results in more rapid regain of birth weight than the use of glucose solutions alone. Significantly greater overall weight gains can also achieved. The case study reviewed on page 584 illustrates this method of management. Complications will include those common to both enteral and IV nutrient delivery. However, oral amounts are small, minimizing the risk of aspiration. There may be a theoretical advantage to initiating natural digestive and absorptive processes early and gradually. The use of breast milk as the oral aliment provides immunologic advantages which may be critical to the underdeveloped infant. Developmental consequences of immaturity likewise involve immune systems.

Nasojejunal Feeding

Successful use of this method of feeding has been reported by Rhea[111] and Cheek and Staub.[112] Nasojejunal approach overcomes sucking and swallowing problems, avoiding regurgitation and aspiration, and overcomes volume limitations due to delayed gastric emptying. A silastic catheter, positioned in the upper jejunum, is used for the passage of glucose initially, followed by gradually increasing volumes of breast milk or formula. A constant infusion pump regulates flow, providing continuous drip. Although metabolic problems have not been reported, incidences of intestinal perforation in VLBW infants in whom polyvinyl catheters were used have occurred. As quickly as 6 to 8 h after insertion into the jejunum, vinyl tubes stiffen, predisposing to perforation. This has been especially true with repositioning of the tube.[113]

Increasing incidence of necrotizing enterocolitis with the use of nasojejunal feeding has also been associated with the smaller prematures. Heird emphasizes the importance of patient selection in the choice of feeding method.[114] Successful use of this method of feeding has involved infants weighing more than 1500 g. As with any feeding method, advantages are not provided to all LBW infants, and the VLBW in particular may require more caution. Perhaps with these infants, insuring sufficient nutriment to support normal cell division is the first order of business, with provision of more concentrated aliment which allows for "catch-up" a later goal. Paralleling intrauterine growth rates in the VLBW infants may create more hazard than advantage.

Conventional Nipple and Gavage

Infants weighing more than 2000 g, in the absence of respiratory distress or other disease, can usually be fed by the bottle, following normal newborn infant feeding procedures. Advantages of breast-milk feeding is discussed on page 582. Infants of lesser weights should be evaluated for evidence of respiratory distress, other disease problems, and ability to suck. Infants less than 34 weeks gestation can be expected to have sucking and swallowing incoordination and inadequate gag reflex. Within reason, a trial at conventional feeding should be given. When there is no respiratory, cardiac, or CNS distress, hydration and nutrition should be begun within 4 to 6 h of birth. Delay in providing energy source can produce hypoglycemia; chilling with its increased energy needs increases risk.

To determine patency of the gastrointestinal tract, an initial feeding of distilled water is recommended, as it is less damaging if aspirated. In general, infants less than 32 weeks gestation will require gavage feeding. Gavage minimizes energy demands. Feedings should always be introduced by gravity and not under pressure. Initial feeding size varies with birth weight and is based on estimation of stomach volume. A suggested early gavage schedule is presented in Table 26-10. Subsequent feedings can be of breast milk or formula; dilution is not

TABLE 26-10 SUGGESTED EARLY GAVAGE FEEDING SCHEDULE

Body weight	Initial feeding	Advancement	Frequency
1000 g	3 ml	1 ml/fdg to 10 ml	q 1–2 h*
1.0–1.5 kg	5 ml	2 ml/fdg to 15 ml	q 2–3 h
1.5–2.0 kg	7 ml	3 ml/fdg to 20 ml	q 3 h
2.0–2.5 kg	9 ml	3 ml/fdg to 25 ml	q 3 h
2.5 kg	15 ml	3–5 ml/fdg to 40 ml	q 4 hr

* q = every.

Source: Newborn Nursery, Children's Hospital Medical Center, Boston, Mass.

recommended. As volumes consumed during the first week are small, formulas with low renal solute load should be chosen. (See Formula Comparison Chart, Table 12-3.)

Most LBW infants will require some IV supplementation the first few days of life while gradual increase in gastrointestinal intake is being achieved. Glucose and electrolyte solutions will satisfy fluid requirements and early maintenance needs, and only when insufficient intake is expected to continue beyond 5 to 7 days should additional nitrogen source and/or lipid be considered. Vomiting, aspiration, and distention require reduction or discontinuance of oral intake. Questions of stomach emptying should be resolved by aspirating the stomach prior to the next feeding. With more than one-quarter retention of previous feeding, volume should be decreased or temporarily discontinued. Sepsis is likewise an indication for ceasing oral intake.[115] When delayed gastric emptying continues to seriously hamper caloric goals, nasojejunal feeding in larger prematures might be considered. Smaller LBW infants will require balancing decreased oral capacity with protein-lipid IV supplement. Only when oral intake is contraindicated should total intravenous alimentation become the method of management.

Table 26-11 summarizes and compares the various feeding approaches.

TABLE 26-11 COMPENDIUM OF FEEDING METHODS

Feeding method	Nutrient delivery	Technique	Complications	Considerations	Advantages
Total Intravenous Alimentation					
Central Line	Amino acid hydrolysates or crystalline amino acids, 2.5 g/(kg · day). 20% glucose sol. Electrolyte, vitamin, and mineral additives	Slow and continuous infusion of approx. 130 ml/(kg · day) into superior vena cava via external or internal jugular vein. Gradual increase from 8 to 20% CHO conc. required to establish tolerance	Hyperglycemia. Increased BUN and hyperammonemia with high protein intakes. Abnormal plasma aminograms. Hyperchloremic metabolic acidosis with crystalline amino acids. Essential fatty acid deficiency. Zinc and copper deficiency. Sepsis	Frequent chemical monitoring. Meticulous aseptic technique in preparation of solutions, placement of catheter, and its subsequent care	Decreased energy expenditure through elimination of digestion and absorption. Eliminates stress of intermittent dietary loads. More rapid weight gain induced earlier, with faster regain of birth weight
Peripheral	Amino acid hydrolysates or crystalline amino acids. 2.5 g/(kg · day). 10% glucose sol. with or without Intralipid. Electrolyte, vitamin, & mineral additives	Slow and continuous infusion into superficial scalp veins. Intralipid infused separately	Sclerosis at infusion site. With use of Intralipid: Lipemia ↑ serum fatty acids ↑ risk of kernicterus	Need for vitamin E with use of Intralipid. Intralipid contraindicated with jaundice. Intralipid should be used cautiously—maximum of 2 g/(kg · day) (adult dose as indicated by manufacturer)	Avoids central line. ↓ Septic complications. Essential fatty acid provided by lipid
Intravenous supplementation of tolerated oral feedings	Breast milk or formula 10% glucose with or without amino acids or lipid	Peripheral infusion oral aliment by gavage or nipple. With increase in oral intake, concomitant decrease in IV	Includes those of IV aspiration		Reduced risk of aspiration due to small size of feeding. Early and gradual stimulation of natural digestive and absorptive processes. Immunological advantages with the use of breast milk
Nasojejunal	Initially glucose. Breast milk or formula	Nasal insertion of small silastic catheter into upper jejunum. Aliment infused at continuous rate. Amount increased slowly until desired caloric level reached	Perforation reported with the use of polyvinyl tubing	Formulas of high osmolality less well tolerated. Assoc. with ↑ incidence of NEC* in presence of hypoxia, acidosis, and hypothermia, and with infants, 1200 g	Bypasses problems of poor suck, uncoordinated swallowing, delayed gastric emptying. No reported metabolic consequences
Nipple or gavage	Initial feeding sterile water. Breast milk or formula	Over 2000 g, likely by nipple. <2000 g, prior to 32 wk, by gavage. Feeding tube passed through nose and mouth into stomach. Removed after each feeding	Aspiration in LBW less than 34 wk. Malabsorption	Within reason, trial at conventional feeding precedes choice of other feeding methods	

* *Necrotizing enterocolitis*

CUSTOMIZING FORMULA

A hypothetical LBW male infant of 34 weeks gestation, weighing 2000 g, has adapted well to extrauterine existence during the first week of life. He is tolerating 25 ml of a casein-lactalbumin adjusted formula every 3 h very well. A review of this infant's nutritional needs according to Tables 26-8 and 26-9 indicates that 230 kcal (966 kJ), 4.4 g protein, and 155 to 320 ml fluid should be provided. The 200 ml of the formula presently tolerated provides approximately 15 g carbohydrate, 3 g protein, and 8 g fat, or 144 kcal (604.8 kJ). (See Formula Comparison Chart, Table 12-3.) The 72 kcal (302 kJ)/kg available meets resting and intermittent activity energy requirements, however, desired growth will not be supported with formula alone at normal 20 kcal (84 kJ)/ounce concentration. If additional intravenous supplements are to be discontinued and the same formula is to be used, increasing volumes and concentrations will become necessary. With an increase in energy density to 25 kcal (105 kJ)/oz, a total volume of 275 ml will be required, or 35 ml per feeding if a schedule of feedings every 3 h is to continue. Maintaining normal formula concentration of 20 kcal (84 kJ)/oz will require 30-ml feedings every 2 h to furnish the required calories.

Energy density of a formula can be increased through addition of carbohydrate, by increasing concentration of all constituents, or by the addition of fat. The carbohydrate used may be corn syrup or dextrose, which will increase osmolarity—or Polycose, a glucose polymer which does not exert as much of an osmolar load. MCT (medium-chain triglycerides), a concentrated source of calories, provides 7.6 kcal (31.9 kJ)/ml. Increasing calories by concentration adds protein to the same volume, raising renal solute load. Table 26-12 provides the ratios of formula to water required to adjust concentrations. Options available for tailoring formula to individual infant tolerance and needs are illustrated in Table 26-13. The initial 25 ml × 8 regimen cited above for our hypothetical infant provides a basis for comparison. Other available premature formulation are also included.

Compositional differences, other than calories and protein, are considered when choosing formulas most suitable for individual premature infant's oral intake. Variations in calcium, electrolyte, protein, and carbohydrate sources are summarized in the Formula Comparison Chart, Table 12-3. Both Similac PM 60/40 and SMA have had demineralized cow's-milk whey added to their formulations. The increased lactalbumin provides a ratio of calcium to lactalbumin which more closely resembles mother's milk. However, compositional differences exist between human and cow's whey. Human whey contains equal amounts of lactoferrin and alpha-lactalbumin. Cow's whey contains no lactoferrin and three-fifths the amount of lactalbumin. Varying opinions exist regarding the actual benefits of the additional whey. Raïhä, unable to demonstrate advantages in high protein intakes,[116] emphasizes qualitative importance. Foman suggests nutritional advantage has not been demonstrated.[117] Low calcium and electrolyte levels of both formulas, while not imposing undue load on the kidney, may not meet mineral needs of growth, and accentuate the problem of hyponatremia. Effects on trace minerals of the electrophoresis process used to demineralize the whey are not known. Amounts of trace minerals provided would appear to be sufficient. Mead Johnson's premature formula provides carbohydrate as both lactose and sucrose, and furnishes fat calories with a blend of MCT, corn, and coconut oil. Initial low lactase activity and the greater degree of malabsorption common to prematures has been considered. As with feeding methods, no one oral formulation addresses all conceivable limitations. Conversely, most formulas—except those of high osmolality, will adequately nourish most prematures when sufficient intakes can be achieved. Older prematures and SFD term infants have greater tolerance for increased caloric density because of their

TABLE 26-12 ADJUSTING FORMULA CONCENTRATIONS

By additions to standard 20 kcal/oz/(84 kJ/oz) concentration:

Karo 4 kcal/ml–60 kcal/tbsp (15 ml) (16.8 kJ/ml–252 kJ/tbsp)
MCT 7.6 kcal/ml–115 kcal/tbsp (31.9 kJ/ml–483kJ/tbsp)
Polycose
    Powder 3.75 kcal/g–30 kcal/tbsp (15.75 kJ/g–126 kJ/tbsp)
    Liquid 2.00 kcal/ml–30 kcal/tbsp (8.4 kJ/ml–126 kJ/tbsp)

By altering standard dilutions:

Powders	*kcal/oz*	*kJ/oz*	*Tbsp powder per 2 oz H_2O*
Standard	20	84	1
Increased conc.	25	105	1¼
	30	126	1½
Decreased conc.	15	63	¾
	10	42	½

Liquid Concentrates			*Ratio of conc. formula: H_2O*
Standard	20	84	1:1
Increased conc.	25	105	5:3
	30	126	3:1
Decreased conc.	15	63	3:5
	10	42	1:3

more mature enzyme systems and renal capacity. Their catch-up growth potential must be encouraged. Formulations of normal dilution with low mineral content are contraindicated for their management.

Foman submits specifications for formula which considers LBW infant characteristics and requirements.[118] He recommends an energy density of 80 to 100 kcal (336–420 kJ)/100 ml, or 24 to 30 kcal (100.8–126 kJ)/oz. Protein, derived from fat-free milk solids, should provide 11 percent of energy or 2.8 g/100 kcal (420 kJ) (2.2–2.8 g/100 ml). He recommends fat blends which are well absorbed—vegetable oils, vegetable oils and lard with or without MCT. Fifty percent of the energy should be derived from fat which would furnish 4.4 to 5.5 g/100 ml. To prevent excessive lactose loads he suggests one-half to one-third of the carbohydrate be lactose, with the remainder derived from corn syrup solids. Calcium supplied in the above formulation would be grossly below estimated needs and would require supplementation. His recommended formula would have an increased renal solute load which would require monitoring for safety. With urine osmolality exceeding 400 mosmol, he suggests increasing intake above 140 kcal (588 kJ)/kg or reducing caloric concentrations.

ROLE OF BREAST MILK IN NUTRITIONAL MANAGEMENT OF LBW INFANTS

Commercial formulas come close but have not been able to improve upon nature's formulation for nurturing the newborn. However, as

TABLE 26-13 OPTIONS FOR CUSTOMIZING STANDARD FORMULAS

| Options | Volume | Energy | | Protein, g/kg | Adequacy* | | Potential renal solute lead |
		kcal/kg	kJ/kg		% energy	% protein	
Casein-lactalbumin adjusted SMA or PM 60/40 20 kcal/oz	25 × 8 200 ml	72	302	1.5	63	67	94 mosmol/l
Continue 20 kcal/oz ↑ Volume	30 × 12 360 ml	120	504	2.8	104	127	94 mosmol/l
↑ Conc. by addit. CHO or MCT to 25 kcal/oz	35 × 8 280 ml	116	487	2.2	101	100	94 mosmol/l
	30 × 10 300 ml	125	525	2.3	109	105	94 mosmol/l
↑ to 25 kcal/oz by conc	35 × 8 30 × 10	116 125	487 525	3.1 3.3	101 109	141 150	127 to 132 mosmol/l (estimated)
Ross Similac 24 kcal/oz	280 ml 300 ml	112 120	470 504	3.1 3.3	97 104	141 150	149 mosmol/l
Mead Johnson Premature 24 kcal/oz	280 ml 300 ml	112 120	470 504	3.1 3.3	97 104	141 150	144 mosmol/l

* Assuming 115 kcal/kg (483 kJ/kg) 2.2 g protein/kg = desirable intake. Lower ranges as presented on Table 26-9. Based on hypothetical LBW infant of 34 weeks gestation, birth weight 2000 g, otherwise well and tolerating oral feedings well.

techniques for premature management make it possible for younger, smaller infants to survive, nature's perfect blend is being evaluated from a different perspective. Foman expresses reservations regarding the use of breast milk for infants less than 1500 g.[119] With seriously ill LBW infants not growing, or growing slowly, advantages of breast milk may indicate its preferential use. The rapidly growing premature, however, has estimated needs substantially in excess of the quantities of nutrients provided by human milk. Foman estimates that breast milk provides the following percentages of advisable intake for a hypothetical 1200-g LBW infant gaining at 20 g/day: 53 percent of the protein, 23 percent of the calcium, and 72 percent of the sodium. Intended for the full-term infant, capable of consuming larger amounts, breast milk is insufficiently concentrated for the decreased intake of the premature infant.

The unique properties of breast milk[120–122] provide many advantages which cannot be discounted. Its higher cystine content is of interest in light of the premature's lack of cystathionase and subsequent inability to synthesize cystine from methionine. Higher percentage of non-protein nitrogen, higher lactalbumin/casein ratio, and different nucleotide patterns may account for better utilization of its lower protein content. Fatty acid differences and presence of lipase in breast milk improve fat digestion and absorption. The higher cholesterol content of human milk may be instrumental in the proper development of enzyme systems necessary for the maintenance of cholesterol homeostasis. To the premature, highly susceptible to sepsis, the bacteriostatic properties may be the most critical advantage. Bifidus factor, a nitrogen-containing polysaccharide found in breast milk, promotes the growth of *Lactobacillus bifidus*. These bacteria produce an acid media which is not conducive to intestinal growth of *Shigella, Escherichia coli,* or yeast. Antistaphylococcal factors, antibodies (particularly IgA), and macrophages have been demonstrated to be present in human milk.

Coincidentally, or as a direct result, the use of more concentrated formulas has been associated with increased incidence of necrotizing enterocolitis (NEC). Various causes have been suggested in addition to intolerance to enteric feeding, including ischemic intestinal damage (possibly the result of perinatal hypotension and hypoxemia) followed by bacterial invasion. Both formula and enteric bacteria are necessary for the production of hydrogen gas, which is a major constituent of the intramural gas found in NEC.[123] Intestinal colonization with *Klebsiella* (an able hydrogen producer) has been found to be increased in NEC patients. Macrophages of breast milk have been found able to kill *Klebsiella.*[124] Decreased carbohydrate absorption has been demonstrated 1 to 4 days prior to onset of gastrointestinal bleeding, abdominal distention, poor feeding, or emesis in 10 of 14 patients who developed NEC.[125] Although withholding of oral feedings in infants with increased fecal reducing substance

has not been shown to prevent development of NEC, formula-fed premature infants with higher than 2+ reducing substance deserve careful observation for signs and symptoms.

The advantages of human milk recommend its use, although its inadequacies for the rapidly growing premature would seem to require protein and mineral supplementation. The psychological indication for utilization of a mother's milk in the care of her infant should not be overlooked. The helplessness experienced by mothers of tiny, critically ill infants, and the separation imposed by long-delayed opportunities for mothering, can be partially assuaged by providing this personal and vital contribution to the infant's care. Early establishment of mother-infant attachment is important. Normal growth and development, and adaptation to extrauterine life, may be impeded by the unstimulating environment of the incubator. Recently more attention has been directed toward enhancing the premature's development by simulating intrauterine environments with rocking waterbeds and tape recordings of heartbeat and woman's voice.[126] Critical care units today are less "off limits" and encourage parent visitation and interaction.

CASE STUDY AND DISCUSSION 26-1

A 964-g infant was delivered by cesarean section at 28 weeks due to abruptio placentae. Her birth weight placed her at the 25th percentile on Lubchenco's intrauterine weight chart (males and females).[127] With an Apgar score of one at 1 min, the infant was immediately intubated and placed on 100 percent oxygen, which was reduced to 35 percent within 8 h. However, the infant was maintained on a respirator for 5 days, and during the early weeks of life continued to experience recurrent episodes of apnea and bradycardia. Her respiratory distress intermittently required nasal CPAP (continuous positive

airway pressure), which compromised ability to feed by mouth.

Initially, 3 ml D_5W pg every 2 h was tolerated, with an IV ($D_{10}W$) running at 4 cc/h. Elevated bilirubin, which peaked on day 5, was treated by phototheraphy. Early episodes of apnea limited intake to less than maintenance energy, and therefore hyperalimentation, using 1.5 percent Freamine (crystalline amino acids) in $D_{10}W$, , was begun on the third day. Mother's milk, by gavage, augmented intake, and energy increased to 70 kcal (294 kJ)/kg. By day 6, weight had fallen to 850 g—a 12 percent loss of birth weight—and intake had reached a marginal 80 kcal (336 kJ)/kg.

Over the next few days, small increases in the intake of breast milk, along with the addition of MCT, raised energy over 100 kcal (420 kJ)/kg. A 2 percent amino acid IV infusate, along with the protein present in the milk, provided 2.5 g protein/kg. However, respiratory problems requiring nasal CPAP continued, and missed feedings decreased total intake. Between the 10th and 15th days, consistent weight gain was not achieved, and the decision was made to institute Intralipid and discontinue gavage feedings. Administration of 5 ml/h of a 2.5 percent Freamine solution in $D_{10}W$ was begun, with 15 ml of Intralipid being infused separately. In this manner, 3 g protein and approximately 80 kcal (366 kJ)/kg were provided.

During the ensuing 5 days, feedings were withheld and gradual increases in total daily volumes of IV and Intralipid were made. By the 20th day, after the achievement of 100 kcal (420 kJ)/kg intake, birth weight had been regained, and a steady weight gain became evident. A

Figure 26-5
Correlation of weight with various feeding methods.

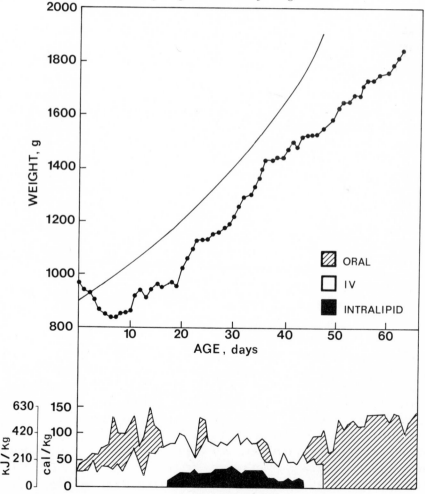

gradual reinstitution of oral feedings was attempted using half-strength breast milk. Again apnea and bradycardia required discontinuance of feedings.

At 5 weeks, with apnea apparently resolved, oral feedings were slowly begun and decreases in daily volumes of IV and Intralipid were planned. For each 10 g of oral fat intake, Intralipid was decreased by 5 g, or 5 ml. The formula being used, Similac PM 60/40, provided 3.5 g fat/100 ml, and the infant tolerated 5 ml every 2 h, or 60 ml/day, without aspiration. Weight steadily increased. Supplements of 25 IU of vitamin E were supplied daily. With recurrence of bradycardic episodes and discontinued oral intake, energy dipped to a low of 50 kcal (210 kJ)/kg on day 39. Poor intake persisted for several days as difficulties were experienced in the placement of IV.

Intralipid was discontinued on the 43d day. During Intralipid administration, weight increased by 570 g (950 to 1520) with an average daily gain of 20 g. During this time, IV and Intralipid provided a maximum of 100 kcal/kg. It is interesting to note in Fig. 26-5, which summarizes the correlation between caloric intake and weight gain, the extent of the decrease in energy required to support growth when it is provided intravenously.

With the resolution of respiratory problems, increasing volumes of formula intake became possible. Within several days of Intralipid discontinuance, IV was replaced totally by Similac PM 60/40 (10 ml every 2 h with 0.6 ml MCT added to each feed). Within 3 days, 125 kcal (525 kJ)/kg was consumed, providing a total of 1.8 g protein, which produced daily weight gains of 15 to 30 g.

By the 50th day, the infant succeeded in taking 30 ml of formula by bottle, and over the next 2 weeks managed to achieve total intake (in excess of 125 kcal (525 kJ)/kg) by bottle. At 72 days of life—the equivalent of 38 weeks gestation—weighing 2100 g, the infant was discharged on an iron-fortified formula, standard 20 kcal (84 kJ)/oz, with additional vitamin supplements. Prior to discharge, and once the infant was tolerating oral feedings, the parents were encouraged to feed their infant on visits to the newborn nursery. Their involvement familiarized them with the feedings and helped them to recognize the components of their infant's feeding behavior. They were able to approach what could have been a tense situation in a more relaxed manner. After discharge, close follow-up, with periodic formula adjustments and much parental support was provided.

STUDY QUESTIONS

1 How are nitrosamines formed in the body?

2 Distinquish between benign and malignant tumors.

3 What nutritional problems can you anticipate when a patient receives radiation to the head and neck area?

4 Why is it essential that inborn errors of metabolism be diagnosed and treated as early as possible?

5 What is the physiological change detected by the Guthrie screening test for PKU.

6 What does dietary treatment of a child with PKU involve? What indices are used to measure success?

7 Describe the interdisciplinary team approach to treatment of inborn errors of metabolism.

8 What do the terms *small for gestational age* (SGA) and *small for dates* (SFD) mean?

9 Under what weight are infants classified as low-birth-weight (LBW)?

10 Cite the nutritional hazards of the SGA and the premature infant.

11 Discuss the energy, protein, fluid, and vitamin-mineral concerns of the LBW infant.

12 What different feeding approaches are used for the low-birth-weight infant? Discuss the advantages and complications of each.

REFERENCES

1 American Cancer Society, *Cancer Statistics,* Professional Education Publications, 1976, p. 4.

2 Ibid., pp. 16–17.

3 American Cancer Society, *Nutrition and Cancer,* Professional Education Publications, 1972, p. 5.

4 John Berg, "Nutrition and Cancer," *Seminars in Oncology,* 3:17–23, 1976.

5 Ibid., p. 18.

6 National Academy of Sciences, *Sweeteners, Issues and Uncertainties,* Washington, D.C., 1975, p. 138.

7 The Committee on Professional Education, International Union Against Cancer, *Clinical Oncology,* 1975, p. 27.

8 Ibid., p. 27.

9 Council for the Analysis and Projection of the American Cancer Society, "Working Conference on Anorexia and Neoplastic Disease," *Cancer and Research,* November 1970, p. 2816.

10 E. Copeland and S. Dudrick, "Cancer: Nutritional Concepts," *Seminars in Oncology,* 2:329, 1975.

11 E. Copeland et al., "Intravenous Hyperalimentation in Patients with Head and Neck Cancer," *Cancer,* March 1975, p. 610.

12 E. Steiger et al., "Effects of Nutrition on Tumor Growth and Tolerance to Chemotherapy," *Journal of Surgical Research,* 18:455–461, 1975.

13 S. Hegedus and M. Pelham, "Dietetics in a Cancer Hospital," *Journal of The American Dietetic Association,* 67:238, 1975.

14 A. Prader, "Inborn Errors of Metabolism," *Bibliotheca Nutritio et Dieta,* no. 18, 1973, p. 179.

15 Neil A. Holtzman, "Dietary Treatment of Inborn Errors of Metabolism," *Annual Review of Medicine,* 21:335, 1970.

16 James S. Thompson and Margaret W. Thompson, *Genetics in Medicine,* 2d ed., W. B. Saunders Company, Philadelphia, 1973, p. 435.

17 H. Ghadimi, "Diagnosis of Inborn Errors of Metabolism," *American Journal of Diseases in Childhood,* 114:435, 1967.

18 Barbara Burton, Albert B. Gerbie, and Henry L. Nadler, "Present Status of Intrauterine Diagnosis of Genetic Defects," *American Journal of Obstetrics and Gynecology,* 118:718, 1974.

19 American Academy of Pediatrics, Committee on Nutrition, "Special Diets for Infants with Inborn Errors of Metabolism," *Pediatrics,* 57:783, 1976.

20 Robert Guthrie and Ada Susi, "Simple Phenylalanine Method for Detecting Phenylketonuria in Large Populations of Newborn Infants," *Pediatrics,* 32:338, 1963.

21 Committee for the Study of Inborn Errors of Metabolism, *Genetic Screening: Programs, Principles, and Research,* National Academy of Sciences, National Research Council, Washington, D.C., 1975, p. 293.

22 Ibid., p. 91.

23 American Academy of Pediatrics, *Standards of Child Health Care,* American Academy of Pediatrics, Evanston, Ill., 1972, p. 23.

24 Carol S. Shear, Nancy S. Wellman, and William L. Nyhan, "Phenylketonuria: Experience with Diagnosis and Management," in William L. Nyhan (ed.), *Heritable Disorders of Amino Acid Metabolism,* John Wiley & Sons, Inc., 1974, p. 143.

25 J. Dobson, R. Koch, M. Williamson, R. Spector, W. Frankenburg, M. O'Flynn, R. Warner, and F. Hudson, "Cognitive Development and Dietary Therapy in Phenylketonuric Children," *New England Journal of Medicine,* 278:1142, 1968.

26 Richard Koch, Milan Blaskovics, Elizabeth Wenz, Karol Fishler, and Graciela Schaeffler, "Phenylalaninemia and Phenylketonuria," in William L. Nyhan (ed.), op. cit., p. 121.

27 L. E. Holt and E. E. Synderman, "Amino Acid Requirements of Children," in W. E. Nyhan, *Amino Acid Metabolism and Genetic Variation,* McGraw-Hill Book Company, New York, 1967, pp. 381–391.

28 Barbara E. Clayton, "Principles of Treatment by Dietary Restriction as Illustrated by Phenylketonuria," in N. Raine (ed.), *The Treatment of Inherited Metabolic Disease,* American Elsevier Publishing Co., Inc., New York, 1975, p. 13.

29 Robert A. MacGready and Harvey L. Levy, "Problem of Maternal Phenylketonuria," *American Journal of Obstetrics and Gynecology,* 113: 121, 1972.

30 Barbara E. Clayton, op. cit., p. 3.

31 R. Koch, N. F. Shaw, P. B. Acosta, K. Fishler, G. Schaeffler, E. Wenz, and A. Wohlers, "Approach to the Management of Phenylketonuria," *Journal of Pediatrics,* 76:826, 1970.

32 R. J. Grand, J. B. Watkins, and F. M. Torti, "Development of the Human Gastrointestinal Tract, A Review," *Gastroenterology,* 70(5):792, 1976.

33 L. O. Lubchenco, C. Hansman, M. Dressler, and E. Boyd, "Intrauterine Growth as Estimated from Liveborn Birth-Weight Data at 24–42 Weeks of Gestation," *Pediatrics,* 32(5):793–800, 1963.

34 J. R. St. Petery, "The High Risk Infant and Family," *Comprehensive Pediatric Nursing,* McGraw-Hill Book Company, New York, 1975, p. 311.

35 L. O. Lubchenco et al., "Long-Term Follow-up Studies of Prematurely Born Infants. I. Relationship of Handicaps to Nursing Routines," *Journal of Pediatrics,* 80:501, 1972.

36 R. G. Grassy, "The Growth and Development of LBW Infants Receiving Intensive Neonatal Care," *Clinical Pediatrics,* 15(6):549, 1976.

37 J. B. Warshaw and R. Uauy, "Identification of Nutritional Deficiency and Failure to Thrive in the Newborn," *Clinics of Perinatology,* 2(2):328, 1975.

38 J. C. Sinclair, S. Saigal, and C. Y. Young, "Early Postnatal Consequences of Fetal Malnutrition," *Nutrition and Fetal Development,* John Wiley & Sons, Inc., 1974, p. 150.

39 J. B. Warshaw, op. cit., p. 327.

40 A. Erenberg, "Hypoglycemia," presented at Intensive Course in Pediatric Nutrition, University of Iowa, June, 1976.

41 S. J. Foman, E. E. Ziegler, and A. M. O'Donnell, "Infant Feeding in Health and Disease," *Infant Nutrition,* W. B. Saunders Company, Philadelphia, 1974, p. 503.

42 R. N. Roy and J. C. Sinclair, "Hydration of the Low Birth-Weight Infant," *Clinics in Perinatology,* 2(2):393, 1975.

43 Ibid., p. 395.

44 Ibid., p. 401.

45 E. E. Ziegler and J. E. Ryu, "Renal Solute Load and Diet in Growing Premature Infants," *Journal of Pediatrics,* 89(4):609–611, 1976.

46 R. N. Roy and J. C. Sinclair, op. cit., p. 401.

47 J. G. Gault, J. A. Sturman, and N. C. R. Raïhä, "Development of Sulfur Metabolism: Absence of Cystathionase in Human Fetal Tissue," *Pediatric Research,* 6:538, 1972.

48 S. E. Snyderman, "Amino Acid Requirements," *Intravenous Nutrition in the High Risk Infant,* John Wiley & Sons, Inc., New York, 1975, p. 210.

49 T. A. Anderson and S. J. Foman, "Vitamins," *Infant Nutrition,* 2d ed., W. B. Saunders Company, Philadelphia, 1974, p. 224.

50 J. C. Sinclair et al., "Supportive Management of the Sick Neonate," *Pediatric Clinics of North America,* 17:836, 1970.

51 J. C. Sinclair, "Thermal Control in Premature Infants," *Annual Review of Medicine,* 23:130, 1972.

52 Ibid., p. 133.

53 Ibid., p. 132.

54 Ibid., p. 140.

55 Ibid., p. 141.

56 J. C. Sinclair, S. Saigal, and C. Y. Young, op. cit., p. 157.

57 H. Ghadimi, K. Arulanantham, and M. Rathi, "Evaluation of Nutritional Management of the Low Birth Weight Newborn," *American Journal of Clinical Nutrition,* 26(5):473, 1973.

58 R. J. Grand, J. B. Watkins, and F. M. Torti, op. cit., p. 794.

59 Ibid., p. 792.

60 Ibid., p. 797.

61 J. B. Watkins, P. Szczepanik, and J. B. Gould, "Bile Salt Metabolism in the Human Premature Infant," *Gastroenterology,* 69(3):706–713, 1975.

62 P. Tantibhedhyang Kul and S. A. Hashim,

"Medium-Chain Triglyceride Feeding in Premature Infants: Effects on Fat and Nitrogen Absorption," *Pediatrics,* 55:359–370, 1975.

63 J. B. Warshaw and R. Uauy, op. cit., p. 331.

64 R. J. Grand, J. B. Watkins, and F. M. Torti, op. cit., p. 804.

65 L. A. Barness, "Nutrition for the Low Birth-Weight Infant," *Clinics in Perinatology,* 2(2):349, 1975.

66 L. O. Lubchenco et al., op. cit.

67 S. J. Foman, E. E. Ziegler, and A. M. O'Donnell, op. cit., p. 499.

68 W. C. Heird and J. M. Driscoll, "Newer Methods for Feeding Low Birth-Weight Infants," *Clinics of Perinatology* 2(2):323, 1975.

69 K. Rickard and E. Gresham, "Nutritional Considerations for the Newborn Requiring Intensive Care," *J.A.D.A.* 66(6):594, 1975.

70 R. N. Roy and J. C. Sinclair, op. cit., p. 405.

71 K. Rickard and E. Gresham, op. cit., p. 595.

72 L. A. Barness, op. cit., p. 346.

73 S. J. Foman, E. E. Ziegler, and A. M. O'Donnell op. cit., p. 505.

74 H. Ghadimi et al., op. cit., p. 474.

75 Ibid., p. 473.

76 H. I. Goldman et al., "Late Effects of Early Dietary Protein Intake on Low Birth-Weight Infants," *Journal of Pediatrics,* 85(6):764–769, 1974.

77 K. Rickard and E. Gresham, op. cit., p. 595.

78 N. C. R. Raïhï et al., "Milk Protein Quantity and Quality in Low Birth Weight Infants," *Journal of Pediatrics,* 86(5):766–772, 1975.

79 S. J. Foman, E. E. Ziegler, and A. M. O'Donnell, op. cit., p. 505.

80 S. E. Snyderman, op. cit., p. 210.

81 C. L. Abitol et al., "Plasma Amino Acid Pattern During Supplemental Intravenous Nutrition of Low-Birth-Weight Infants," *Journal of Pediatrics* 86(5): 770, 1975.

82 D. R. Brown, R. C. Tsang, and I. U. Chen, "Oral Calcium Supplementation in Premature and Asphyxiated Neonates," *Journal of Pediatrics,* 89(6):976, 1976.

83 A. W. Root and H. E. Harrison, "Recent Advances in Calcium Metabolism, II Disorders of Calcium Homeostasis," *Journal of Pediatrics,* 88(2):178, 1976.

84 A. W. Root and H. E. Harrison, "Recent Advances in Calcium Metabolism, I Mechanisms of Calcium Homeostasis," *Journal of Pediatrics,* 88(1):11, 1976.

85 D. R. Brown, R. C. Tsang, and I. U. Chen, op. cit., pp. 973–977.

86 G. M. Chance et al., "Growth and Mineral Metabolism in Very Low Birth Weight Infants, II Effects of Calcium Supplementation on Growth and Divalent Cations," *Pediatric Research,* 9(7):568–575, 1975.

87 _____"Neonatal Calcium Homeostasis, Vitamin

D and Parathyroid Function," *Nutrition Reviews,* **34**(4):113, 1976.

88 _____"Renal Handling of Salt by Preterm Infants," *Nutrition Reviews,* **33**(4):105–107, 1975.

89 D. K. Melhorn and S. Gross, "Vitamin E-dependent Anemia in the Premature Infant II Relationships between Gestational Age and Absorption of Vitamin E," *Journal of Pediatrics,* **79**:581, 1971.

90 P. R. Dallman, "Iron, Vitamin E, and Folate in the Preterm Infant," *Journal of Pediatrics,* **85**(6): 742–752, 1974.

91 J. E. Graeber, M. L. Williams, and F. A. Oski, "The Use of Intramuscular Vitamin E in the Premature Infant," *Journal of Pediatrics,* **90**(2):282–284, 1977.

92 Ibid., p. 284.

93 P. R. Dallman, op. cit., pp. 742–752.

94 Ibid., p. 746.

95 Ibid., p. 749.

96 S. Gross and D. K. Melhorn, "Vitamin E-dependent Anemia in the Premature," *Journal of Pediatrics,* **85**(6):753, 1974.

97 J. J. Bullen, H. J. Rogers, and E. Griffith, "Iron-binding Proteins and Infections," *British Journal of Haematology,* **23**:387, 1972.

98 P. R. Dallman, op. cit., pp. 742–752.

99 W. C. Heird and R. W. Winters, "Total Parenteral Nutrition—The State of the Art," *Journal of Pediatrics,* **86**(1):2–16, 1975.

100 G. W. Chance, "Results in VLBW Infants (<1300 gram birth weight)", *Intravenous Nutrition in the High Risk Infant,* John Wiley & Sons, Inc., New York, pp. 39–50.

101 J. M. Driscoll, "A Preliminary Study of Total Intravenous Alimentation in Low Birth Weight Infants," *Intravenous Nutrition in the High Risk Infant,* John Wiley & Sons, Inc., New York, pp. 51–63.

102 M. T. Stahlman, "Alimentation and Growth Patterns in Small Prematures and Infants with Hyaline Membrane Disease," *Intravenous Nutrition in the High Risk Infant,* John Wiley & Sons, Inc., New York, pp. 35–73.

103 H. L. Greene, "Trace Elements and Vitamins," *Intravenous Nutrition in the High Risk Infant,* John Wiley & Sons, Inc., New York, pp. 274–276.

104 L. D. Steginck, "Amino Acid Metabolism," *Intravenous Nutrition in the High Risk Infant,* John Wiley & Sons, Inc., New York, pp. 181–203.

105 C. L. Abitol et al., op. cit., pp. 766–772.

106 L. D. Steginck, "Sources of Intravenous Nitrogen," presented at Intensive Course in Pediatric Nutrition, University of Iowa, June 1976.

107 R. H. Winters, "Introduction to the Conference" *Intravenous Nutrition in the High Risk Infant,* John Wiley & Sons, Inc., New York, 1975, p. 4.

108 L. H. Victorin, "Intralipid Metabolism in Low Birth Weight Infants," *Intravenous Nutrition in the High Risk Infant,* John Wiley & Sons, Inc., New York, pp. 357–367.

109 G. Andrew, G. Chan, and D. Schiff, "Lipid Metabolism in the Neonate," *Journal of Pediatrics,* **88**(2):279–284, 1976.

110 W. C. Heird and J. M. Driscoll, op. cit., p. 319.

111 J. W. Rhea, M. S. Ahmid, and E. S. Mange, "Nasojejunal (transpyloric) Feeding: A Commentary," *Journal of Pediatrics* **86**:451, 1975.

112 J. A. Cheek and G. F. Staub, "Nasojejunal Alimentation for Premature and Full Term Infants," *Journal of Pediatrics,* **82**:955, 1973.

113 S. J. Boros and J. W. Reynolds, "Duodenal Perforation: A Complication of Neonatal Nasojejunal Feeding," *Journal of Pediactrics,* **85**(1):107–108, 1974.

114 W. C. Heird, "Nasojejunal Feeding: A Commentary," *Journal of Pediatrics,* **85**(1):111–112, 1974.

115 L. A. Barness, op. cit., p. 347.

116 N. C. R. Raïhä, op. cit., pp. 766–772.

117 S. J. Foman and L. J. Filer, "Milks and Formulas," *Infant Nutrition,* 2d edition, W. B. Saunders Company, Philadelphia, 1974, p. 370.

118 S. J. Foman, E. E. Ziegler, and A. M. O'Donnell, op. cit., p. 507.

119 S. J. Foman, E. E. Ziegler, and H. D. Vazquez, "Human Milk and the Small Premature," unpublished address, Department of Pediatrics, University of Iowa.

120 D. B. Jelliffe, "Unique Properties of Human Milk," *Journal of Reproductive Medicine* **14**(4):133–136, 1975.

121 P. Gyorgy, "Biochemical Aspects," *American Journal of Clinical Nutrition,* **24**:970–975.

122 B. Hall, "Changing Composition of Human Milk and Early Development of an Appetite Control," *The Lancet,* April 5, 1975, 779–781.

123 I. D. Frantz, "Necrotizing Enterocolitis," *Journal of Pediatrics,* **86**(2):259–263, 1975.

124 J. Pitt, B. Barlow, W. C. Heird, and T. V. Santulli, "Macrophages and the Protective Action of Breast Milk in Necrotizing Enterocolitis," *Pediatric Research,* **8**:384, 1974.

125 J. J. Herbst, "CHO Malabsorption in NEC," *Pediatrics,* **57**:201–204, 1976.

126 L. I. Kramer and M. E. Pierpont, "Rocking Waterbeds and Auditory Stimuli to Enhance Growth of Preterm Infants," *Journal of Pediatrics,* **88**(2):297–299, 1976.

127 L. O. Lubchenco et al., op. cit., p. 795.

APPENDIXES

CASE DISCUSSIONS

TABLES

CASE
DISCUSSIONS

CASE DISCUSSION 2-1

Scoring P's diet using the basic four food groups revealed a diet score of 6½. The diet had no representatives from the fruit and vegetable groups and insufficient representatives from the milk and meat groups. This placed P in the high-risk category for deficiencies of vitamin A, vitamin C, and fiber, and moderate-risk for calcium, phosphorus, protein, iron, zinc, and riboflavin. His diet is high in empty calories (Coke, potato chips, candy). The following dietary changes were recommended:

1 Morning
   Inclusion of juice and easy-to-prepare protein food such as yogurt, cereal and milk, peanut butter sandwich; also addition of milk in coffee.
2 Lunch and dinner
   At fast-food restaurants, lettuce, tomato, cole slaw, salad additions. Milk for beverage.
3 Snack
   Fruits, especially easy-to-store dried fruits, nuts, seeds.

Planning meals, shopping, and preparing foods within such an environment was the central issue in helping P toward a better diet. When the money spent on food was compared to the nutrients bought in vending machines and fast-food restaurants P was more motivated to coordinate his efforts with those of his roommates, and to plan and shop ahead. This enabled them to utilize sales and to purchase in quantity. The success of their joint effort led to participation in a local food cooperative and a better diet for all.

CASE DISCUSSION 3-1

Treatment
While breast feeding, S. G. seemed to be receiving an adequate intake of protein and cal-

TABLE 2-8   P's BASIC FOUR SCORING RECORD

Food group	Amount consumed	Total no. servings consumed	Total possible points	Score for food group
Milk Milk			2 adults (non-pregnant and nonlactating) 3 children 4 teenagers	1½
Cheese	1½ oz pizza	1½		
Yogurt				
Ice cream				
Others				
Meat Meat, fish, poultry	3 oz hamburger	1	3	
Eggs				1
Nuts or legumes				
Others				
Fruit and vegetable Vitamin C–rich			1	0
Vitamin A–rich			1	0
Others			2	0
Grain Bread	Hamburger roll	2		
Cereal			4	4
Others	Pizza	3		
Other Sweets	1 candy bar sugar			
Fats and oils	Potato chips		0	0
Beverages; e.g., coffee, tea, Coke, Kool-Aid, alcohol	24 oz Coke			
Others				
Grand total				6½

NOTE: Optimum points: Children 13, teenagers 14, adults 12 ories from breast milk, supplemented by vegetables and grains. Evidence of this is S. G.'s consistent growth along the 10th percentile for both height and weight for his first 10 months of life, which was consistent with his familial pattern. When S. G. stopped breast feeding, his growth problems began. On a diet consisting of only grains, vegetables, nuts, and seeds, S. G. was unable to consume an intake of protein and energy adequate to sustain growth. His weight loss is evidence of an inadequate energy intake. This would suggest that the protein consumed was used primarily to meet energy needs.

Children who follow vegan diets are consuming proteins which have lower biological value, are less readily digested, and are more difficult to chew. These problems, coupled with rapid growth, which causes an increased need for protein in young children, may result in protein-calorie (joule) deficiencies.

Treatment involves increasing both protein and energy in the diet. The G.'s were referred to the nutritionist at the health center for careful dietary evaluation and nutritional counseling.

Nutritional Education

The parents were counseled on the nutritional value of animal and vegetable proteins. Since the G.'s are strict vegetarians, they were not amenable to including animal foods in the child's diet. Careful instruction in the mechanics of protein complementarity was the primary focus of nutritional education. The parents were also encouraged to include some soy products and a well-processed commercial soy formula.

Follow-up Plans

The patient was seen weekly by the nurse and nutritionist for weight checks, growth monitoring, and supportive nutritional care to ensure adequate protein and calorie (joule) intakes and developmental feeding progress.

CASE DISCUSSION 4-1

Review of the diet shows the excessive use of refined carbohydrate in the form of baked goods, candy bars, and soft drinks. The lack of fruits, vegetables, whole-grain breads and cereals, and nuts makes the diet low in polysaccharides (cellulose, hemicellulose, lignin, and pectin) and thus low in dietary fiber.

Dietary fiber promotes intestinal function by its ability to take up water and swell, to absorb organic molecules such as bile salts, to exchange cations, and to form a gel. Therefore, Susan was encouraged to increase dietary fiber by including more fresh fruits, vegetables, whole grains (especially bran), and nuts in meals and snacks. In addition, foods with special laxative effect (prunes, apricots, and raisins) were encouraged, along with water and fruit juices. She was also encouraged to increase her activity and incorporate a daily exercise program into her life style. The following plan was devised.

Breakfast	4 oz prune juice
	½ grapefruit
	raisin bran or granola with milk
Midmorning	bran muffin
Lunch	tuna fish sandwich on whole-wheat bread with lettuce and tomato
	apple
	milk
Midafternoon	juice
	soy nuts
Dinner	meat, fish, or poultry
	2 vegetables
	salad
	fruit

CASE DISCUSSION 5-1

This infant shows the classic signs of essential fatty acid deficiency. Since essential fatty acids are necessary to maintain the function and integrity of the cellular and subcellular membranes, changes in the skin manifest the deficiency state. It is speculated that the change in the fatty acid composition of the phospholipid of the membranes is the primary lesion of the EFA deficiency.*

All of these symptoms were reversed within a 2-week period by the administration of linoleic acid. The infant was gaining steadily and thriving on iron-fortified Similac, in which linoleic acid constitutes 15 percent of the total calories, providing more than the 1 to 3 percent of the total calories recommended to be fed as linoleic acid. The parents were counseled regarding baby-food additions and the hazards of using skim milk during the first year of life.

CASE DISCUSSION 6-1

Assuming there was no other biochemical abnormality, the patient's yellow skin was caused by the ingestion of 9 or 10 carrots per day. β-carotene, the yellow pigment contained in both yellow and dark green vegetables, imparts a yellow tinge to the skin when blood levels are elevated; blood data supported this hypothesis. The serum alkaline phosphatase level is an indicator of bone metabolism, and serum levels are elevated during times of bone resorption, which occurs when there is an inadequate intake of vitamin D or calcium. Because estrogen has an effect on bone metabolism, many postmenopausal women are prone to osteoporosis and osteomalacia, which may be manifested as aching bones; susceptibility to fractures is another concern. The patient's serum riboflavin levels were probably decreased because of an inadequate intake of the vitamin; omission of milk from the diet severely compromises the availability of this vitamin.

You should recommend that she eliminate her intake of carrots until her skin returns to

---

* E. F. A. Sinclair, in R. Paoletti (ed.), *Lipid Pharmacology*, Academic Press, New York, 1964, p. 237.

its normal color, and then eat them only in moderation. She would be well advised to consume some milk products for their calcium, riboflavin, and vitamin D content. If this is not acceptable to her, a calcium supplement plus an increase in green leafy vegetables will provide additional calcium and riboflavin, but not vitamin D. This fat-soluble vitamin would have to be supplied by either supplementation, or by the patient's spending more time outdoors to take advantage of the sun. She should also be counseled that to ensure adequate intake of all nutrients, diet planning becomes more important when energy intake is decreased, since some food groups may be completely (and unwisely) restricted in an unsupervised weight reduction program.

CASE DISCUSSION 7-1

On the basis of clinical and laboratory findings, the diagnosis of iron-deficiency anemia was made. An oral supplement of ferrous sulfate was prescribed with specific instructions regarding administration. The recommended dose was 3 ml per day (the daily dose should give 4.5 to 6 mg of elemental iron/kg of body weight), given between meals in fruit juice or water (never milk).

Within 7 days, the hemoglobin began to rise, and after 8 weeks values had returned to normal. Therapy was continued for 8 months. (A common error is to discontinue iron after 2 or 3 months, but therapy should be continued for 6 to 12 months to replete stores.) Since food intake was only providing 4.5 mg of iron (the recommended dietary allowance is 15 mg), iron-containing foods including lean red meat, liver, iron-fortified cereals, and whole-grain breads were encouraged. Citrus juices and vitamin C–rich foods were recommended to enhance iron absorption.

Since Jeremy had very definite food preferences, his parents were counseled about normal developmental feeding issues (i.e., toddler feeding behavior; see Chap. 11) and weaning was suggested. With respect to Jeremy's constipation, his parents were advised that since iron medication can also cause constipation, it was important to include prunes, juices, water, and bran in Jeremy's diet on a daily basis. Milk was curtailed to 24 oz per day, enough to provide requirements without interfering with appetite for solid foods. Also, the parents were counseled against the hazards of leaving the iron medication within easy reach of the child. Follow-up well-child care with laboratory analysis occurred at 3-month intervals over the next year.

CASE DISCUSSION 8-1

The child was diagnosed as having hypertonic dehydration and metabolic acidosis resulting from losses of water, sodium, potassium, and bicarbonate caused by the diarrhea and further complicated by the use of a concentrated high "renal solute load" formula of boiled skim milk. The serum levels of potassium, sodium, and bicarbonate reflect the electrolyte imbalance. The increase in urine specific gravity shows the decrease in extracellular fluid which prompted the hypothalamus to stimulate pituitary secretion of antidiuretic hormone (ADH). In turn, the ADH signaled the kidneys to facilitate the reabsorption of water. However, the extreme losses of electrolytes from the diarrhea were worsened by the use of the concentrated boiled skim milk formula, which has a renal solute load of 308 mosmol/l (whole cow's milk has a renal solute load of 221 mosmol/l). Adequate fluid intake is needed in order to excrete the solute load. Since the infant's body was unable to maintain homeostasis, the infant became dehydrated and developed metabolic acidosis, because of an accumulation of strong acid in the extracellular fluid.

The infant was admitted to the hospital and rehydrated with intravenous therapy. Since 150/ml/kg of body weight per day is an infant's normal fluid requirement, fluid replacement of sodium involved giving 15 to 30 meq of sodium per liter of fluid each day, in a 5 percent dextrose solution. Potassium was withheld until adequate fluid volume was assured, and was then added to the intravenous fluid. Replacement therapy was monitored by serum electrolyte levels. The patient was discharged after 4 days, by which time the laboratory findings had returned to normal and the diarrhea had subsided. The parents were advised against the hazards of using a boiled milk formula.

CASE DISCUSSION 9-1

The most active site of nutrient absorption in the gastrointestinal tract is the small intestine. Disaccharidases, peptidases, and intestinal lipase are secreted by the mucosa of the small intestine and are responsible for nutrient breakdown. Intestinal absorption of most nutrients occurs in the upper portion of the intestine where the mucosal enzymes are able to act on complex carbohydrate, protein, and fat molecules and break them into more easily absorbable forms.

However, the jejunal and ileal mucosa is active in the absorption of monosaccharides, amino acids, monoglycerides, and some diglycerides. In the presence of a diseased mucosa, or with a bypass of the jejunum and ileum as in the case of S. J., nutrient absorption becomes incomplete for two reasons:

1 Although some breakdown of nutrients occurs at the gastric level and in the duodenum, the lack of contact with enzymes from the lower section of the small bowel results in incomplete nutrient breakdown.

2 Malabsorption results in the quick loss of partially digested nutrients in the form of diarrhea. Because fats require a longer time in the small bowel for enzymatic breakdown and are considered to be the most complex nutrient molecules for digestion, the consequent lack of mucosal surface contact results in a massive loss of partially digested fats in the form of steatorrhea.

Because of the contribution of carbohydrate-, protein-, and fat-specific enzymes, all nutrients are affected in a bypass of the jejunum and ileum. The absorption of water, vitamins, and minerals is also affected. Rapid loss of partially digested fats result in the loss of significant fat-soluble vitamins and warrants close attention in malabsorption.

In lieu of surgical intervention for obesity, many authorities feel that a balanced calorie-deficient diet will result in sufficient weight loss to prevent further weight gain.

In determining the actual caloric needs of an individual many factors must be considered. Age, sex, height, current weight, basal energy requirements, and activity level must be considered in determining actual caloric needs.

S. J. is a 35-year old described as sedentary. With a height of 5 ft 7 in (170 cm) and a weight of 280 lb (127 kg), it is obvious that her energy intake far exceeds her output.

The National Research Council suggests that the optimal weight for a female 5 ft 7 in tall should be 135 lb (61.4 kg). Therefore basal metabolic requirements for S. J.'s ideal weight are 1474 kcal/day (6191 kJ/day).

$$BMR = 61.4 \text{ kg} \times 24 \text{ kcal/day}$$
$$= 1474 \text{ kcal/day}$$
$$= 6191 \text{ kJ/day}$$

To determine caloric needs for a sedentary life style, an allowance of 30 percent of the BMR caloric requirements is added to the BMR caloric needs:

$$\text{Sedentary activity} = 30\% \text{ BMR}$$
$$= 30\% \times 1474$$
$$= 442.2 \text{ kcal/day}$$
$$= 1857 \text{ kJ/day}$$
$$\text{Total energy needs} = \text{BMR} + \text{calculated activity requirement}$$
$$= 1474 + 442$$
$$= 1916 \text{ kcal/day}$$
$$= 8084 \text{ kJ/day}$$

Total energy needs are the sum total of the basal requirement plus the calculated energy requirements for activity. Therefore, S. J. will require approximately 1916 kcal (8084 kJ) to maintain an optimal weight of 135 lb (61.4 kg).

However, if the energy expenditure is increased (e.g., because of increased activity or illness), the estimated caloric needs to maintain her ideal weight will change proportionately.

CASE DISCUSSION 10-1

A team comprising a physical therapist, psychologist, pediatrician, nurse, speech pathologist, and nutritionist then met and devised a program to begin oral feeding that might be best accomplished in a very structured environment. The goal was to wean Teddy and to provide food by the oral route. It was decided to admit Teddy to the hospital since the attempt at gradual weaning on an outpatient basis had not been successful.

Changing Teddy's behavior toward food required very careful planning. Before his hospitalization the program for Teddy was discussed with the nurses and physicians who would be in contact with Teddy so that their behavior would be in concert with the program. It was decided that the most effective way to make oral food reinforcing for him was to have him be hungry before oral feeding was attempted. Heretofore he had always been tube-fed when he refused food presented orally. He had become quite adept at handling anyone, especially his mother, who tried to get him to sample food orally. He had no need to try food, for his tube feeding would always occur regardless of his behavior. In order to facilitate his learning to eat orally the tube was entirely discarded and no one in the hospital was to feed him this way. A very important concern was that without the tube feeding he could become dehydrated and begin to lose weight if he did not start eating. We decided the risk was worth taking since no other approach had shown any sign of working. Everyone connected with Teddy had to be reassured that we would not let him starve to death and within the hospital environment fluid balance could be reestablished intravenously if the need arose.

Initially we wished to involve his mother in getting him to eat in the hospital but she felt that the situation would be very stressful for her, although she agreed with the intent of the program. She therefore left town for the first week of the program. Because of Teddy's difficulties she tended to be overprotective toward him and could not bear to see him unhappy or distressed. For about the first 3 years of his life she alone could feed Teddy. They were inseparable and literally tied by the tube.

To get him eating as quickly as possible a program with the highest amount of consistency was implemented. One person, the physical therapist, was selected to feed him at the same times each day and in the same place. The physical therapist already had had positive experiences with Teddy, as she had been the one encouraging and promoting the development of his motor skills. Teddy was given baby food with Isomil. At first he refused to try the food but after several sessions when he obviously was becoming hungrier he began to try it. Because he was no longer being tube-fed the food he received orally served as a primary reinforcement as it assuaged his hunger. The physical therapist also responded with praise and attention each time he ate a spoonful or drank a mouthful of food. He did, however, present a great deal of negative behavior such as crying and fussing when the food was offered. This behavior was extinguished by removal of the physical therapist's attention. The therapist would turn away from Teddy until the negative behavior stopped. Within 1 week, Teddy was drinking Isomil from a cup and had begun to accept baby food on a spoon with a notable decrease in negative behavior.

After an initial weight loss, Teddy's weight stabilized and he began to regain weight. When his mother returned she was trained in the feeding procedures that the physical therapist had used and she was instructed never to return to tube feeding. Teddy was then discharged from the hospital and followed at biweekly intervals. Although he was now eating orally at home he demonstrated many negative, manip-

ulative, and controlling food behaviors with his mother to the extent that he would only eat foods he preferred and not try any others. His mother found it difficult to be consistent in her attempts to get him to try new foods.

The behavior modification program had demonstrated success in helping Teddy to learn to eat orally and his growth began to improve. The development of completely appropriate eating habits was not accomplished at that time because that part of the program depended upon his mother, who found it difficult to maintain the program at home despite supportive counseling. With his new feeding pattern Teddy has also showed general developmental gains in many areas and the degree of his developmental retardation was significantly reduced.

CASE DISCUSSION 12-1

Growth needs and the onset of menstruation have a negative effect upon iron stores and hemoglobin level, as evidenced by Jennie's low hematocrit, which is diagnostic of iron-deficiency anemia. However, anthropometric data (height/weight ratio) and the clinical state do not support the presence of other nutrient deficiencies.

Jennie has been surreptitious in her eating behavior and has been able to cache food without her parents' knowledge. She exhibits, through her negative and manipulative food refusals, a desire to control—an exercise of the will, hitherto denied by her overly restrictive parents.

Normalization of mealtimes depended upon her parents' acceptance of the fact that Jennie's eating habits had evolved over a period of 14 years and at this point were no longer subject to their influence; and furthermore, that her food choices were her own personal choices and that their reactions further reinforced Jennie's own negative behavior.

Jennie was assured by the nutritionist that she was proportionate for her size and that she could improve an already good figure by exercise. She was further advised that her brittle nails and lethargy were related to the lack of iron, a result of her poor eating habits and increased menstrual loses. Her concern for her body image was used as the motivating force to encourage a better diet and exercise program. She was initially reluctant to join the program at the local youth club, but with counseling at the local mental health facility she overcame her fears of peer rejection. She was maintained on an iron supplement for the next six months.

CASE DISCUSSION 13-1

A weight-reducing regimen is not appropriate during pregnancy, especially during the third trimester when the fetus is growing most rapidly and energy demands are greatest.

An appropriate energy level would be approximately 40 kcal/kg (168 kJ/kg) of ideal body weight. C.P.'s ideal weight is 53 kg. Therefore, energy requirements would be:

$$53 \text{ kg} \times 40 \text{ kcal} = 2120 \text{ kcal} = 8904 \text{ kJ}$$

There has been much controversy over sodium and its role in preeclampsia. However, it has been shown that there is an increased need for sodium during pregnancy. If sodium is not supplied via the diet, the renin-angiotensin system will conserve sodium and less will be excreted, thereby defeating the purpose. Sodium restriction may even exacerbate toxemia; therefore, no restriction should be initiated.

A thorough nutritional history should be taken to evaluate C. P.'s dietary intake. C. P. should be encouraged to consume the following if she is not already doing so:

4 servings of milk and milk products
4 servings of protein foods

3 servings of grain products
1 serving of vitamin C–rich fruits and vegetables
2 servings of leafy green vegetables
1 serving of other fruits and vegetables

CASE DISCUSSION 14-1

Since S. C.'s diet contains no milk or milk products it appears to be inadequate in calcium and vitamin D. Milk is not generally consumed as a beverage by many Chinese individuals; however, it is acceptable when used on cereal. S. C. was also encouraged to use tofu and soybeans, a good source of calcium and protein. Greens such as mustards, collards, and kale were also recommended for their calcium content.

By increasing the amount of milk in S. C.'s diet and encouraging exposure to sunlight the amount of vitamin D will most likely be adequate.

S. C.'s protein intake may be low, depending upon the amount of meat, fish, or chicken used in mixed dishes.

The nutritionist informed S. C. that she probably was eligible for food stamps and told her where she could apply. The nutritionist also enrolled S. C. and her baby in the WIC program at the health center, as she met the criteria for limited income and she also had an inadequate dietary intake.

CASE DISCUSSION 15-1

#1 Poor nutritional status due to resectable cancer of the pancreas

Assessment

1 Significant weight loss due to inadequate food intake and malabsorption

2 Diarrhea caused by lactose intake which exacerbates the electrolyte imbalance; also related to malabsorption of fat

3 Elevated blood glucose resulting from post-operative diabetes.

Plan

1 Recommend 2200 kcal (9240 kJ), lactose-free, 100-mg fat diet six small feedings. Gradual reintroduction of milk products to determine tolerance

2 Increase potassium-rich foods. Push fluids

3 Carefully chart food and fluid intake for review by doctor

4 Continual dietary counseling during hospitalization in preparation for discharge. Follow-up counseling during outpatient visits, especially upon initiation of radiation therapy

_____R.D.

CASE DISCUSSION 16-1

According to Waterlow's standards the infant was classified as having third-degree malnutrition since his height for age was 86 percent of the expected value and his weight had dropped significantly from his birth weight because of an inadequate supply of breast milk, although the child was placed at the breast every 2 hours throughout the day.

On admission, the child was rehydrated with Ringer's lactate and subsequently with 5 percent dextrose and 0.2% saline, and was given potassium supplementation and magnesium intramuscularly. He was also treated with ampicillin and gentamicin for 10 days because of clinical suspicion of sepsis. After 48 h, he was started on one-half-strength Similac with Iron and then gradually advanced to full-strength Similac with Iron. He was also given additional vitamins and minerals (B complex, K, multivitamins, folic acid, and iron). After 4 weeks of hospitalization, the infant was discharged weighing 3160 g. Parents were advised on the amount of formula to give per feeding (4½ to 5 oz) and were given suggestions about the type of nipple to use (since the infant was formerly breast-fed, he initially experienced difficulties getting accustomed to the bottle). Additional information was provided on the introduction of baby food. The child was followed up routinely in the well-child clinic and after 1 month the supplementary vitamins were discontinued.

Malnutrition occurring during this critical period of rapid brain and body growth placed this child at risk. In addition his condition was further compromised by the depression of the immune response system, leaving him susceptible to infection, allowing the sepsis to develop. This child shows the effect of the synergism between nutritional status, the body's immune response, and infection.

CASE DISCUSSION 17-1

Mr. Smith was diagnosed as having type II hyperlipoproteinemia after baseline cholesterol, triglyceride, and electrophoresis results were determined. Other risk factors present included smoking, lack of activity (until he had initial feelings of chest pressure), and a positive family history.

The first step in treatment of this disorder is the institution of the correct diet. A dietary history revealed that Mr. Smith had already made many alterations in his dietary intake. He was given instructions on a diet low in cholesterol (250 mg or less) and low in saturated fat (polyunsaturates/saturates ratio of 2 to 1), with calories unrestricted as long as he maintained his weight. He had a drop of approximately 20 percent in both serum cholesterol and triglycerides with strict adherence to this diet.

Drug therapy was instituted when the plasma lipids were not lowered to the desired level with diet alone. The importance of continued dietary restriction was emphasized also. Several different doses and forms of medication were prescribed to achieve an optimal lowering of his plasma lipids to acceptable levels.

Mr. Smith has continued to follow the same diet for the last 6 years. He knows and understands the dietary principles involved very well. He has good support from his family and does not feel that the diet imposes restrictions on them.

Mr. Smith will continue to be followed on infrequent visits with periodic review of his diet. He has found many of the new products for fat-controlled diets very useful, such as egg substitutes, textured vegetable protein, etc., so continued adherence to his diet is expected.

CASE DISCUSSION 18-1

S. suffered from ulcerative colitis, an illness affecting the transit time of the small bowel and the absorptive capacities of the colon, with consequent malabsorption of ingested vitamins, minerals, and some nutrients.

Characteristic of ulcerative colitis is the presence of an inflamed intestinal mucosa with the occurrence of lesions and haustrations in the colon. Evident from S.'s admission laboratory data is a significant loss of red blood cells because of these lesions, resulting in a secondary anemia. There is no interference with the initial process of digestion, nor are amylase and gastric secretions affected in ulcerative colitis. However, the malabsorption and diarrhea that are evident in the early stages of the low serum calcium, magnesium, and folic acid levels, and to the generalized malnourished state of the afflicted patient. S. experienced an 8-kg weight loss during the early stages of his disease due primarily to a loss of healthy, functioning intestinal mucosa and consequent malabsorption of ingested nutrients. Dehydration developed as a result of the massive stooling and dysfunctioning colon; however, not in significant enough degree to affect the fluid and electrolyte characteristics.

The presence of a diseased intestinal mucosa often interferes with the colitis patient's ability to properly digest and absorb lactose because of interference with the production and functioning of the intestinal disaccharidases. However, mucosal damage does not usually affect sucrose hydrolysis, probably because of the high levels of sucrase that usually are present. Lactase deficiency is commonly believed to be responsible for the colitis patient's intolerance to dairy products. S. is in a critical period for growth and development of skeletal tissue. He requires a high supply of dietary calcium, which is perhaps the greatest mineral contribution of the dairy and milk food group (his recommended dietary allowance is 1200 mg of calcium daily). Therefore, Tums, an antacid containing calcium bicarbonate, was prescribed to compensate for the decreased dietary calcium intake. One tablet provides 195 mg of utilizable calcium.

Dietary fiber and spices such as black pepper and chili powder have been found to affect the absorptive capacity of the normal intestinal mucosa, and therefore aggravate the diseased mucosa of the colitis patient. Elimination of these items from the diet and establishment of a bland, low-residue regimen achieves the purpose of resting the small bowel and eliminating potential mucosal irritation. However, with the elimination of all raw and most processed fruits and vegetables because of their fiber content, the dietary supply of water-soluble vitamins and minerals is critically low. Since the nutritional status of the colitis patient is significant in recuperation from the illness, multivitamins were necessary to compensate for decreased cellular resistance to infection and to help in the regulatory process during the healing stage.

To aid in tissue regeneration of the inflamed mucosa and colonic lesions, as well as to improve hemoglobin levels, a high-protein diet was ordered simultaneously with the administration of ferrous sulfate, folate, and prednisone. High-protein snacks coupled with high-protein meals of low fat constitution will improve the body's ability to regenerate diseased cells and expedite the recuperative process. Consequently with improved absorption because of decreased stress to the small bowel, S. was able to gain in height and weight.

Recuperation from the initial onset of colitis is a slow process requiring strict dietary monitoring and compliance with the drug regimen. As the patient's symptoms subside, food items are gradually reintroduced into the daily diet and the individual is able to liberalize his diet as tolerated, with the ultimate dietary restrictions dependent on the status of mucosal integrity and functioning.

CASE DISCUSSION 19-1

Sara's problem of fluid overload is evident by three criteria: shortness of breath, hypertension, and an admission weight 8 kg above her normal weight. Dialysis was initiated immediately in an attempt to reduce Sara's fluid weight, and there were important routine procedures, relating to her admission diagnosis, which the nursing staff also initiated.

Daily weights were obtained every A.M. along with accurately recorded intake and output records. (A fluid restriction of 500 to 800 ml total per 24 h was ordered since Sara is essentially anuric and fluid-overloaded.) With fluids identified precisely as to the precentage of the total fluid allowance to be sent on the patient's tray, the nursing staff was then responsible for administering the remaining fluids with medications and as nourishments (although Sara was not receiving intravenous therapy; this would have been another avenue of fluid entry). The dietitian determined from the diet history that Sara had overindulged in both sodium and fluid while at a weekend party (as reflected by a serum sodium of 150 meq/l and weight gain) and attempted to understand the reason for this indiscretion and to motivate Sara accordingly in dietary principles as related to her own kidney function.

Sara's diet prescription included 2100 kcal (882 kJ), 52 g of protein, and 2 g of sodium. This was determined by using the energy requirements for an adult receiving hemodialysis: 30 to 45 kcal (126–189 kJ)/kg of "dry" or ideal body weight. Sara's dry weight was 52 kg [52 kg × 40 kcal/kg = 2080 kcal (8736 kJ) or, rounded off, 2100 kcal (8820 kJ)]. Her protein requirements were 1 to 1½ g/kg of body weight or 52 g (52 × 1 g). Sodium was restricted to 1.5 to 2 g since she manifested symptoms of fluid overload and had an elevated serum sodium level.

CASE DISCUSSION 20-1

Obesity and adult-onset diabetes often go hand in hand, and often weight reduction alone will lower blood sugar and ameliorate symptoms, controlling the diabetes, not curing it. The major aim of therapy for R. G. was weight reduction. Using the criteria outlined in the chapter, his caloric and nutrient requirements approximate 1750 kcal, or 7350kJ (70 kg × 25 kcal or 70 kg × 105kJ); and carbohydrate, 219 g; protein, 66 g; and fat, 70 g. Emphasis on a low saturated fat and low cholesterol intake was included in dietary counseling, because of the presence of risk factors, (questionable hypertension and obesity) associated with cardiovascular disease, since diabetes often affects the small and large vessels, causing atherosclerosis and circulatory complications.

R. G. was given specific advice on how to follow his diet when eating out in restaurants. His wife was present during dietary counseling to help her learn how to modify her gourmet recipes. R. G.'s physician has recommended that he limit alcohol to 1½ oz per day, which was calculated into his total calories, with no sweet mixed drinks. R. G.'s physician discontinued the Orinase when R. G. had lost 51 lb. R. G. was motivated by the fact that he wanted to discontinue this medication since he noted a flushing sensation on drinking alcohol.

Gradual exercise was instituted, with proper conditioning under the physician's supervision. Periodic dietary follow-up was arranged.

CASE DISCUSSION 21-1

The increments in weight appeared to date from the mother's return to work and Chris's entrance into preschool. Examination of the family dynamics showed that Chris had been a somewhat overprotected, infantilized child whose dependency had been fostered until that time. Thus, Chris had to cope with the stress of separation and the parents' expectation that he achieve academically, which heightened when he entered the first grade. He turned increasingly to food to relieve his anxiety. Another factor promoting the obese state was his extreme inactivity; he rode the bus to and from school, and read or watched television or went to sedentary types of lessons after school.

Intervention was based on the multidisciplinary team's decision that counseling which centered around family dynamics was imperative before dietary measures could be introduced. The fact that the parents' denial was so strong that it was the school nurse and teacher who initiated the referral was a significant issue. Food could not be taken away from the child without establishing the family support system that he needed. Alterations in the family's life style to allow time for attention and activity for Chris meant that family cooperation was mandatory. In addition, the parents would have to overcome their negative and rejecting attitudes about obesity and look to "the person within" Chris.

Unfortunately, this did not happen. Despite the extensive endocrine (laboratory analysis) the parents could not accept the diagnosis. Chris was lost to follow-up.

If Chris had continued in the program, a 1300-kcal (5460-kJ) diet, which provided 500 kcal (2100 kJ) less than the 1800 kcal he needed on the basis of his height, would have been introduced, along with a gentle exercise program that included daily walks. With Chris's increasing physical tolerance and a stimulation of interest in activities by family example, more exercise would have been incorporated. Also, behavior modification techniques would have been simultaneously introduced as part of management.

Early recognition of Chris's problems by the parents and an open rather than a negative attitude might have prevented the problem. It is an amazing paradox that these otherwise liberal and intelligent parents could not accept the diagnosis. In this respect, much to the detriment of their child, they mirror our American hostile cultural attitude which regards even a mild degree of obesity with disdain and repulsion.

CASE DISCUSSION 22-1

The goals of treatment as outlined by the feeding team were as follows:

1 To reestablish C.'s nutritional status
2 To introduce remediation techniques in order to:
   a Inhibit extensor hypertonus
   b Facilitate postural control, beginning with head control
   c Inhibit the asymmetrical tonic neck reflex
   d Decrease oral hypersensitivity
   e Decrease tongue protrusion
3 To help provide a pleasant and successful mealtime experience for the child and her parents.

In order to assist in achieving the first goal, the nutritionist designed a diet that aimed at gradually increasing C.'s intake until she was ingesting 700 kcal (2940 kJ) a day, including foods in all four basic food groups. She suggested thickening the texture of the foods by adding wheat germ, yogurt, or fortified baby cereal, since children who are having difficulty with swallowing are frequently more successful with food of a thickened texture. A vitamin-mineral supplement with fluoride was prescribed.

The nurse began discussions with the parents about the mealtime experiences at home. She supported the family in their efforts to help C. and agreed with them that feeding a child with poor postural control and constant thrusting is extremely difficult.

In order to accomplish either of the outlined goals, the physical and speech therapists determined that the first need was to achieve inhibition of the extensor hypertonus and facilitation of head control. In addition it was necessary to decrease C.'s oral sensitivity to stimuli and facilitate oral control. The therapists felt that achieving these two goals would facilitate feeding, and that with a more successful feeding experience parental anxiety would be relieved.

Treatment

To inhibit extensor hypertonus, C. was held in a flexed posture with her head brought forward. At times she would thrust out of the position and it was not possible to hold her. When this occurred, C. was placed in a hammock made from a bed sheet. With a person holding each end of the sheet, C. was gently rocked back and forth, gradually flexing her body. After the extensor tone was inhibited she was placed on her side on a mat or bed. C.'s parents were shown how to rock her from this side position toward prone and supine positions while holding her at the hip. This gentle rolling encouraged rotation in C.'s trunk, which further helped to inhibit her extensor hypertonus. Once C. had been "prepared" in this way she could maintain a sitting position more easily.

To facilitate head control C. was held in an upright position with only partial support given to her head so that she would help in its control. Oral stimulation and food were then given, in the center of her mouth so that asymmetrical responses were not facilitated (see Fig. 24-4). This encouraged motor activity which would help to promote symmetry in the use of her extremities and assisted in bringing the child's extremities toward the midline of the body, thus helping to inhibit the asymmetrical tonic neck reflex.

A decrease in oral hypersensitivity may occur in response to increasing stimulation of the oral area. The child may adapt to the sensory stimulation if the stimulation occurs in a planned sequence. C.'s parents were shown techniques of oral stimulation to be carried out before and during feeding. The techniques included stroking C.'s upper and lower lip, beginning at the center of her mouth and moving outward toward the corners of the mouth, so that four separate stroking motions occurred. The gums were then similarly stroked, again starting medially and working laterally. Once C. tolerated this type of oral stimulation (after 2 sessions), stimulation was given to the tongue in order to assist in reducing tongue protrusion. Pressure was applied with the therapist's finger on the front half of the tongue, starting at the lip and working back. When the spoon was introduced, the same pressure was applied to the tongue.

The treatment program was carried out before and during every mealtime. This meant organization and cooperation between the feeding team and the hospital staff responsible for her daily care. This relationship was critical to the success of treatment.

Results of Treatment

C. began feeding more successfully. She had no recurring incidences of aspiration pneumonia. At the time of discharge (2 weeks after admission), her caloric intake had increased from 450 kcal (1890 kJ) a day to 600 kcal (2520 kJ) a day and she was beginning to eat textured food. She had gained weight (going from 6 kg to 7 kg) and her parents were becoming skilled at feeding and handling C. This made the mealtime experience pleasant.

CASE DISCUSSION 23-1

The stagnation of milk, fruit juice, or sweetened beverages (Kool-Aid, cola) around Mary's teeth for a 10-h sleep interval led to lactic acid production and the subsequent destruction of the tooth structure, known as "bottle-caries" syndrome. Although brushing the teeth is not started before the third year of life because of the thin oral mucosa, Mary's parents could have gently cleansed her teeth with gauze pads to remove the plaque and prevent the problem.

Mary was 2½ and drinking well from a cup but because of overdependency continued to take a bottle to bed at nap and bed time. Water was advised as a replacement for the milk in the bottle, along with a gradual reduction in the frequency of bottles. Milk was curtailed to 24 oz, given only by cup. Since Mary would only take milk from her bottle, an alternate source of calcium and phosphorus (yogurt, cheese) and the addition of evaporated milk and dried milk solids to soups and puddings had to be utilized during this immediate period of adjustment. Because Mary refused vegetables, meats, and fruits, her diet was low in iron, folic acid, vitamin C, and zinc.

Iron medication was prescribed and Mary's parents were given suggestions about including easy-to-chew foods containing the missing nutrients and about excluding sugar-containing ones. They were also counseled regarding food behavior problems, weight control, and the hazards of leaving the iron medication within easy reach of the child. They were advised to give the iron medication through a straw in order to prevent tooth stains.

Mary was scheduled for periodic dental visits at 6-month intervals and topical fluoride treatments were given; a fluoride-containing toothpaste was recommended. She continued to take iron medication for the next 6 months, and during her well-child visits her parents periodically met with the nutritionist.

CASE DISCUSSION 24-1

Crohn's disease, an inflammatory disease of the bowel, is a sclerosing, granulomatous disease of unknown etiology. It infiltrates all layers of the intestinal wall, with the lower terminal ileum the prime area of the disease.

In the acute phase, the disease is manifested by the presence of abscesses, fistulas, severe cramping, diarrhea, nausea, and vomiting. Food intake is inadequate and the patient is unable to fully digest food.

The severe stress of the disease results in muscle proteolysis for energy needs. This results in marked muscle wasting, loss of strength, and easy fatigability.

Lack of adequate food intake and diminished protein reserves result in hypoalbuminemia, and decreased hemoglobin and hematocrit. The patient is predisposed to infection, edema, and anemia.

Mrs. R. I. shows the classic symptoms of Crohn's disease: a 10-lb weight loss, anemia, and infection. Preoperative and postoperative management focused on nutritional rehabilitation.

During the preoperative period, Vivonex, an elemental diet, was used. Since elemental diets are predigested and easily absorbed, they provide full nutritional support for nitrogen repletion [50 kcal (210 kJ)/1 g protein] to optimize utilization, while reducing fecal output. This allows the lower bowel to rest. Also, drainage from the fistula is reduced. Mrs. R. I. received the standard Vivonex preparation, which was administered half-strength for a total volume of 2400 ml per day, and provided 1200 kcal or 5040 kJ. As the patient's tolerance increased, the strength of the Vivonex was increased to 1 kcal (4.2 kJ)/ml. She also received 1 unit of packed cells and 3 units of salt-poor albumin (SPA) intravenously to help correct the low hemoglobin and low serum albumin.

After surgical incision and drainage of the abscess, the patient was maintained on D_5W (5 percent dextrose solution) until she was fully awake and reactive. She then progressed to clear liquids, then to half-strength Vivonex, and then to full-strength as tolerated. Within 7 days she was discharged with a prescription for 25 mg prednisone per day (a steroid preparation to control the inflammatory process) and 2400 ml of full-strength Vivonex.

On discharge, the patient was instructed on the rationale of an elemental diet, with the added caution to include adequate water (2400 ml). In addition, recipes were given for

Vivonex Jello, slush, and broth. She was informed about signs of intolerance (cramping, diarrhea) and was asked to keep a daily weight record.

During the follow-up visit 10 days later, the patient was given a low-residue, low-lactose diet, high in energy and protein, to ensure maximum weight gain and further replenish nitrogen stores.

CASE DISCUSSION 25-1

The history and the physical and laboratory studies ruled out infection, metabolic disease, bowel obstruction, tumor, and cystic fibrosis. Since the onset of symptoms coincided with the introduction of cow's milk, milk allergy was suspected. Julie was started on a soy protein formula (which is processed with supplementary vitamins and iron) and all cow's milk was excluded from her diet. She showed rapid improvement, and by the end of 1 week there were no symptoms of vomiting or diarrhea.

One month later, Julie was seen for follow-up in the allergy clinic. She had made excellent gains both in weight and height, and her parents reported that she was again a contented baby with none of the former symptoms. At 8 months her weight was 7.8 kg and her length was 70.5 cm (both between the 50th and 75th percentiles). She was tolerating the soy formula and enjoying a variety of cereals, fruits, vegetables, and meats. Her caloric intake averaged 825 calories (3465 kJ)/day, or 105 Kcal (441 kJ)/kg of body weight. It was decided that the milk-free diet should be continued but that Julie should receive regular medical follow-up with a periodic review of the diet.

TABLES

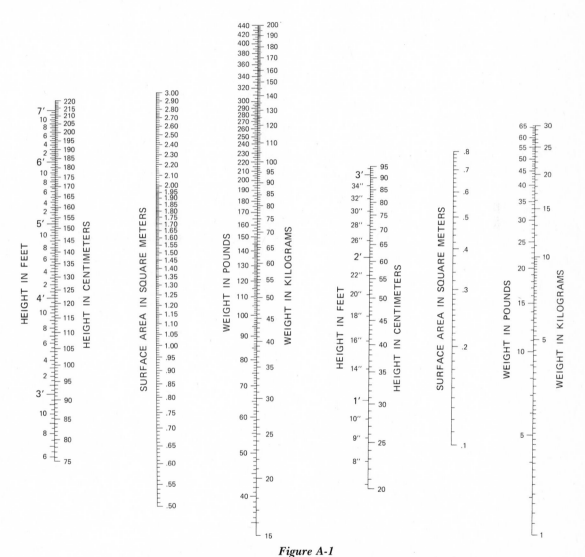

Figure A-1

Nomograms for estimating body surface area from height and body weight. The patient's body surface area is found by drawing a straight line between the point representing his weight and the point representing his height. (From J. D. Crawford, M. E. Terry, and G. M. Rourke, Pediatrics, **5**:783, 1950.)

TABLE A-1 RECOMMENDED DAILY DIETARY ALLOWANCES,[a] REVISED 1974

Food and Nutrition Board, National Academy of Sciences—National Research Council

Designed for the maintenance of good nutrition of practically all healthy people in the U.S.A.

	Age (years)	Weight (kg)	Weight (lbs)	Height (cm)	Height (in)	Energy (kcal)[b]	Protein (g)	Vitamin A Activity (RE[c])(IU)	Vitamin A Activity[d] (IU)	Vitamin D (IU)	Vitamin E Activity[e] (IU)	Ascorbic Acid (mg)	Folacin[f] (µg)	Niacin[g] (mg)	Riboflavin (B₂)(mg)	Thiamin (B₁)(mg)	Vitamin B₆ (mg)	Vitamin B₁₂ (µg)	Calcium (mg)	Phosphorus (mg)	Iodine (µg)	Iron (mg)	Magnesium (mg)	Zinc (mg)
Infants	0.0–0.5	6	14	60	24	kg × 117	kg × 2.2	420[a] 1,400	400	4	35	35	50	5	0.4	0.3	0.3	0.3	360	240	35	10	60	3
	0.5–1.0	9	20	71	28	kg × 108	kg × 2.0	400 2,000	400	5	35	35	50	8	0.6	0.5	0.4	0.3	540	400	45	15	70	5
Children	1–3	13	28	86	34	1300	23	400 2,000	400	7	40	40	100	9	0.8	0.7	0.6	1.0	800	800	60	15	150	10
	4–6	20	44	110	44	1800	30	500 2,500	400	9	40	40	200	12	1.1	0.9	0.9	1.5	800	800	80	10	200	10
	7–10	30	66	135	54	2400	36	700 3,300	400	10	40	40	300	16	1.2	1.2	1.2	2.0	800	800	110	10	250	10
Males	11–14	44	97	158	63	2800	44	1,000 5,000	400	12	45	45	400	18	1.5	1.4	1.6	3.0	1200	1200	130	18	350	15
	15–18	61	134	172	69	3000	54	1,000 5,000	400	15	45	45	400	20	1.8	1.5	2.0	3.0	1200	1200	150	18	400	15
	19–22	67	147	172	69	3000	54	1,000 5,000	400	15	45	45	400	20	1.8	1.5	2.0	3.0	800	800	140	10	350	15
	23–50	70	154	172	69	2700	56	1,000 5,000		15	45	45	400	18	1.6	1.4	2.0	3.0	800	800	130	10	350	15
	51+	70	154	172	69	2400	56	1,000 5,000		15	45	45	400	16	1.5	1.2	2.0	3.0	800	800	110	10	350	15
Females	11–14	44	97	155	62	2400	44	800 4,000	400	12	45	45	400	16	1.3	1.2	1.6	3.0	1200	1200	115	18	300	15
	15–18	54	119	162	65	2100	48	800 4,000	400	12	45	45	400	14	1.4	1.1	2.0	3.0	1200	1200	115	18	300	15
	19–22	58	128	162	65	2100	46	800 4,000	400	12	45	45	400	14	1.4	1.1	2.0	3.0	800	800	100	18	300	15
	23–50	58	128	162	65	2000	46	800 4,000		12	45	45	400	13	1.2	1.0	2.0	3.0	800	800	100	18	300	15
	51+	58	128	162	65	1800	46	800 4,000		12	45	45	400	12	1.1	1.0	2.0	3.0	800	800	80	10	300	15
Pregnant						+300	+30	1,000 5,000	400	15	60	60	800	+2	+0.3	+0.3	2.5	4.0	1200	1200	125	18+[h]	450	20
Lactating						+500	+20	1,200 6,000	400	15	80	80	600	+4	+0.5	+0.3	2.5	4.0	1200	1200	150	18	450	25

a The allowances are intended to provide for individual variations among most normal persons as they live in the United States under usual environmental stresses. Diets should be based on a variety of common foods in order to provide other nutrients for which human requirements have been less well defined. See text for more detailed discussion of allowances and of nutrients not tabulated. See Table I (p. 6) for weights and heights by individual year of age.

b Kilojoules (kJ) = 4.2 × kcal.

c Retinol equivalents.

d Assumed to be all as retinol in milk during the first six months of life. All subsequent intakes are assumed to be half as retinol and half as β-carotene when calculated from international units. As retinol equivalents, three fourths are as retinol and one fourth as β-carotene.

e Total vitamin E activity, estimated to be 80 percent as α-tocopherol and 20 percent other tocopherols. See text for variation in allowances.[*]

f The folacin allowances refer to dietary sources as determined by *Lactobacillus casei* assay. Pure forms of folacin may be effective in doses less than one fourth of the recommended dietary allowance.

g Although allowances are expressed as niacin, it is recognized that on the average 1 mg of niacin is derived from each 60 mg of dietary tryptophan.

h This increased requirement cannot be met by ordinary diets; therefore, the use of supplemental iron is recommended.

* National Research Council. Food and Nutrition Board. 1974. *Recommended Dietary Allowances.* 8th rev. ed. Washington, D.C.: National Academy of Sciences.

TABLE A-2 ADULT HEIGHT AND WEIGHT TABLES

Desirable weights in pounds according to height and frame (in indoor clothing)

	Height (with shoes on; 1-in heels), ft	in	*Small frame*	*Medium frame*	*Large frame*
Men	5	2	112–120	118–129	126–141
age	5	3	115–123	121–133	129–144
25 and	5	4	118–126	124–136	132–148
over	5	5	121–129	127–139	135–152
	5	6	124–133	130–143	138–156
	5	7	128–137	134–147	142–161
	5	8	132–141	138–152	147–166
	5	9	136–145	142–156	151–170
	5	10	140–150	146–160	155–174
	5	11	144–154	150–165	159–179
	6	0	148–158	154–170	164–184
	6	1	152–162	158–175	168–189
	6	2	156–167	162–180	173–194
	6	3	160–171	167–185	178–199
	6	4	164–175	172–190	182–204

	Height (with shoes on; 2-in heels), ft	in	*Small frame*	*Medium frame*	*Large frame*
Women	4	10	92–98	96–107	104–119
age	4	11	94–101	98–110	106–122
25 and	5	0	96–104	101–113	109–125
*over**	5	1	99–107	104–116	112–128
	5	2	102–110	107–119	115–131
	5	3	105–113	110–122	118–134
	5	4	108–116	113–126	121–138
	5	5	111–119	116–130	125–142
	5	6	114–123	120–135	129–146
	5	7	118–127	124–139	133–150
	5	8	122–131	128–143	137–154
	5	9	126–135	132–147	141–158
	5	10	130–140	136–151	145–163
	5	11	134–144	140–155	149–168
	6	0	138–148	144–159	153–173

* For girls between 18 and 25, subtract 1 lb for each year under 25

Source: Metropolitan Life Insurance Company, New York.

TABLE A-3   TRICEPS SKINFOLD OF CHILDREN BY SEX AND AGE AT LAST BIRTHDAY

Age	Percentile						
yr	5th	10th	25th	50th	75th	90th	95th
Male							
6	5.0	5.0	6.0	8.0	9.0	12.0	13.0
7	4.5	5.0	6.0	8.0	9.5	12.0	14.0
8	4.5	5.0	6.5	8.0	11.0	13.5	17.0
9	5.0	6.0	7.0	8.5	12.0	16.0	20.0
10	5.0	6.0	7.0	9.0	12.0	16.0	20.0
11	5.0	6.0	7.0	9.5	14.0	19.0	22.0
12	5.1	5.5	6.8	9.4	13.3	19.6	23.3
13	4.5	5.2	6.7	9.1	12.9	19.3	22.6
14	4.2	4.7	6.0	7.8	12.0	17.1	20.8
15	4.3	4.7	5.8	7.6	10.7	15.8	20.7
16	4.2	4.7	5.8	7.5	11.1	15.8	20.2
17	4.1	4.6	5.5	7.5	11.4	15.6	20.5
Female							
6	5.5	6.0	7.0	9.0	11.0	14.0	16.0
7	6.0	6.5	8.0	10.0	12.0	16.0	17.0
8	6.0	6.5	8.0	10.5	13.5	18.0	20.0
9	6.0	7.0	9.0	11.0	14.5	19.0	22.0
10	6.0	7.0	9.0	12.0	15.0	20.0	23.0
11	6.0	7.0	9.0	12.0	15.0	20.0	23.0
12	6.1	7.0	8.8	11.8	16.0	22.2	25.2
13	6.4	7.3	9.2	12.4	17.1	22.8	25.5
14	7.1	8.3	10.7	14.0	18.5	23.3	26.7
15	7.4	8.6	11.6	14.8	19.5	25.1	29.4
16	7.7	9.2	11.8	15.6	20.8	25.5	29.7
17	8.1	9.6	12.1	15.8	20.5	25.0	29.1

Source: Adapted from U.S. Department of Health, Education, and Welfare, Public Health Service, Health Resources Administration, vital and health statistics data from the *National Health Survey,* ser. 11, no. 132, 1974, p. 20.

TABLE A-4 OBESITY STANDARDS FOR ADULT CAUCASIAN AMERICANS

	Skinfold measurements, mm	
Age, yr	Males	Females
18	15	27
19	15	27
20	16	28
21	17	28
22	18	28
23	18	28
24	19	28
25	20	29
26	20	29
27	21	29
28	22	29
29	23	29
30–50	23	30

Source: Adapted from C. C. Seltzer and J. Mayer, "A Sample Criterion of Obesity," *Postgraduate Medicine,* **38:**101–107, 1965.

TABLE A-5 COMMON METRIC EQUIVALENTS

1 U.S. fluidounce	= 29.573 milliter
1 U.S. liquid pint	= 0.47317 liter
1 U.S. liquid quart	= 0.94633 liter
1 U.S. gallon	= 3.78533 liter
1 U.S. dry quart	= 1.1012 liter
1 avoirdupois ounce	= 28.350 grams
1 avoirdupois pound	= 0.45359 kilogram
1 pound	= 2.2 kilograms
1 inch	= 2.54 centimeters

TABLE A-6 NUTRITIONAL ASSESSMENT TOOL FOR USE WITH CHILDREN

Patient _____ Date _____

Birth date _____ Age _____

Informant _____

Presenting nutritional problem(s) _____

_____

Current concern (parental) _____

_____

Growth

Height _____ (_____%)   Head circumference _____ (_____%)

Weight _____ (_____%)   Fat-fold measure _____

Birth weight _____lb _____oz   Birth length _____ inches

Has weight gain since birth been: Satisfactory? _____ Slow? _____

Fluctuating? _____

Has there been recent weight: Gain? _____ Loss? _____ Neither _____

Mother's height _____ft _____in   Weight _____lb

Father's height _____ft _____in   Weight _____lb

As compared to siblings at the same age, patient is: Larger _____

Same size _____ Smaller _____

Pertinent laboratory findings

Nutrition History

Has the patient taken vitamin-mineral supplements? Yes _____ No _____

Kind _____ At what age? _____

Has the patient been prescribed medication(s)? Yes _____ No _____

Kind _____ Reason _____

At what age? _____

Indicate if there have been problems with the following:

	Patient	Family	Comment
Colic	_____	_____	_____
Spitting up	_____	_____	_____
Appetite	_____	_____	_____
Food allergies	_____	_____	_____
Diarrhea	_____	_____	_____

(continued)

	Patient	Family	Comment
Constipation	———	———	———————————————
Vomiting	———	———	———————————————
Anemia	———	———	———————————————
Dehydration	———	———	———————————————
Failure to thrive	———	———	———————————————
Unusual cravings	———	———	———————————————
Overweight	———	———	———————————————
Need for special diet	———	———	———————————————

Feeding history

Who fed the child? ——————

Was the child difficult to feed? Yes ——— No ———

How long did feedings take? ———

Was there any early feeding intervention? Yes ——— No ———

Was the child: Breast-fed? ——— Formula-fed? ——— Formula: ——————

Was the child fed: On demand? ——— On hourly schedule? ———

At what age was the child weaned: From breast? ——— From bottle? ———

Did the child suck his/her thumb? Yes ——— No ——— Did the child use

a pacifier? Yes ——— No ———

Indicate if there were early difficulties with the following:

		Comment
Sucking	———	———————————————
Swallowing	———	———————————————
Chewing	———	———————————————
Tongue control	———	———————————————
Lip control	———	———————————————

Developmental feeding milestones

	Age	Comment
Baby food introduction	———	———————————————
Junior foods	———	———————————————
Finger feeding	———	———————————————
Cup drinking	———	———————————————

(continued)

	Age	Comment
Weaning	_____	_____
Whole table foods	_____	_____
Use of spoon	_____	_____
Independent feeding	_____	_____
Self-preparation of food	_____	_____

Feeding environment

Is the child fed: Alone? _____ With family? _____

Who feeds the child: _____ Others that may feed or care for the child at mealtime: _____

The child eats: Alone _____ With family _____

Does the child care for himself/herself at the table? Yes _____ No _____

Does the child serve himself/herself food? Yes _____ No _____

Does the child generally finish all food served? Yes _____ No _____

Does the child ask for second helpings? Yes _____ No _____

How long is the usual eating period? _____

Where does the child eat: Breakfast? _____ Lunch? _____

Dinner? _____

Number of persons eating together at: Breakfast _____ Lunch _____

Dinner _____

Who prepares: Breakfast? _____ Lunch? _____

Dinner? _____

Is the child's behavior during mealtimes: Acceptable? _____ Disruptive? _____

Dawdling? _____ Distractible? _____

Is the rule for eating: Clean plate? _____ Taste everything? _____

Other: _____

How many times does the family dine out during the month? _____

How often is shopping done for food? _____

How much money is spent on food each week: _____

Are food stamps used? Yes _____ No _____

Present eating habits

Child's appetite is: Excellent _____ Fair _____ Poor _____ Fluctuating _____

Has there been recent appetite: Increase? _____ Decrease? _____

(continued)

When is the child most hungry? _____

Does the child know when he/she is full? Yes _____ No _____

What is the usual snacking pattern? _____

Are the child's food habits similar to those of other family members?

Yes _____ No _____

Does the child get up during the night or early morning to eat or drink?

Yes _____ No _____

Is the child's acceptance of foods: Good? _____ Fair? _____ Poor? _____

Rigidly selective? _____

What are the child's food dislikes? _____

What is the child's favorite food? _____

Dental

Does the child have regular dental check-ups? Yes _____ No _____

Does the child brush and floss teeth regularly? Yes _____ No _____

Is the local water supply fluoridated? Yes _____ No _____

Is a fluoride supplement taken? Yes _____ No _____ Age _____

Kind _____

Does the child receive topical fluoride applications? Yes _____ No _____

Are sweets included as: Part of meals? _____ Snacks? _____

Present food intake

24-h recall
1 to 3-day food record
General recall of usual food pattern

Time	*Amount*	*Type of food*

(continued)

Frequency of foods:

	Number of times eaten per week		
	Daily	Occasionally	Seldom
Milk	_____	_____	_____
Cheese, ice cream	_____	_____	_____
Cold or hot cereal	_____	_____	_____
Sweet rolls or doughnuts	_____	_____	_____
Sandwiches	_____	_____	_____
Soup	_____	_____	_____
Fruit or fruit juice	_____	_____	_____
Peanut butter or nuts	_____	_____	_____
Dried peas or beans	_____	_____	_____
Meat in casseroles	_____	_____	_____
Red meat, fish, or poultry	_____	_____	_____
Cooked or raw vegetable	_____	_____	_____
Potato, rice, or noodles	_____	_____	_____
Cookies or crackers	_____	_____	_____
Pie, cake, or brownies	_____	_____	_____
Potato chips or corn chips	_____	_____	_____
Candy	_____	_____	_____
Soft drinks or Kool-Aid	_____	_____	_____

Does the weekend food pattern vary from the usual food intake during the week?

Yes _____ No _____ Comment _____

Comments regarding food intake: _____

_____

_____

_____

Analysis of food intake:

Total fluid _____

Cal _____ Cal/kg _____ Cal/cm _____

Protein, g _____ Protein, g/kg _____

Vitamins/minerals _____

(continued)

Impressions:

Recommendations:

Summary:

Source: Developmental Evaluation Clinic, Children's Hospital Medical Center, Boston, Mass.

TABLE A-7 COMMON MEDICAL ABBREVIATIONS

a	ante, before		LMP	last menstrual period
ad lib	ad libitum, as desired		lytes	electrolytes
ASHD	arteriosclerotic heart disease		MI	myocardial infarction
Ba	barium		ml	milliliters
bid	bis in die, twice daily		MOM	milk of magnesia
BMR	basal metabolic rate		MS	multiple sclerosis
BP	blood pressure		NG	nasogastric
BUN	blood urea nitrogen		NPO	nothing per os, nothing by mouth
BS	Blood sugar		NTG	nitroglycerin
c̄	cum, with		Ob or OBS	obstetrics
Ca	carcinoma		OPD	outpatient department
cath	catheter		OR	operating room
CBC	complete blood count		OT	occupational therapy
CC	chief complaint		P	post, after
CHF	congestive heart failure		pc	post cibos, after meals
Cl	chloride		PE	physical exam
CNS	central nervous system		PID	pelvic inflammatory disease
CVA	cardiovascular accident		PKU	phenylketonuria
D&C	dilatation and curettage		po	per os, by mouth
Dx	diagnosis		PP	postprandial, after eating
D/C	discharge		prn	pro renata, as needed
DOA	dead on arrival		pt	patient
DT	delirium tremens		PT	physical therapy
ECG or EKG	electrocardiogram		PTA	prior to admission
EDC	expected date of confinement		q	quod, every
EEG	electroencephalogram		qd	every day
ENT	ear, nose, and throat		qh	every hour
ER or EW	emergency room or emergency ward		qid	4 times a day
FBS	fasting blood sugar		qod	every other day
FTT	failure to thrive		qoh	every other hour
FUO	fever of unknown origin		RBC	red blood cell
Fx	fracture		re	concerning
GI	gastrointestinal		RHD	rheumatic heart disease
GTT	glucose tolerance test		R/O	rule out
GU	genitourinary		Rx	treatment
Gyn	gynecology		s̄	sine, without
Hgb	hemoglobin		SOB	shortness of breath
Hct	hematocrit		sp gr	specific gravity
hem	blood		Staph	staphylococcus
hs	hora sommi, at bedtime		stat	statim, immediately
Hx	history		Sx	symptoms
ICU	intensive care unit		T&A	tonsils and adenoids
IM	intramuscular		TB	tuberculosis
Imp	impression		tid	ter in die, 3 times a day
I&O	intake and output		trach	tracheostomy
IV	intravenous		URI	upper respiratory infection
IVP	intravenous pyelogram		UTI	urinary tract infection
K	potassium		VD	veneral disease
l	liter		WBC	white blood count
Lat	lateral		WNL	within normal limits
LLQ	left lower quadrant		×	times

TABLE A-8 FOODBORNE ILLNESSES

Microorganism	Name of illness	Onset of symptoms	Symptoms	Duration	Foods susceptible
Salmonella	Salmonellosis	12 h	Cramps, fever, nausea, vomiting, diarrhea (sick people, infants and elderly are more susceptible because of decreased resistance)	2–6 days	Poultry, Eggs and egg products, Milk, Pork
Clostridium perfringens	Pefringens poisoning	10–20 h	Cramps, diarrhea, nausea	24 h	Meat
Staphylococcus aureus	Staphylococcus poisoning	2–8 h	Vomiting, diarrhea	1–2 days	Custards, Sauces, Gravies, Soups, Salads (chicken, tuna)
Clostridium botulinum	Botulism	12–36 h	Double vision, paralysis of respiratory muscles; can be fatal	3–8 days	Canned low-acid food, Creamed soups, Canned meat, mushrooms, etc.
Trichinella spiralis	Trichinosis	24–72 h	Nausea, vomiting, diarrhea, muscle pain, chest pain	Can be as long as 1 year	Pork and pork products

Food and approximate measure		Weight, g	Food energy		Protein, g	Fat (total lipids), g	Fatty acids			Carbohydrate, g	Calcium, mg	Iron, mg	Vitamin A value, IU	Thiamine, mg	Riboflavin, mg	Niacin, mg	Ascorbic acid, mg
							Saturated (total), g	Unsaturated									
			kcal	kJ				Oleic, g	Lino-leic, g								
Milk, cream, cheese (related products)																	
Milk, cow's																	
Fluid, whole (3.5% fat)	1 cup	244	160	672	9	9	5	3	trace	12	288	0.1	350	0.08	0.42	0.1	2
Fluid, nonfat (skim)	1 cup	246	90	378	9	trace				13	298	0.1	10	0.10	0.44	0.2	2
Cheddar, process	1 oz	28	105	441	7	9	5	3	trace	1	219	0.3	350	trace	0.12	trace	0
Cottage, creamed	1 cup	225	240	1008	31	9	5	3	trace	7	212	0.7	380	0.07	0.56	0.2	0
Ice cream, plain, factory packed container	8 fl oz	142	295	1239	6	18	10	6	1	29	175	0.1	740	0.06	0.27	0.1	1
Yogurt, from partially skimmed milk	1 cup	246	120	504	8	4	2	1	trace	13	295	0.1	170	0.09	0.43	0.2	2
Eggs																	
Whole, without shell	1 egg	50	80	336	6	6	2	3	trace	trace	27	1.1	590	0.05	0.15	trace	0
Meat, poultry, fish, shellfish (related products)																	
Hamburger (ground beef), broiled, regular	3 oz	85	245	1029	21	17	8	8	trace	0	9	2.7	30	0.07	0.18	4.6	—
Steak, broiled, lean and fat	3 oz	85	330	1386	20	27	13	12	1	0	9	2.5	50	0.05	0.16	4.0	—
Chicken, cooked																	
Flesh only, broiled	3 oz	85	115	483	20	3	1	1	1	0	8	1.4	80	0.05	0.16	7.4	—
With bone	3.3 oz	94	155	651	25	5	1	2	1	0	9	1.3	70	0.04	0.17	11.2	—
Lamb leg roasted, lean and fat	3 oz	85	235	987	22	16	9	6	trace	0	9	1.4	—	0.13	0.23	4.7	—
Pork, fresh, trimmed to retail basis, cooked																	
Chop, thick, with bone	3.5 oz	98	260	1092	16	21	8	9	2	0	8	2.2	0	0.63	0.18	3.8	—
Bluefish, baked or broiled	3 oz	85	135	567	22	4		3		0	25	0.6	40	0.09	0.08	1.6	—
Haddock, fried	3 oz	85	140	588	17	5	1	3		5	34	1.0	—	0.03	0.06	2.7	2
Tuna, canned in oil	3 oz	85	170	714	24	7				0	7	1.6	70	0.04	0.10	10.1	—
Mature dry beans and peas, nuts, peanuts (related products)																	
Red beans	1 cup	256	230	966	15	1				42	74	4.6	trace	0.13	0.10	1.5	—
Lima beans, cooked	1 cup	192	260	1092	16	1				48	56	5.6	trace	0.26	0.12	1.3	trace
Cashew nuts, roasted	1 cup	135	760	3192	23	62	10	43	4	40	51	5.1	140	0.58	0.33	2.4	—
Peanut butter	1 tbsp	16	95	399	4	8	2	4	2	3	9	0.3	—	0.02	0.02	2.4	0
Peas, split, dry, cooked	1 cup	250	290	1218	20	1				52	28	4.2	100	0.37	0.22	2.2	—
Vegetables and vegetable products																	
Asparagus, canned green	6 spears	96	20	84	2	trace				3	18	1.8	770	0.06	0.10	0.8	14

Snap beans, green, cooked short time in small amount of water	1 cup	125	30	126	2	trace	—	—	—	7	62	0.8	680	0.08	0.11	0.6	16
Broccoli spears, cooked	1 cup	150	40	168	5	trace	—	—	—	7	132	1.2	3750	0.14	0.29	1.2	135
Carrots, cooked, diced	1 cup	145	45	189	1	trace	—	—	—	10	48	0.9	15,220	0.08	0.07	0.7	9
Peas, green, cooked	1 cup	160	115	483	9	1	—	—	—	19	37	2.9	860	0.44	0.17	3.7	33
Potato, baked, peeled after baking	1	99	90	378	3	trace	—	—	—	21	9	0.7	trace	0.10	0.04	1.7	20
Spinach, cooked	1 cup	180	40	168	5	1	—	—	—	6	167	4.0	14,580	0.13	0.25	1.0	50
Squash, winter, baked, mashed	1 cup	205	130	546	4	1	—	—	—	32	57	1.6	8610	0.10	0.27	1.4	27
Sweet potatoes, boiled, peeled after boiling	1	147	170	714	2	1	—	—	—	39	47	1.0	11,610	0.13	0.09	0.9	25
Tomato juice, canned	1 cup	242	45	189	2	trace	—	—	—	10	17	2.2	1940	0.13	0.07	1.8	39
Fruits and fruit products																	
Apple, raw, 2½ in diameter	1	150	70	294	trace	trace	—	—	—	18	8	0.4	50	0.04	0.02	0.1	3
Fruit cocktail, canned in heavy syrup	1 cup	256	195	819	1	1	—	—	—	50	23	1.0	360	0.04	0.03	1.1	5
Grapefruit, white, raw, medium, 4½ in diameter	½	285	55	231	1	trace	—	—	—	14	22	0.6	10	0.05	0.02	0.2	52
Orange, raw California, naval, 2⅘ in diameter	1	180	60	252	2	trace	—	—	—	16	49	0.5	240	0.12	0.05	0.5	75
Orange juice, frozen concentrate, diluted with 3 parts water, by volume	1 cup	248	110	462	2	trace	—	—	—	27	22	0.2	500	0.21	0.03	0.8	112
Raisins, dried	1 cup	160	460	1932	4	trace	—	—	—	124	99	5.6	30	0.18	0.13	0.9	2
Strawberries, raw, capped	1 cup	149	55	231	1	1	—	—	—	13	31	1.5	90	0.04	0.10	1.0	88
Tangerine raw, medium	1	114	40	168	1	trace	—	—	—	10	34	0.3	350	0.05	0.02	0.1	26
Bread (related products)																	
White bread, enriched	1 slice	23	60	252	2	1	trace	trace	trace	12	16	0.6	trace	0.06	0.04	0.5	trace
Whole-wheat bread, made with 2% nonfat dry milk	1 slice	23	55	231	2	1	trace	trace	trace	11	23	0.5	trace	0.06	0.03	0.7	trace
Macaroni, enriched, cooked, firm stage (8–10 min; undergoes additional cooking in a food mixture)	1 cup	130	190	798	6	1	—	—	—	39	14	1.4	0	0.23	0.14	1.9	0
Rice, white (fully milled or polished) cooked, common commercial	1 cup	168	185	777	3	trace	—	—	—	41	17	1.5	0	0.19	0.01	1.6	0
Wheat flakes, with added nutrients	1 oz	28	100	420	3	trace	—	—	—	23	12	1.2	0	0.18	0.04	1.4	0
Fats, oils																	
Butter, pat or square (64 per pound)	1 pat	7	50	210	trace	6	3	2	1	trace	1	0	230	—	—	—	0
Margarine, pat or square (64 per pound)	1 pat	7	50	210	trace	6	1	3	1	trace	1	0	230	—	—	—	0

(continued)

Food and approximate measure		Weight, g	Food energy kcal	Food energy kJ	Protein, g	Fat (total lipids), g	Fatty acids Saturated (total), g	Fatty acids Unsaturated Oleic, g	Fatty acids Unsaturated Linoleic, g	Carbohydrate, g	Calcium, mg	Iron, mg	Vitamin A value, IU	Thiamine, mg	Riboflavin, mg	Niacin, mg	Ascorbic acid, mg
Corn oil	1 tbsp	14	125	525	0	14	1	4	7	0	0	0	—	0	0	0	0
Mayonnaise	1 tbsp	15	110	462	trace	12	2	3	6	trace	3	0.1	40	trace	0.01	trace	—
Sugars, sweets																	
Candy, fudge plain	1 oz.	28	115	483	1	3	2	1	trace	21	22	0.3	trace	0.01	0.03	0.1	trace
Jellies	1 tbsp	20	55	231	trace	trace	—	—	—	14	4	0.3	trace	trace	0.01	trace	1
Sugar, cane or beet, granulated	1 tbsp	12	45	189	0	0	—	—	—	12	0		0	0	0	0	0
Beverages																	
Carbonated																	
Cola type	1 cup	240	95	399	0	0	—	—	—	24	—	—	0	0	0	0	0
Ginger ale	1 cup	230	70	294	0	0	—	—	—	18	—	—	0	0	0	0	0
Coffee	1 cup	180	2	8	trace	trace	—	—	—	trace	4	0.2	0	0	trace	0.5	0

Source: U.S. Department of Agriculture, *Nutritive Values of Food*, Home and Garden Bulletin No. 72, 1971.

TABLE A-10 AMINO ACID CONTENT OF FOODS PER 100 g, EDIBLE PORTION

Food item	Nitrogen conversion factor	Protein content, percent	Phenylalanine, mg	Isoleucine, mg	Leucine, mg	Valine, mg	Methionine, mg	Cystine, mg	Total, mg	Tryptophan, mg	Threonine, mg	Lysine, mg	Tyrosine, mg	Arginine, mg	Histidine, mg
							Sulfur-containing								
Milk, milk products															
Fluid, whole	6.38	3.5	170	223	344	240	86	31	117	49	161	272	178	128	92
Human milk	6.38	1.4	48	68	100	70	25	22	47	18	50	73	61	45	22
Isomil	6.38		105	107	153	92	29	—	29	19	69	91	—	—	53
Cheese, cheddar, processed	6.38	23.2	1244	1563	2262	1665	604	131	735	316	862	1702	1109	847	756
Eggs, whole															
fresh or stored	6.25	12.8	739	850	1126	950	401	299	700	211	637	819	551	840	307
Meat, poultry, fish															
Hamburger, regular	6.25	16.0	658	837	1311	888	397	202	599	187	707	1398	543	1032	556
Rib roast	6.25	17.4	715	910	1425	590	432	220	652	203	768	1520	590	1122	604
Lamb leg	6.25	18.0	732	933	1394	887	432	236	668	233	824	1457	625	1172	501
Pork loin	6.25	16.4	646	842	1207	853	409	192	601	213	761	1346	585	1005	567
Chicken, fryer	6.25	20.6	811	1088	1490	1012	537	277	814	250	877	1810	725	1302	567
Haddock, raw	6.25	18.2	676	923	1374	930	530	245	775	181	789	1596	492	1025	593
Legumes, dry, and nuts															
Bean, red kidney, canned	6.25	5.7	315	324	490	346	57	57	114	53	247	423	220	343	162
Peanuts	5.46	26.9	1557	1266	1872	1532	271	463	734	340	828	1099	1104	3296	749
Grains and grain products															
Bread, white, 4% milk solids	5.70	8.5	465	429	668	435	142	200	342	91	282	225	243	340	192
Rice, white or converted	5.95	7.6	382	356	655	531	137	103	240	82	298	300	347	438	128
Vegetables															
Beans, lima, canned	6.25	3.8	197	233	306	246	41	42	83	49	171	240	131	230	125

Sources:

1 M. L. Orr and B. K. Watt, *Amino Acid Content of Foods*, Home Economics Research Report No. 4, U.S. Dept. of Agriculture, Washington, D.C. 1957.

2 S. J. Foman, *Infant Nutrition*, 2d ed., W. B. Saunders Company, Philadelphia, 1974, p. 362.

3 *Handbook of Infant Formulas*, 6th ed., J. B. Roerig Division, Charles Pfizer & Co. Inc., New York, 1969.

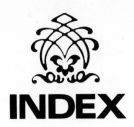

INDEX

Page numbers in *italic* indicate illustrations or tables.

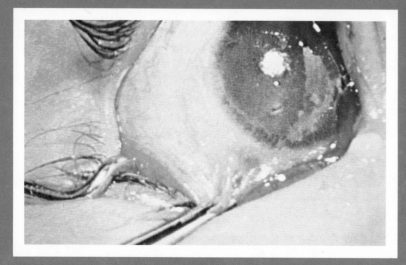

COLOR PLATES OF THE PHYSICAL SIGNS OF NUTRITIONAL DEFICIENCY.

(Courtesy of *Nutrition Today.*)

**Figure B-1.
Xerosis. Cause:
Lack of vitamin A.**

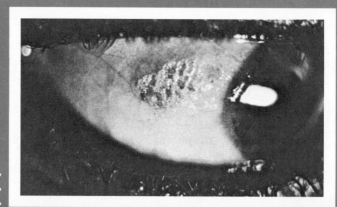

**Figure B-2.
Bitot's spots.
Cause: Lack of vitamin A.**

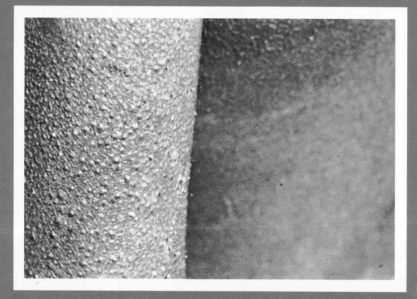

**Figure B-3.
Follicular hyperkeratosis
(of the arm). Cause:
Lack of vitamin A.**